Medicine Morning Report Subspecialties

Medicine Morning Report Subspecialties

Beyond the Pearls

Series Editors

RAJ DASGUPTA, MD, FACP, FCCP, FAASM
Associate Professor of Clinical Medicine
Division of Pulmonary/Critical Care/Sleep Medicine
Associate Program Director of the Sleep Medicine Fellowship
Assistant Program Director of the Internal Medicine Residency
Keck School of Medicine of the University of Southern California
Los Angeles, California

R. MICHELLE KOOLAEE, DO, CCD
Assistant Professor of Clinical Medicine
Division of Rheumatology
Keck School of Medicine of the University of Southern California
Los Angeles, California

Volume Editors

RAJ DASGUPTA, MD, FACP, FCCP, FAASM
SOPHIA LI, MD
HELEN YANG, MD, MPH
DARREN WONG, MD
HUI YI SHAN, MD

Section Chiefs

SHEILA SAHNI, MD, FACC, FSCAI
CLAY WU, DO

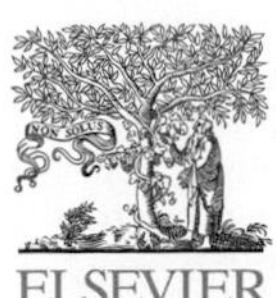

Elsevier
1600 John F. Kennedy Blvd.
Suite 1800
Philadelphia, PA 19103-2899

MEDICINE MORNING REPORT SUBSPECIALTIES:
BEYOND THE PEARLS

ISBN: 978-0-323-83136-9

Director, Content Development: Ellen Wurm-Cutter
Executive Content Strategist: James Merritt
Publishing Services Manager: Shereen Jameel
Senior Project Manager: Manikandan Chandrasekaran
Design Direction: Bridget Hoette

Printed in India

Last digit is the print number: 9 8 7 6 5 4 3 2 1

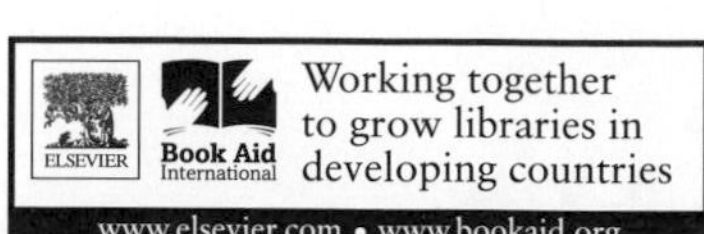

Michelle and I would like to dedicate this book to my parents, Tita and Arabinda Dasgupta. They fell in love and have been together for 54 years. Through the good times and the bad, they always stood strong together and supported one another. Their journey to come to the United States to make a better life for themselves and me, their only child, is an amazing story, and one that I never get tired of hearing. My parents love my wife, Michelle, like the daughter they never had and are always proud of her many accomplishments, but especially for bringing our family together and giving them 3 precious grandkids. We are honored to dedicate this book to them as a symbol that their hard work, positive attitude, and love paid off.

– Raj Dasgupta and R. Michelle Koolaee

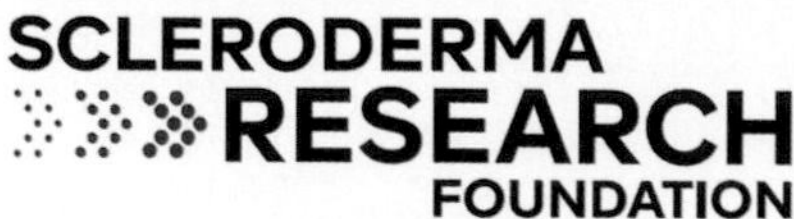

About Scleroderma Research Foundation (SRF)

Established in 1987 by patient-turned-activist Sharon Monsky, when research on this potentially life-threatening illness was nearly nonexistent, the Scleroderma Research Foundation is focused on bringing the best minds in science together to find a cure for scleroderma. Led by a Scientific Advisory Board of world-renowned scientists, the SRF's collaborative research program enables scientists from leading institutions across the nation and around the world to work together and develop an understanding of how the disease begins, how it progresses, and what can be done to slow, halt, or reverse the disease process.

Guided by Sharon's passion for a cure, we have become the largest nonprofit investor in scleroderma research in the United States. Sharon lost her battle to the disease in 2002, but her vision lives on today, as the SRF remains committed to funding the most promising research aimed at improved therapies and finding a cure.

CONTRIBUTORS

Brandon L. Adler, MD
Clinical Assistant Professor, Dermatology
Keck School of Medicine of the University of Southern California
Los Angeles, California

Daniel Aldea, MD
Resident Physician
Department of Internal Medicine
Keck School of Medicine of the University of Southern California
Los Angeles, California

Shamili Allam, MD
Cardiology Fellow
Department of Internal Medicine
UC Davis
Sacramento, California

Nancy Baker, MD, MS
Assistant Professor of Neurology
Loma Linda University School of Medicine
Loma Linda, California

Braden Barnett, MD
Clinical Assistant Professor of Medicine
Division of Endocrinology, Department of Medicine
Keck School of Medicine of the University of Southern California
Los Angeles, California

Rachel Bartash, MD
Assistant Professor
Medicine/Infectious Diseases
Montefiore Medical Center
Albert Einstein College of Medicine
Bronx, New York

Neil Bhambi, MD
General Cardiology Fellow
Department of Cardiology
Kaiser Permanente Los Angeles Medical Center
Los Angeles, California

Emily Blodget, MD, MPH
Associate Professor of Clinical Medicine
Division of Infectious Diseases
Keck School of Medicine of the University of Southern California
Los Angeles, California

Christopher Bradley, MD
Resident Physician
Department of Internal Medicine
Keck School of Medicine of the University of Southern California
Los Angeles, California

Esther Byun, MD
Assistant Professor of Neurology
Veterans Affairs Hospital Loma Linda
Loma Linda, California

John David Carmichael, MD
Associate Professor of Clinical Medicine
Keck School of Medicine of the University of Southern California
Los Angeles, California

Patrick Chan, MD
Pulmonary Critical Care Fellow
Department of Pulmonary, Critical Care, and Sleep Medicine
University of Southern California
Los Angeles, California

Daniel Chao, MD
Staff Physician, Gastroenterology
VA Loma Linda Healthcare System
Loma Linda, California

Dafang Chen, MD
Division of Pulmonary, Critical Care, and Sleep Medicine
University of Southern California
Los Angeles, California

Jonathan Cheng, MD
Nephrology Fellow
Division of Nephrology–Hypertension
University of California, San Diego
San Diego, California

Shankar Chhetri, MBBS, MD
Internal Medicine
Raritan Bay Medical Center
Perth Amboy, New Jersey;
MBBS, General Medicine
UCMS
Bhairahawa, Rupandehi, Nepal

Kristal Choi, MD
Assistant Clinical Professor
Rheumatology
University of California, Los Angeles
Los Angeles, California

Maggie Chow, MD, PhD, FAAD
Mohs Surgeon and Dermatologist
Skin and Beauty Center
Glendale, California

Nasim Daoud, MD
Rheumatologist
Valley Oaks Medical Group;
Clinical Assistant Professor
Loma Linda University
Loma Linda, California

Raj Dasgupta, MD, FACP, FCCP, FAASM
Associate Professor of Clinical Medicine
Division of Pulmonary/Critical Care/Sleep Medicine
Associate Program Director of the Sleep Medicine Fellowship
Assistant Program Director of the Internal Medicine Residency
Keck School of Medicine of the University of Southern California
Los Angeles, California

Lillian Dawit, MD
Resident Physician
Department of Internal Medicine
Keck School of Medicine of the University of Southern California
Los Angeles, California

Tyler Degener, MD
Internal Medicine Resident
Keck School of Medicine of the University of Southern California
University of Southern California
Los Angeles, California

An H. Do, MD
Associate Professor
Department of Neurology
University of California, Irvine
Orange, California

Fernando Dominguez, MD
Infectious Diseases Attending
LAC+USC Medical Center
Los Angeles, California

Christina Downey, MD
Assistant Professor of Medicine
Division of Rheumatology
Loma Linda University Health
Loma Linda, California

Benjamin A. Emanuel, DO
Neurointensivist/Neurologist
Department of Neurology
Keck School of Medicine of the University of Southern California
Los Angeles, California

Michael Fong, MD, FACC
Associate Professor of Clinical Medicine
Keck School of Medicine of the University of Southern California
Los Angeles, California

Christina S. Gainey, MD
Resident Physician
Department of Internal Medicine
Keck School of Medicine of the University of Southern California
Los Angeles, California

Sivagini Ganesh, MD
Attending Physician
Pulmonary and Critical Care Medicine
University of Southern California
Los Angeles, California

Percy Genyk, MD
Resident Physician
Department of Internal Medicine
Keck School of Medicine of the University of Southern California
Los Angeles, California

Jean Gibb, MD
Assistant Clinical Professor of Infectious Disease
Keck School of Medicine of the University of Southern California
Los Angeles, California

Noopur Goel, MD
Consultant Rheumatologist
Department of Rheumatology
Arogya Rheumatology PLLC
Apex, North Carolina

David J. Goldstein, MD
Department of Dermatology
Kaiser Permanente West Los Angeles Medical Center
Los Angeles, California

Gregory Grandio, MD
Pulmonary and Critical Care Medicine Fellow
University of Southern California
Los Angeles, California

Arezoo Haghshenas, MD
Physician
Department of Rheumatology
Kaiser Permanente Eastbay
Oakland, California

Semi Han, MD
Internal Medicine
University of Southern California
Los Angeles, California

Liam Hilson, MD
Resident Physician
Department of Internal Medicine
Keck School of Medicine of the University of Southern California
Los Angeles, California

Antreas Hindoyan, MD
Assistant Professor of Clinical Medicine
Department of Cardiology
Keck School of Medicine of the University of Southern California
Los Angeles, California

Diana Homeier, MD
Associate Professor, Family Medicine
Geriatric Fellowship Director
Geriatric, Hospital, Palliative, and General Internal Medicine
Keck School of Medicine of the University of Southern California
Los Angeles, California

Patil Injean, DO
Resident, Medicine
Loma Linda University
Loma Linda, California

Kelli Kam, BA, MD
Resident Physician, Internal Medicine
Loma Linda University
Loma Linda, California

Kevin Kaplowitz, MD
Associate Clinical Professor, Ophthalmology
VA Loma Linda
Loma Linda University
Loma Linda, California

Talha Khawar, MD, RhMSUS
Assistant Professor of Medicine
Loma Linda University
University of California, Riverside
Division of Rheumatology
VA Loma Linda
Loma Linda, California

Chongiin Kim, MD
Department of Medicine
LAC+USC Medical Center
Los Angeles, California

Jackson Kim, MD
Nephrology Fellow
Division of Nephrology
Stanford University School of Medicine
Stanford, California

Justine Ko, MD, MPH
Resident Physician
Internal Medicine
LAC+USC Medical Center
Los Angeles, California

Yash Kothari, MD
Fellow
Department of Pulmonary, Critical Care, and Sleep Medicine
University of Southern California
Los Angeles, California

Wilson Kwan, MD, MS
Fellow Physician, Cardiology
Department of Cardiology
Keck School of Medicine of the University of Southern California
Los Angeles, California

Anna Lafian, DO, MS
Physician, Rheumatology
The Healing Rheum
Glendale, California

Alyssa Lampe Dominguez, MD
Assistant Professor of Clinical Medicine
Division of Endocrinology, Diabetes and Metabolism
Keck School of Medicine of the University of Southern California
Los Angeles, California

Joan Leavens, MD
Dermatopathologist and Dermatologist
Cascade Eye & Skin Centers
University Place, Washington

Arnold Lee, MD, PhD
Chief, Dermatology
Kaiser West Los Angeles Medical Center
Los Angeles, California

Chih-Han Lee, MD
Endocrinology and Diabetes Fellow
Keck School of Medicine of the University of Southern California
Los Angeles, California

Joseph Lee, MD
Nephrology Fellow
Johns Hopkins University School of Medicine
Baltimore, Maryland

Patrick Lee, MS, MD
Resident Physician
Department of Internal Medicine
Keck School of Medicine of the University of Southern California
Los Angeles, California

Shiqian Li, MD
Pulmonary and Critical Care Fellow
Keck School of Medicine of the University of Southern California
Los Angeles, California

Sophia Li, MD
Assistant Professor of Clinical Medicine
Division of Rheumatology
VA Loma Linda
Loma Linda University
Loma Linda, California

Maria Magar, MD
Department of Endocrinology
Kaiser Permanente
Los Angeles, California

Toby Maher, MD, PhD
Pulmonary and Critical Care Medicine Attending
University of Southern California
Los Angeles, California

Thin Thin Maw, MBBS, MS
Assistant Professor of Clinical Medicine
Division of Nephrology and Hypertension
Keck School of Medicine of the University of Southern California
Los Angeles, California

Colin M. McCrimmon, MD, PhD
Resident Physician
Department of Neurology
University of California, Los Angeles
Los Angeles, California

Christine McElyea, DO
Pulmonary Critical Care Fellow
Pulmonary and Critical Care
University of Southern California
Los Angeles, California

Neha Mehta, DO
Pulmonary, Critical Care, and Sleep Medicine
Keck School of Medicine of the University of Southern California
Los Angeles, California

Araz Melkonian, MD
Fellow in Geriatric Medicine
Division of Geriatric, Hospital, Palliative and General Internal Medicine
Keck School of Medicine of University of Southern California
Los Angeles, California

Teodulo (Jun) Meneses, MD
Pathology/Cytopathology
Department of Pathology and Laboratories
Kaiser Permanente West Los Angeles Medical Center
Los Angeles, California

Evan Mosier, MD
Physician, Gastroenterology
VA Loma Linda Healthcare System
Loma Linda, California

Ashwini Mulgaonkar, MS, MD
Internal Medicine
LAC+USC Medical Center
Los Angeles, California

Swathi Nallapa, MD
Internal Medicine
LAC+USC Medical Center
Los Angeles, California

Binh Ngo, MD
Clinical Associate Professor of Dermatology
Keck School of Medicine of the University of Southern California
Los Angeles, California

Caroline T. Nguyen, MD
Assistant Professor of Clinical Medicine, Obstetrics, and Gynecology
Division of Endocrinology, Diabetes, and Metabolism
Keck School of Medicine of the University of Southern California
Los Angeles, California

Priya Nori, MD
Medical Director
Antimicrobial Stewardship Program
Division of Infectious Diseases
Department of Medicine
Montefiore Medical Center
Albert Einstein College of Medicine
Bronx, New York

James Onwuzurike, MD
Resident Physician
Department of Internal Medicine
Keck School of Medicine of the University of Southern California
Los Angeles, California

Anish R. Patel, MD
Sleep Medicine Fellow, Pulmonary/Sleep Medicine
Neurocritical Care Fellow, Neurology
University of Southern California
Los Angeles, California

Reshma Patel, MD
Clinical Endocrinology Fellow
Division of Endocrinology, Department of Medicine
Keck School of Medicine of the University of Southern California
Los Angeles, California

Caroline I. Piatek, MD
Associate Professor of Clinical Medicine
Jane Anne Nohl Division of Hematology and Center for the Study of Blood Diseases
University of Southern California
Norris Comprehensive Cancer Center
Los Angeles, California

Chitra Punjabi, MD
Director of Tuberculosis and Communicable Disease Control
Rockland County DOH
Pomona, New York

Samantha Quon, MD, BA
Resident Physician
Department of Internal Medicine
University of Southern California
Los Angeles, California

Sahar Rabiei-Samani, MD
Fellow, Pulmonary, Critical Care, and Sleep Medicine
University of Southern California
Los Angeles, California

Soroush Rabiei-Samani, MD
Endocrinology Fellow
Department of Endocrinology, Diabetes, and Metabolism
Michigan State University College of Human Medicine
Lansing, Michigan

Ravi M. Rao, MD, MBA
Cardiology Fellow
University of California, Riverside
Riverside, California

Rennie L. Rhee, MD, MSCE
Assistant Professor of Medicine
Department of Medicine
Division of Rheumatology
Hospital of the University of Pennsylvania
Philadelphia, Pennsylvania

Mateen Saffarian, MD
Resident Physician
Department of Internal Medicine
Keck School of Medicine of the University of Southern California
Los Angeles, California

Ara Sahakian, MD
Assistant Professor of Medicine
Internal Medicine; Division of Gastrointestinal and Liver Diseases
University of Southern California
Los Angeles, California

Sheila Sahni, MD, FACC, FSCAI
Director of the Women's Heart Program
Sahni Heart Center
Hackensack Meridian Health
Clark, New Jersey

Vaneet K. Sandhu, MD
Associate Professor, Rheumatology
Loma Linda University Health
Loma Linda, California;
Assistant Professor, Medicine
University of California, Riverside
Riverside, California

Michael T. Schmidt, DO
Medical Director of Autopsy Services
Department of Pathology
Kaiser Permanente-West Los Angeles Medical Center
Los Angeles, California

Prabhdeep S. Sethi, MD, MPH, FACC, FSCAI, FSVM
Health Science Associate Clinical Professor
Program Director, Internal Medicine Residency
University of California, Riverside
Riverside, California

Hui Yi Shan, MD
Assistant Professor of Clinical Medicine
Director, Nephrology Fellowship Program
Division of Nephrology and Hypertension
Keck School of Medicine of the University of Southern California
Los Angeles, California

Sarah Sheibani, MD
Assistant Professor of the Division of Gastrointestinal and Liver Diseases
Keck School of Medicine of the University of Southern California
Los Angeles, California

Drew Sheldon, MD
Pulmonary and Critical Care Medicine Fellow
University of Southern California
Los Angeles, California

Chelsea Stone, DO, MA
Clinical Assistant Professor of Neurology (Clinician Educator)
Keck School of Medicine of the University of Southern California
Los Angeles, California

Shahid Syed, MD
Nephrologist, Internist
California Kidney Specialists
Physicians of Southern California
San Dimas, California

Diego Tabares, MD
Resident Physician
Department of Family Medicine
Kaiser Permanente Los Angeles Medical Center
Los Angeles, California

Justin Tiulim, MD
Fellow Physician
Hematology and Oncology
University of Southern California
LAC+USC Medical Center
Los Angeles, California

Chuong Tran, MD
Fellow Physician, Gastroenterology
Loma Linda University
Loma Linda, California

Hien T. Tran, MD, PhD
Seaside Dermatology and Skin Cancer Center
Irvine, California

Maria E. Vergara-Lluri, MD
Assistant Professor of Clinical Pathology
Department of Pathology and Laboratory Medicine, Hematopathology Section
Keck School of Medicine of the University of Southern California
LAC+USC Medical Center
Los Angeles, California

Christopher Vo, MD
Division of Infectious Diseases
Department of Medicine
Icahn School of Medicine at Mount Sinai
New York, New York

Noah Wald-Dickler, MD, FACP
Clinical Assistant Professor of Medicine
University of Southern California Keck School of Medicine
Associate Hospital Epidemiologist
LAC+USC Medical Center
Los Angeles, California

Michelle Walters, MD
Resident Physician
Division of Dermatology
Harbor-UCLA Medical Center
Torrance, California

Darren Wong, MD
Assistant Professor of Medicine
Medicine/Infectious Diseases
University of Southern California
Los Angeles, California

Clay Wu, DO
Fellow, Pulmonary/Critical Care
University of Southern California
Los Angeles, California

Patrick Wu, DO, MPH
Assistant Professor of Medicine
Loma Linda University
Loma Linda, California

Viktoriya Yanchuk, DO
Nephrologist
Arrowhead Regional Medical Center
Northridge, California

Howard Yang, MD, RhMSUS
Assistant Clinical Professor
Internal Medicine, Rheumatology
University of California, Los Angeles
Los Angeles, California

Katharine Yang, MD
Clinical Instructor
Department of Hospital Medicine
University of California, San Francisco
San Francisco, California

Michelle Yim, DO
Geriatric Medicine Fellow
Division of Geriatric, Hospital, Palliative, and General Internal Medicine
Keck School of Medicine of the University of Southern California
Los Angeles, California

Diana H. Yu, MD
Assistant Professor of Clinical Medicine
Director, Interventional Pulmonology Research
Division of Pulmonary, Critical Care and Sleep Medicine
Keck School of Medicine of the University of Southern California
Los Angeles, California

Micah Yu, MD
Rheumatologist
Arrowhead Regional Medical Center
Colton, California

Liyun Yuan, MD, PhD
Assistant Professor of Clinical Medicine
Gastroenterology and Liver Diseases
University of Southern California
Los Angeles, California

Meiling L. Fang Yuen, MD
Associate Program Director, Department of Medicine/Dermatology
Associate Staff, Department of Medicine/Dermatology
Harbor-UCLA Medical Center
Torrance, California

FOREWORD

I had the pleasure of first meeting Dr. Dasgupta when he approached me to be on his podcast to raise awareness about scleroderma, a disease that eventually took my sister's life. Soon into the recording I quickly realized that Raj and I share common beliefs and qualities. I don't think he'll stop practicing medicine and join a comedy tour, but his desire to help others, being selfless, and just being a positive person who loves to smile and bring happiness to others is what I saw in him throughout the interview. I am honored that Raj wanted to dedicate this book to the Scleroderma Research Foundation and my sister. I know this book will reflect Dr. Dasgupta's knowledge and passion for patients and teaching.

Bob Saget

PREFACE

It is with great pleasure that we present to you our sixth book in the Morning Report: Beyond the Pearls series, *Medicine Morning Report Subspecialties: Beyond the Pearls*. Writing the "perfect" case-based review text has been a dream of mine ever since I was a first-year medical student. Dr. Koolaee and I envisioned a text that integrates a United States Medical Licensing Examination (USMLE) Steps 1, 2, and 3 focus with up-to-date, evidence-based clinical medicine. We wanted the platform of the text to be drawn from a traditional theme that many of us are familiar with from residency—the "morning report" format. This book is written for a wide audience, from medical students to attending physicians practicing Internal Medicine and its subspecialties. The cases have been carefully chosen, and each case was written and reviewed by a subspecialist in Internal Medicine. The cases in the book cover scenarios and questions frequently encountered on the USMLE, Internal Medicine boards, shelf exams, and wards, integrating both basic science and Clinical Pearls.

We sincerely thank all the many contributors who have helped to create this text. Their insightful work will be a valuable tool for medical students and physicians to gain an in-depth understanding of Internal Medicine. It should be noted that while a variety of clinical cases in Internal Medicine were selected for this book, it is not meant to substitute a comprehensive Internal Medicine reference.

Dr. Koolaee and I would like to thank our volume editors Dr. Shan, Dr. Wong, Dr. Yang, and Dr. Li for all their hard work and dedication to this book. It was truly a pleasure to work with everyone associated with the book, and we look forward to our next project together.

CONTENTS

SECTION 1 Nephrology 1

1 A 50-Year-Old Male With Lethargy, Vomiting, and Pruritis 3
Viktoriya Yanchuk ■ Hui Yi Shan

2 A 40-Year-Old Male With Abdominal Distention and Decreased Urine Output 13
Jonathan Cheng ■ Hui Yi Shan

3 A 28-Year-Old Male With Left Flank Pain and Bloody Urine 19
Joseph Lee ■ Hui Yi Shan

4 A 62-Year-Old Male With Worsening Peripheral Edema 27
Jackson Kim ■ Hui Yi Shan

5 A 56-Year-Old Male With Acquired Immunodeficiency Syndrome With Nausea and Weakness 32
Shahid Syed ■ Thin Thin Maw

SECTION 2 Hematology 39

6 A 58-Year-Old Female With Syncope 41
Justin Tiulim ■ Maria E. Vergara-Lluri ■ Caroline I. Piatek

7 A 24-Year-Old Male With Easy Bruising and Mucosal Bleeding 49
Justin Tiulim ■ Maria E. Vergara-Lluri ■ Caroline I. Piatek

SECTION 3 Geriatrics 59

8 An 87-Year-Old Male With Acute Onset of Confusion 61
Diana Homeier ■ Araz Melkonian

9 A 78-Year-Old Female With a Ground-Level Fall 68
Michelle Yim ■ Diana Homeier

SECTION 4 Dermatology 75

10 A 57-Year-Old Female With Burning Red Rash on Lower Legs 77
Arnold Lee ■ Hui Yi Shan ■ Teodulo (Jun) Meneses ■ David J. Goldstein

11 A 70-Year-Old Female With Chronic Unilateral Rash on Left Nipple 85
Arnold Lee ■ Michael T. Schmidt ■ Hien T. Tran

12 A 58-Year-Old Female With Progressive Facial Lesions 90
Brandon L. Adler ■ Binh Ngo

13 A 79-Year-Old Male With a Fungating Mass on the Left Lower Extremity 100
Maggie Chow ▪ Binh Ngo

14 A 38-Year-Old Female With a Diffuse Rash and Mucositis 108
Joan Leavens ▪ Binh Ngo

15 A 62-Year-Old Woman With an 8-Year History of a Pruritic Rash 118
Michelle Walters ▪ Meiling L. Fang Yuen

SECTION **5 Neurology 125**

16 A 28-Year-Old Male With Progressive Lower Back Pain, Paraplegia, and Urinary Incontinence 127
Colin M. McCrimmon ▪ An H. Do

17 A 23-Year-Old Male With Severe Headache Behind the Right Eye 134
Chelsea Stone ▪ Esther Byun

18 A 61-Year-Old Female With Right-Hand Numbness 139
Nancy Baker ▪ Esther Byun

19 A 21-Year-Old Male With Sudden Onset of Right-Sided Hemiparesis and Aphasia 145
Anish R. Patel ▪ Benjamin A. Emanuel

SECTION **6 Cardiology 155**

20 A 62-Year-Old Female With Progressively Worsening Shortness of Breath, Fatigue, and Lower Extremity Edema 157
Neil Bhambi ▪ Michael Fong

21 A 77-Year-Old Female With Worsening Shortness of Breath and Leg Swelling 169
Shamili Allam ▪ Michael Fong

22 A 54-Year-Old Male With Bilateral Leg Pain 177
Ravi M. Rao ▪ Prabhdeep S. Sethi

23 A 58-Year-Old Female With Recurrent Chest Pain With Exertion 186
Mateen Saffarian ▪ Daniel Aldea ▪ Shankar Chhetri ▪ Sheila Sahni

24 A 59-Year-Old Male With Sudden, Burning Chest Pain 196
Christopher Bradley ▪ Percy Genyk ▪ Wilson Kwan ▪ Antreas Hindoyan

25 A 55-Year-Old Female With Retrosternal Chest Pain 206
Shankar Chhetri ▪ Sheila Sahni

26 A 48-Year-Old Male With Acute Shortness of Breath 218
James Onwuzurike ▪ Katharine Yang ▪ Shankar Chhetri ▪ Sheila Sahni

SECTION 7 Rheumatology 229

27 A 32-Year-Old Female With Right Lower Extremity Edema 231
Arezoo Haghshenas ■ Vaneet K. Sandhu

28 A 35-Year-Old Female With Dry Eyes and Dry Mouth 242
Micah Yu ■ Kevin Kaplowitz ■ Sophia Li

29 A 36-Year-Old Male With 3 Years of Worsening Joint Pain 251
Anna Lafian ■ Nasim Daoud

30 A 55-Year-Old Female With Muscle Weakness 259
Howard Yang

31 A 46-Year-Old Female With Purpura and Arthralgia 266
Kristal Choi ■ Talha Khawar

32 A 65-Year-Old Male With Acute Monoarticular Arthritis 275
Noopur Goel ■ Sophia Li

33 A 22-Year-Old Female With Easy Bruising, Joint Hypermobility, and Arthralgia 281
Patil Injean ■ Christina Downey

34 A 70-Year-Old Female With Bilateral Shoulder Pain 293
Kelli Kam ■ Kevin Kaplowitz ■ Sophia Li

SECTION 8 Gastroenterology 305

35 A 44-Year-Old Female With Acute Onset Epigastric Pain 307
Evan Mosier ■ Daniel Chao

36 A 26-Year-Old Female With Chronic Hepatitis B 316
Chuong Tran ■ Daniel Chao

37 A 24-Year-Old Male With Elevated Liver Function Tests 324
Daniel Chao

38 A 54-Year-Old Female With Dysphagia 331
Lillian Dawit ■ Christina S. Gainey ■ Ara Sahakian

39 A 25-Year-Old Male With Chronic Diarrhea 345
Patrick Lee ■ Liam Hilson ■ Sarah Sheibani

SECTION 9 Infectious Diseases 351

40 A 29-Year-Old Male With a Headache 353
Fernando Dominguez ■ Emily Blodget

41 A 45-Year-Old Male With Knee Pain 358
Chitra Punjabi ■ Priya Nori

42 A 70-Year-Old Male With Fever and Diarrhea 363
Rachel Bartash ■ Priya Nori

43 A 30-Year-Old Female With Neutropenia and Fever 369
Patrick Wu ■ Darren Wong

44 A 42-Year-Old Male With Fever and Malaise 378
Katharine Yang ■ Noah Wald-Dickler

45 A 19-Year-Old Female With Acute Abdominal Pain 386
Christopher Vo ■ Noah Wald-Dickler

46 A 30-Year-Old Male With Shortness of Breath, Fatigue, and Weight Loss 392
Tyler Degener ■ Jean Gibb

SECTION **10 Hepatology 403**

47 A 60-Year-Old Female With Elevated Alkaline Phosphatase and Hypercalcemia 405
Ashwini Mulgaonkar ■ Liyun Yuan

48 A 77-Year-Old Male With Progressive Jaundice and Pruritus 412
Ashwini Mulgaonkar ■ Liyun Yuan

SECTION **11 Endocrine 419**

49 A 49-Year-Old Male With Polyuria and Polydipsia 421
Maria Magar ■ Braden Barnett

50 A 48-Year-Old Male With Bitemporal Hemianopsia 430
Chih-Han Lee ■ John David Carmichael

51 A 32-Year-Old Female With Recurrent Pregnancy Loss 442
Reshma Patel ■ Caroline T. Nguyen

52 A 60-Year-Old Female Presents for Wellness Visit 449
Diego Tabares ■ Braden Barnett

53 A 19-Year-Old Female With Oligomenorrhea and Facial Hair Growth 461
Alyssa Lampe Dominguez ■ Caroline T. Nguyen

SECTION **12 Pulmonary 473**

54 A 67-Year-Old Male With Sudden Onset of Dyspnea and Pleuritic Chest Pain 475
Anish R. Patel ■ Raj Dasgupta

55 A 27-Year-Old Male Who Experienced a Seizure 484
Chongiin Kim ■ Neha Mehta ■ Raj Dasgupta

56 A 73-Year-Old Female With Dysphagia and Cough 490
Christine McElyea ■ Semi Han ■ Raj Dasgupta

57 A 58-Year-Old Male With Occupational Lung Disease 497
Gregory Grandio ■ Drew Sheldon ■ Raj Dasgupta ■ Toby Maher

58 A 68-Year-Old Male With Progressively Worsening Dyspnea and Dry Cough 505
Drew Sheldon ▪ Clay Wu ▪ Raj Dasgupta ▪ Toby Maher

59 A 47-Year-Old Female With Shortness of Breath 515
Samantha Quon ▪ Yash Kothari ▪ Clay Wu ▪ Drew Sheldon ▪ Raj Dasgupta ▪ Sivagini Ganesh

60 A 64-Year-Old Male With a 3-Month History of Worsening Cough 523
Swathi Nallapa ▪ Shiqian Li ▪ Raj Dasgupta ▪ Diana H. Yu

61 A 58-Year-Old Female With Acute-on-Chronic Abdominal Pain 530
Justine Ko ▪ Shiqian Li ▪ Raj Dasgupta ▪ Diana H. Yu

62 A 55-Year-Old Female With Chronic Cough 538
Patrick Chan ▪ Clay Wu ▪ Raj Dasgupta

63 A 64-Year-Old Female With Fevers 546
Dafang Chen ▪ Clay Wu ▪ Raj Dasgupta

64 A 53-Year-Old Male With Fever, Fatigue, and Myalgia 553
Sahar Rabiei-Samani ▪ Raj Dasgupta ▪ Soroush Rabiei-Samani ▪ Rennie L. Rhee

Index 567

SECTION 1

Nephrology

CASE 1

A 50-Year-Old Male With Lethargy, Vomiting, and Pruritis

Viktoriya Yanchuk ■ Hui Yi Shan

A 50-year-old male without significant medical history presents with 3 weeks of lethargy, nausea, vomiting, and pruritis. His wife reports that his mentation is slower from his baseline. He had a recent root canal and was taking daily ibuprofen for pain relief prior to the procedure.

What is uremia and its signs and symptoms?
Blood urea nitrogen (BUN) elevation alone is termed azotemia. When this elevation is coupled with a constellation of symptoms, it is termed uremia. Uremic syndrome is due to renal failure, acute or chronic, with subsequent buildup of toxins causing symptoms summarized in Table 1.1.

CLINICAL PEARL **STEP 2/3**

Causes of an elevated BUN in the absence of renal failure include fever and increased catabolism (steroid use), high protein intake such as tube feeds, total parenteral nutrition, or gastrointestinal bleed (autodigestion of red blood cells), and hypovolemic states.

What aspects of medical history and physical examination should be included in the evaluation of this patient's uremia?
History gathering should be thorough and needs to include medical history (specifically history of kidney disease, urologic disorders, trauma, or cancer) and surgical/procedural history. Furthermore, it must include family history of kidney disease and hypertension or systemic

TABLE 1.1 ■ **Signs and Symptoms of Uremia**

Uremic Symptoms	Uremic Signs
Vomiting	Asterixis (flapping tremor)
Fatigue	Mental status changes
Anorexia	Foot or wrist drop (due to uremic motor neuropathy)
Weight loss	Uremic frost
Muscle cramps	Pericardial friction rub
Pruritus	
Visual disturbances	
Increased thirst	

autoimmune disease, as well as toxin exposure, medications including recent changes and over the counter or herbal supplement use, contrasted imaging studies, and work exposures. Lastly, one must inquire about recent viral or bacterial illnesses, recent fevers, or rashes. Patients may not be able to ascertain what history is important; thus, organized and comprehensive history can provide necessary clues to narrow the differential for renal dysfunction.

Physical examination should be systematic and include evaluation of the retina (looking for signs of diabetic retinopathy or hypertensive vascular changes), neck exam evaluation for jugular venous distention, pulmonary exam, cardiac exam (looking for murmurs or pericardial friction rub), abdominal exam (evaluating for suprapubic tenderness and distended bladder by percussion), skin evaluation, and lower extremity exam for edema.

Further history reveals that the patient has anorexia, a bitter taste in his mouth, and decreased urine output. He also reports his shoes feel tighter than usual. He denies any personal or family history of renal disease or systemic autoimmune disease.

On exam, vital signs are significant for blood pressure of 167/95. You note the patient has bruising on his shins and the dorsal aspects of his hands. On further questioning, the patient also admits to having increased gum bleeding, which started in the last 3 weeks. You also note 2+ pitting edema to the shins bilaterally. Palpation over the bladder is unremarkable.

BASIC SCIENCE PEARL **STEP 1**

Uremic bleeding is thought to be due to circulating toxin interference with platelets. This has been observed by mixing normal platelets with uremic serum leading to platelet dysfunction and mixing uremic platelets with normal serum without clotting abnormalities. Urea itself is not the culprit and BUN level in the serum cannot predict bleeding time in a patient with renal failure. Uremic bleeding can be temporarily treated by infusing desmopressin, which releases the von Willebrand factor from the endothelial cells.

How can one distinguish chronic kidney disease (CKD) from acute kidney injury (AKI)?

Anemia, small sclerosed kidneys, and waxy casts (from distended tubules) point to CKD. Hyperkalemia, elevation of phosphate, and even elevation of parathyroid hormone (PTH) can occur in AKI as well as echogenic kidneys, which can be seen both in AKI and CKD if the kidneys appear of normal size.

BASIC SCIENCE PEARL **STEP 1**

On ultrasonography (US), a substance that reflects most of the sound waves appears white or echogenic. Fat and fibrous tissue are very echogenic and appear white, which is why usually echogenic kidneys are associated with CKD, assuming the cause of the bright appearance is fibrosis; however, inflammatory infiltrates can cause a bright appearance of the kidneys on US as seen with AIN and GN.

AIN, Allergic interstitial nephritis; *GN*, glomerulonephritis.

What is the differential for AKI?

See Table 1.2.

What renal conditions can be caused by nonsteroidal antiinflammatory drugs (NSAIDs)?

See Table 1.3.

TABLE 1.2 ■ **Acute Kidney Injury**

Prerenal (↓ECV)	Intrarenal	Postrenal
↑TBV • Hepatorenal syndrome • Cardiorenal syndrome	**Glomerular** • Nephritic syndrome (hematuria) • Nephrotic syndrome (proteinuria)	**Kidney** (B/L or single kidney [anatomic or functionally]) • RCC (severe tumor burden) • Struvite stones
↓TBV • Bleeding • Nonbleeding: GI: NVD Renal: diuretics, polyuria ↑ Insensible losses: flu, fevers, heat stroke	**Tubular** • Ischemic ATN: Prolonged prerenal state • Direct endogenous nephrotoxicity: Protein deposits: paraproteinemias (MM, Waldenstrom, amyloid) heme pigment, amyloid Nonprotein deposits: ↑phos, ↑calcium, ↑bilirubin, ↑uric acid (urate nephropathy, TLS) Endotoxemia in sepsis and pancreatitis • Direct exogenous nephrotoxicity: Vancomycin, tenofovir, aminoglycosides, contrast, ACEI/ARB, amphotericin, platins, sulfa drugs, tacrolimus	**Ureter** (B/L or single kidney [anatomic or functionally]) • Obstructive stones • Strictures (BK virus in renal transplant) • Kink in renal transplant
	Interstitial (WBC) • Acute interstitial nephritis • Leukemia/lymphoma • Amyloidosis	**Bladder** • Tumor • Bleeding/clots • Neurogenic bladder
↔TBV • Shocks (non-hemorrhagic): Distributive: anaphylaxis, Addison's, sepsis cardiogenic obstructive neurogenic • Renal vein thrombosis • Abdominal compartment syndrome	**Vascular** • TMA: TTP, HUS/aHUS, DIC, antiphospholipid antibody syndrome, CNI • Atheroembolic renal disease **Miscellaneous** • Warfarin • NSAIDs	**Urethra** • Benign prostate hypertrophy • Foley obstruction/ Foley balloon out of place • Stricture/tumor invasion

aHUS, Atypical hemolytic uremic syndrome; *ATN*, acute tubular necrosis; *B/L*, bilateral; *CNI*, calcineurin inhibitor toxicity; *DIC*, disseminated intravascular coagulopathy; *ECV*, effective circulating volume; *HUS*, hemolytic uremic syndrome; *RCC*, renal cell carcinoma; *TBV*, total body volume; *TMA*, thrombotic microangiopathy.

TABLE 1.3 ■ **Diseases Caused by Nonsteroidal Antiinflammatory Drug Use**

AKI	Prerenal azotemia Acute tubular necrosis Acute papillary necrosis
Glomerular disease	Minimal change disease Membranous nephropathy
Tubulointerstitial disease	Acute interstitial nephritis Chronic interstitial nephritis
Electrolyte disorders	Hypertension and edema from sodium retention

AKI, Acute kidney injury.

BASIC SCIENCE PEARL **STEP 1**

NSAIDs obtain their analgesic, antiinflammatory, and antipyretic function through suppression of prostaglandin (PG) synthesis via inhibition of cyclooxygenase 1 and 2. The PGs most pertinent to the kidneys are E2 and I2. PG-E2 regulates sodium and chloride transport in the thick ascending loop of Henle and has diuretic and natriuretic effects. PG-I2 regulates vascular tone and increases potassium secretion by increasing renin and activating RAAS. Collectively, PGs increase renal blood flow and glomerular filtration rate (GRF) via vasodilation of afferent arterioles in patients with reduced effective circulating volume. In healthy, normotensive individuals, PGs seem to play a small role in renal function or blood pressure, but patients with underlying comorbidities are at risk for renal dysfunction from NSAIDs.

RAAS, Renin-angiotensin-aldosterone system.

CLINICAL PEARL **STEP 2/3**

Acute renal papillary necrosis (Fig. 1.1) is the death and sloughing of the renal papilla caused by ischemia, which may be due to a variety of etiologies. A commonly used mnemonic for causes of papillary necrosis is POSTCARDS: pyelonephritis, obstruction of the urogenital tract, sickle cell disease, tuberculosis, cirrhosis of the liver, analgesia/alcohol abuse, renal vein thrombosis, diabetes mellitus, and systemic vasculitis. Paracetamol poses more risk for this disorder than other NSAIDs or aspirin. A classic diagnostic feature is ring-shaped renal calcification on plain radiography, which is more common with analgesic nephropathy than other causes. Computerized tomography may show a "ball-in-tree" sign (Fig. 1.2).

What is the appropriate workup to order at this time?

Complete blood count (CBC), basic metabolic panel (BMP), phosphate, albumin, PTH, urine analysis (UA) with microscopy, renal ultrasound with postvoid residual.

Lab results showed white blood cell count (WBC) of 7, hemoglobin (Hg) of 13, platelets of 170; sodium of 132, potassium of 5.1, chloride of 99, bicarbonate of 19, BUN 96, creatinine of 5.8; phosphate 6.8, albumin 3.6, PTH 176; UA with specific gravity of 1.010, negative nitrites, positive leukocyte esterase, 10+ protein, 11–40 WBC, 0–2 (red blood cell count) RBC, white cell casts, no bacteria, and 1–2 granular casts. Renal ultrasound noted bilateral echogenic kidneys of normal size.

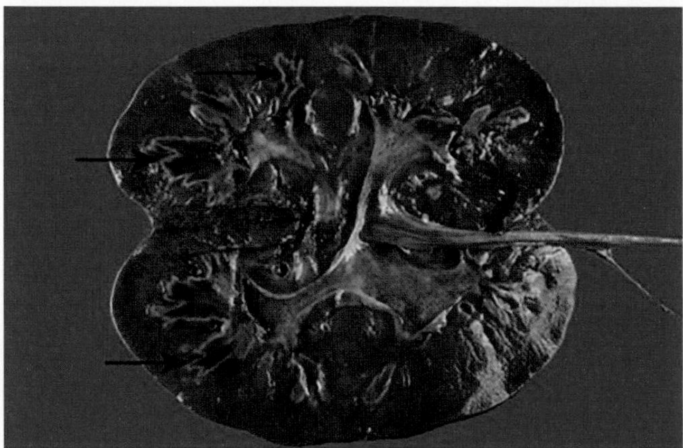

Fig. 1.1 Transected kidney showing papillary necrosis notable by brown discolored papillae *(arrows)*.

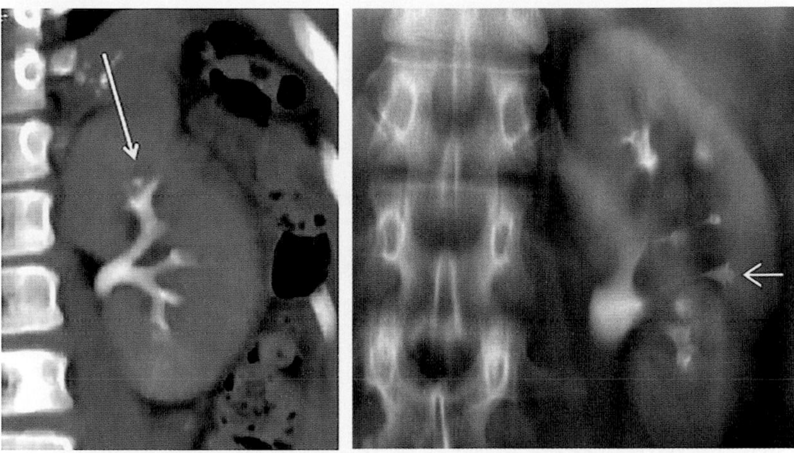

Fig. 1.2 Renal papillary necrosis on computer tomography. (Tublin M, Nelson, *J. Imaging in Urology*. p161. 2018 Elsevier.)

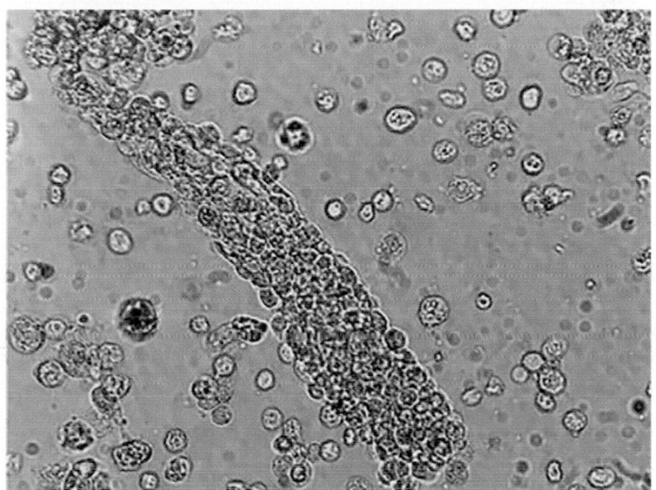

Fig. 1.3 White blood cell urinary cast.

Based on the laboratory results, what further workup should be ordered?

White cell casts are suggestive of either urinary tract infection or allergic interstitial nephritis; thus, urine culture and eosinophil microscopy in urine should be obtained (Figs. 1.3 and 1.4).

Urine culture is negative. Urine microscopy shows eosinophils.

What is the most likely diagnosis at this time?

The patient has renal insufficiency. Based on the lab values, it appears to be an acute process: hemoglobin is normal, no waxy casts are seen, and the kidneys appear normal size on

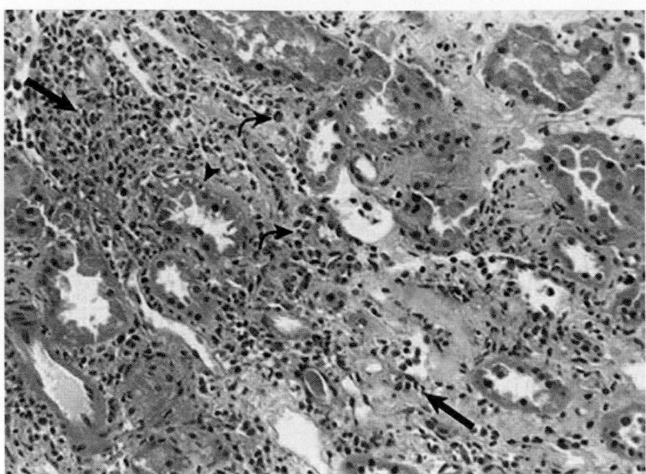

Fig. 1.4 Kidney biopsy showing acute interstitial nephritis. A diffuse interstitial infiltrate is present *(arrows)* along with severe tubular injury and tubulitis *(arrowhead)*, where lymphocytes have crossed the tubular basement membrane. Also present are eosinophils *(curved arrows)* (hematoxylin and eosin ×40).

ultrasound—all arguing against chronic renal disease. The etiology appears to be intrarenal as the specific gravity (the measure of urine concentration) is 1.010, termed isosthenuria, suggesting an inability of the kidney to either dilute or concentrate the urine. The UA also shows 1–2 granular casts, which suggests tubular damage and necrosis and can been seen with virtually any process that causes microvascular renal ischemia or direct toxicity to the tubules and should not be confused with "acute tubular necrosis" (ATN) as a diagnosis. As seen in Table 1.2, ATN is a broad term with many possible etiologies. The presence of "muddy-brown" casts or a heavy burden of granular casts suggests the diagnosis of ATN, which this patient does not have. Glomerulonephritis in this case is unlikely given absences of significant proteinuria and hematuria). In the absence of significant, gross, or heavy microscopic hematuria, a lack of flank pain and fever argue against acute papillary necrosis and short-term use of ibuprofen argues against analgesic nephropathy, both discussed in more detail later in the chapter. The UA showing sterile pyuria, white cell casts, and urine eosinophils, coupled with the history of ibuprofen use suggests allergic interstitial nephritis.)

What is allergic interstitial nephritis (AIN)?

Inflammation and infiltration of the interstitium with acute inflammatory cells including polymorphonucleocytes (PMNs), eosinophils, and lymphocytes. Somewhere between 75%–90% of all cases of AIN are caused by drug exposure. Initially, AIN was described primarily with beta-lactam antibiotics, although now we know that a variety of medications can cause AIN, and nearly any drug has the potential to cause AIN much like nearly any drug has the potential to cause an allergic reaction. The remainder of the AIN cases are linked to autoimmune systemic diseases and infections.

What are common causes of allergic interstitial nephritis?

See Tables 1.4 and 1.5.

TABLE 1.4 ■ **Drugs Known to Cause Allergic Interstitial Nephritis**

Class	Examples
Antibiotics	Beta-lactams, sulfonamides, fluoroquinolones, macrolides, antituberculins (rifampin)
Antiviral	Indinavir
Diuretics	Loop diuretics, thiazide-like diuretics
Analgesics	NSAIDs, selective COX-2 inhibitors
GI medications	PPIs, H2-receptor blockers, mesalamine
Anticonvulsants	Phenytoin, carbamazepine, phenobarbital
Miscellaneous	Allopurinol, Chinese herbs

COX, Cyclooxygenase; *PPI*, proton pump inhibitor.

TABLE 1.5 ■ **Common Nondrug Causes of Allergic Interstitial Nephritis**

Bacterial infections	Legionella, Staphylococcus, Streptococcus, Yersinia
Viral infections	Hantavirus, CMV, EBV, HIV, HSV, hepatitis C
Autoimmune	Systemic lupus erythematosis, Sjögren syndrome, sarcoidosis
Neoplastic diseases	Lymphoproliferative disorders, plasma cell dyscrasias
Other	TINU (tubulointerstitial nephritis and uveitis)

CMV, Cytomegalovirus; *EBV*, Epstein-Barr virus; *HIV*, human immunodeficiency virus; *HSV*, herpes simplex virus.

CLINICAL PEARL **STEP 2/3**

Tubulointerstitial nephritis and uveitis (TINU) is a rare condition usually seen in adolescent girls, which, like the name suggests, involves both the kidneys and eyes. Pathogenesis and etiology of the syndrome are not known. TINU presents with weight loss, fever, anemia, nausea, vomiting, anorexia, and hyperglobulinemia, which occur before ocular and kidney manifestations. The initial kidney dysfunction manifestation is Fanconi syndrome with glucosuria, proteinuria, and aminoaciduria followed by a tubulointerstitial infiltrate, sometimes with granulomas.

BASIC SCIENCE PEARL **STEP 1**

In leptospirosis the spirochete enters the bloodstream through the skin or mucosa, and eventually invades glomerular capillaries before migrating into the tubulointerstitium. Once there, the organism induces inflammation and direct tubular injury that with time manifests as large, edematous kidneys. Eradication of infection resolves the renal failure.

CLINICAL PEARL **STEP 2/3**

Hantavirus is an RNA virus that can cause interstitial edema with infiltration of PMNs, eosinophils, and monocytes. Notably, interstitial hemorrhage follows renal inflammation and is associated with gross or microscopic hematuria.

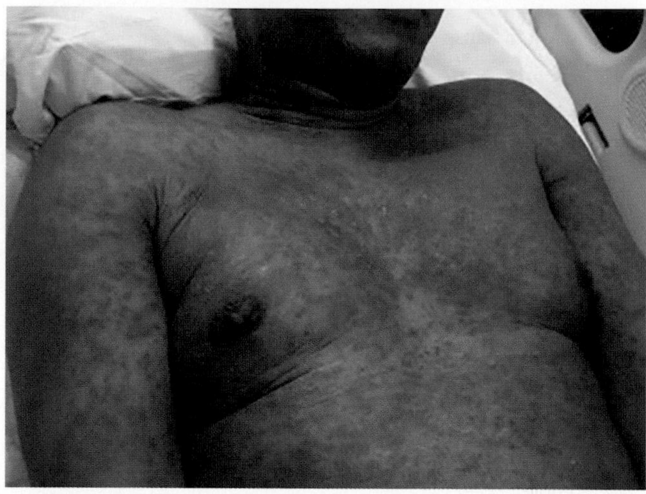

Fig. 1.5 A patient with a morbilliform eruption secondary to allopurinol with peripheral eosinophilia.

What is the typical presentation of allergic interstitial nephritis?

The classic presentation of AIN is the triad of rash (maculopapular) (Fig. 1.5), fever, and peripheral eosinophilia (absolute eosinophil count >500/μL) but this is seen in 5%–10% of cases. Most presentation is nonspecific with malaise, nausea, and vomiting. Patients may also be asymptomatic and only abnormal lab results are noted. Eosinophiluria is defined by eosinophils that account for more than 1% of urinary white cells by Hansel stain. This finding is neither very sensitive nor specific, and presence or absence alone does not clinch the diagnosis. Fever is seen in 50% of drug induced–AIN (DI-AIN). For DI-AIN, the prodrome can range anywhere from 1 day to 18 months. Usually, AKI is nonoliguric but oliguria can occur.

What is the management of allergic interstitial nephritis?

Treatment of the underlying cause or withdrawal of the provoking drug is the main treatment. Controversy exists over use of steroids to treat AIN. Limited, retrospective studies suggest that early use of corticosteroids is associated with better outcomes. Regimens suggested include 250–500 mg IV methylprednisolone followed by 1 mg/kg per day of oral prednisone or 1 mg/kg per day of oral prednisone continued for 1–1.5 months.

The patient stopped taking NSAIDs. On his one month follow up visit with primary care physician, the patient's serum Cr was back to 1.1.

Case Summary

- **Complaint/History:** A 50-year-old male without significant medical history presents with 3 weeks of lethargy, nausea, vomiting, and pruritis after ingesting ibuprofen daily for a toothache.
- **Findings:** Hypertension, lower extremity pitting edema, bruising.
- **Lab Results/Tests:** Acute renal failure with UA with sterile pyuria, white cell casts, and eosinophils.

Diagnosis: Drug associated acute interstitial nephritis.

- **Treatment:** Withdrawal of the offending agent (ibuprofen) with return to baseline renal function.

BEYOND THE PEARLS

- Incidence of NSAID-related renal disease in the United States is 2.5 million cases annually with the same potential for untoward effects for both selective and nonselective NSAIDs. AKI in NSAID use appears to be dose dependent and is negatively synergistic with intravenous contrast as radiocontrast can cause vasoconstriction, reducing renal blood flow. Patients should be informed to hold NSAIDs for 48 hours prior to contrast studies.
- Long-term use of NSAIDs can induce analgesic nephropathy (AN), the most common form of chronic interstitial nephritis (CIN) worldwide. AN can present as slowly progressive CKD as CIN is difficult to diagnose without a biopsy and a high index of suspicion.
- One NSAID implicated as a causative agent of AN no longer on the market is phenacetin, an acetaminophen-like analgesic, which metabolizes into the active drug paracetamol (still widely used in Europe). In 1983 phenacetin was banned by the United States Food and Drug Administration as it caused hemolytic anemia in patients with glucose-6-phosphate dehydrogenase deficiency, urothelial carcinoma of the renal pelvis, and renal papillary necrosis and AN in all comers. The culprit metabolite is believed to be p-phenetidine. Interestingly, Howard Hughes is believed to have died of renal failure due to analgesic nephropathy because of prolonged use of phenacetin for chronic pain. The phenacetin-acetaminophen combination required to cause CIN has been estimated to be at least 2–3 kg over many years. While the drug is off the market, this piece of history can still be clinically relevant to older patients who may have used this drug extensively while it was available, and it is important to extract this history from patients with CKD.
- Initially AN was observed only with phenacetin-containing analgesic combinations; however, it is now known that other combinations may also induce this disease. CIN is caused by daily use of a combination of two or more analgesics for multiple years in combination with central nervous system active dependence-inducing substances (caffeine, opiates, barbiturates).
- The population most affected by AN are women in their 60s and 70s with history of chronic pain such as lower back pain or migraines. One should inquire about any episodes suggesting papillary necrosis such as fever, flank pain, or gross hematuria or urinary outflow obstruction (from the sloughing papilla). The clinical presentation of AN includes a prolonged history of combination analgesic use as previously described, renal failure (chronic and progressive), sterile pyuria (eosinophiluria), anemia (from CKD), proteinuria (papillae loss), and may have hypertension. The classic imaging finding on plain radiograph is papillary or medullary calcification (Fig. 1.6). Patients with AN should be screened for transitional cell carcinoma if presenting with painless hematuria as the source of bleeding may be from the bladder as well.

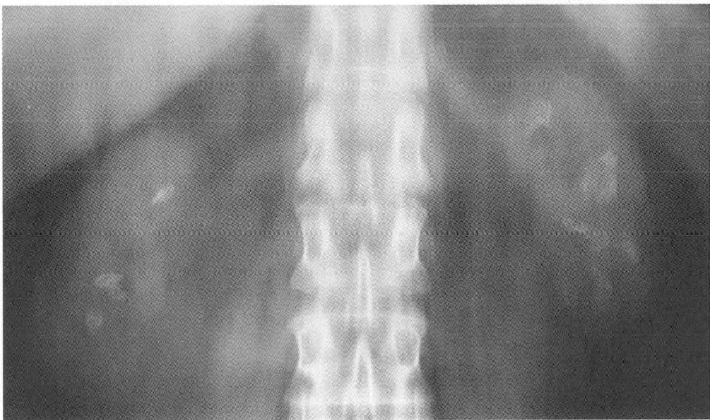

Fig. 1.6 Plain radiograph of the abdomen showing multiple medullary calcifications.

Bibliography

Arend, L. (2013). Tubulointerstitial diseases. In: *Practical renal pathology*. Elsevier. pp. 127–158.

Ahmed, A., Pritchard S., et al. (2013). A review of cutaneous drug eruptions. *Clinics in Geriatric Medicine, 29*(2), 527–545.

Brewster, U., & Luciano, R. (2018). Acute interstitial nephritis. In: *National kidney foundation primer on kidney disease*, 7th edition. Elsevier. pp. 320–325.

Hendericks, M. et al. (2017). Renal papillary necrosis in patients with sickle cell disease: how to recognize this 'forgotten' diagnosis. *Journal of Pediatric Urology, 13*(3), 250–256.

Zagoria, R., et al. (2016). The kidney: Diffuse parenchymal abnormality. In: *Genitourinary imaging: The requisites*, 3rd edition. Elsevier. pp. 107–145.

CASE 2

A 40-Year-Old Male With Abdominal Distention and Decreased Urine Output

Jonathan Cheng ■ Hui Yi Shan

A 40-year-old male with a history of alcohol-induced cirrhosis presents with 2 weeks of worsening jaundice, nausea, and vomiting. He also reports increased abdominal distention and decreased urine output. His current medications include ciprofloxacin, metronidazole, pantoprazole, lactulose, pentoxifylline, and tamsulosin. He says he is not suffering from fever, chills, chest pain, shortness of breath, hematuria, hematemesis, or hematochezia. He has been drinking three beers a day for the last 6 years and denies illicit drug use.

What is cirrhosis and what are the signs and symptoms of decompensation?

Cirrhosis is a form of chronic liver disease in which healthy liver tissue is replaced with scar tissue. The most common causes of cirrhosis include long-term viral infections (hepatitis B and C), fatty liver associated with obesity and diabetes, and alcohol abuse. The signs and symptoms of decompensated cirrhosis include jaundice, edema (more commonly involving the lower extremities), ascites, variceal hemorrhage, and encephalopathy (see Fig. 2.1). This patient is manifesting signs and symptoms of decompensated cirrhosis.

What is the significance of decreased urine output in a patient with decompensated cirrhosis?

Decreased urine output may signify urinary obstruction or acute kidney injury (AKI). Patients with decompensated cirrhosis undergo physiological changes that place them at a higher risk for AKI.

Portal hypertension from cirrhosis leads to increased splanchnic vasodilation with subsequent compensatory activation of the vasoconstrictor system (see Fig. 2.2). Initially, the heart can increase cardiac output to restore effective arterial blood volume to perfuse the kidneys. Over time, the sustained activation of the vasoconstrictor system leads to decreased renal perfusion. This mechanism along with changes in fluid shifts can lead to AKI.

CLINICAL PEARL **STEP 2/3**

Of hospitalized cirrhotic patients, 20% present with AKI and 70% develop AKI during hospitalization. Mortality is increased in cirrhotic patients with AKI.

CLINICAL PEARL **STEP 2/3**

AKI Definition: Rise in serum creatinine $\geq$ 0.3 mg/dL within 48 hours, or 50% increase within 7 days, or urine output less than 0.5 mL/kg/h for 6 hours.

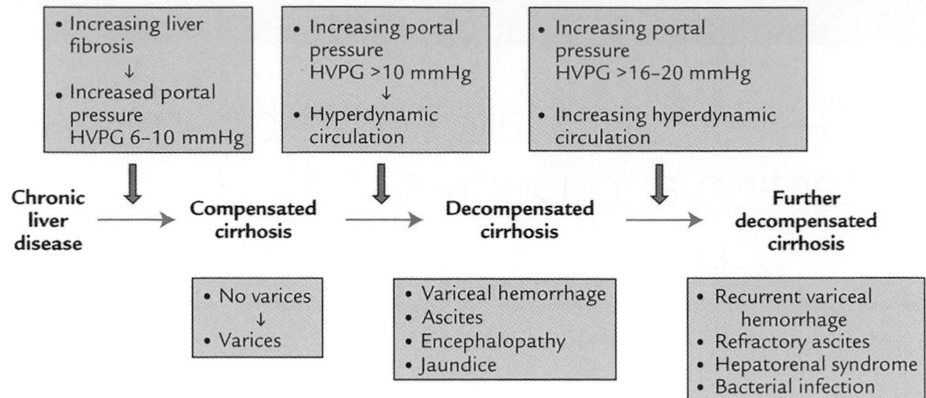

Fig. 2.1 Symptoms of decompensated cirrhosis. (From Muir, A. J. (2015). Understanding the complexities of cirrhosis. *Clinical Therapeutics*, *37*(8), 1822–1836.)

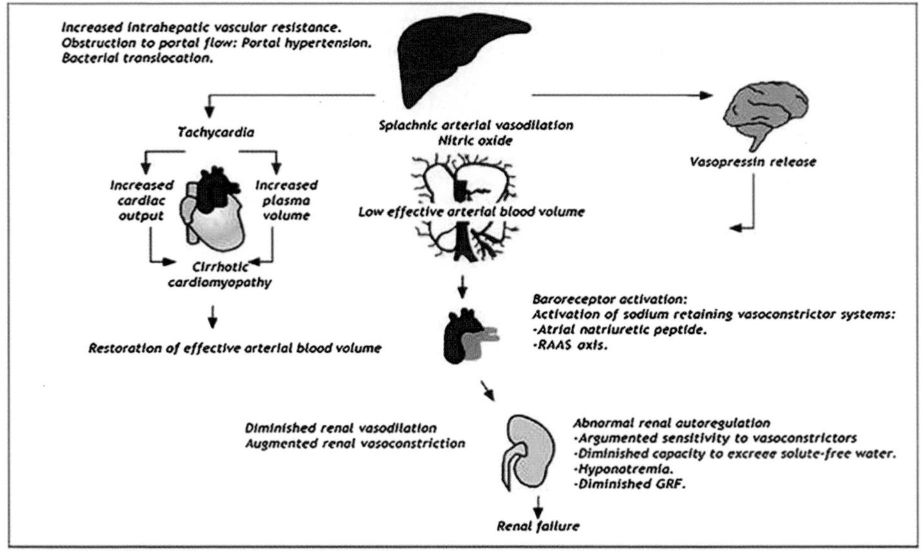

Fig. 2.2 Portal hypertension leads to higher chance of acute kidney injury. *GRF*, Glomerular filtration rate; *RAAS*, renin-angiotensin-aldosterone system. (From Lullo, L., Bellasi, A., Barbera, V., Russo, D., Russo, L., Iorio, B., Cozzolino, M., & Ronco, C. (2017). Pathophysiology of the cardio-renal syndromes types 1–5: An uptodate. *Indian Heart Journal*, *69*(2):255–265.)

Which aspects of medical history and physical examination should be included in the evaluation of this patient's decreased urine output?

Factors that may lead to intravascular volume depletion are important questions to review with the patient. These include diuretic usage; oral intake; presence of nausea, vomiting, and diarrhea; gastrointestinal bleed; and recent large volume paracentesis. In addition, inquiry about the patient's blood pressure is an essential part of history taking. Patients with decompensated cirrhosis frequently have low blood pressure, which leads to further reduction in blood flow to the kidneys. Nephrotoxins that can lead to intrinsic damage to the renal parenchyma should also be reviewed.

These include medications such as NSAIDs, proton pump inhibitors, antibiotics, and contrast dye used for diagnostic studies. Lastly, it is important to review symptoms of conditions such as benign prostate hyperplasia, neurogenic bladder, and nephrolithiasis that can lead to urinary obstruction and decreased urine output.

In addition to a detailed history, a complete physical examination is needed. Special attention should focus on evaluation of the patient's vital signs, the presence and degree of abdominal distention, presence of ascites, and a careful assessment of the patient's volume status.

On physical examination, blood pressure is 98/59 mmHg, pulse rate is 87 beats per minute, respiration rate is 18 breaths per minute, and oxygen saturation is 98% on room air. He is calm and oriented to name, place, and time. He has bilateral scleral icterus and his entire body is jaundiced. Mucous membranes are dry. Abdomen is soft, nontender, and moderately distended with fluid waves. He has 1+ pitting edema bilaterally in the lower extremities. The remainder of the physical examination is within normal limits.

What are the potential causes of AKI in patients with cirrhosis?

See Fig. 2.3.

What is the appropriate initial workup for the cause of AKI?

Appropriate initial laboratory workup includes complete blood count (CBC), complete metabolic panel, amylase, lipase, and urinalysis. Because the patient reported decreased urine output, a renal ultrasound is recommended to assess for presence of urinary obstruction and hydronephrosis.

The results for laboratory testing were as follows: leukocyte count 9100 cells/μL, hematocrit 26.6%, platelet count 59,000 cells/μL, sodium 126 mg/dL, potassium 3.9 mg/dL, chloride 86 mg/dL, bicarbonate 23 mg/dL, BUN 76 mg/dL, creatinine 3.61 mg/dL, glucose 82, calcium 9.1 mg/dL, PT/INR 32.4/3.13, bilirubin 25 mg/dL, and a urine study notable for no protein, 0–3 red blood cells, 0–3 white blood cells, large bilirubin, and a few bilirubin casts.

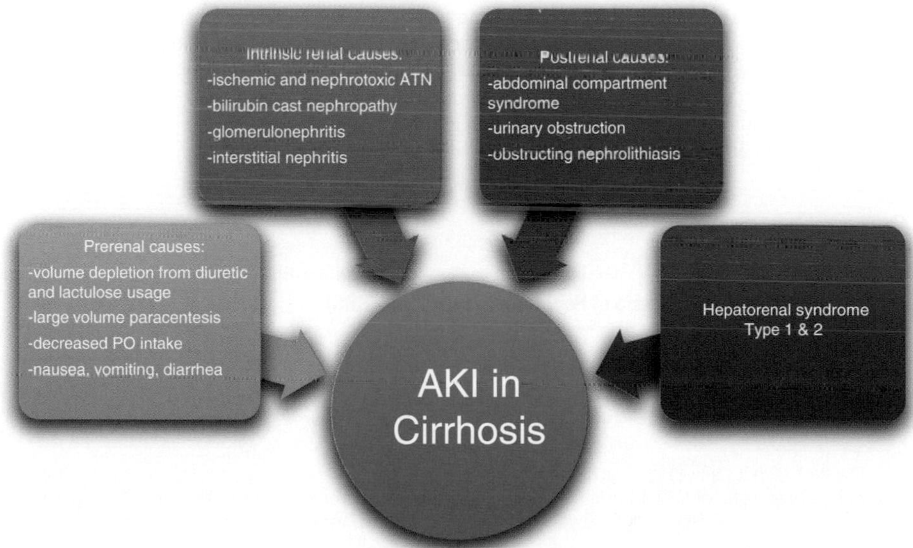

Fig. 2.3 Potential causes of acute kidney injury (AKI) in patients with cirrhosis.

The ultrasound examination showed that both kidneys were normal in size (left kidney 10.8 cm and right kidney 10.8 cm), shape, and echogenicity. There were no renal masses or calcifications. There was no intra- or extrarenal collecting system dilatation.

CLINICAL PEARL **STEP 2/3**

Creatinine is converted from creatine, which is produced by the liver and stored in muscle cells. Baseline creatinine production is lower in patients with cirrhosis because of impairment of liver function, decreased creatinine synthesis, muscle wasting, and increased tubular secretion of creatinine. The increased volume of distribution in cirrhotic patients also may lead to dilute creatinine measurements. Despite creatinine not being an accurate marker for determining renal function in cirrhotic patients, an increase in serum creatinine level still signifies AKI.

What is the differential diagnosis of this patient's AKI?

His physical examination does not support abdominal compartment syndrome. Glomerular disorders are not likely given a lack of proteinuria and cells in the urinalysis. Urinary obstruction is ruled out by renal ultrasound.

Intravascular volume depletion is high on our differential diagnosis because it is supported by history, physical examination, and urine findings. In the setting of an elevated bilirubin level and the presence of a few bilirubin casts in the urine sediment, bile cast nephropathy should also be included in the differential diagnosis for this patient. Finally, hepatorenal syndrome, a diagnosis of exclusion, needs to be considered in a patient with decompensated cirrhosis (see Table 2.1).

CLINICAL PEARL **STEP 2/3**

For patients with decreased urine output and ascites that is tense on physical examination, it is important to evaluate for abdominal compartment syndrome. Abdominal compartment syndrome represents the pathophysiologic consequence of a raised intra abdominal pressure. An estimate of the patient's intra abdominal pressure can be obtained by measuring bladder pressure via an indwelling urinary catheter. Normal bladder pressure is 0–5 mmHg. When intra abdominal pressure is between 15 and 25 mmHg, abdominal compartment syndrome may be observed due to a compromised perfusion of intra abdominal organs.

TABLE 2.1 ■ **Diagnostic Criteria of Hepatorenal Syndrome (HRS)**

Criteria
Presence of cirrhosis and ascites
Diagnosis of AKI by ICA-AKI Criteria
No improvement of serum creatinine after at least 48 h of diuretic withdrawal and volume expansion with albumin (recommended dose of 1 g/kg body weight per day to maximum of 100 g albumin/day
Absence of shock
No current or recent use of nephrotoxic drugs
No macroscopic signs of structural kidney disease as defined as absence of proteinuria >500 mg/day, microhematuria (>50 RBCs/high power field), and/or abnormal renal ultrasound scanning.

AKI, Acute kidney injury.

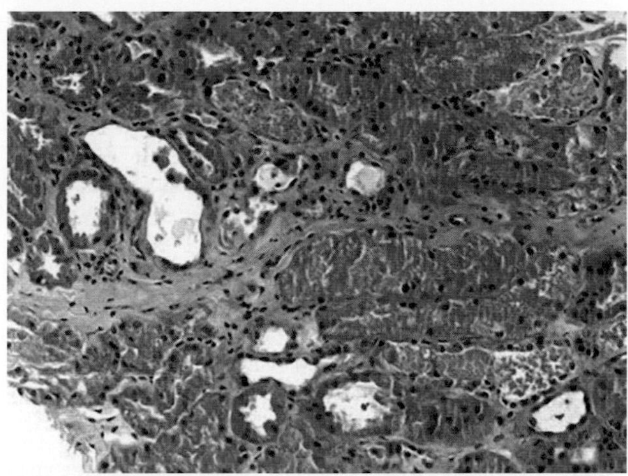

Fig. 2.4 Bile cast in the renal tubules. Hematoxylin and eosin stain. (From Chan, S., Spraggon, E. S., Francis, L., & Wolley, M. J. (2019). Bile cast nephropathy in a patient with obstructive jaundice. *Kidney International Reports*, *4*(2):338–340.)

CLINICAL PEARL **STEP 2/3**

Prerenal injury and acute tubular necrosis account for more than 70% of AKI in cirrhotic patients.

CLINICAL PEARL **STEP 2/3**

To diagnose hepatorenal syndrome, intravascular volume depletion needs to be first ruled out with adequate volume expansion. Normal saline, albumin, and blood are good volume expanders for cirrhotic patients (see also Table 2.1).

What is bile cast nephropathy?

Bile cast nephropathy is a condition of renal dysfunction in the setting of hyperbilirubinemia. It represents a spectrum of renal injury from proximal tubulopathy to intrarenal bile cast formation. Elevated total bilirubin levels, typically greater than 20 mg/dL, are reported in cases of bile cast nephropathy. AKI is probably caused by renal epithelial cell damage and tubular obstruction caused by the bile casts (Fig. 2.4).

What is the appropriate management at this time?

This patient was given 2 units of packed red blood cells to correct his anemia and volume depletion. His serum creatinine on the next day improved to 2.5 mg/dL. His diagnosis is AKI secondary to intravascular volume depletion, worsened by bile cast nephropathy. Hepatorenal syndrome (HRS) is unlikely because his renal function responded to volume repletion.

Case Summary

- **Complaint/History:** A 40-year-old male with a history of alcohol-induced cirrhosis presents with worsening jaundice, nausea and vomiting, increased ascites, and decreased urine output.
- **Findings:** Diffuse jaundice, scleral icterus, dry mucous membranes, soft ascites, 1+ pitting edema in lower extremities.

- **Lab Results/Tests:** Labs reveal thrombocytopenia, hyponatremia, and elevated blood urea nitrogen/creatinine (BUN/Cr). Urinalysis is notable for no protein, 0–3 red blood cells, 0–3 white blood cells, large bilirubin, and a few bilirubin casts.

Diagnosis: AKI secondary to intravascular volume depletion, worsened by bile cast nephropathy.

- **Treatment:** The patient was given 2 units of packed red blood cells to correct his anemia and volume depletion, which resulted in improved creatinine and urine output.

BEYOND THE PEARLS

- First-line treatment of ascites is a combination of diuretics that consists of furosemide and spironolactone. Patients with refractory ascites require second-line treatment of large-volume paracentesis or insertion of transjugular intrahepatic portosystemic shunt (TIPS). Complications of TIPS include hemorrhage, hepatic encephalopathy, and decompensation of liver or cardiac function.
- Paracentesis-induced circulatory dysfunction is a complication of large volume paracentesis. It occurs when more than 5 L of ascetic fluid is removed without albumin replacement. This leads to faster reaccumulation of ascites, hyponatremia, and renal function impairment.
- Hepatorenal syndrome (HRS) is a serious complication of liver cirrhosis that is associated with extremely poor prognosis. The pathophysiologic hallmark of HRS is severe renal vasoconstriction. There are two main types of HRS: HRS type 1 and HRS type 2. HRS type 1 presents as an acute renal failure and HRS type 2 is associated with more gradual decline of renal function.
- Treatment of HRS usually involves albumin, vasoconstrictors such as terlipressin, noradrenaline, and midodrine to counteract splanchnic vasodilation. Renal replacement therapy can be used if all else fails.
- In the future, biomarkers may help distinguish between HRS and acute tubular necrosis (ATN). These biomarkers include neutrophil gelatinase-associated lipocalin (NGAL), interleukin-18 (IL-18), kidney injury molecule-1 (KIM-1), and liver-type fatty acid binding protein (L-FABP).

Bibliography

Belcher, J. M., Garcia-Tsao, G., Sanyal, A. J., et al. (2013). Association of AKI with mortality and complications in hospitalized patients with cirrhosis. *Hepatology*, *57*(2), 753–762.

Chan, S., Spraggon, E. S., Francis, L., & Wolley, M. J. (2019). Bile Cast nephropathy in a patient with obstructive jaundice. *Kidney International Reports*, *4*(2), 338–340.

Di Lullo, L., Bellasi, A., Barbera, V., et al. (2017). Pathophysiology of the cardio-renal syndromes types 1–5: An up to date. *Indian Heart Journal*, *69*(2), 255–265.

du Cheyron, D., Bouchet, B., Parienti, J. -J., Ramakers, M., & Charbonneau, P. (2005). The attributable mortality of acute renal failure in critically ill patients with liver cirrhosis. *Intensive Care Medicine*, *31*(12), 1693–1699.

Muir. A. J. (2015). Understanding the complexities of cirrhosis. *Clinical Therapeutics*, *37*(8), 1822–1836.

Russ, K. B., Stevens, T. M., & Singal, A. K. (2015). Acute kidney injury in patients with cirrhosis. *Journal of Clinical and Translational Hepatology*, *3*(3), 195–204.

Tsochatzis, E. A., Bosch, J., & Burroughs, A. K. (2014). Liver cirrhosis. *The Lancet.*, *383*(9930), 1749–1761.

CASE 3

A 28-Year-Old Male With Left Flank Pain and Bloody Urine

Joseph Lee ■ Hui Yi Shan

A 28-year-old male presents to your office with 1 day of left flank pain and bloody urine. He was in his usual state of health until the day prior to presentation, when he was elbowed in the back while playing in a pickup basketball game.

What is the significance of hematuria?

Hematuria is the presence of blood in the urine. When visible to the naked eye it is known as gross hematuria. It can also be microscopic, in which case, the red blood cells are only detectable under microscopic examination of the urine. The source of hematuria can come from anywhere in the genitourinary tract, which includes the kidneys, ureters, bladder, prostate, and urethra. Disease conditions involving the blood vessels supplying the kidneys can also cause hematuria (Fig. 3.1).

CLINICAL PEARL **STEP 1/2/3**

False hematuria can occur as a result of the presence of myoglobin in the urine from rhabdomyolysis or hemoglobin in the urine from hemolysis. Menstruation is another cause of false hematuria. Medications (e.g., rifampin) and food products such as beets can also cause dark discoloration of the urine, which can be mistaken for hematuria.

How do you diagnose hematuria?

The first step in the evaluation of hematuria is to perform a thorough history and physical examination. History should focus on obtaining a detailed description of the hematuria, including its onset, duration, urine color, initiating or exacerbating factors, and the presence of associated symptoms such as fever, dysuria, or flank pain. Physical examination should be comprehensive and include a thorough examination of the genitourinary system.

On review of systems, the patient denies any history of hematuria. He denies any recent upper respiratory tract infection or sore throat. He is not experiencing shortness of breath, joint ache, or rash. The patient also denies any symptoms of urinary retention, dysuria, or frequent urination. He describes the color of his urine as red. The remainder of the review of systems is unremarkable.

On physical examination, blood pressure is 160/100 mmHg, pulse rate is 71 bpm, respiratory rate is 16, and temperature is 36.6°C.

The patient is not in acute distress. Examination is notable for left-sided costovertebral angle tenderness. The patient has no supra-pubic tenderness. The rest of the physical examination is unremarkable.

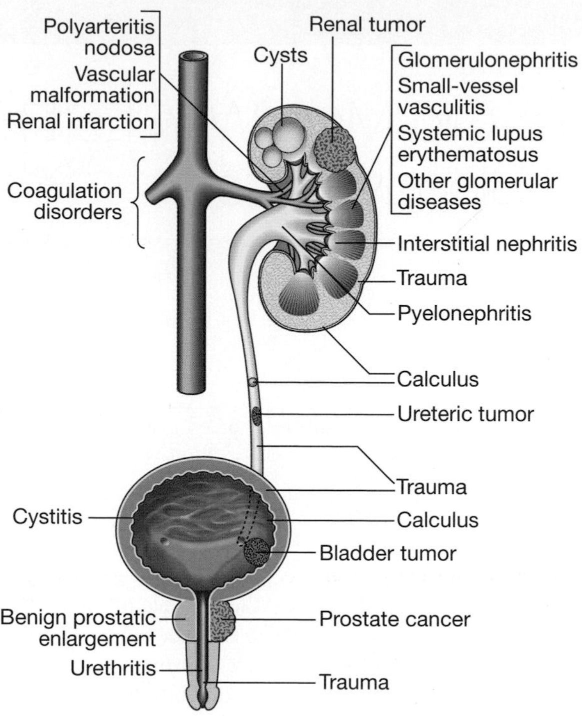

Fig. 3.1 Causes of hematuria. (From Conway, B. (2018). In *Davidson's principles and practice of medicine* (23rd ed.) (pp. 381–440). London: Elsevier.)

What is the appropriate initial laboratory workup for hematuria?

The initial laboratory workup includes a complete blood count, complete metabolic panel, urinalysis with microscopy, and urine culture. Imaging studies such as a renal ultrasound or computed tomography scan of the abdomen and pelvis can also be part of the workup to detect structural abnormalities.

The patient's complete blood count and complete metabolic panel are unremarkable. Serum creatinine is 0.8 mg/dL. Urinalysis is notable for 4+ blood, negative protein, >50 red blood cells, and 0 white blood cells per high power field. Microscopic examination of the urine sediment reveals the presence of nondysmorphic erythrocytes. Urine culture is negative.

What is the next step in the assessment of hematuria based on the laboratory results?

In the assessment of hematuria, it is important to determine whether the hematuria is the result of a glomerular or a nonglomerular bleed. This can help guide the subsequent workup and correct subspecialty referral.

Urinalysis provides essential information that helps distinguish a glomerular bleed from a nonglomerular bleed. Concurrent proteinuria, the presence of irregularly shaped red blood cells (RBCs) in the urine, or RBC casts would be suggestive of a glomerular hematuria. Table 3.1 summarizes the etiologies of glomerular hematuria. Because the kidneys are affected, hypertension and peripheral edema are often present in a patient with glomerular hematuria.

TABLE 3.1 ■ **Causes of Glomerular Bleeding**

Causes of Glomerulonephritis (Glomerular Bleeding)			
Primary	Multisystem	Infectious	Hereditary
IgA nephropathy	Lupus nephritis	Poststreptococcal glomerulonephritis	Alport's syndrome
Thin basement membrane nephropathy	Microscopic polyangiitis		Fabry's disease
MPGN	Goodpasture's disease		
Fibrillary GN	Granulomatosis with polyangiitis		
	Thrombotic microangiopathy		
	Henoch-Schönlein purpura		

GN, Glomerulonephritis; *MPGN*, membranoproliferative glomerulonephritis.

TABLE 3.2 ■ **Features Distinguishing Glomerular Versus Nonglomerular Causes of Hematuria**

Features	**Glomerular Bleed**	**Nonglomerular Bleed**
Physical Examination		
Hypertension	Often	Unlikely
Peripheral edema	Sometimes	No
Rash, arthritis	Sometimes (i.e., lupus)	No
Abdominal mass	No	Renal tumor, polycystic kidney disease
Urinalysis		
Color	Brown, tea-colored, cola-colored	Bright red or pink
Proteinuria	Often	No
Dysmorphic RBCs	Yes	No
RBC casts	Yes	No
Crystals	No	Sometimes

RBC, Red blood cells.

This patient has hematuria confirmed by urinalysis. His urine microscopy is negative for dysmorphic RBCs and RBC casts and there is a lack of concurrent proteinuria. This suggests that the cause of this patient's hematuria is more likely caused by a nonglomerular bleed. His urine culture is negative, which helps rule out a significant infection of the urinary tract. Imaging of the urinary tract is the appropriate next step to evaluate for structural abnormalities that may be the cause of this patient's hematuria (Table 3.2 and Fig. 3.2).

A renal ultrasound is obtained, which demonstrates innumerable cysts in both kidneys, consistent with a diagnosis of autosomal dominant polycystic kidney disease. (See Figs. 3.3–3.5and Table 3.3.)

CLINICAL PEARL **STEP 2/3**

Kidney imaging studies remain the mainstay for diagnosing autosomal dominant polycystic kidney disease (ADPKD). The characteristic findings include enlarged kidneys and the presence of multiple cysts in the renal parenchyma. Renal ultrasound is the initial imaging modality of choice. Diagnostic criteria are based on familial genotype, patient's age, and number of cysts (see Table 3.3).

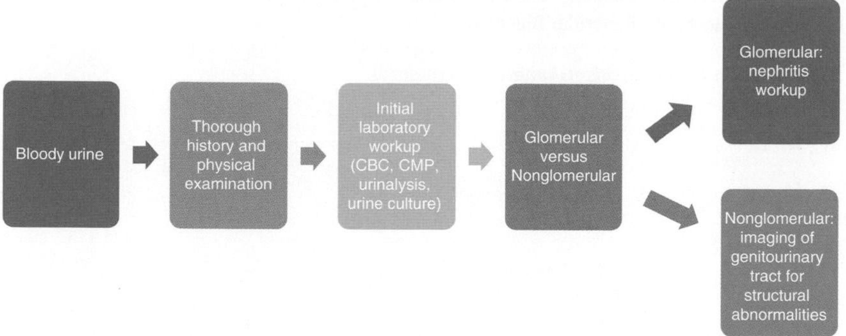

Fig. 3.2 Summary of hematuria workup. *CBC*, Complete blood count; *CMP*, comprehensive metabolic panel.

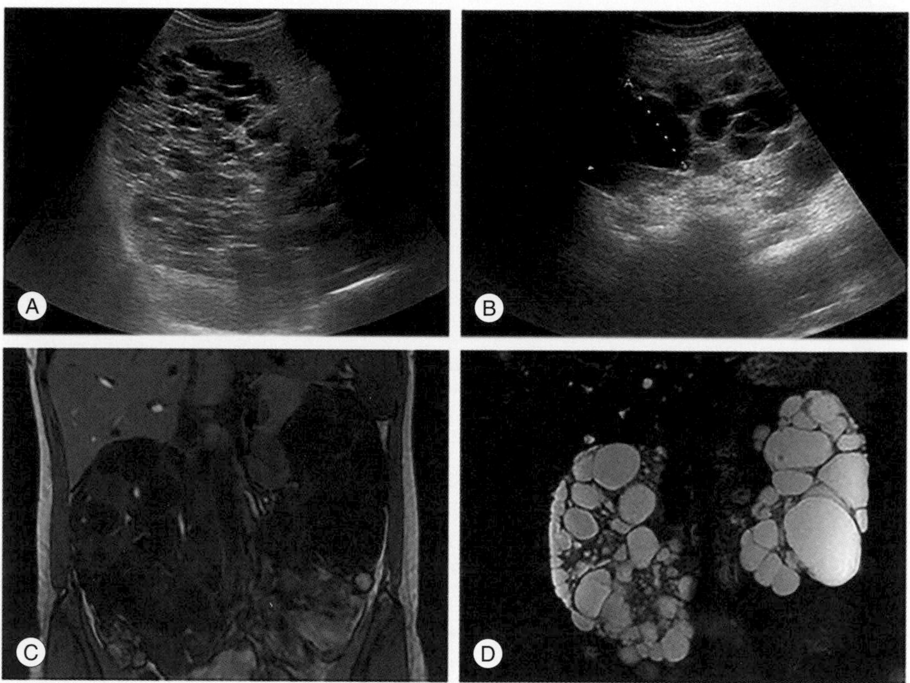

Fig. 3.3 Imaging of autosomal dominant polycystic kidney disease using renal ultrasound (A and B) and MRI (C and D). (From Bouleti, C. *American Journal of Cardiology*, *123* (3), 482–488.)

BASIC SCIENCE/CLINICAL PEARL **STEP 1/2/3**

ADPKD is the most common inherited kidney disorder, occurring in 1 of 400 to 1000 live births. It has equal representation in all ethnic groups and accounts for about 5% of the end-stage renal disease (ESRD) cases in the United States. Two genes have been implicated in the pathogenesis of ADPKD. PKD1 mutation accounts for 85% of cases, whereas PKD2 mutation accounts for the remaining 15% of cases. Patients with Type 1 ADPKD have a mean age of ESRD incidence of 58 years. Type 2 ADPKD has a later onset of symptoms and a slower rate of progression to renal failure, with a mean age of ESRD incidence of 79 years. Knowing the family history of ADPKD and ESRD helps provide diagnostic and prognostic information for the patient.

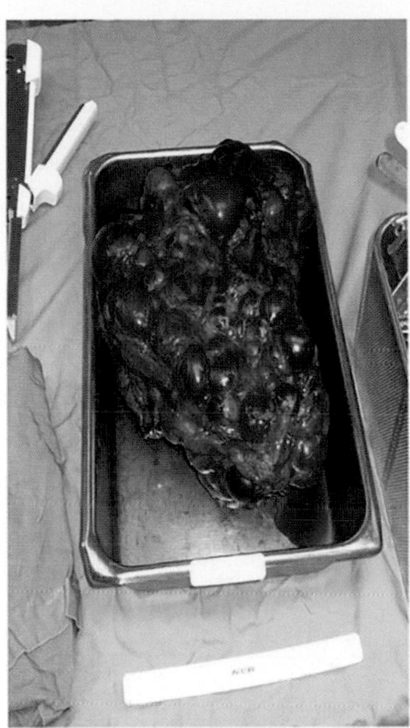

Fig. 3.4 Gross specimen of a kidney affected by autosomal dominant polycystic kidney disease. (From Nash, N.A., *Injury Extra*, *41* (10), 109–111.)

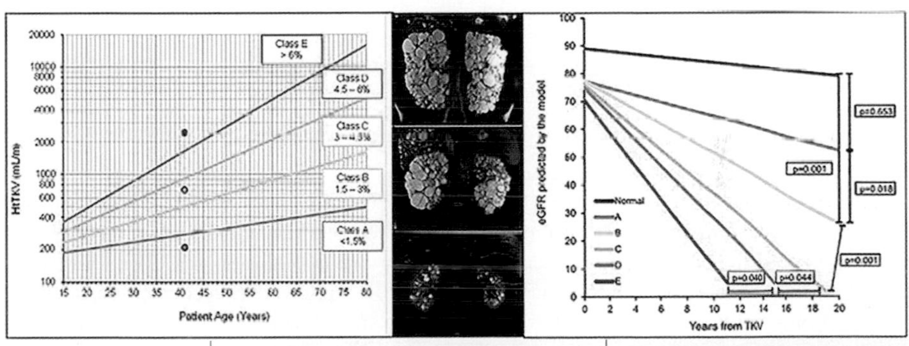

Class	Estimated kidney growth rate: yearly percentage increase	Risk for eGFR decline
1A	<1.5%	Low risk
1B	1.5%-3%	Intermediate risk
1C	3%-4.5%	High risk
1D	4.5%-6%	High risk
1E	>6%	High risk

Fig. 3.5 Total kidney volume and age together help predict the change in glomerular filtration rate over time in patients with autosomal dominant polycystic kidney disease. (From Chebib, F.T. *American Journal of Kidney Diseases*, *67* (5), 792–810.)

TABLE 3.3 ■ **Diagnostic Criteria for Autosomal Dominant Polycystic Kidney Disease**

Radiographic Diagnostic Criteria for Autosomal Dominant Polycystic Kidney Disease	
Age (years)	Number of Cysts
Ultrasound (At Risk of Adpkd Type 1)	
<30	≥ 2 in one or both kidneys
30 to 59	≥ 2 in each kidney
≥60	≥ 4 in each kidney
Ultrasound (At Risk and Unknown Genotype)	
15 to 39	≥ 3 in one or both kidneys
40 to 59	≥ 2 in each kidney
≥60	≥ 4 in each kidney

What are the common renal and extrarenal manifestations of ADPKD?

Renal manifestations of ADPKD include:

- Nephrolithiasis
- Polyuria
- Hematuria
- Urinary tract infections
- Hypertension

Extrarenal manifestations of ADPKD include:

- Polycystic liver disease
- Intracranial aneurysm
- Mitral valve prolapse
- Left ventricular hypertrophy
- Pancreatic cysts
- Diverticulosis

It is important to be aware of these renal and extrarenal manifestations of ADPKD for early detection and treatment.

How would you manage this patient's gross hematuria?

Hematuria, gross or microscopic, occurs in about 35% to 50% of patients with ADPKD. It is associated with increased kidney size and with worse kidney outcomes. Hematuria is often precipitated by an acute event such as trauma, heavy exercise, cyst rupture, nephrolithiasis, or a UTI. This patient's hematuria was probably caused by cyst hemorrhage caused by trauma during contact sports.

The management of uncomplicated cyst hemorrhage and hematuria is supportive and includes hydration, rest, and pain control.

CLINICAL PEARL **STEP 2/3**

Pain is a common symptom found in patients with ADPKD. It can be acute or chronic. Acute pain is often caused by cyst rupture, cyst infection, and nephrolithiasis. Chronic pain is often related to the stretching of the renal capsule caused by massive enlargement of the kidneys.

What is the significance of hypertension in this patient with ADPKD?

Hypertension is one of the earliest manifestations of ADPKD and is associated with progression to ESRD. Renal ischemia and activation of the renin-angiotensin-aldosterone system (RAAS) induced by cyst compression of renal vasculature is thought to play a role in the development of hypertension in patients with ADPKD.

What is recommended for the treatment of hypertension in patients with ADPKD?

The results of a clinical study (HALT-PKD trial) comparing a standard (<130/80) versus rigorous (<110/70) blood pressure target demonstrated that aggressive blood pressure control was associated with a slower increase in total kidney volume.

If there are no contraindications, an angiotensin-converting enzyme (ACE) inhibitor should be used as the initial antihypertensive agent. If a patient cannot tolerate an ACE inhibitor, an angiotensin receptor blocker (ARB) should be considered.

The patient was instructed to increase his fluid intake and avoid heavy exercise or contact sports. His gross hematuria and flank pain resolved after 1 week of rest.

Case Summary

- **Complaint/History:** A 28-year-old male patient with 1 day of left flank pain and bloody urine after being elbowed in the back during a basketball game.
- **Findings:** Blood pressure is 160/100 mmHg. Examination of the back reveals left-sided costovertebral angle tenderness.
- **Lab Results/Tests:** The complete blood count and comprehensive metabolic panel are normal. The patient has a creatinine of 0.8. Urinalysis is notable for 4+ blood, negative protein, >50 red blood cells, and 0 white blood cells. A renal ultrasound is obtained, which demonstrates innumerable cysts in both kidneys, consistent with autosomal dominant polycystic kidney disease.

Diagnosis: Autosomal dominant polycystic kidney disease.

- **Treatment:** The management of uncomplicated cyst hemorrhage and hematuria was supportive and includes hydration, rest, and pain control. Hypertension was managed with an angiotensin-converting enzyme inhibitor.

BEYOND THE PEARLS

- ADPKD is caused by mutations in the genes coding for polycystin-1 and polycystin-2. Polycystin complexes act as mechanosensors that transduce extracellular signals into intracellular responses that regulate kidney proliferation and morphogenesis. Disruption of the gene coding for polycystin leads to cyst development and eventual destruction of kidney parenchyma.
- Cerebral aneurysm is the most dangerous extrarenal renal manifestation of ADPKD. Magnetic resonance angiography is recommended for patients with ADPKD who have a family history of aneurysm or stroke in order to screen for cerebral aneurysms. Screening is also recommended for any patient with known ADPKD who develops a new onset of severe headaches and for patients in high-risk occupations such as those who operate heavy machinery, including bus drivers and airplane pilots.
- Approximately 30% to 50% of patients with ADPKD will have a UTI during their lifetime. An infected cyst and acute pyelonephritis are the most common kidney infections. The infections are typically caused by Gram-negative organisms. *Escherichia coli* accounts for approximately 75% of cyst infections.
- Ciprofloxacin and trimethoprim sulfamethoxazole are the preferred antibiotics for patients with PKD and urinary tract infections because they can achieve therapeutic concentrations within the cysts. Patients with a cyst infection are typically treated for 4–6 weeks. In cases of an extremely large cyst infection, antibiotic therapy alone may not be sufficient for treatment and cyst drainage may be required for source control.
- Tolvaptan, a vasopressin V2 receptor blocker, reduces intracellular cAMP accumulation and has been shown to slow the increase in total kidney volume and the decline in kidney function in patients with ADPKD who are at risk of rapid progression.

Bibliography

Grantham, J. J. (2008). Autosomal dominant polycystic kidney disease. *New England Journal of Medicine*, *359*(14), 1477–1485.

Gilbert, S. J., Weiner, D. E., Bomback, A. S., Perazella, M. A., Tonelli, M., Rizk, D. V., Reddy, B., & Chapman, A. B. (2018). Polycystic and Other Cystic Kidney Diseases. In *National Kidney Foundation's Primer on Kidney Diseases*, pp. 375–384. chapter, Elsevier.

Wilson, P. D. (2004). Polycystic kidney disease. *New England Journal of Medicine*, *350*(2), 151–164.

CASE 4

A 62-Year-Old Male With Worsening Peripheral Edema

Jackson Kim ■ Hui Yi Shan

A 62-year-old male with a history of poorly controlled diabetes mellitus for 20 years and chronic kidney disease due to diabetic nephropathy presents to the clinic with a complaint of worsening bilateral lower extremity swelling for 3 weeks.

What is the differential diagnosis of chronic bilateral leg edema?

Differential diagnosis includes:

- Congestive heart failure
- Renal disease
- Decreased capillary oncotic pressure:
  - Protein malnutrition
  - Protein losing enteropathy (examples include celiac disease, inflammatory bowel disease, and giardiasis)
- Increased capillary hydrostatic pressure:
  - Venous obstruction causes localized swelling.
- Liver cirrhosis:
  - Genetic disorders (alpha-1 antitrypsin deficiency, cystic fibrosis, and Wilson disease)
  - Infectious etiologies
  - Structural problems of the biliary tree
- Increased capillary permeability: angioedema

On physical examination, blood pressure is 160/110, heart rate is 85 beats per minute, and oxygen saturation is 97% on room air. Cardiac exam is normal; lungs are clear to auscultation. There is bilateral symmetrical pitting edema up to the knees. The remainder of the physical examination is within normal limits.

Laboratory findings are notable for hemoglobin of 11.2, serum creatinine of 1.3 mg/dL, and hemoglobin A1c 9%. Urinalysis reveals 3+ protein, no blood, 2+ glucose, negative leukocyte esterase, and negative nitrite. Twenty-four-hour urine protein collection is 10 g.

What are common tests used to evaluate for proteinuria and their limitations?

- Urinalysis:
  - Advantage: quick and easy to perform
  - Limitations:
    (1) Test becomes unreliable at the extreme of urine concentration and pH.
    (2) Test only picks up negatively charged protein such as albumin. This test will miss the positively charged light chains in the urine from patients with multiple myeloma.

- Urine protein/creatinine
  - Advantage: easy to perform and has strong correlation to the 24-hour urine protein excretion
  - Limitations:
    (1) When creatinine excretion is not close to 1 gram per day (examples include people at the extreme of muscle mass), this test becomes unreliable.
    (2) When creatinine excretion fluctuates such as in acute kidney injury, this test becomes unreliable.
- 24-hour urine protein
  - Advantage: accounts for daily fluctuating urinary protein excretion
  - Limitations: cumbersome to do; this test is prone to error due to under- or over-collection of urine.

What is the clinical significance of proteinuria?

Clinical evaluation of proteinuria provides significant diagnostic and prognostic information. Proteinuria is one of the earliest markers for diagnosing kidney injury and is a useful therapeutic target for clinicians. Increasing levels of proteinuria have been associated with faster kidney disease progression, higher cardiovascular events, and mortality. This result leads to clinicians' effort to reduce proteinuria and improve a patient's overall prognosis.

What is diabetic nephropathy?

The diabetic milieu leads to the generation of advanced glycation end products (AGEs), growth factors, and hemodynamic and hormonal changes. These promote the release of reactive oxygen species and inflammatory mediators. These changes result in functional and structural changes in the kidneys, which are manifested clinically as albuminuria and hypertension (Fig. 4.1). Pathologically, the kidneys undergo several changes, including deposition (in primarily the mesangium) of the extracellular matrix, glomerular basement membrane thickening, and tubular atrophy, ultimately resulting in interstitial fibrosis and glomerulosclerosis (Fig. 4.2).

Kidney ultrasound shows bilateral kidneys measuring 12 cm and 13 cm, with normal echogenicity. There are no renal masses or calcifications. No hydronephrosis is present.

CLINICAL PEARL **STEP 2/3**

With the onset of diabetes mellitus, kidney size and weight increase by an average of 15%. An examination of kidney tissue reveals thickening of the glomerular basement membrane and expansion of the mesangium.

CLINICAL PEARL **STEP 2/3**

Diabetic nephropathy is one of the common causes of enlarged kidneys. Other clinical conditions that cause enlarged kidneys include HIV nephropathy, multiple myeloma, lymphoma with renal involvement, bilateral renal cell carcinoma, leukemia, infiltrative disease such as sarcoidosis or amyloidosis, vasculitis or autoimmune disease, polycystic kidney disease, pyelonephritis, acute nephritis, von Hippel–Lindau disease, nephroblastomatosis, tuberous sclerosis, and obstruction.

Can diabetic nephropathy be reversed?

In type 1 diabetics, the rate of progression or the chance of regression are strongly linked to the intensity of glycemic control. In contrast, type 2 diabetics experience a higher chance of progression from microalbuminuria to end-stage renal disease. In these patients, although aggressive

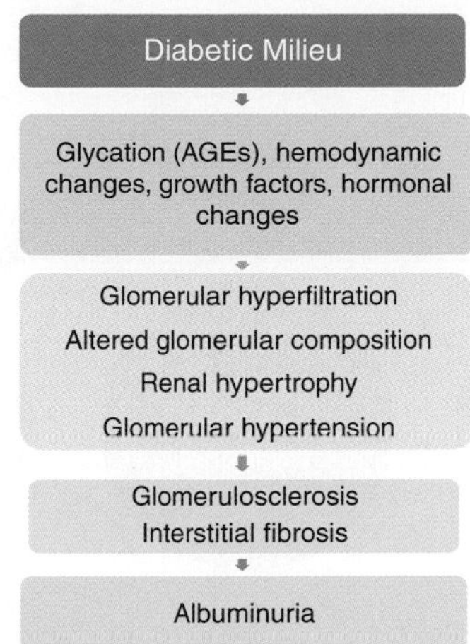

Fig. 4.1 Pathophysiology of diabetic nephropathy.

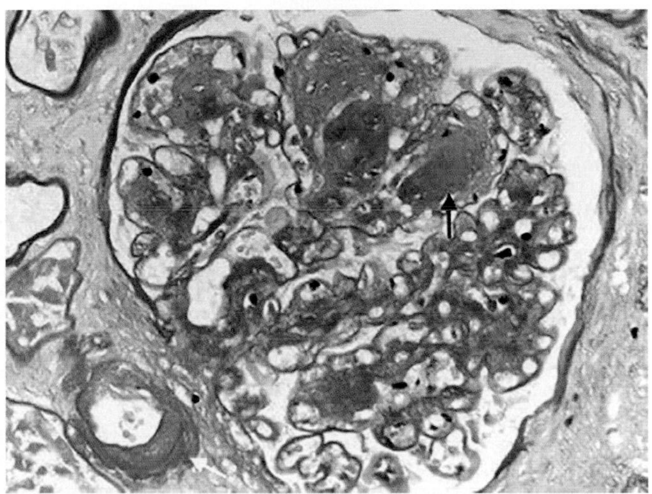

Fig. 4.2 Histology of diabetic nephropathy. Features of diabetic nephropathy include prominent nodular mesangial sclerosis (Kimmelstiel-Wilson nodule, *black arrow*). (From Henriksen, K. (2017). Assessment of kidneys in adult autopsies. *Diagnostic Histopathology 23*(3), 117–125.)

insulin therapy, protein restriction, and renin-angiotensin-aldosterone system (RAAS) blockade may slow or halt progression of diabetic nephropathy, durable evidence of diabetic nephropathy reversal has yet to be found.

How is diabetic nephropathy managed?

The cornerstone of diabetic nephropathy management consists of intensive glycemic control, antihypertensive treatment via RAAS blockade, and lipid-modifying statin therapy to reduce cardiovascular disease risk. It is also recommended to educate patients on low salt intake to slow kidney function decline (Fig. 4.3).

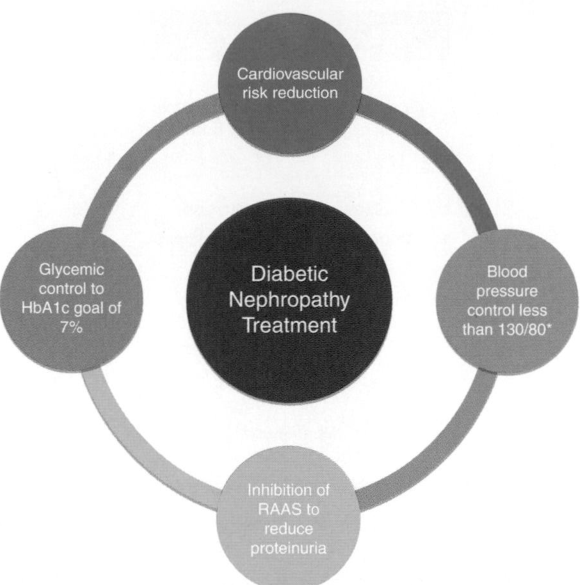

Fig. 4.3 Diabetic nephropathy treatment recommendation. *KDOQI (Kidney Disease Outcomes Quality Initiative) guideline.

How would you manage this patient's lower extremity swelling?

In this patient with significant lower extremity edema, a loop diuretic such as furosemide is a good initial therapeutic choice. If a patient develops diuretic tolerance after being on furosemide for long periods of time, the addition of thiazide can be considered. While sequential blockade with thiazide and a loop diuretic promotes increased fluid losses and helps reduce hypertension, these benefits are counteracted with the risk of rise in serum creatinine, hypokalemia, and other electrolyte disturbances. A reasonable alternative approach is to switch to a more potent loop diuretic. Bumetanide and torsemide are more potent as compared to furosemide due to their increased bioavailability.

CLINICAL PEARL **STEP 1/2/3**

In contrast to most diuretics, ethacrynic acid is not a sulfonamide; therefore, it can be used in patients with sulfa drug allergy. Ethacrynic acid is a loop diuretic. The side effect profile is like other loop diuretics, including frequent urination, hypokalemia, and ototoxicity. Ethacrynic acid may also cause liver damage when used in high dosages.

The most likely cause of the patient's leg edema is nephrotic syndrome secondary to diabetic nephropathy. The patient is started on an insulin regimen, atorvastatin, amlodipine, lisinopril, and furosemide with subsequent improvement in lower extremity edema. Blood pressure is maintained at less than 130/80. With improved glycemic and blood pressure control, his proteinuria is reduced to 5 g. Patient is discharged home with close follow-up.

Case Summary

- **Complaint/History:** A 62-year-old man presents with progressively worsening lower extremity swelling for 3 weeks.
- **Findings:** Blood pressure is 160/110, heart rate is 85 beats per minute, oxygen is 97% on room air, and cardiopulmonary exam is normal. Bilateral symmetrical pitting lower extremity edema is present to the knees.
- **Lab Results/Tests:** Labs reveal anemia, serum creatinine 1.3, HbA1c 9%, and urinalysis significant for 3+ protein, no blood, 2+ glucose, negative leukocyte esterase, and negative nitrite. Twenty-four-hour urine protein collection is 10 g.

Diagnosis: Nephrotic syndrome secondary to diabetic nephropathy.

- **Treatment:** The patient is started on a statin, insulin regimen, and three antihypertensive medications including a diuretic.

BEYOND THE PEARLS

- Most patients with diabetes will require two or more drugs for adequate blood pressure management to target <130/80.
- ACE inhibitors may reduce the risk for end-stage kidney disease and reduce all-cause mortality in diabetic patients.
- Patients with diabetes may have impaired immune systems with associated high risk of complications, hospitalizations, and death from influenza and pneumococcal disease; therefore, immunization is an important part of preventative diabetic patient care.
- Deaths due to cardiovascular events are more frequent than progression from CKD to ESRD; therefore, appropriate cardiovascular risk modification is an important part of diabetic patient care.

Bibliography

Balafa, O., Liapis, G., Pavlakou, P., Baltatzis, G., Kalaitzidis, R., & Elisaf, M. (2016). "Diabetic nephropathy" in a non-diabetic patient. *Pathology - Research and Practice*, *212*(12), 1199–1201.

Craig Brater. D. (1986). Disposition and response to bumetanide and furosemide. *The American Journal of Cardiology*, *57*(2), A20–A25.

Makino, H., & Nakamura, Y. (2003). Wada J. Remission and Regression of Diabetic Nephropathy. *Hypertension Research*, *26*(7), 515–519.

Somberg, J., & Molnar, J. (2009). The Pleiotropic Effects of Ethacrynic Acid. *American Journal of Therapeutics*, *16*(1), 102–104.

Umanath, K., & Lewis, J. B. (2018). Update on Diabetic Nephropathy: Core Curriculum 2018. *American Journal of Kidney Diseases*, *71*(6), 884–895.

Wei, M., Gaskill, S. P., Haffner, S. M., & Stern, M. P. (1998). Effects of Diabetes and Level of Glycemia on All-Cause and Cardiovascular Mortality: The San Antonio Heart Study. *Diabetes Care*, *21*(7), 1167–1172.

A 56-Year-Old Male With Acquired Immunodeficiency Syndrome With Nausea and Weakness

Shahid Syed ■ Thin Thin Maw

A 56-year-old Hispanic male with a history of acquired immunodeficiency syndrome (AIDS), CD4 count of 52, presents to the primary care physician for nausea and weakness that have been progressively worsening for a month. These symptoms started shortly after restarting his anti-human immunodeficiency virus (HIV) medications, after being off them for several months because of insurance issues. His medications include. emtricitabine/tenofovir combination, dolutegravir, Bactrim prophylaxis dose, and azithromycin prophylaxis dose.

Laboratory testing reveals a cell count showing pancytopenia that is at baseline. His metabolic panel is as follows: sodium 132 mmol/dL, potassium 6.3 mmol/dL, chloride 107 mmol/dL, CO_2 13 mmol/dL, BUN 58 mmol/dL, and creatinine 2.41 mg/dL.

What are the leading causes of this patient's acute kidney injury (AKI) at this time?

AKI in a patient with HIV leads to an expansive differential diagnosis (see Table 5.1). However, the differential can be weaned down with a thorough history, physical examination, and analysis of available lab results.

On physical examination, this patient's vitals are significant for blood pressure 93/46 mmHg, with pulse rate 68 beats/min, respiratory rate 16/min, and oxygen saturation 100% on room air. He is a thin Hispanic male in no acute distress with dark skin pigmentation throughout his body. The rest of the physical examination is within normal limits.

His laboratory tests are significant for hyperkalemia, low bicarb with elevated BUN and Cr. The urinalysis shows a pH of 7.0, specific gravity of 1.011, negative blood, and negative protein, with 0–4 hyaline casts. No other casts or crystals are present.

The differential diagnosis of his AKI is:

1. Prerenal cause from volume depletion given history of nausea, vomiting, and hypotension.
2. Acute tubular injury either drug induced or resulting from hypoperfusion.
3. Crystal-induced nephropathy from medications.
4. Glomerular disease is less likely given no proteinuria nor hematuria.

TABLE 5.1 ■ **Causes of Acute Kidney Injury in Patients with HIV**

Functional Compartment	Injury

Glomerulus	• HIVICK
	  • MPGN
	  • IgA nephropathy
	  • Lupus-like GN
	  • Cryoglobulinemia
	  • Postinfectious GN
	• HIVAN (podocytopathy)
	• Thrombotic microangiopathy

Tubules	• Drug-induced
	  • Acute tubular necrosis
	  • Renal tubular acidosis
	  • Crystal nephropathy
	• HIVAN (tubuloreticular inclusion bodies)
	• Rhabdomyolysis

Interstitium	• Drug-induced
	  • Acute interstitial nephritis
	  • Immune reconstitution syndrome
	• Infiltrative disease
	  • Kaposi's sarcoma
	  • Lymphoma
	• Opportunistic infections of the parenchyma
	  • Viral infections (CMV, Parvovirus, EBV, HSV)
	  • Mycobacterial
	  • Fungal

CMV, Cytomegalovirus; *EBV*, Epstein-Barr virus; *GN*, glomerulonephritis; *HIVAN*, HIV-associated nephropathy; *HIVICK*, HIV immune complex disease of the kidney; *HSV*, herpes simplex virus; *MPGN*, membranoproliferative glomerulonephritis.

BASIC SCIENCE/CLINICAL PEARL **STEP 1/2/3**

Apolipoprotein 1, or APOL1, is a gene that encodes for a constituent of the APO lipoprotein. Through in vitro studies, it has been found that variant alleles for this gene confer protection against *Trypanosoma brucei* infection, in much the same way that sickle cell variants confer protection against malaria. However, it has been well studied that APOL1 variants also carry an increased risk of HIVAN, as well as chronic kidney disease in general. Approximately 50% of West Africans have these risk variants, as do 35% of all Black Americans.

What is the significance of the lack of proteinuria and hematuria on urinalysis?

The glomerulus is the functional unit of the kidney responsible for generating the initial filtrate that eventually becomes urine. As blood courses through the capillary bed of the glomerulus, solutes and water are filtered through the pores in the endothelial cells, through the glomerular basement membrane, and eventually through the slit diaphragms of the podocyte fingers. If there is damage to any part of this structure, large solutes such as blood cells and protein can fall into the filtrate and eventually end up in the urine, showing up as hematuria and proteinuria. The absence of either of these entities makes glomerular disease low on the differential. Should this patient have significant proteinuria and hematuria, HIV-associated immune complex kidney disease (HIVICK) should be higher on the differential.

CLINICAL PEARL **STEP 2/3**

HIVICK is an umbrella term that is used to categorize a set of glomerular disease in patients with HIV that is caused by the deposition of immune complexes at specific parts of the glomerulus. HIVICK presents with hematuria and sub-nephrotic proteinuria. It can manifest as IgA nephropathy, membranoproliferative glomerulonephritis, lupus-like glomerulonephritis, cryoglobulinemic vasculitis, and postinfectious glomerulonephritis. The mechanism behind this disease entity is not fully understood, but it is thought that an antibody response to HIV epitopes and polyclonal gammopathy are responsible for the creation and deposition of immune complexes in the glomerulus. Coinfection with other pathogens, such as hepatitis C virus, may influence the pathogenesis of HIV immune-mediated kidney disease.

HIV-associated nephropathy (HIVAN), on the other hand, is a broad category of glomerular diseases that involve specifically the destruction of podocytes. The resulting manifestation is heavy proteinuria and nephrotic syndrome. HIVICK subnephrotic Since HIVAN is associated with only podocyte destruction, an patient with HIVAN will present with nephrotic range proteinuria, decreased renal function, and little to no hematuria. Other functional components of the nephron are also affected with HIVAN. Microcystic tubular dilation can be seen, in addition to tubuloreticular inclusion bodies (Fig. 5.1), interstitial inflammation, and fibrosis.

Which other drug-related AKIs can be seen in a patient with HIV/AIDS?

The sulfamethoxazole component of Bactrim can cause an acute interstitial nephritis (AIN). In the setting of sterile pyuria, eosinophilia, and rash, acute interstitial nephritis should be chief on the differential. Immune reconstitution syndrome (IRIS) can manifest as AIN and dense interstitial infiltrates can form as a result of immune reactivation in the kidney. Certain protease inhibitors such as indinavir and atazanavir can crystallize in alkaline urine and promote crystal nephropathy.

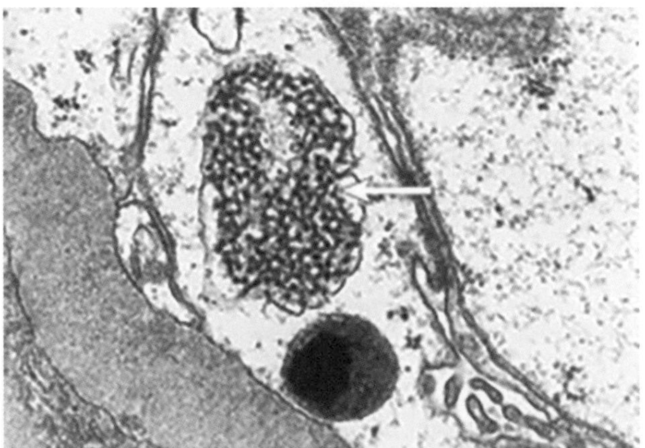

Fig. 5.1 HIV-associated nephropathy. The glomerular endothelial cell pictured here contains a large intracytoplasmic tubuloreticular inclusion (also known as the "interferon footprint," *arrow*) composed of inter-anastomosing tubular structures within a dilated cisterna of endoplasmic reticulum. (Electron micrograph, ×15,000.) (From Floege, J., Johnson, R. J., & Feehally, J. (2018). *Comprehensive clinical nephrology*. (6th ed.). Philadelphia: Elsevier Saunders.)

Given the lack of proteinuria or hematuria on urinalysis, glomerular disease is lower on the differential and other possibilities for this patient's AKI should be considered. An AKI from a tubular dysfunction is possible, even in the absence of granular casts on urinalysis.

CLINICAL PEARL **STEP 2/3**

Patients with severe AIDS from HIV may present to the hospital with multiple coinfections and infections with opportunistic infections. It is common to see the patient's inpatient drug list includes multiple antibiotics that are nephrotoxic. Vancomycin, piperacillin/tazobactam, and amphotericin are some of the broad-spectrum antibiotics and antifungal medications that patients can be started on empirically. Be cognizant of initiation dates of these nephrotoxic agents with relation to when a patient develops an AKI.

What is the significance of this patient's normal anion gap metabolic acidosis?

A normal gap acidosis signifies that the patient is probably losing bicarbonate from the body, rather than consuming bicarbonate, which is the mechanism behind an anion gap acidosis. The patient can either lose bicarbonate through gastrointestinal (GI) losses or through a renal dysfunction as seen in renal tubular acidosis. A urine anion gap can help determine the source of bicarbonate loss. A negative urine anion gap indicates a probable GI source for the loss, but a positive urine anion gap indicates a renal tubular loss of bicarbonate is likely.

Urine sodium is 89 mEq/L, urine potassium is 7 mEq/L, and urine chloride is 88 mEq/L.

What is significant of these urine electrolytes for this patient?

The urine anion gap is positive, indicating that the patient has a problem in producing ammonium chloride to excrete H+ ions. This indicates a renal tubular acidosis as the likely cause of this patient's normal anion gap acidosis. In addition, this patient's urine potassium is low relative to his hyperkalemia. This further indicates that the renal tubules are not appropriately excreting potassium into the urine in response to the high serum potassium.

What is the cause of this patient's renal tubular acidosis (RTA)?

Antiretroviral therapy and HIV-associated medications are associated with various nephrotoxic affects. Protease inhibitors such as tenofovir are associated with proximal or Type 2 RTA, which presents with Fanconi's syndrome. Trimethoprim, which is a key component of Bactrim used as PCP prophylaxis, can cause a distal Type 4 RTA by blocking the ENaC channel in the collecting duct, rendering aldosterone ineffective at this level. This manifests predominantly as a normal anion gap acidosis with hyperkalemia and often hyponatremia. Hypotension can also be seen in extreme cases.

This patient probably has type 4 RTA from trimethoprim given hyperkalemia, normal anion gap with low bicarbonate, and positive urine anion gap.

The patient received IV fluid and Bactrim and lisinopril were held. The infectious disease team was consulted to aid in changing this patient's medication regimen given nephrotoxicity. His AKI was probably caused by acute tubular injury from hypoperfusion resulting from prolonged prerenal state and medication induced (tenofovir, lisinopril). Furosemide was started to help increase potassium excretion in the urine after the patient was fluid resuscitated. With Bactrim and lisinopril held, as well as a change in highly active antiretroviral therapy (HAART), his renal function improved. The patient was discharged with nephrology and infectious disease follow-up as outpatient.

Case Summary

- **Chief Complaint:** Weakness and Nausea.
- **Lab Findings:** Lab Findings: Hyponatremia, Hyperkalemia, Metabolic Acidosis, AKI.

Diagnosis: Medication induced Type 4 RTA

- **Treatment:** Withdraw bactrim and lisinopril, fluid resuscitate patient with steroids must not be taken lightly.

BEYOND THE PEARLS

- Proximal renal tubular acidosis, also known as type 2 RTA, is synonymous with Fanconi's syndrome. The proximal tubule is responsible for most of the resorption of solutes after the filtrate is created from the glomerulus. With proximal RTA, the proximal tubular epithelial cells are affected and, therefore, the kidney has a hard time resorbing sodium, glucose, phosphorus, and magnesium. The carbonic anhydrase II is also adversely affected, which destroys the proximal tubules' ability to resorb bicarbonate. These problems manifest as a normal anion gap metabolic acidosis, phosphaturia, glycosuria in the setting of normal serum glucose, hyponatremia, and hypomagnesemia. These electrolyte abnormalities constitute Fanconi's syndrome.
- Primary focal segmental glomerulosclerosis (FSGS) is a podocytopathy that causes scarring of portions of a number of glomeruli in the kidney. Because the podocytes are destroyed in FSGS, the filtration barrier for protein is lost and patients will present with nephrotic syndrome. There are five histological variants of FSGS: tip, collapsing (Fig. 5.2), cellular, perihilar, and not otherwise specified (NOS). HIVAN presents as the collapsing variant of FSGS, which is also, prognostically, the worst variant.
- Acute interstitial nephritis is an immune reaction in the interstitium of the kidney to an offending agent, whether that be an infection of a certain organism, or an offending drug. Identification of the triad of fever, rash, and peripheral eosinophilia can lead the investigator to a possible AIN diagnosis. However, the gold standard method of diagnosis is by renal biopsy, showing increased lymphocyte and neutrophils in the interstitium of the kidney. A renal biopsy is often needed to commit to the diagnosis of AIN because the definitive treatment of AIN, other than withdrawing the offending agent, is to treat with high-dose steroids. Because patients with HIV/AIDS usually present with coinfections, the decision to immunosuppress the patient.

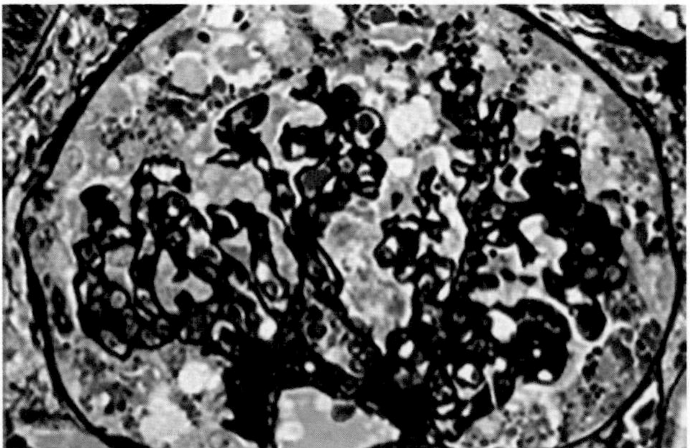

Fig. 5.2 Focal segmental glomerulosclerosis, collapsing variant. In this example, exuberant proliferation of glomerular epithelial cells forms a pseudocrescent that obliterates the urinary space. The pseudocrescent lacks the spindle cell morphology, ruptures of the Bowman capsule, or pericellular matrix typically seen in true inflammatory crescents of parietal epithelial origin. (Jones methenamine silver, ×400.) (From Floege, J., Johnson, R. J., & Feehally, J. (2018). *Comprehensive clinical nephrology*. (6th ed.). Philadelphia: Elsevier Saunders.)

Bibliography

Cohen, S. D., Kopp, J. B., & Kimmel, P. L. (2017). Kidney diseases associated with human immunodeficiency virus. *N Engl J Med*, *377*, 2263–2274.

Floege, J., Johnson, R. J., & Feehally, J. (2018). *Comprehensive clinical nephrology* (6th ed.). Philadelphia: Elsevier Saunders.

Gilbert, S., Weiner, D., et al. (2014). *National kidney foundation's primer on kidney disease* (6th ed.). Philadelphia: Elsevier/Saunders;.

Taal, M. W., Chertow, G. A., Marsden, P. A., Skorecki, K., Yu, A. S. L., & Brenner, B. M. (2011). *Brenner and Rector's; The kidney* (9th ed.). Philadelphia: Elsevier.

Zaidan, M., Lescure, F. X., Brocheriou, I., & Dettwiler, S. (2013). Tubulointerstitial nephropathies in HIV-infected patients over past 15 years. *Clinical Journal of the American Society of Nephrology*, *8*(6), 930–938.

SECTION 2

Hematology

CASE 6

A 58-Year-Old Female With Syncope

Justin Tiulim ■ Maria E. Vergara-Lluri ■ Caroline I. Piatek

A 58-year-old female presents to the emergency room after evaluation for syncope by her primary care doctor revealed significant anemia with a hemoglobin of 6.0 g/dL. Her medical history is significant for type 2 diabetes for which she takes metformin.

What are key questions for patients presenting with anemia?

- Is the patient having symptoms of lightheadedness, dizziness, fainting, chest pain, or dyspnea on exertion?
  - Qualify anemia as symptomatic versus asymptomatic. Patients who have symptomatic anemia may need a transfusion of packed red blood cells.
- Does the patient report bleeding, such as dark stools (melena), frank red blood in the stools (hematochezia), or blood in the urine (hematuria)?
  - Patients with anemia should be asked about blood loss.
- How long has the patient had anemia? Does anyone else in the family have anemia? What is the patient's ethnic background?
  - A patient with a lifelong history of anemia may have an inherited cause of anemia, such as thalassemia. An inherited cause of anemia is further supported by a family medical history of anemia and certain ethnic backgrounds.
- Presence of menorrhagia?
  - In premenopausal women, the most prevalent cause of iron deficiency is heavy menstrual bleeding.
- Does the patient have any dietary restrictions?
  - Certain dietary restrictions may lead to nutritional deficiencies.
  - Vitamin B_{12} (cobalamin) is present in many animal products, including meats, dairy products, and eggs. Therefore, reduced intake of animal products or a strict vegan diet are risk factors for vitamin B_{12} deficiency.
  - Folate is present in many plant and animal products, especially dark-green leafy vegetables. Thus, decreased intake of fresh vegetables and fortified grains, especially in alcoholics, leads to folate deficiencies. However, the prevalence of folate deficiency in healthy people with normal dietary intake has declined progressively due to food fortification with folic acid.
  - Certain foods can cause malabsorption of other nutrients. Dietary iron absorption is impaired with foods with high content of tannates, phosphates, phytates (found in whole grains and seeds), and calcium.
- Does the patient have a history of gastric surgery or inflammatory bowel disease?
  - Vitamin B_{12} absorption is dependent on gastric cells in the stomach to produce acid and intrinsic factor, as well as in the terminal ileum, where absorption occurs. Therefore, any surgery or process affecting these areas may result in B_{12} deficiency.

- Folate is absorbed in the jejunum, and an absence of this part of the small intestine will lead to a predilection toward folate deficiency.
- Iron is absorbed in the upper gastrointestinal tract with the duodenum being the site of maximal absorption.
- A history of gastric bypass surgery is a risk factor for developing deficiencies in all three of the aforementioned nutrients.

- Has the patient received prior transfusions?
  - A history of transfusions can help to gauge the severity of anemia because transfusion thresholds are typically for hemoglobin less than 7 g/dL.
- Does the patient report pica (i.e., cravings for ice, clay, or dirt)?
  - These symptoms are highly concerning for iron deficiency anemia.
- Does the patient report yellowing of the skin or sclera (i.e., presence of jaundice)?
  - The presence of jaundice indicates elevated bilirubin levels in the blood. The combination of anemia and jaundice is suggestive of a hemolytic process.
- Does the patient report a history of weight loss?
  - Weight loss may result from inadequate nutrition intake or increased basal metabolic rate from an underlying inflammatory condition. Thus, malignancy or malabsorption should be considered.
  - Anemia, weight loss, and a change in bowel habits is highly concerning for GI cancer and would prompt an urgent GI workup.
- Is the patient up-to-date on routine healthcare maintenance?
  - If there is a lack of age-appropriate screening, consider an underlying malignancy.

The patient reports a 3-week history of general malaise, progressive dyspnea on exertion, external chest discomfort, and lightheadedness. One day prior to presentation, the patient experienced a syncopal episode while walking. She denies dark urine, gross hematuria, hematochezia, or melena. There is no jaundice or skin discoloration. She reports no recent medication changes, travel, or sick contacts. On review of systems, she has noted an unintentional weight loss of 30 pounds over the last 2 years. She is postmenopausal. She is not a vegetarian or vegan. She denies any cravings for ice, clay, or dirt. Her last colonoscopy was at the age of 50 years, which was normal. The patient has never received a blood transfusion. She denies any other past medical problems apart from diabetes. She denies any surgical history. There is no family history of anemia, easy bruising, or bleeding.

What are typical findings in a patient with anemia?

The signs and symptoms of anemia are dependent upon the severity of the anemia and the rate at which the anemia occurs. Symptoms may be less pronounced if the anemia develops chronically because of the body's ability to compensate. Patients with mild or moderate anemia are often asymptomatic. Fatigue and dyspnea on exertion or at rest are common symptoms. Tachycardia and systolic flow murmur can develop as a result of a compensatory hyperdynamic state from a lower blood volume and lower oxygen carrying capacity. In severe cases, patients can develop lethargy, confusion, and angina, and might even die. Anemic patients normally present with pallor found in the palms, nail beds, face, or conjunctiva as a result of blood shunting away from the skin to allow adequate perfusion to vital organs. The presence of jaundice is suggestive of hemolysis or ineffective erythropoiesis.

On physical examination, the patient's temperature is 37°C, pulse rate is 80/min, blood pressure is 113/60 mmHg, and respiration rate is 21 with an oxygenation saturation of 98% on room air. Orthostatic vital signs are negative. There is conjunctival pallor on the head/eyes/ears/nose/throat/neck examination. Her cardiopulmonary exam is normal. The abdominal exam has normal bowel sounds, with no tenderness to palpation, and no organomegaly. The pelvic exam is normal with no vaginal or cervical discharge. No skin lesions, oral ulcers, or lower extremity edema are present. The neurological exam reveals no focal neurological deficits.

TABLE 6.1 ■ **Laboratory Data**

		Reference Ranges
White blood cell	4.1 K/μL	4.0–11.0 K/μL
Absolute neutrophil count	1.4 K/μL	1.8–8.0 K/μL
Absolute lymphocyte count	2.4 K/μL	1.2–3.3 K/μL
Absolute monocyte count	0.2 K/μL	0.3–1.0 K/μL
Absolute eosinophil count	0.1 K/μL	0.0–0.4 K/μL
Absolute basophil count	0.0 K/μL	0.0–0.1 K/μL
Hemoglobin	6.6 g/dL	12.0–16.0 g/dL
Hematocrit	19.3%	35.0%–47.0%
Mean corpuscular volume	124 fL	82–97 fL
Red blood cell distribution width	25%	12%–15%
Platelets	108 K/μL	140–440 K/μL
Absolute reticulocyte count	34 x 10^9/L	29–116 x 10^9/L
Prothrombin time	14.5 seconds	11.5–14.4 seconds
INR	1.15	0.86–1.14
Total bilirubin	1.5 mg/dL	<1.0 mg/dL
Direct bilirubin	0.4 mg/dL	<0.3 mg/dL
Lactate dehydrogenase	2297 U/L	90–220 U/L
Haptoglobin	<10 mg/dL	30–200 mg/dL
Iron	220 μg/dL	50–160 μg/dL
Iron binding capacity	283 μg/dL	250–430 μg/dL
Iron saturation	78%	15%–50%
Vitamin B_{12}	<150 pg/mL	232–1245 pg/mL
Folate	Unable to obtain due to hemolysis	>4.6 ng/mL
Homocysteine	136 μmol/L	<15 μmol/L
Methylmalonic acid	6933 nmol/L	87–318 nmol/L
Gastrin	1534 pg/mL	<100 pg/mL
Intrinsic factor antibody	Positive	Negative
HIV antibody/antigen	Negative	Negative
Hepatitis panel	Negative	Negative
Direct antiglobulin test	Negative	Negative

The results of laboratory testing are shown in Table 6.1.

How do you interpret the laboratory results?

The laboratory results are most notable for a profound macrocytic anemia with concomitant thrombocytopenia. There is also evidence of ineffective erythropoiesis/hemolysis with an elevated lactate dehydrogenase (LDH) and indirect bilirubin and low haptoglobin. Iron studies are not consistent with iron deficiency anemia. Folate could not be determined; however, it is uncommon to have folate deficiency in the United States with food fortification. The serum vitamin B_{12} level is low, and homocysteine and methylmalonic acid levels are elevated; overall, the findings confirm biochemical vitamin B_{12} deficiency.

BASIC SCIENCE PEARL **STEP 1**

Methylmalonic acid (MMA) and homocysteine (HCY) may be checked to confirm a suspected vitamin B_{12} deficiency. MMA and HCY are substrates in the reaction that uses vitamin B_{12} as a cofactor; thus, MMA and HCY will be elevated in the setting of vitamin B_{12} deficiency. MMA is more sensitive and specific for vitamin B_{12} deficiency than HCY. In folate deficiency, the HCY level will be elevated, but the MMA will be normal.

How do you define macrocytic and megaloblastic anemia?

The mean corpuscular volume (MCV) is a weighted measure of the size/volume of red blood cells, as an average. Fig. 6.1 shows the breakdown of anemia based on the MCV. Macrocytosis refers to the increased average red cell volume, typically defined as an MCV greater than 100 fL.

BASIC SCIENCE/CLINICAL PEARL STEP 1/2

The most common cause of mild elevations (101–109 fL) in MCV is reticulocytosis, which may be compensatory as a result of hemolysis or blood loss.

However, megaloblastic anemia refers to a subgroup of macrocytic anemias in which megaloblasts can be seen. Megaloblasts are erythroid and/or granulocytic precursors that display nuclear-to-cytoplasmic dyssynchrony because of impaired DNA synthesis. This results in a delay in nuclear (in contrast to cytoplasmic) maturation; cytoplasmic maturation (in contrast to nuclear maturation) proceeds unimpeded because the cytoplasm relies mostly on protein and RNA synthesis. The most common causes of megaloblastic anemia are alcoholism, vitamin B_{12} deficiency (most frequently from pernicious anemia), folate deficiency, and medication.

What are symptoms and signs of vitamin B_{12} deficiency?

Vitamin B_{12} is a cofactor for the enzyme methionine synthase, which is necessary for the development and myelination of the central nervous system. Therefore, vitamin B_{12} deficiency may present with neuropsychiatric symptoms—most commonly, symmetric paresthesia or numbness and gait problems.

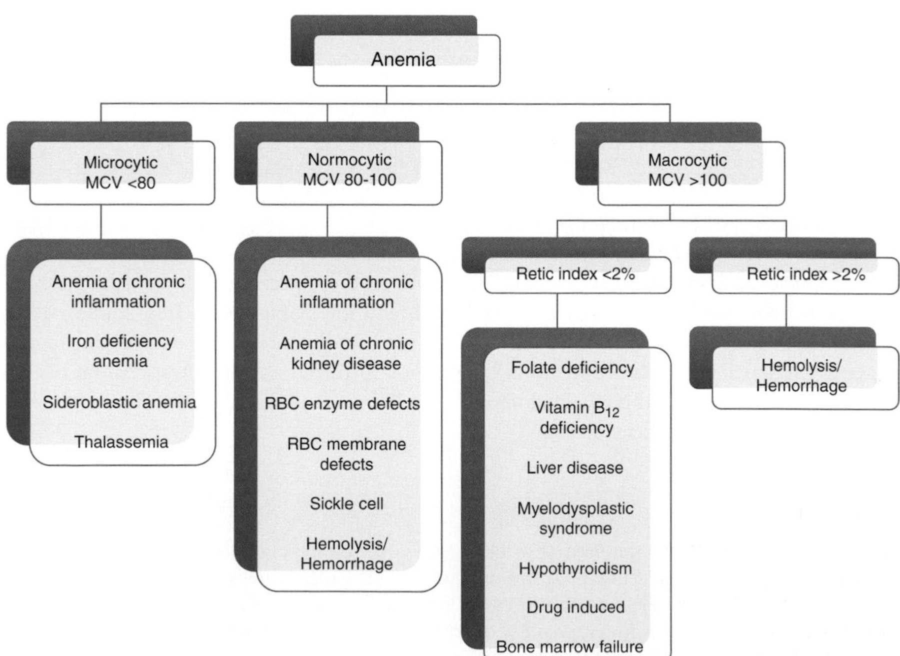

Fig. 6.1 Anemia differential by mean corpuscular volume (MCV). *RBC*, Red blood cells.

CLINICAL PEARL **STEP 2/3**

Vitamin B_{12} neuropathy is typically symmetrical and affects the legs more than the arms. These symptoms can manifest even in the absence of anemia or macrocytosis.

Lack of vitamin B_{12} also leads to a nuclear-to-cytoplasmic dyssynchrony. In the peripheral blood and bone marrow, it can be observed in the form of red cell macro-ovalocytosis, gigantism in myeloid precursors ("giant bands"), and/or hypersegmentation in granulocytes. Ineffective erythropoiesis results in hemolysis within the bone marrow, which may show some peripheral smear features similar to that of microangiopathic hemolytic anemia. Other associated clinical features of vitamin B_{12} deficiency include glossitis, malabsorption, infertility, and thrombosis (because of increased HCY).

CLINICAL PEARL **STEP 2/3**

Macrocytosis is the most common clinical finding in vitamin B_{12} deficiency, and it can precede the anemia by months.

Potential causes for vitamin B_{12} deficiency are highlighted in Table 6.2.

Concordant with the CBC finding of striking red cell macrocytosis (with MCV of 124 fL), the peripheral blood smear demonstrates a profound macrocytic anemia with oval macrocytes, basophilic stippling, and hypersegmented neutrophils (see Fig. 6.2). Where vitamin B_{12} deficiency and positive intrinsic factor antibody are present, the diagnosis would be pernicious anemia.

What is pernicious anemia?

Pernicious anemia is an autoimmune disorder that prevents formation of the vitamin B_{12}–intrinsic factor complex, leading to decreased vitamin B_{12} absorption. Intrinsic factor is a protein that binds ingested vitamin B_{12} in the gut and is necessary for absorption in the ileum. Common autoantibodies in individuals with pernicious anemia are those directed against intrinsic factor or gastric parietal cells. However, only the antibodies against intrinsic factor are important in the pathogenesis of pernicious anemia.

BASIC SCIENCE PEARL **STEP 1**

A positive test for anti-intrinsic factor antibody (sensitivity of 50% and specificity of 100%) confirms the diagnosis of pernicious anemia. Antiparietal cell antibodies are less specific for pernicious anemia (sensitivity of 80% and specificity of 50%–100%).

TABLE 6.2 ■ **Differential Diagnosis for Causes of Vitamin B_{12} Deficiency**

Malabsorption
- Pernicious anemia (autoimmune gastritis)
- Total or partial gastrectomy
- Inflammatory bowel disease/tropical sprue
- Imerslund-Grasbeck syndrome
- Use of metformin
- Use of drugs that block stomach acid

Dietary deficiency
- Vegan or vegetarian diet low in meat and dairy products

Recreational occupational abuse of nitrous oxide

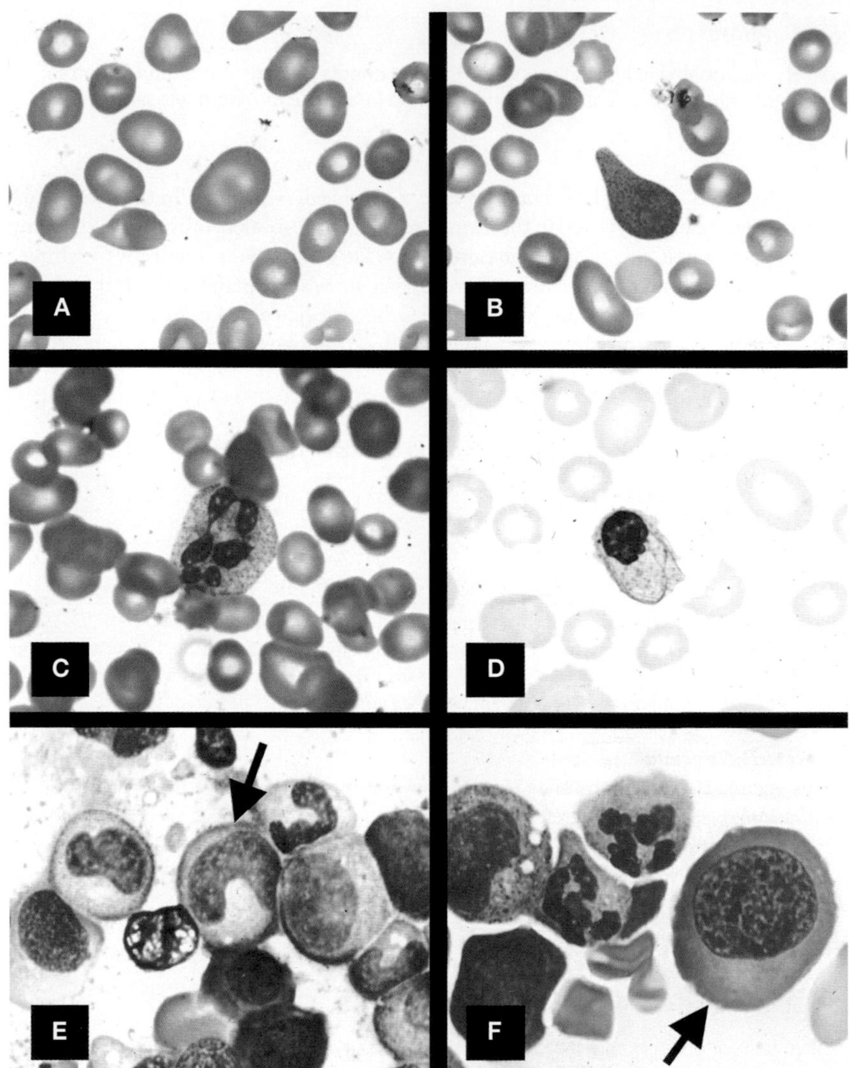

Fig. 6.2 Pernicious anemia. Peripheral blood smear (A–D); bone marrow aspirate smear (E–F), Wright-Giemsa stained slides; 1000× magnification. (A) An oval macrocyte (or macro-ovalocyte) is seen in the center, an indication of abnormal red cell maturation. It is most commonly associated with vitamin B_{12} or folic acid deficiency. Note that this red cell is much larger than its neighbors, even though it has the same color as the surrounding mature red blood cells (RBCs). This contrasts with one of its look-alikes, the polychromatophilic red cell (a presumptive reticulocyte), which has a slightly darker, gray-blue cytoplasmic color compared with mature RBCs. (B) Coarse basophilic stippling, representing ribosomal aggregates, can also be observed in megaloblastic anemia. (C) A hypersegmented neutrophil can be identified in cases of megaloblastic anemia. To be considered hypersegmented, the neutrophil must have six or more nuclear lobes, a sign of megaloblastic change in leukocytes. (D) A Cabot ring is rare and is a thin, thread-like, red cell cytoplasmic inclusion that forms either twisted loops or figures-of-eight. These are remnants of the mitotic spindle, which are left over after cell division; their presence indicates abnormal erythropoiesis (as can be seen in megaloblastic anemias or myelodysplastic syndromes). (E) In the bone marrow, another sign of megaloblastic maturation is giant bands *(arrow)*, which are 1.5 times larger than normal bands. (F) A megaloblastic erythroid precursor is identified in this bone marrow, a manifestation of nuclear-to-cytoplasmic dyssynchrony *(arrow)*, where the nuclear chromatin appears to be at an earlier stage, whereas the cytoplasm is at a later stage of maturation.

Pernicious anemia is also associated with other autoimmune disorders, such as thyroid disease, type 1 diabetes mellitus, and vitiligo. The median age at diagnosis is approximately 70 to 80 years, but all age groups are affected. It is more common in persons of African or European ancestry. Pernicious anemia can lead to chronic atrophic gastritis, which will show elevated levels of fasting serum gastrin and low levels of serum pepsinogen-1.

CLINICAL PEARL **STEP 2/3**

Upper endoscopy with biopsy is recommended to confirm gastritis and exclude gastric cancer in all patients diagnosed with pernicious anemia.

The patient received intramuscular vitamin B_{12}. Her Hgb improved and she was discharged with outpatient hematology follow-up. Because the patient has pernicious anemia, she will need lifelong vitamin B_{12} treatment.

What is the treatment for vitamin B_{12} deficiency?

The treatment for vitamin B_{12} deficiency is either intramuscularly or high-dose oral repletion of vitamin B_{12}. About 10% of the injected vitamin B_{12} (cyanocobalamin) is retained. Patients with severe deficiency often initially receive injections of 1000 µg at least several times a week for 1 to 2 weeks, then weekly, then monthly. About 0.5% to 4% of oral vitamin B_{12} can be absorbed by passive diffusion without the need of intrinsic factor. Thus, high doses of daily vitamin B_{12} (> 500 µg) may also be given.

CLINICAL PEARL **STEP 2/3**

Hematologic response is rapid with a reticulocyte count rise in 1 week and correction of megaloblastic anemia in 6 to 8 weeks. Neurologic symptoms may take weeks to months to subside.

Case Summary

- **Complaint/History:** A 58-year-old female presents with a 3-week history of general malaise, progressive dyspnea on exertion, external chest discomfort, and lightheadedness.
- **Findings**: Eye exam reveals conjunctival pallor.
- **Lab Results/Tests:** Lab results reveal a profound macrocytic anemia (MCV >120 fL) with concomitant thrombocytopenia. There is also evidence of ineffective erythropoiesis and hemolysis, including elevated LDH and indirect bilirubin, and low haptoglobin. The serum vitamin B_{12} level is low; the homocysteine and methylmalonic acid are elevated. The anti-intrinsic factor antibody test is positive. Peripheral blood smear reveals oval macrocytes, basophilic stippling, and occasional hypersegmented neutrophils.

Diagnosis: Vitamin B_{12} deficiency caused by pernicious anemia.

- **Treatment:** The patient received intramuscular vitamin B_{12} injections.

BEYOND THE PEARLS

- Vitamin B_{12} deficiency presents with neurological symptoms, megaloblastic anemia, and markers of ineffective erythropoiesis, and with peripheral blood smear findings showing hypersegmented neutrophils, macro-ovalocytes, basophilic stippling, and, rarely, Cabot rings.
- A bone marrow biopsy is not indicated for the evaluation of vitamin B_{12} deficiency.
- Treatment duration of vitamin B_{12} deficiency depends on the cause of the deficiency. In the case of pernicious anemia, the treatment is lifelong.

Bibliography

Bunn, H., & Heeney, M. Megaloblastic anemias. In J. C. Aster & H. Bunn (Eds.), *Pathophysiology of Blood Disorders* (2nd ed.) New York, NY: McGraw-Hill. http://accessmedicine.mhmedical.com.libproxy1.usc.edu/content.aspx?bookid=1900§ionid=137394859.

Glassy, E. F. (Ed.). (1918). Color Atlas of Hematology: An Illustrated Field Guide Based on Proficiency Testing (Peripheral Blood), (2nd ed.) *Erythrocytes* (pp. 76–79). Erythrocyte Inclusions (pp. 134–143). College of American Pathologists; Northfield, IL.

Gnanaraj, J., Parnes, A., Francis, C. W., Go, R. S., Takemoto, C. M., & Hashmi, S. K. (2018 Sepp). Approach to pancytopenia: Diagnostic algorithm for clinical hematologists. *Blood Reviews*, *32*(5), 361–367.

Green, R. (2017). Vitamin B12 deficiency from the perspective of a practicing hematologist. *Blood*, *129*(19), 2603–2611.

Hariz, A., & Bhattacharya, P. T. (2019). Megaloblastic anemia. [Updated 2019 Jan 23]: In: *StatPearls [Internet]*. Treasure Island (FL): StatPearls Publishing. https://www.ncbi.nlm.nih.gov/books/NBK537254/.

Kaferle, J., & Strzoda, C. E. (2009). Evaluation of macrocytosis. *American Family Physician*, *79*(3), 203–208.

Stabler, S. P. (2013). Clinical practice. Vitamin B12 deficiency. *The New England Journal of Medicine*, *368*(2), 149–160.

Weinzierl, E. P., & Arber, D. A. (2013). The differential diagnosis and bone marrow evaluation of new-onset pancytopenia. *American Journal of Clinical Pathology*, *139*(1), 9–29.

CASE 7

A 24-Year-Old Male With Easy Bruising and Mucosal Bleeding

Justin Tiulim ■ Maria E. Vergara-Lluri ■ Caroline I. Piatek

A 24-year-old male presents with 2 weeks of progressive fatigue and gum bleeding, which has worsened acutely over the past day. On the morning of presentation, he awoke with a large amount of blood in his mouth. He states that he has been having subjective fevers for the past day. He notes easy bruising and headaches. He denies chills, shortness of breath, chest pain, abdominal pain, and joint pain or swelling. He denies epistaxis, gross hematuria, hematochezia, or melena. He denies any recent travel or sick contacts. He has no significant past medical history.

Vital signs include a temperature of 38.9°C, pulse rate of 102/min, blood pressure of 110/71 mmHg, and respiration rate of 18 with an oxygenation saturation of 94% on room air. On physical examination, there is dried blood in the oral cavity and presence of multiple blood-filled blisters on his oral mucosa. Neck exam reveals an enlarged 2-cm lymph node in the submandibular region. His cardiopulmonary exam is significant for borderline tachycardia with a normal rhythm. His abdominal exam demonstrates normal bowel sounds, no tenderness to palpation, and no organomegaly. Diffuse ecchymoses are present over his abdomen and bilateral upper and lower extremities, as well as widespread petechiae. He exhibits no focal neurological deficits.

How do you approach symptoms of bleeding and ecchymoses?

Platelet and vascular disorders are generally characterized by mucosal bleeding (e.g., mouth, nose, urinary tract, gastrointestinal tract) and immediate bleeding upon a hemostatic challenge. In contrast, coagulation factor disorders are generally characterized by bleeding into muscles and joints and delayed bleeding after a hemostatic challenge. Other medical conditions, such as cancer, cirrhosis, renal failure, and infection, may also lead to acquired bleeding disorders. Table 7.1 compares platelet function defects with clotting factor deficiencies or inhibitors.

Ask the patient about the use of medications that are associated with easy bruising or increased bleeding. A family history of bleeding should be obtained to help determine the likelihood of an inherited condition. Inherited disorders tend to present in childhood if the genetic defect results

TABLE 7.1 ■ **Platelet Dysfunction Versus Clotting Factor Dysfunction/Deficiency**

Bleeding Characteristics	Platelet Function Defects	Clotting Factor Deficiencies or Inhibitors
Major sites of bleeding	Mucocutaneous (mouth, nose, gastrointestinal tract, urinary tract, menorrhagia)	Deep tissue (joint, muscle) or soft tissue hematoma
Petechiae	Common	Uncommon
Excessive bleeding after minor cuts	Yes	Not usually
Excessive bleeding after surgery	Often immediate	Often during procedure, some may experience delayed bleeding (factor VII deficiency)

in a clinically severe phenotype, but inherited bleeding disorders of milder severity may only become apparent in adulthood.

CLINICAL PEARL **STEP 2/3**

Common medications that cause increased risk for bleeding are antiplatelet agents such as aspirin and non-steroid antiinflammatory drugs (NSAIDs), or the use of anticoagulants such as warfarin or anti-Xa inhibitors.

The results of laboratory testing are shown in Table 7.2.

How should laboratory results be interpreted?

The complete blood count with differential shows pancytopenia with severe neutropenia. Table 7.3 shows a broad differential for causes of pancytopenia. The preliminarily reported white blood cell differential shows the presence of suspicious "other cells" (pending further pathologist review) and occasional left-shifted neutrophils (i.e., myelocytes and metamyelocytes). Elevated prothrombin time (PT), international normalized ratio (INR), partial thromboplastin time (PTT), and D-dimer in combination with low fibrinogen levels indicate a coagulopathy. Low haptoglobin, increased total bilirubin (with significant contribution from indirect bilirubin), and high lactate dehydrogenase levels are suggestive of hemolysis.

The laboratory results are compatible with disseminated intravascular coagulation (DIC), with an additional concern for an associated leukemia/lymphoma given the suspicious "other cells" seen by the laboratory technologist.

What is disseminated intravascular coagulation?

DIC is a life-threatening coagulopathy that may lead to thrombosis and hemorrhage. DIC results from the release of either tissue factor or exposure of blood to procoagulants, which activates the clotting cascade leading to the consumption of coagulation factors and platelets. Furthermore, plasmin is also activated, resulting in secondary fibrinolysis. The overall clinical picture of thrombosis versus bleeding is determined by the balance of prothrombotic and antithrombotic abnormalities. Table 7.4 shows some of the causes of DIC.

A diagnosis of DIC is based on an appropriate clinical suspicion supported by relevant laboratory tests. Lab abnormalities in DIC include thrombocytopenia, elevated D-dimer, prolonged PT, prolonged aPTT, and low fibrinogen. The peripheral blood smear will show thrombocytopenia; there may be larger platelet forms noted. The peripheral blood smear in about a fourth of patients with DIC will show schistocytes, which are red cells with irregular size and shape, often with sharp pointed ends, and lacking central pallor.

BASIC SCIENCE PEARL **STEP 1**

The larger platelet forms seen in the peripheral blood smears of DIC cases indicate peripheral destruction of platelets – prompting compensatory release of younger and larger platelets from the bone marrow – as opposed to impaired platelet production.

TABLE 7.2 ■ **Laboratory Results**

		Reference Ranges
White blood cell	1.2 K/μL	4.0–11.0 K/μL
Absolute neutrophil count	0.2 K/μL	1.8–8.0 K/μL
Absolute lymphocyte count	0.7 K/μL	1.2–3.3 K/μL
Absolute monocyte count	0.0 K/μL	0.3–1.0 K/μL
Absolute eosinophil count	0.0 K/μL	0-0.4 K/μL
Absolute basophil count	0.0 K/μL	0.0–0.1 K/μL
Neutrophils	17%	Reference range not defined
Lymphocytes	58%	Reference range not defined
Myelocytes	5%	<0%
Metamyelocytes	1%	<0%
"Other cells," pending pathologist review	19%	<0%
Hemoglobin	8.3 g/dL	12.0–16.0 g/dL
Hematocrit	23.6%	35.0%–47.0%
Mean corpuscular volume	95 fL	82–97 fL
Platelets	26 K/μL	140–440 K/μL
Sodium	139 mmol/L	135–145 mmol/L
Potassium	3.7 mmol/L	3.5–5.1 mmol/L
Chloride	105 mmol/L	100–110 mmol/L
Bicarbonate	21 mmol/L	20–30 mmol/L
Blood urea nitrogen	12 mg/dL	10–20 mg/dL
Creatinine	1.04 mg/dL	0.5–1.3 mg/dL
Glucose	98 mg/dL	65–99 mg/dL
Calcium	9.8 mg/dL	8.5–10.3 mg/dL
Phosphorus	3.9 mg/dL	2.5–4.5 mg/dL
Magnesium	2.0 mg/dL	1.7–2.3 mg/dL
Alkaline phosphatase	63 U/L	40–129 U/L
Total protein	7.8 g/dL	6 8 g/dL
Albumin	5.1 g/dL	3.5–5.0 g/dL
Aspartate aminotransferase	51 U/L	10–40 U/L
Alanine aminotransferase	51 U/L	10–55 U/L
Total bilirubin	1.5 mg/dL	<1.0 mg/dL
Direct bilirubin	0.3 mg/dL	<0.3 mg/dL
Activated partial thromboplastin time	35.4 seconds	24.7–35.3 seconds
Prothrombin time	17.9 seconds	12–14.2 seconds
INR	1.49	0.9–1.11
Fibrinogen	157 mg/dL	239–439 mg/dL
D-dimer	>20 μg/mL	<0.49 μg/mL
Haptoglobin	11 mg/dL	30–200 mg/dL
Lactate dehydrogenase	582 U/L	90–220 U/L
Uric acid	6 mg/dL	4–8.1 mg/dL

BASIC SCIENCE PEARL **STEP 1/2**

Schistocytes are red blood cells that have been sheared by fragmentation through a meshwork of fibrin strands in the vessels in thrombotic microangiopathy. These red cell fragments indicate the presence of hemolysis.

Given the clinical and laboratory evidence of DIC, the patient received transfusions of fresh frozen plasma and platelets to decrease the risk of further bleeding.

TABLE 7.3 ■ **Differential Diagnosis of Pancytopenia**

Hematological Processes	Systemic Illnesses and Other Etiologies
Bone marrow failure syndromes/aplastic anemia	Hypothyroidism
Hematological malignancies	Anorexia nervosa
• Myelodysplastic syndrome, leukemia, lymphoma	
Paroxysmal nocturnal hemoglobinuria	Systemic lupus erythematosus
Myelofibrosis	Hypersplenism (caused by liver disease)
	Sepsis
	Alcoholism
	Vitamin deficiencies (vitamin B_{12}, folate)
	Infections
	Tuberculosis, Q fever, ehrlichiosis, brucellosis
	Metastatic carcinomas and sarcomas
	Medications

TABLE 7.4 ■ **Causes of Disseminated Intravascular Coagulation**

Vascular Damage Leading to Release of Tissue Factor

Bacterial sepsis
- Gram negative organisms
  - Meningococcus
  - Pneumococcus
- Gram positive organisms

Metabolic stress
- Acidosis
- Shock
- Heat stroke

Release of Tissue Factor From Injured or Pathologic Tissue

Obstetrical complications
- Placental abruption
- Retained placenta/fetus
- Placenta previa
- Amniotic fluid embolism
- Preeclampsia/eclampsia

Malignancies
- Solid tumors, mucin-secreting adenocarcinomas
- Acute myeloid leukemias, especially acute promyelocytic leukemia

Severe burns

What is the management of DIC?

The treatment for DIC is ultimately to treat the underlying cause. For patients who are bleeding (or are at high risk of bleeding), supportive management is recommended, which includes transfusions with platelets, fresh frozen plasma, cryoprecipitate, and red blood cells. For patients with DIC and active bleeding, platelet transfusions should be given to maintain platelet count >50 K/μL, fresh frozen plasma (FFP) transfusion to maintain INR <1.5, and cryoprecipitate transfusion to maintain fibrinogen >150 mg/dL.

BASIC SCIENCE PEARL **STEP 1/2**

FFP includes all clotting factors and other proteins present in the original unit of blood. However, cryoprecipitate is derived from FFP and includes only fibrinogen, von Willebrand factor, and factors VIII and XIII. FFP is primarily indicated when there is bleeding caused by a deficiency of multiple coagulation factors (e.g., reversal of warfarin, liver disease, and DIC, and as part of a massive transfusion protocol). Cryoprecipitate has fewer indications and is primarily used for the management of bleeding with fibrinogen disorders and DIC.

Because the patient was found to be febrile with an absolute neutrophil count of 400, he was started on cefepime for neutropenic fever.

What is neutropenic fever?

Neutropenic fever is a fever occurring in the setting of neutropenia (absolute neutrophil count [ANC] of 0.5 K/μL or expected ANC <0.5 K/μL in the next 48 hours). Neutropenic fever is most commonly encountered as a complication of cancer therapy but may also been seen when there is decreased neutrophil production resulting from bone marrow infiltration by a hematological cancer.

CLINICAL PEARL STEP 2/3

In 50%–70% of patients with neutropenic fever, there is no clinical or microbiologically documented infection.

A bacterial cause for infection is the most common etiology. Gram negative bacteremia is associated with worse outcomes compared with Gram positive bacteremia. Thus, empiric antibiotic treatment is targeted to cover Gram negative bacteria, with antibiotics such as cefepime or piperacillin-tazobactam. Vancomycin is normally added in patients with severe sepsis, septic shock, catheter-related infection, known colonization with methicillin-resistant *Staphylococcus aureus* (MRSA) or penicillin-resistant *Streptococcus pneumoniae*, severe mucositis, and pneumonia.

The hematopathologist reviewed the peripheral blood smear and notes key morphologic findings that are compatible with leukemic/abnormal promyelocytes with concern for possible acute promyelocytic leukemia (APL), despite the absence of numerous Auer rods (see Fig. 7.1). The patient was immediately started on all-trans retinoic acid (ATRA) while awaiting genetic confirmation. The hematology service was emergently consulted and a bone marrow biopsy was performed.

When do you suspect acute promyelocytic leukemia?

APL should be suspected when there are abnormal promyelocytes on the peripheral blood smear (see Fig. 7.1) and laboratory evidence of DIC. It is important to recognize the characteristic nuclear features of leukemic/abnormal promyelocytes; some cases may not have abnormal promyelocytes containing many Auer rods in peripheral blood smears. The presentation of acute promyelocytic leukemia (APL) is considered a medical emergency because of its association with DIC, which can lead to life-threatening hemorrhage in what is a curable cancer for the vast majority of patients. Once the diagnosis of APL is suspected, the case should be treated as a medical emergency and treatment should be started urgently.

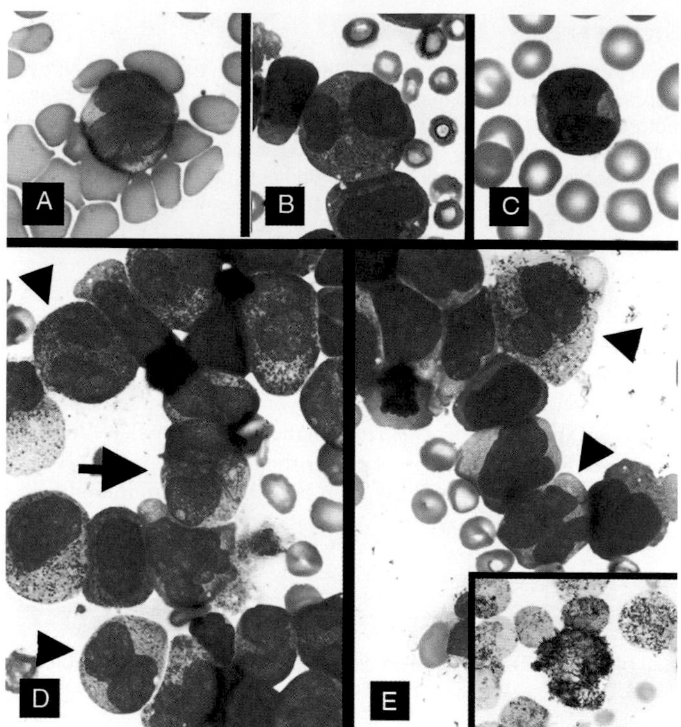

Fig. 7.1 (1000× magnification). Peripheral blood smear, Wright-Giemsa stain (A–C). Bone marrow aspirate smears, Wright-Giemsa stain (D, E). Myeloperoxidase stain positivity in microgranular variant of acute promyelocytic leukemia (APL) (*inset*, E). Even in the absence of numerous Auer rods in the abnormal cells seen in the peripheral blood, note the characteristic twisted (A), bilobed (B), and kidney-shaped (C) nuclear morphology of these leukemic promyelocytes. The nuclei of abnormal/leukemic promyelocytes (which are considered "blast equivalents") have also been described as "butterfly wings," "French windows," "sliding plates," or "cottage loaf" (a traditional type of bread originating in the UK). In contrast, normal promyelocytes are unilobed, with smooth and round to oval nuclear contours, and with prominent perinuclear Golgi hofs (not shown). In the bone marrow aspirate smear of this typical hypergranular APL case (D), the bilobed nuclei of the abnormal promyelocytes are easily seen *(arrowheads)*, and others have numerous azurophilic granules. The leukemic promyelocyte in the center (D) contains stacks of many Auer rods *(arrow)*, denoting it as a faggot cell, derived from the British term for bundles of wood. In this microgranular variant of APL (E), cells with numerous Auer rods and/or prominent azurophilic granules are very rare; however, notice that the abnormal nuclear morphology of "butterfly wings" in these blast equivalents is still evident. The inset photo in (E) reveals the strikingly intense myeloperoxidase expression that is characteristic of all APLs, even in this microgranular variant (myeloperoxidase cytochemical stain).

CLINICAL PEARL **STEP 1/2/3**

ATRA should promptly be initiated with high suspicion for APL based on clinical and morphological analysis while awaiting genetic confirmation by chromosomal analysis, fluorescence in situ hybridization (FISH), and/or reverse transcription polymerase chain reaction (RT-PCR).

Bone marrow biopsy showed a markedly hypercellular bone marrow with the presence of numerous abnormal promyelocytes (blast equivalents) and presence of Auer rods. There is a marked decrease in maturing hematopoietic cells. Ancillary studies (flow cytometry, oncologic chromosomal analysis, and FISH and RT-PCR for PML-RARa fusion) confirm the morphologic diagnosis of APL (see Fig. 7.2).

Diagnosis: Acute promyelocytic leukemia (APL).

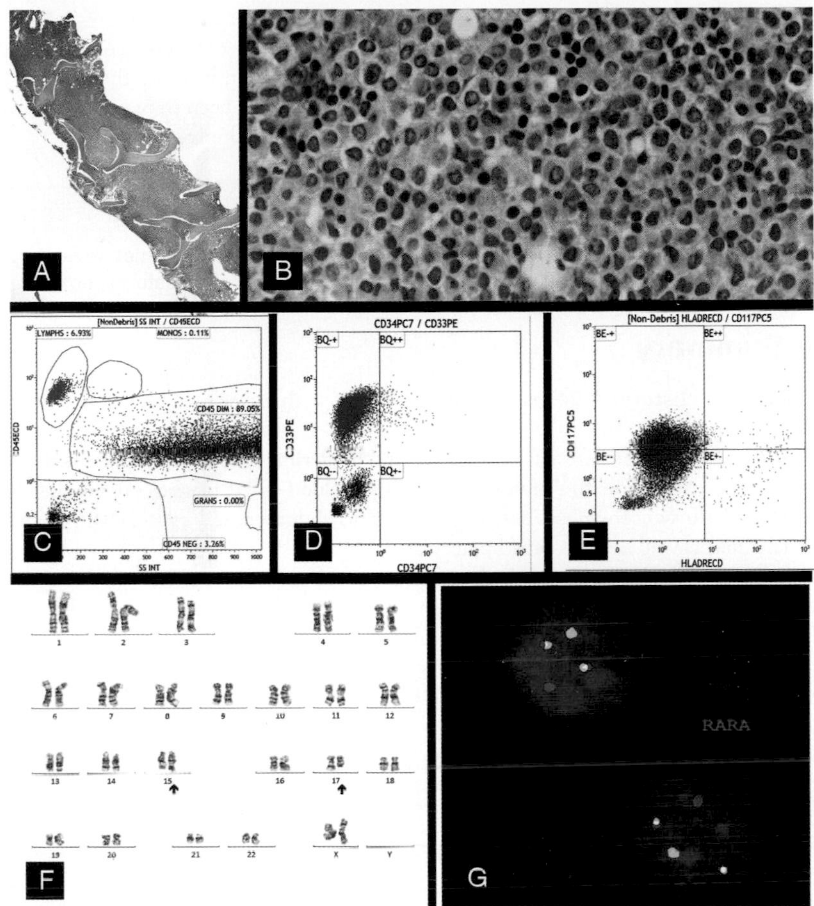

Fig. 7.2 Bone marrow trephine biopsy and ancillary studies in acute promyelocytic leukemia (APL). (A and B) Bone marrow biopsy, hematoxylin and eosin stain, reveals a 100% cellular bone marrow (20× magnification) with near-complete effacement by numerous abnormal promyelocytes (blast equivalents) in this "typical" hypergranular acute promyelocytic leukemia (APL) case. Note that other normal hematopoietic elements such as maturing erythroid, granulocytic, and megakaryocytic precursors are sparse or absent. (C–E) Flow cytometry graphs demonstrate a characteristic APL phenotype: dim expression of CD45 and heterogeneous intermediate to high side scatter (due to complexity of cells) seen in (C), with expression of myeloid markers, CD33 and CD117, yet absence of CD34 and HLA-DR, respectively seen in (D) and (E) in the leukemic promyelocytes. Results of chromosomal analysis (F) and fluorescence in situ hybridization (FISH) (G) provide genetic confirmation of the diagnosis of APL and are positive for the PML-PARA t(15;17) fusion.

What is acute promyelocytic leukemia?

APL is a subtype of acute myeloid leukemia (AML) and represents approximately 5%–15% of adult AML patients. In the vast majority of APL cases, there is a balanced reciprocal translocation between chromosomes 15 and 17, resulting in the product of promyelocytic leukemia (PML) and retinoic acid receptor-α *(RARα)* genes, which affects normal differentiation. APL blasts contain granules with proteolytic enzymes, which induce a hyperfibrinolytic form of DIC.

Once the diagnosis of APL was genetically confirmed, arsenic trioxide was added to the treatment. The patient's cell counts recovered over the next few days and the patient was discharged to follow-up in the hematology clinic.

What is the treatment of acute promyelocytic leukemia?

Although APL was previously one of the most lethal subtypes of AML, complete response rates are now attained in 90% of patients and complete remission in more than 80% with the introduction of ATRA. Prompt treatment of APL with ATRA has been shown to minimize early death from catastrophic hemorrhage, differentiation syndrome, and infection.

BASIC SCIENCE PEARL **STEP 1/2**

ATRA promotes the terminal differentiation of malignant promyelocytes to mature neutrophils, allowing the marrow and peripheral blood to repopulate with normal hematopoietic cells.

Case Summary

- **Complaint/History:** A 24-year-old male presents with 2 weeks of progressive fatigue and gum bleeding.
- **Findings:** The patient presents with fever and borderline tachycardia. There is dried blood in the oral cavity and the presence of multiple blood-filled blisters on his oral mucosal surfaces. Diffuse ecchymoses are present over his abdomen and bilateral upper and lower extremities, as well as widespread petechiae.
- **Lab Results/Tests:** Lab results show pancytopenia with severe neutropenia. The white blood cell differential shows abnormal promyelocytes (i.e., blast equivalents). Elevated PT/INR and PTT and low fibrinogen indicate a coagulopathy. A low haptoglobin and an elevated indirect bilirubin are suggestive of hemolysis. Bone marrow shows a markedly hypercellular marrow extensively infiltrated by abnormal promyelocytes, with occasional blast equivalents with many Auer rods; there is a strikingly decreased number of maturing hematopoietic cells in all three erythroid, granulocytic, and megakaryocytic lineages.

Diagnosis: Acute promyelocytic leukemia (APL) with disseminated intravascular coagulation (DIC) complicated by neutropenic fever.

- **Treatment:** The patient was started on all-trans retinoic acid (ATRA) once the diagnosis of APL was suspected. Arsenic trioxide was added once the diagnosis was genetically confirmed. DIC was supported with blood products. Neutropenic fever was treated with appropriate antibiotics until the fever resolved and the counts recovered.

BEYOND THE PEARLS

- In neutropenic fever with severe sepsis or septic shock, dual coverage therapy for Gram negative bacteria is recommended with a β-lactam + aminoglycoside/fluoroquinolone.
- If the fever resolves in neutropenic fever, the antibiotics are typically continued until the ANC >0.5 K/µL.
- For patients with DIC and bleeding, red blood cell transfusions for a hemoglobin >7 g/dL and platelet transfusions should be given to maintain platelet count >50/µL, FFP transfusion to maintain INR <1.5, and cryoprecipitate transfusion to maintain fibrinogen >150.
- APL should be suspected when there is laboratory evidence of DIC and the presence of abnormal promyelocytes on the peripheral blood smear.
- APL is a medical emergency and ATRA should be started prior to genetic confirmation.

Bibliography

Bunn, H., & Furie, B. Acquired coagulation disorders In: Aster J.C., Bunn H. eds. Pathophysiology of BloodDisorders, 2e New York, NY: McGraw-Hill; http://accessmedicine.mhmedical.com.libproxy1.usc.edu/content.aspx?bookid=1900§ionid=137395412

Glassy, E.F., ed. (2018). Color Atlas of Hematology: An Illustrated Field Guide Based on Proficiency Testing (Peripheral Blood) *Promyelocyte, Abnormal.* 2nd ed. Northfield, IL: College of American Pathologists; 226–227.

Levi, M. (2016). Management of cancer-associated disseminated intravascular coagulation. *Thromb Res, 140*(Suppl 1):S66–70.

National Comprehensive Cancer Network. Prevention and Treatment of Cancer-Related Infections (Version 1.2019). https://www.nccn.org/professionals/physician_gls/pdf/infections.pdf.

Sanz, M. A., Fenaux, P., Tallman, M. S., et al. (2019). Management of acute promyelocytic leukemia: updated recommendations from an expert panel of the European Leukemia Net. *Blood, 133*(15),1630–1643.

SECTION 3

Geriatrics

An 87-Year-Old Male With Acute Onset of Confusion

Diana Homeier ■ Araz Melkonian

An 87-year-old male with history of mild Alzheimer's dementia, cervical stenosis, and atrial fibrillation presents with 3 days of confusion, left-sided gait instability, and left-sided body pain. His daughter reports that he has been having increased confusion from his baseline for 3 days with intermittent agitation. She also reports that he has had low-grade fevers for 2 days prior to admission. At baseline, patient is alert and oriented to person and place.

What is the differential diagnosis of confusion in an elderly patient?

Differential diagnosis includes:

1. Delirium (also called acute confusional state, toxic or metabolic encephalopathy, altered mental status)
2. Dementia
3. Depression
4. Acute psychiatric syndromes

Be aware that several of these conditions can also coexist in the same patient.

Social history is negative for smoking, alcohol, and illicit drug use. Current medications include donepezil 10 mg daily, apixiban 2.5 mg twice a day, mirtazapine 15 mg nightly, and tramadol 50 mg, 2 tablets every 12 hours for pain.

What is delirium?

Delirium is an acute disorder of attention and global cognitive functioning. It is a common, serious, and potentially preventable source of morbidity and mortality for hospitalized older persons. Up to one-third of hospitalized patients 70 years or older admitted to a medicine ward experience delirium (half of these develop delirium in the hospital). Delirium is associated with many complex underlying medical problems and may be difficult to recognize; thus, less than half of cases are recognized in routine care.

CLINICAL PEARL **STEP 3**

In US hospitals today, five older patients become delirious every minute; 2.6 million older adults develop delirium each year (US Department of HHS, AoA Report, Profile of Older Americans 2011).

TABLE 8.1 ■ **Risk Factors for Delirium**

Predisposing Factors	Precipitating Factors
Dementia/cognitive impairment	Acute medical problem
Advanced age >70 years	New medications
Other central nervous system disease	Exacerbation of chronic medical problem
Multi-morbidity	Surgery
Polypharmacy	Pain
Impaired vision/hearing	Use of physical restraints
History of prior delirium	Dehydration
History of alcohol use	Poor nutritional status
Functional impairment	

The development of delirium is dependent upon the interaction of multiple risk factors. Several consistent risk factors for delirium have been identified and classified into two groups: baseline factors that predispose patients to delirium and acute factors that can precipitate delirium (Table 8.1).

What are the causes of delirium?

Because there are often multiple contributing factors, a patient with a diagnosis of delirium requires a thorough history, physical examination, and targeted laboratory testing to search for any treatable causes. The history should focus on the time course of the mental status changes and any other symptoms the patient may have. Some historical clues to the underlying etiologies may include recent fever, shortness of breath, complaints of pain, history of organ failure, current medications, changes in medications, use of alcohol or drugs, and recent depression. The mnemonic DELIRIUM can help to consider common reversible causes of delirium.

CLINICAL PEARL **STEP 2/3**

- D : Drugs, alcohol (medications)
- E : Electrolyte abnormalities
- L : Lack of drugs (pain, withdrawal)
- I : Infection (urinary tract infection, aspiration pneumonia)
- R : Restraints/reduced sensory input (hearing, vision)
- I : Injury (pain)/intracranial (rare)
- U : Unfamiliar environment/urinary retention/fecal impaction
- M: Metabolic/myocardial

Medications are the most common treatable cause of delirium. It is important to ensure that all medications being used (including over-the-counter and herbal medications) are reviewed. A list of medications that are commonly implicated in delirium is shown in Box 8.1.

How do you diagnose delirium?

The American Psychiatric Association's *Diagnostic and Statistical Manual*, 5th edition (DSM-V) lists five key features that characterize delirium (Box 8.2).

Some additional features that may accompany delirium include psychomotor behavioral disturbances (such as hypoactivity, hyperactivity, and impairment in sleep duration and architecture) and emotional disturbances (fear, depression, euphoria, or perplexity).

There are multiple instruments that can aid in the identification of delirium. The most widely used is the Confusion Assessment Method (CAM). It has been recommended as the most useful bedside assessment tool for delirium. The CAM helps a clinician establish the diagnosis of delirium by assessing a patient for four diagnostic features shown in Box 8.3.

BOX 8.1 ■ Medications/Drugs Predisposing to Delirium

- Alcohol
- Anticholinergics: oxybutynin, belladonna, cyclobenzaprine, hyoscyamine, meclizine, scopolamine
- Anticonvulsants: phenobarbital, phenytoin
- Antidepressants: amitriptyline, imipramine, doxepin, paroxetine
- Antihistamines: diphenhydramine, chlorphenamine
- Antiparkinsonian agents: levodopa-carbidopa, dopamine agonists, amantadine
- Antipsychotics: chlorpromazine, thioridazine, clozapine
- Benzodiazepines: diazepam, lorazepam
- H2-blocking agents: cimetidine
- Nonbenzodiazepine hypnotics: zolpidem
- Pain medications: meperidine, propoxyphene, opioids
- Any medication

BOX 8.2 ■ Clinical Characteristics of Delirium

- Acute onset of mental status change with fluctuating course
- Attentional deficits
- Confusion or disorganized thinking
- Altered level of consciousness
- Perceptual disturbances
- Disturbed sleep/wake cycle
- Altered psychomotor activity
- Disorientation and memory impairment
- Other cognitive deficits
- Behavioral and emotional abnormalities

From Jankovic J et al, Bradley and Daroff's neurology in clinical practice, ed 8. Philadelphia, Elsevier, 2022.

BOX 8.3 ■ Confusion Assessment Method (CAM)

1. Acute change in cognition and/or fluctuating course
2. Inattention
3. Disorganized thinking
4. Altered level of consciousness
   Delirium diagnosis: 1 and 2 and either 3 or 4

The CAM has also been adapted for use in other settings, including the intensive care unit (CAM-ICU), nursing home (NH-CAM), and emergency department (CAM-ED and ED-CAM). Although one can use the criteria of the CAM to diagnose a patient with delirium from their observations of the patient, several brief mental status tools have been developed to help operationalize the CAM. Some examples are the 3D-CAM (3-Minute Diagnostic Interview for Delirium Using the Confusion Assessment Method) and bCAM (Brief Confusion Assessment Method) calculator.

CLINICAL PEARL **STEP 2/3**

Hypoactive Delirium	Hyperactive Delirium
Cognitive changes	Cognitive changes
Lethargy	Agitation
Excess somnolence	Hallucinations

Hypoactive form is more common in older persons (75%) and associated with higher mortality.

On examination, the patient is agitated, trying to get out of the bed, confused, and not cooperative with history or physical examination. He has physical restraints in place to prevent him from falling or getting out of the bed. Vitals are significant for a blood pressure of 145/80 mmHg, heart rate of 94 beats/minute, respiratory rate of 22 breaths/minute, oxygen saturation of 98%, and temperature of 100.4 °F. He is alert and oriented × 1 (oriented to self), well developed, and well nourished.

Which aspects of the history and physical examination should be included in the evaluation?

Any older adult with a change in cognition requires a careful history and physical examination. The history should gather information about the underlying medical illnesses and any medications being taken as well as the time course of the cognitive changes and any associated symptoms (fever, cough, swelling). The physical examination must include vital signs and oxygen saturation. A comprehensive physical examination should take note of hydration status, skin condition, and any possible signs of infection or inflammation. A neurological examination should assess for any focal findings.

What is the appropriate initial workup?

Targeted laboratory tests and imaging should be done based on the findings from the history and physical examination. Laboratory tests might include complete blood count, electrolytes, glucose, kidney function tests, and urinalysis. Patients may require urine culture, toxicology screen, alcohol level, medication levels, arterial blood gas, and blood cultures depending upon the physical examination findings. Radiological and other studies that may be considered in delirious patients include chest radiograph, EKG, and neuroimaging. Neuroimaging (head CT) may be used selectively rather than routinely for most patients with delirium. If there is a history of head trauma or focal findings on the neurologic examination, neuroimaging is recommended. The need for imaging should be guided by patient history and findings on neurologic examination. Neuroimaging should be considered if the neurologic examination is confounded by diminished patient responsiveness or cooperation or if the patient does not improve as expected. Further tests that can be considered include cerebrospinal fluid analysis (if you suspect meningitis or if the delirium remains unexplained) and electroencephalogram (if seizure activity is considered).

A thorough physical and neurological examination was difficult because of the patient's confusion. However, the examination was unremarkable except for a swollen, warm, and moderately tender left ankle joint. Laboratory studies were completed and results are displayed in Table 8.2. Radiograph of the left ankle revealed no fracture or other acute changes. Rheumatology was consulted to evaluate and aspirate the left ankle. The ankle joint fluid analysis is shown in Table 8.3.

What is the recommended approach to manage delirium?

Virtually any medical condition can precipitate delirium in a susceptible patient and multiple underlying conditions are often found. A delirious patient is at risk of hospital complications, immobility (which can lead to functional decline), and poor outcomes. There are often many factors involved in the delirium and management therefore requires a multifactorial approach (Table 8.4).

TABLE 8.2 ■ **Laboratory Results**

Leukocyte count	12,200/nL
Hematocrit	45.6%
Platelet count	187,000/nL
Sodium	136 mmol/L
Serum creatinine	0.82 mg/dL
BUN	18 mg/dL
Glucose	134 mg/dL
Urinalysis	Normal
Liver function test	Normal

TABLE 8.3 ■ **Left Ankle Fluid Analysis**

Color	Cloudy, yellow
WBC	56,700
RBC	3000
Culture	No growth
Positive calcium pyrophosphate crystals	

TABLE 8.4 ■ **Delirium Management**

Treat underlying conditions	Treat infection, dehydration, electrolyte disturbances Simplify medication regimen Stop or wean all dangerous medications
Manage behaviors	Nonpharmacologic measures Medications (low dose antipsychotics preferred) only when necessary
Prevent and treat complications	Mobilize the patient Physical therapy Enhance sleep without sedatives
Preserve and enhance function	Frequent orientation Safe hospital environment Physical therapy/occupational therapy Education

The most important step is to identify and treat all potentially reversible causes and contributors of delirium. This includes treating infection, metabolic problems, electrolyte abnormalities, pain, and any other organ system involvement. Eliminating medications that might be contributing is essential. Simplifying the medication regimen (taking care to wean medications that can cause withdrawal) to only those medications necessary or safer substitutes is recommended. Managing behaviors, particularly agitation and combative behavior, is a challenging aspect of delirium therapy. Nonpharmacologic interventions should be attempted in all delirious patients. Mild confusion and agitation may respond to interpersonal and environmental manipulations. Physical restraints should be avoided if possible (unless needed for a patient trying to remove lines or tubes in the ICU) because they can increase agitation and the potential for injury. For patients who are severely agitated or whose behavior is a risk to their safety, pharmacologic intervention can be considered (although studies show little benefit and some risk). If pharmacologic intervention is necessary, low doses of high-potency antipsychotics are preferred. (No antipsychotics are FDA approved for delirium and the use of these

TABLE 8.5 ■ **Pharmacologic Treatment for Agitation in Delirium**

Drug	Dose range	
Haloperidol	0.25–0.5 mg IV, IM, or PO	
Risperidone	0.25–0.5 mg PO	
Olanzapine	2.5–5 mg PO, SL, or IM	
Quetiapine	12.5–25 mg PO	
Ziprasidone	5–1 mg PO or IM	
Lorazepam	0.25–0.5 mg PO or IV	Benzodiazepine; used for alcohol withdrawal delirium

agents for such an indication is therefore off label). Table 8.5 lists some of the medications that can be used and the dose ranges.

Because delirium can be associated with longer hospital stays and complications, preventing and managing these complications is important. A patient with delirium may spend more time in a hospital bed and thus becomes deconditioned. Physical therapy helps mobilize the patient and prevents pressure ulcers. Staff can also work to preserve and enhance the patient's function by employing a nonpharmacologic sleep regimen, providing frequent orientation, and educating the patient and family about delirium.

The rheumatology consultant injects the patient's ankle with intra-articular corticosteroids. His pain improves and is better controlled. His left ankle tenderness and swelling decrease over the next 24 hours. He is slowly weaned off tramadol and the hospital ward is kept quiet at night to enhance his sleep. He has a bedside sitter who speaks with him and orients him frequently. Physical therapy is involved to assist in maintaining his mobility. Patient returns to his baseline cognitive function within 3 days and is discharged home to his daughter's care.

How can delirium in elderly patients be prevented?

As delirium can cause increased morbidity and mortality for older adults, there is much interest in preventing delirium in hospitalized older adults. Some simple, nonpharmacologic measures have been shown to decrease the incidence of delirium. These measures include early mobilization, adequate hydration, enhancing sleep without sedatives (preserving the sleep-wake cycle), frequent orientation, hearing and vision improvement (use of hearing aids and glasses), and avoiding dangerous medications.

CLINICAL PEARL **STEP 3**

Avoid physical restraints to manage behavioral symptoms of hospitalized older adults with delirium. Do not use benzodiazepines or other sedative-hypnotics in older adults as the first choice for insomnia, agitation, or delirium.

Case Summary

- **Complaint/History:** An 87-year-old male with a history of mild Alzheimer's disease presented with increased confusion from his baseline for 3 days with intermittent agitation. He had low-grade fevers for 2 days prior to admission. At baseline, the patient was alert and oriented to person and place.
- **Findings:** On examination, the patient was agitated, trying to get out of the bed, confused, and not cooperative. He was alert and oriented ×1 (oriented to self). The examination was also remarkable for a swollen, warm, and moderately tender left ankle joint. Left ankle aspiration was performed at bedside; aspirate showed positive calcium pyrophosphate crystals.

Diagnosis: Delirium precipitated by pseudogout.

- **Treatment:** The rheumatology consultant injected the patient's ankle with intra-articular corticosteroids. The patient's pain improved. His left ankle tenderness and swelling decreased over the next 24 hours. He was weaned off tramadol and became calmer with nonpharmacologic delirium interventions. He was able to work with physical therapy to assist in maintaining his mobility. He returned to his baseline cognitive function within 3 days and was discharged home to his daughter's care.

BEYOND THE PEARLS

- Delirium can present with a hyperactive state (25%) or a hypoactive state (75%). The hypoactive state is associated with the same or worse prognosis as the hyperactive state (possibly because it is more difficult to recognize).
- Delirium is a transient (reversible) change in cognition. However, the delirium can persist for weeks to months. Additionally, delirium may permanently impact long-term cognitive function.
- Postoperative delirium can occur in 15% (elective noncardiac surgery) to 50% (high-risk surgeries) of older adults. The greatest risk factors for postoperative delirium include advanced age, cognitive impairment, physical functional impairment, alcohol abuse, abnormal serum chemistries, intrathoracic surgery, and aortic aneurysm surgery.
- Benzodiazepines should not be used as first-line treatment of agitation in delirium. In fact, medications should be avoided if possible. If medications are required for the patient's safety or to target symptoms that are disrupting the patient's care, a high-potency antipsychotic drug might be utilized.
- A proactive geriatric consultation preoperatively for older adults admitted for surgery has been shown to decrease the incidence of delirium postoperatively.
- Multiple nonpharmacologic measures performed by the members of the health care team in older hospitalized patients can potentially prevent delirium in these patients. These include frequent orientation, enhancing sleep without sedatives, avoiding dangerous medications, preventing dehydration, and mobility, hearing, and vision improvement.

Bibliography

American Psychiatric Association. (2013). *Diagnostic and Statistical Manual* (5th ed).

Oh, E. S., Fong, T. G., Hshieh, T. T., & Inouye, S. K. (2017). Delirium in older persons: advances in diagnosis and treatment. *JAMA*, *318*(12), 11611174.

Marcantario. E. R. (2017). Delirium in hospitalized older adults. *N Engl J Med*, *377*(15), 1456–1466.

Harper, G. M., Lyons, W. L., & Potter, J. F. (Eds.) (2019). *Geriatrics review syllabus: a core curriculum in geriatric medicine* (10th ed.). New York: American Geriatrics Society.

Halter, J. B., Ouslander, J. G., & Studenski, S. (Eds.), (2017). *Hazzard's geriatric medicine and gerontology*. New York: McGraw-Hill Education.

Oh, E. S., Needham, D. M., Nikooie, R., et al. (2019). Antipsychotics for preventing delirium in hospitalized adults: a systematic review. *Ann Intern Med*, *171*(7), 474–484.

CASE 9

A 78-Year-Old Female With a Ground-Level Fall

Michelle Yim ■ Diana Homeier

A 78-year-old female with a history of hypertension, diabetes mellitus type 2, urinary incontinence, insomnia, coronary artery disease, and knee osteoarthritis presents with her daughter after a ground-level fall. This is her second fall in the last 12 months.

How common are falls in community dwelling older adults?

Falls are very common in community dwelling older adults. Approximately 30% of older adults fall each year, resulting in 29 million falls and 7 million fall injuries in the United States. The incidence is even higher in those with increased age and among nursing-home residents. In fact, 50% of persons >80 years old or in a nursing home fall each year. For older adults who had a prior fall in the last year, the incidence of falls in the next year is 60%.

CLINICAL PEARL **STEP 3**

Falls are common in older adults
30% of community dwelling older adults fall every year.
50% of those over 80 years of age fall every year.
50% of those in nursing homes fall every year.

What are the risk factors for falls in older adults?

Falls are known to be a geriatric syndrome that result from the interaction of multiple risk factors. Risk factors for falls are generally divided into intrinsic risk factors (those intrinsic to the older adult), extrinsic risk factors (those related to the outside environment), and situational risk factors (those related to the current situation or activity). Table 9.1 outlines these risk factors. In multiple prospective cohort studies, several risk factors have been consistently associated with falls: older age, cognitive impairment, female gender, past fall history, arthritis, foot disorders, balance problems, hypovitaminosis D, psychotropic medication use, pain, Parkinson disease, and stroke.

CLINICAL PEARL **STEP 3**

Falls are usually multifactorial and result from the interaction of intrinsic risk factors, extrinsic risk factors, and situational factors.

What are the outcomes linked to falls?

Fall-related injuries range from minor scratches and bruises to severe, life-threatening injuries. Most falls cause only minor injury, but 5%–10% of falls in older adults result in fracture or a more serious soft-tissue injury or head trauma. Falls are the leading cause of injury-related visits to

TABLE 9.1 ■ **Risk Factors for Falls in Older Adults**

Intrinsic risk factors	**Demographic risk factors**	Advanced age
	Physiologic risk factors	History of falls
	Pathologic risk factors	Inactivity/limitations in mobility
		Female
		Alterations in gait and balance • Muscle weakness • Sensory loss • Cerebral microvascular disease • Peripheral neuropathy
		Abnormalities in blood pressure (BP) regulation • Reduced baroreflex sensitivity • Decreased cerebral blood flow • Decreased diastolic filling • Vascular stiffness
		Sensory deficits • Cataracts • Hearing loss • Peripheral neuropathy
		Orthopedic • Arthritis • Spinal stenosis
		Cardiovascular • Arrythmia • Valvular disease • Hypotension-postprandial, postural • Carotid sinus syndrome
		Neuromotor • Stroke • Parkinson disease • Depression • Sciatica • Myopathy • Normal pressure hydrocephalus
		Foot problems
		Medications
		Acute illness
Extrinsic risk factors	**Home environment**	Poor lighting
	Outdoor environment	Low or elevated bed heights
	Facility/hospital	Low toilet seats
		Upended carpet or rug edges or loose rugs
		Stairs
		Poor fitting shoes
		Uneven sidewalks or curb edges
		Icy or wet walkways
		Stairs
		Highly polished or wet floors
		Restraint use
Situational risk factors	**Activity**	High risk activities (ladder climbing)
		Nonuse or improper use of assist devices

emergency departments in the United States and the primary etiology of accidental deaths in persons over 65 years of age. The mortality for falls in older adults increases with increasing age. Even without physical injury, falls are associated with subsequent decline in functional status, increased likelihood of nursing home placement, increased use of medical services, and increased fear of falling. Additionally, increased fear of falling can also lead to self-restriction of physical activity, which leads to decreased physical function, and results in increased risk and vulnerability to falls. Almost one-half of older adults who fall are unable to get up off the floor on their own and may experience a "long lie" on the floor associated with further complications.

CLINICAL PEARL **STEP 3**

Falls are the leading cause of injury-related visits to the emergency room among older adults and the leading cause of accidental death in this age group.

On examination, the patient's blood pressure when sitting is 135/65 mmHg, pulse 74/min, temperature 98.2°F, and weight 150 pounds. Orthostatic vital signs are measured. When lying down, her blood pressure is 135/68 mmHg and her pulse is 74/min. When standing her blood pressure is 140/68 mmHg and her pulse is 75/min, and she denies any dizziness.

What type of evaluation should be done for an older adult after a fall?

An older adult who has had a fall should be evaluated for any injuries and undergo a multifactorial fall evaluation. This includes considering the potential intrinsic, extrinsic, and situational risk factors that might have contributed to the fall and finding ways to mitigate those factors in the future. A detailed fall history, physical examination, medication review, and gait and balance testing will guide the provider to determine whether further medical evaluation is needed. The physical examination should include orthostatic vital signs (see following Clinical Pearl), with special emphasis on the evaluation of skin, cardiac, neurologic, musculoskeletal, and cognitive function. Additionally, an evaluation of visual acuity, feet, and footwear can identify possible risks for falls.

CLINICAL PEARL **STEP 1/2/3**

Orthostatic vital sign measurements are blood pressure and heart rate of patient while supine and when standing up (sitting can also be included). A positive result occurs when the blood pressure decreases ≥20 in systolic BP or ≥10 in diastolic BP within 3 minutes of standing or heart rate increases ≥20 bpm while standing.

An abnormal test indicates possible fluid loss or malfunction of the cardiovascular or neurologic system.

The patient states that she fell after tripping on the sidewalk. She has been feeling unsteady for some time now when standing and walking and attributes that to her worsening knee osteoarthritis.

What are important components of taking a fall history?

For older adults presenting after a fall, the important components of the fall history include determining the activity at the time of the fall, the presence of any prodromal symptoms (lightheadedness, dizziness, weakness), the location and time of the fall, and the occurrence of loss of consciousness. Loss of consciousness is rare, but it could suggest orthostatic hypotension or cardiac or neurologic etiologies. When discussing the location and timing of the fall, the clinician should try to determine whether any environmental factors contributed to the fall. It is important to ask about gait, balance, and history of prior falls when taking a fall history. Witnesses to a fall can also contribute information about how the fall occurred. A complete medication history is essential to the evaluation of a fall. The clinician should be aware of all of the medications being used, including over-the-counter and herbal substances. Newly added medications and recent dose changes should be noted.

CLINICAL PEARL **STEP 3**

A complete medication review, including over-the-counter and herbal medications, is essential to the fall evaluation. Be mindful of newly added or recently changed medications.

Her medications include metformin, losartan, and aspirin. In addition, she takes acetaminophen and cyclobenzaprine for chronic back pain and oxybutynin for urinary incontinence. She reluctantly admits that almost every night she takes diphenhydramine to help her sleep.

Which medications increase the risk of falls in older adults?

Medications are one of the most modifiable risk factors for falls. The 2019 American Geriatrics Society Beers Criteria were developed as a guide to improve medication safety in older patients. Polypharmacy frequently occurs in older patients as they have increased medical comorbidities. Many commonly used medications increase the risk of falls in older adults. See Table 9.2 for a list of drugs that increase the fall risk based on the 2019 American Geriatrics Society Beers Criteria.

Which laboratory and diagnostic studies should be included in the workup after a fall?

A detailed history and physical examination provide the initial guide for further laboratory testing. Hemoglobin, blood urea nitrogen (BUN), creatinine level, and serum glucose level help exclude anemia, volume depletion, and hypoglycemia or hyperglycemia as causes of a fall. Because of the high prevalence in older patients and potentially treatable conditions, other useful laboratory tests include serum electrolyte levels, vitamin B_{12} and vitamin D levels, thyroid function tests, and urinalysis. A clinician might also consider urine toxicology or specific drug levels if there is a suspicion that the patient is taking medications whose levels need to be assessed.

Further diagnostic testing should also be guided by the fall history and physical examination. This might include further cardiac evaluation with electrocardiogram, Holter monitor, or echocardiography. If evaluation suggests neurologic etiology, brain imaging or spine imaging may be considered.

How does a clinician evaluate gait and balance in an older adult?

A balance and gait assessment is a crucial part of a fall evaluation. There are various balance and gait tests that can be used. The most commonly used test is the Up and Go Test (see Table 9.3).

TABLE 9.2 ■ **Medication Classes Associated With an Increased Risk of Falls in Older Adults (Based on Beers Criteria)**

Medication Classes Associated With an Increased Risk of Falls in Older Adults
Nonselective peripheral alpha-1-blockers
Amiodarone
Anticholinergics
Antispasmodics (e.g., scopolamine)
Antidepressants (selective serotonin reuptake inhibitors, tricyclic antidepressants)
First-generation antihistamine drugs (e.g., diphenhydramine)
Antiepileptics
Antimuscarinics/incontinence agents
Benzodiazepines
Nonbenzodiazepine hypnotics (i.e., “Z-drugs”)
Acetylcholinesterase inhibitors
Opioids
Muscle relaxants (i.e., cyclobenzaprine)
Diuretics

TABLE 9.3 ■ **Up and Go Test**

Direct Patient to Do the Following

1. Rise from sitting position (without using arms if possible)
2. Walk across the examination room (approximately 10 feet)
3. Turn around
4. Walk back to the chair
5. Turn around
6. Sit down
7. *If timed, >12 seconds suggests increased risk of falls.*

TABLE 9.4 ■ **Evidence-Based Interventions to Decrease Fall Risk in Older Adults**

Risk Factor	Intervention to Decrease Falls
Gait/balance abnormality	Muscle strengthening or balance training Physical therapy Tai Chi (or other evidence-based fall prevention program)
Potential home hazards	Home hazard assessment • Home hazard checklist • Home physical therapy or occupational therapy
Medication risks	Review all medications Withdrawal of medications that increase fall risk
Vitamin D deficiency	Vitamin D supplementation
Visual impairment	Referral to ophthalmologist/cataract surgery if indicated Proper eyewear
Orthostatic hypotension (OH)	Decrease medications that can increase risk of OH Appropriate blood pressure goals
Foot/footwear abnormality	Podiatry referral Education about proper footwear
Heart/rhythm abnormality	Management of heart rate and rhythm

This test can be performed with or without timing. It can grade muscle weakness, balance problems, and gait abnormalities. If an older adult needs to use their arms to stand, this could indicate hip extensor weakness. If the test is timed (Timed Up and Go), inability to complete the test within 12 seconds suggests increased fall risk.

The patient was advised to stop diphenhydramine and cyclobenzaprine. Additionally, the oxybutynin was discontinued and she was started on an alternative medicine for urinary incontinence with a less sedating side effect. When she returned to the clinic 2 weeks later, she admitted feeling less unsteady, but was still worried that she might fall.

What interventions have been found to decrease falls in older adults?

There is strong evidence to support interventions for preventing falls in older people. Because falls are usually multifactorial, the management approach must be individualized and address multiple risk factors. Table 9.4 lists evidence-based interventions for lowering fall risk. The prescribed interventions may be different for each patient who has had a fall.

TABLE 9.5 ■ **CDC Screening Questions for Falls in Older Adults**

1. Feels unsteady when walking?
2. Worries about falling?
3. Has fallen in the past year?

The patient was referred to a physical therapist and took part in a regular exercise program. A home hazard assessment was performed: a nightlight was added to her bathroom and a grab bar added to her bathtub. She was found to have visual impairment and after referral to an ophthalmologist she underwent cataract surgery. At 3-month follow-up, she felt much more confident walking on her own and was steadier on her feet.

Should older adults be screened for fall risk?

The Centers for Disease Control and Prevention (CDC) has published an algorithm for fall risk assessment and interventions (CDC STEADI Algorithm). The STEADI (Stopping Elderly Accidents, Deaths and Injuries) Algorithm can be found at https://www.cdc.gov/steadi/. The CDC recommends that all older adults should be screened yearly for fall risk. This screening can be done using a questionnaire or asking the patient three key questions (Table 9.5).

If an older adult answers no to these questions, they should still receive education about falls and referral to community-based fall prevention program. If they answer yes to any of the fall risk questions, they should undergo the multifactor assessment and interventions previously described. The CDC STEADI website has many resources for clinicians and older adults to aid in fall prevention.

Case Summary

- **Complaint/History:** A 78-year-old female with history of hypertension, diabetes, mixed urinary incontinence, insomnia, coronary artery disease, and knee osteoarthritis presents after a ground level fall after tripping on the sidewalk.
- **Findings:** On examination, blood pressure is 135/65 mmHg, pulse 74 beats/minute, temperature 98.2°F. Patient's medications include cyclobenzaprine, diphenhydramine, and oxybutynin.

Diagnosis: Patient is on medications that increased her risk of fall. She was also found to have visual impairment due to cataract.

- **Treatment:** Patient stopped taking medications that increases her fall risk. She was referred to a physical therapist and takes part in a regular exercise program. A home hazard assessment was performed: a nightlight was added to her bathroom and a grab bar was added to her bathtub. She also underwent cataract surgery. At 3-month follow-up, she felt much more confident walking on her own and is steadier on her feet.
  - On medication review, Ms. F. reveals that she has been taking metformin for diabetes, losartan for hypertension, aspirin for her heart, acetaminophen for arthritis pain, oxybutynin for incontinence, and cyclobenzaprine for chronic back pain. She also reluctantly admits that almost every night she takes diphenhydramine to help her sleep.
  - Several of Ms. F.'s medications are high risk with concern for falls. Ms. F. agrees to stop using diphenhydramine and cyclobenzaprine. Additionally, the oxybutynin is discontinued and she is started on a bladder medicine with fewer side effects for her incontinence. When she returns to the clinic 2 weeks later, she admits to feeling less unsteady, but still worries that she might fall.

- Ms. F. was referred to a physical therapist and takes part in a regular exercise program. A home hazard assessment was performed: a nightlight was added to her bathroom and a grab bar was added to her bathtub. She was found to have visual impairment and after referral to an ophthalmologist she underwent cataract surgery. At 3-month follow-up, she felt much more confident walking on her own and is steadier on her feet.

BEYOND THE PEARLS

- In multiple prospective cohort studies, several risk factors have been consistently associated with falls, including older age, cognitive impairment, female gender, past fall history, arthritis, foot disorders, balance problems, hypovitaminosis D, psychotropic medication use, pain, Parkinson disease, and stroke.
- Intensive home safety interventions in the home by an occupational therapist can decrease risk of falls by 21%.
- The amount of total body water is reduced with aging, which places older adults at increased risk of dehydration with acute illness, diuretic use, or hot weather.
- Older adults may be more vulnerable to falls in the days or weeks after a new medication is started or the dosage of an existing medication is increased.
- Recommended shoes for older adults to decrease fall risk should have thin, slip-resistant soles, low heel height, supported heel collars, beveled heels, and a fastening mechanism.
- The evidence for effectiveness of vitamin D supplementation on fall prevention is mixed and may be dose dependent. The recommended dose is 800–1000 IU (international units) daily. High dose vitamin D supplementation (500,000 IU once a year or 60,000 IU per month) has been associated with an increased risk of falls.

Bibliography

2019 American Geriatrics Society Beers Criteria Update Expert Panel American Geriatrics Society 2019 updated AGS Beers Criteria® for potentially inappropriate medication use in older adults. *J Am Geriatr Soc. 67*(4), 674–694.

Centers for Disease Control and Prevention (2021) STEDI—*older adult fall prevention*. https://www.cdc.gov/steadi/

Harper, G. M., Lyons, W. L., & Potter, J. F. (Eds.). (2019). *Geriatrics review syllabus: a core curriculum in geriatric medicine* (10th ed.). New York: American Geriatrics Society.

Hirth, V., Wieland, D., & Dever-Bumba, M. (Eds.). (2011). *Case based geriatrics: a global approach* (1st ed.). New York: McGraw Hill.

Ham, R. J., Sloane, P. D., et al. (2007). *Primary care geriatrics: a case based approach* (5th ed.). Philadelphia: Elsevier.

Halter, J. B., Ouslander, J. G., & Studenski, S. (Eds.). (2017). *Hazzard's geriatric medicine and gerontology*. New York: McGraw-Hill Education.

SECTION 4

Dermatology

CASE 10

A 57-Year-Old Female With Burning Red Rash on Lower Legs

Arnold Lee ■ Hui Yi Shan ■ Teodulo (Jun) Meneses ■ David J. Goldstein

A 57 year-old healthy Hispanic woman was referred to the dermatology clinic from the Emergency department for red to violaceous macules and papules on her right and left lower legs. This rash has been present for more than 1 week and is extending up her legs. She reports experiencing intermittent itching and burning sensation and tried topical diphenhydramine cream without relief. A review revealed no other symptoms. This patient denies taking any oral medications including over-the-counter supplements. Her physical examination is notable for palpable purpura on the right and left lower legs with mild edema of the ankles.

What is the differential diagnosis for this patient with petechial or purpuric eruption on the lower legs?
The differential diagnosis of cutaneous purpuric eruptions is extensive.

- Palpable purpura is the hallmark of cutaneous leukocytoclastic vasculitis (LCV) (Fig. 10.1). The size of the lesions can range from pinpoint to several centimeters. Annular, bullous, pustular, or ulcerated lesions may develop. These skin lesions are often asymptomatic but can be associated with itching, pain, or burning sensation. They most commonly occur in a symmetrical distribution on the ankles and lower legs, on dependent areas, or on areas under local pressure (such as constrictive clothing).
- Senile purpura is caused by chronic sun exposure, trauma, age, anticoagulants, or oral/topical corticosteroid use (Fig. 10.2). This condition affects about 10% of people over age 50. Lesions commonly present as red to dark violaceous, irregularly shaped macules and patches ranging from 1 to 4 cm. They typically last 1–3 weeks before fading. The surrounding skin is typically thin and shows signs of sun damage and aging. Senile purpura usually is distributed on the extensor forearms and dorsal hands. This condition is benign although cosmetically displeasing.
- Pigmented purpuric dermatoses is also known as capillaritis. It is a harmless skin condition caused by leaky capillaries, resulting in red-brown ("cayenne pepper") dots and patches resulting from hemosiderin deposition in the dermis (Fig. 10.3). For unknown reasons, the capillaries become inflamed and leak.
- Stasis dermatitis affects one or both lower legs in association with chronic venous insufficiency. It is most often seen in middle-aged and older patients. Itchy, red, blistered and crusted plaques, or dry fissured and scaly thin plaques, on one or both lower legs are characteristic lesions. There is often pitting edema and brown macular pigmentation caused by hemosiderin deposition on the affected leg.
- Cellulitis is bacterial infection of the skin. Characteristic lesions show localized areas of redness, swelling, pain, and induration. Possible site of origin may show ulcer or purulent discharge. The affected skin is usually hot or warm to touch. The extent of redness usually spreads over time. Bilateral lower leg cellulitis is uncommon.

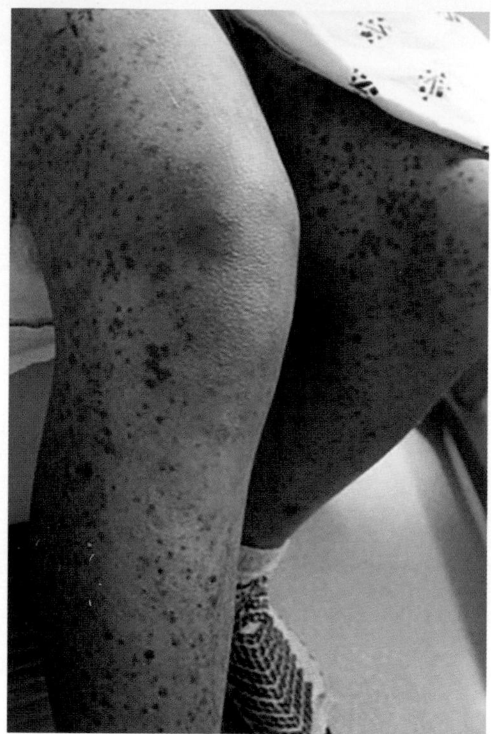

Fig. 10.1 Leukocytoclastic vasculitis. Palpable purpura coalescing into large plaques on the thigh. (From Brinster, N. K., Liu, V., Diwan, H., & McKee, P. H. (2011). *Dermatopathology: High-yield pathology*. Saunders.)

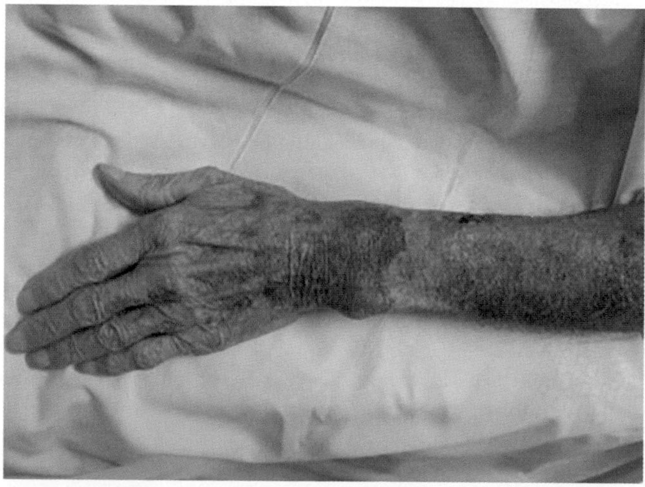

Fig. 10.2 Senile purpura. The skin of this man's forearm is very thin; the tendons in his hand are visible. The skin can easily be torn away. The purpura consists of sheets of extravasated red cells. It is not palpable. (From Kitchens, C.S., Konkle, B., & Kessler, C. (2019). *Consultative hemostasis and thrombosis* (4th ed.). Elsevier.)

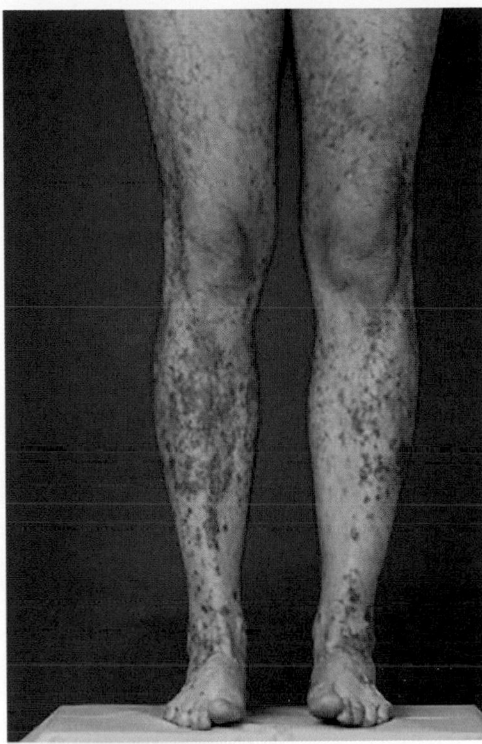

Fig. 10.3 Capillaritis (pigmented purpuric dermatoses). (From Sunderkotter, C. (2018). *Treatment of skin disease: comprehensive therapeutic strategies* (5th ed.). Elsevier.)

What is purpura?

Purpura is defined to be nonblanchable, hemorrhagic skin lesions that result from the extravasation of red blood cells into the skin. Palpable purpura is the classic and common manifestation of cutaneous small vessel vasculitis (LCV).

CLINICAL PEARL **STEP 3**

How can you tell whether or not the skin lesion is blanchable?

The application of pressure to a skin lesion with a glass slide is called diascopy. It is a very helpful clinical tool. If the lesion does not disappear under diascopy, it is nonblanchable. Blanchable erythematous lesions are common in nonvasculitic dermatologic inflammatory es.

What should you do next?

A skin punch biopsy should be performed in all patients being evaluated for vasculitis to differentiate between vasculitic and nonvasculitic skin diseases. It is important to note that the clinical characteristics of skin lesions cannot reliably distinguish the different types of cutaneous vasculitis.

Although direct immunofluorescence (DIF) study is not essential for diagnosis of LCV, it is highly recommended because it can assess for immunoglobulin A (IgA) predominance. Only the identification of perivascular IgA deposits with DIF confirms the diagnosis of IgA vasculitis (Henoch-Schönlein purpura).

CLINICAL PEARL **STEP 3**

Shave biopsy should not be performed when evaluating for vasculitis because it prevents the evaluation of blood vessels in the mid- to deep dermis. The skin punch biopsy of petechial or palpable purpura should be taken from within the lesion.

Because the histologic appearances of vasculitic lesions evolve over time, lesions that are between 24 and 48 hours old are most likely to demonstrate the diagnostic findings of vasculitis. Therefore, it is recommended to ask patients to help identify a lesion that has been present approximately 24 hours for biopsy.

Ideally, DIF should also be performed on a lesion less than 24 hours old because the inflammatory reaction stimulated by the immunoglobulin deposition in blood vessel walls quickly results in the destruction of both the vessel walls and the immune complexes. This can result in a negative DIF.

For this patient, a skin punch biopsy was performed from a recent violaceous papule on her left lower leg. A DIF test was also performed.

BASIC SCIENCE PEARL **STEP 3**

The skin specimen from a punch biopsy can be fixed in formalin and stained with hematoxylin and eosin. In contrast, the specimen for DIF must be placed in a special Michel's transport medium or normal saline, or flash frozen with liquid nitrogen. Tissue submitted in normal saline must be processed within 24 hours.

What is the histology of cutaneous leukocytoclastic vasculitis?

Because leukocytoclastic vasculitis is a dynamic process, not all features will be present at all disease stages. The epidermis can vary from normal to necrotic, sometimes with vesicles or pustules. The hallmark histologic features include fibrinoid necrosis and endothelial swelling. The characteristic pattern is a neutrophilic small-vessel vasculitis involving dermal vessels, but the infiltrate can be polymorphic and includes lymphocytes, eosinophils, or histiocytes. Karyorrhexis or leukocytoclasia (which is the destructive fragmentation of the nucleus of the dying neutrophil) leads to the appearance of nuclear dust. The damage to the vessel wall (typically postcapillary venules) results in the extravasation of red blood cells. Thrombi can sometimes be seen (Fig. 10.4).

For cutaneous LCV, a DIF test can be helpful but findings depend on the age of the lesion. In early lesions, the DIF test reveals IgM, fibrinogen, or complement (C3) in a granular pattern in the superficial blood vessels (Fig. 10.5). Fully developed lesions are often positive for fibrinogen, albumin, and IgG. Late lesions demonstrate fibrinogen with some C3. In contrast, for IgA vasculitis (Henoch-Schönlein purpura), the DIF will show granular IgA in the superficial dermal blood vessels.

This patient's skin biopsy is consistent with leukocytoclastic vasculitis. The DIF is positive for vascular/perivascular IgG, IgM, C3, and fibrinogen staining. No IgA staining is detected.

BASIC SCIENCE PEARL **STEP 1/2/3**

It has been suggested that circulating immune complexes cause cutaneous small vessel vasculitis. They lodge and deposit in the small blood vessels and activate complement. Various inflammatory mediators are then produced and result in endothelial damage.

What are possible etiologies of leukocytoclastic vasculitis?

A vast number of conditions may result in cutaneous LCV. It is often idiopathic but may be caused by infections, medications, rheumatologic disorders, or malignancy.

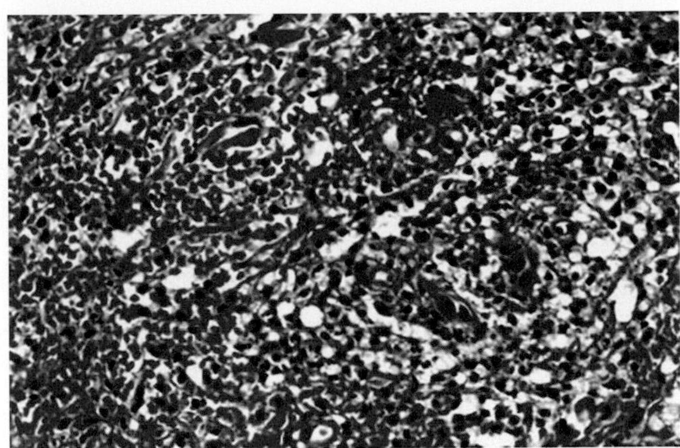

Fig. 10.4 Leukocytoclastic vasculitis. Note the red cell extravasation and mixed inflammatory cell infiltrate with leukocytoclasis. (From Brinster, N. K., Liu, V., Diwan, H., & McKee, P. H. (2011). *Dermatopathology: High-yield pathology*. Saunders.)

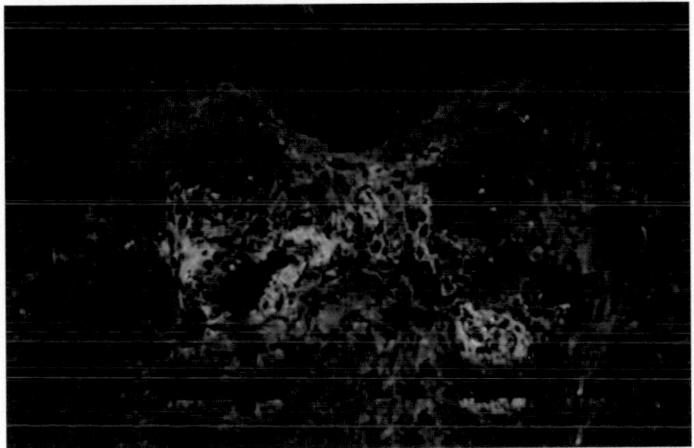

Fig. 10.5 Leukocytoclastic vasculitis. Direct immunofluorescence (DIF) staining. There is C3 deposition around superficial vessels. (From Brinster, N. K., Liu, V., Diwan, H., & McKee, P. H. (2011). *Dermatopathology: High-yield pathology*. Saunders.)

Medications most often implicated for causing cutaneous vasculitis include penicillin, sulfonamides, cephalosporins, phenytoin, and allopurinol. Infections such as hepatitis B or C, HIV, β-hemolytic *Streptococcus* group A, and herpes viruses (HSV or VZV) can also be associated with cutaneous LCV. Lymphoproliferative neoplasms (Hodgkin's disease, mycosis fungoides, and multiple myeloma) and solid cell malignancies (lung, colon, breast, renal, ovarian, prostate, and head and neck) may also cause cutaneous vasculitis during the disease course.

How can clinical assessment help you identify the possible cause of cutaneous vasculitis?

Inquiries regarding new medications and symptoms of infection (especially upper respiratory infection) are an important aspect of patient evaluation. Asking about joint pain, sicca symptoms, oral or nasal ulcerations, photosensitivity, and Raynaud's phenomenon suggests the need to evaluate for possible connective tissue disorders. Fevers, chills, night sweats, and unexplained weight loss may point to an underlying malignancy.

For this patient, a review of systems was negative except for the skin rash on her lower legs.

What is the primary concern regarding leukocytoclastic vasculitis?

LCV can involve only the skin (cutaneous small vessel vasculitis) versus skin and other internal organs, most often the kidney. If the vasculitis involves the kidneys, lungs, brain, or other internal organs, it is called systemic vasculitis.

Which signs or symptoms can suggest systemic vasculitis?

Fever, chills, night sweats, myalgia, arthralgia, hematuria, abdominal pain or melena, chest pain, cough, hemoptysis, and peripheral neuropathy are signs/symptoms that can suggest systemic vasculitis.

This patient only reports itching and a burning sensation on her lower legs.

Which additional laboratory tests should you order?

Reasonable initial screens for patients with cutaneous vasculitis include a complete blood count; urinalysis; liver function tests; blood urea nitrogen (BUN); creatinine; strep throat culture or ASO titer; hepatitis B and C serologies; human immunodeficiency virus (HIV) antibody; antinuclear antibodies (ANA); anti-dsDNA, anti-Ro, anti-La, anti-RNP, and anti-Smith antibodies; rheumatoid factor; serum protein electrophoresis (SPEP); serum complements (C3, C4, CH50); antineutrophil cytoplastic antibodies (ANCAs); and serum cryoglobulins.

In patients with pulmonary symptoms, a chest X-ray is recommended.

Lab results from our patient are all within normal limits.

What is Henoch-Schönlein purpura (IgA vasculitis)?

Henoch-Schönlein purpura (HSP) is a subtype of small vessel vasculitis. It is characterized by a tetrad of clinical presentations: palpable purpura, arthralgia, abdominal pain, and renal disease. Over 90% of HSP occurs in the pediatric age group; however, adults may also be affected. Male gender is predominant among both children and adults with HSP. Although HSP tends to occur more often in children, kidney involvement is more likely in older children and adults.

The usual triggering event is a viral infection or streptococcal pharyngitis. In about 40% of the cases, the skin manifestations are preceded by mild fever, headache, joint symptoms, and abdominal pain for up to 2 weeks. There may be pulmonary hemorrhage, which can be fatal.

Renal involvement manifesting as microscopic or gross hematuria may occur in 25% or more of the patients. Ninety percent of children who develop renal involvement in HSP usually do so within 2 months of onset and 97% within 6 months. Adults are at increased risk of renal disease both early in the disease course and longer term as manifested by a higher frequency of nephrotic syndrome, hypertension, and elevated serum creatinine. Therefore, close follow-up for patients with renal involvement is necessary as a small subset of these patients can progress to chronic kidney disease.

How do you treat HSP?

Treatment of HSP is supportive as the majority of patients recover spontaneously. The usual duration is 6–16 weeks. Edema of the lower legs, buttocks, and genital area improves with bed rest and/or elevation of the affected areas. Dapsone or colchicine can be used initially if treatment is required and skin lesions are the primary concern. An H2 blocker or prednisone can be effective for abdominal pain. NSAIDs are best avoided because they can cause renal or gastrointestinal issues.

The value of systemic corticosteroids in treating renal disease is controversial but may be used preventively or to treat active nephritis. Treatment of HSP nephritis depends on whether the patient is a child or an adult and upon the severity of the kidney disease. For children with limited kidney involvement (e.g., hematuria, proteinuria <1 g/day, and normal serum creatinine), a systemic corticosteroid, ACE (angiotensin-converting enzyme) inhibitor, or ARB (angiotensin II receptor blocker) is not recommended because such patients typically fully recover. In adults with limited kidney involvement, immunosuppressive therapy is not recommended; an ACE inhibitor or ARB can be used to treat those with proteinuria >0.5 g/day. For those children with more severe kidney involvement (e.g., proteinuria >1 g/day, elevated serum creatinine), initiation of systemic corticosteroid therapy has been suggested. In adults with more severe kidney involvement, immunosuppressive therapy with IV and oral corticosteroids combination with an ACE inhibitor or ARB is recommended.

Diagnosis: Leukocytoclastic vasculitis (cutaneous small vessel vasculitis).

Which treatments are available for cutaneous leukocytoclastic vasculitis?

The majority of LCV are acute and self-limited, affect only the skin, and do not involve internal organs. Rest and elevation of the legs are helpful. For disease limited to the skin, NSAIDs can be considered for arthralgia because a brief course of systemic corticosteroids usually leads to resolution. Colchicine or dapsone has also been reported to be beneficial.

For this patient, due to the extensive symptomatic nature of the cutaneous leukocytoclastic vasculitis, a 2-week course of oral prednisone was prescribed. Improvement was detectable within 1 week after starting therapy. At follow-up after 3 weeks, the rash had completely disappeared.

Case Summary

- **Complaint/History:** A 57-year-old woman with burning red rash on her lower legs.
- **Lab Results/Tests:** A skin biopsy was performed.

Diagnosis: Leukocytoclastic vasculitis.

- **Treatment:** A 2-week course of oral prednisone was prescribed with resolution of the rash.

BEYOND THE PEARLS

- Most causes of cutaneous LCV are idiopathic. Infections, medications, connective tissue diseases, and malignancy have been estimated to account for 23%, 20%, 12%, and 4% of cases of cutaneous vasculitis.
- Detailed knowledge of temporal association of the development of vasculitis can be helpful; medication-induced vasculitis most often occurs 7–10 days after the introduction of the inciting drug.
- A DIF test showing IgA predominance increases the risk of renal involvement.
- Cocaine use may also cause cutaneous leukocytoclastic vasculitis. More specifically, tender retiform purpura on the ear and necrotic purpura on the trunk or extremities in the setting of recent cocaine use suggest the possibility of vasculitis secondary to the use of levamisole-tainted cocaine. Urine toxicology can help in this case. Testing for levamisole in serum or urine is commercially available but its detection is limited by the short half-life of levamisole (5.6 hours).
- Gram, viral, and fungal special stains can be performed on a formalin-fixed biopsy specimen from vasculitic lesion tissue to identify possible infectious etiology.
- Approximately 10% of cutaneous leukocytoclastic vasculitis can recur; a persistent underlying reason must be sought for chronic cases.
- Prior to prescribing dapsone, a glucose-6-phosphate dehydrogenase (G6PD) deficiency screening should be performed to avoid the risk of severe hemolytic anemia.

Bibliography

Alalwani. N., Billings S.D., Gota C.E. Clinical significance of immunoglobulin deposition in leukocytoclastic vasculitis: a 5-year retrospective study of 88 patients at Cleveland Clinic. *Am J Dermatopatholo.* 2014;36:723.

Audemard- A., Terrier B., Dechartres A., et al. Characteristic and Management of IgA Vasculitis (Henoch-Schönlein) in adults: data from 260 patients included in a French multicenter retrospective survey. *Arthritis Rheumatol.* 2017;69:1862.

Blanco R., Martinez-Taboada V.M., Rodriguez-Valverde V., et al. Henoch-Schönlein purpura in adulthood and childhood: two different expressions of the same syndrome. *Arthritis Rheum.* 1997;40:859.

Calvo-Rio V., Loricera J., Mata C., et al. Henoch-Schönlein purpura in northern Spain: clinical spectrum of the disease in 417 patients from a single center. *Medicine (Baltimore).* 2014;93:106.

Carlson J.A., Ng B.T., Chen K.R. Cutaneous vasculitis update: diagnostic criteria, classification, epidemiology, etiology, pathogenesis, evaluation and prognosis. *Am J Dermatopathol.* 2005;27:504.

Chung C., Tumeh P.C., Birnbaum R., et al. Characteristic purpura of the ears, vasculitis, and neutropenia—a potential public health epidemic associated with levamisole-adulterated cocaine. *J Am Acad Dermatol.* 2011;65:722.

Gross R.L., Brucker J., Bahce-Altuntas A., et al. A novel cutaneous vasculitis syndrome induced by levamisole-contaminated cocaine. *Clin Rheumatol.* 2011;30:1385.

Hahn D., Hodson E.M., Willis N.S., et al. Interventions for preventing and treating kidney disease in Henoch-Schönlein purpura (HSP). *Cochrane Database Syst Rev.* 2015;8:CD005128.

James W.D., Berger T.G., Elston D.M. Andrews' diseases of the skin clinical dermatology. 10th ed. Canada: Saunders Elsevier; 2006.

Narchi H. Risk of long-term renal impairment and duration of follow up recommended for Henoch-Schonlein purpura with normal or minimal urinary findings: a systematic review. *Arch Dis Child.* 2005;90:916.

Paller A.S., Kelly K., Sethi R. Pulmonary hemorrhage: An often fatal complication of Henoch Schonlein purpura. *Pediatr Dermatol.* 1997;133:438.

Rapini R.P. *Practical Dermatopathology.* China: Elsevier Mosby; 2005.

Ullrich K., Koval R., Koval E., et al. Five consecutive cases of a cutaneous vasculopathy in users of levamisole-adulterated cocaine. *J Clin Rheumatol.* 2011;17:193.

Uppal S.S., Hussain M.A., Al-Raqum H.A., et al. Henoch-Schonlein purpura in adults versus children/adolescents: a comparative study. *Clin Exp Rheumatol.* 2006;24:S26.

Weiss P.F., Feinstein J.A., Luan X., et al. Effects of corticosteroids on Henoch-Schonlein purpura: a systematic review. *Pediatrics.* 2007;120:1079.

CASE 11

A 70-Year-Old Female With Chronic Unilateral Rash on Left Nipple

Arnold Lee ■ Michael T. Schmidt ■ Hien T. Tran

A 70-year-old healthy female was referred to the dermatology clinic for a crusted erythematous thin plaque on her left nipple. It has been present for 1 year and is associated with intermittent pruritis. She had seen her primary care physician for this and was prescribed a topical antifungal cream and powder. The rash has not improved.

What additional information should be requested?

A detailed history should also include any other additional symptoms, such as pain, nipple discharge, bleeding, or burning sensation. Also, it is critical to ask the patient whether any medications (topical or oral) completely resolved this rash. Further, the history should inquire about the patient's personal or family history of breast cancer.

What should be done on a physical examination for this patient?

Examination of both breasts should be performed, including palpation for possible masses. It is important to note if there is any nipple retraction. Further, axillary lymphadenopathy needs to be examined.

This patient's physical examination was unremarkable. Except for the eczematous thin plaque, no breast mass or axillary lymphadenopathy was palpated.

What is the differential diagnosis for a unilateral nipple rash/lesion?

The differential diagnosis includes both benign causes (eczema, contact dermatitis, tinea corporis, papillary adenoma of the breast) and malignant etiologies (squamous cell carcinoma, basal cell carcinoma, malignant melanoma, and Paget's disease of the breast).

What is the appropriate management at this time?

Because this rash failed to improve on topical antifungal cream, it is reasonable to try a brief course of medium- to high-potency topical steroids if eczema or contact dermatitis is suspected. However, a close follow-up is necessary to ensure resolution of this cutaneous abnormality. At follow-up, if the rash persists, a skin punch biopsy or full-thickness wedge of the nipple is indicated.

A more detailed history for this patient revealed that she had also tried a medium-strength topical steroid ointment for several months. This did not ameliorate her rash. A 4-mm skin punch biopsy was performed.

The skin biopsy showed a malignant infiltrate of adenocarcinoma cells (Paget's cells) within the epidermis (Fig. 11.1).

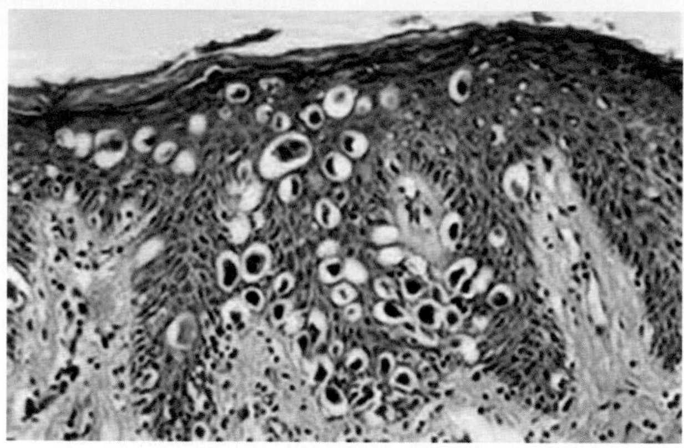

Fig. 11.1 Paget's disease of the nipple. (From Brunhuber, T., Haybaeck, J., Schäfer, G., Mikuz, G., Langhoff, E., Saeland, S., Lebecque, S., Romani, N., & Obrist, P. (2008). Immunohistochemical tracking of an immune response in mammary Paget's disease, *Cancer Letters, 272* (2), 206–220.)

BASIC SCIENCE PEARL **STEP 3**

Examined sections show a malignant infiltrate of single to small groups of large, polygonal, atypical cells with abundant cytoplasm and large nuclei with an occasional prominent nucleolus and irregular nuclear membranes scattered throughout all levels of the epidermis that are positive for cytokeratin 7 as well as another breast specific marker such as GCDFP-15, mammaglobin, or GATA3. The cytologic atypia and positive staining with breast specific markers help distinguish Paget's disease from benign Toker cells of the nipple, which will also show positive staining for cytokeratin 7 (Fig. 11.1).

Diagnosis: Paget's disease of the breast (Fig. 11.2).

How can Paget's disease be differentiated from the other entities in the differential diagnosis?
This can be done based on histomorphologic features and immunohistochemical characterization of the malignant cells.

The staining profile of Paget's cells is distinct. It stains negative for S-100 and cytokeratin 5/6, allowing differentiation from melanoma and squamous cell carcinoma, respectively.

In basal cell carcinoma, small groups to large nests of atypical basaloid cells are formed and demonstrate horizontal growth along the dermoepidermal junction or can become infiltrative and show vertical growth with extension into the underlying dermis. There is often peripheral palisading of the nuclei with retraction artifact (stromal separation from tumor globules).

Although nipple adenoma can clinically mimic Paget's disease, its biopsy shows papillary and adenomatous growth in the dermis with connection to the surface. A lining of apocrine-type secretory epithelium is present.

For eczema or contact dermatitis, acanthosis and spongiosis of the epidermis with superficial perivascular lymphocytic infiltrate in the dermis are found on histology. Occasionally, eosinophils can be identified.

For dermatophyte infection of the skin such as tinea corporis, annular lesions with active scaly borders are often clinically found. PAS stain of the skin biopsy will reveal fungal hyphae elements within the stratum corneum.

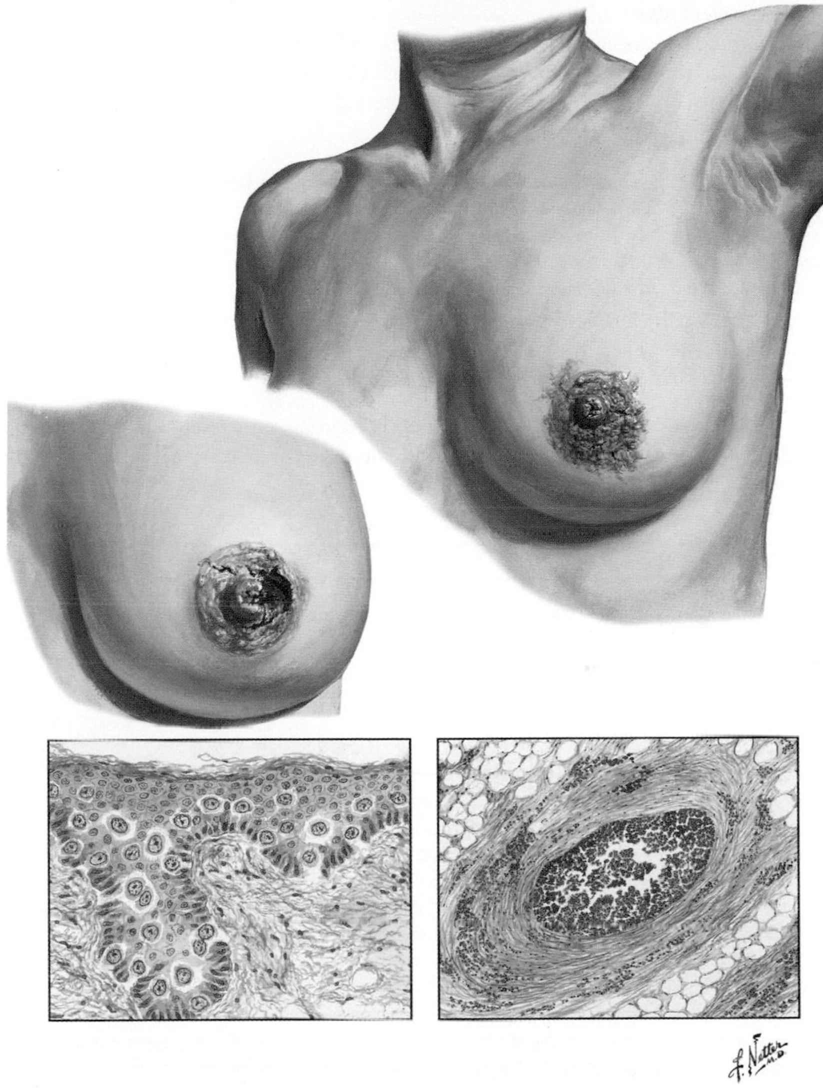

Fig. 11.2 Paget's disease of the breast. (From Smith, R.P. (2018). *Netter's obstetrics and gynecology* (3rd ed.). Elsevier.)

CLINICAL PEARL **STEP 1/2/3**

The presence of a unilateral rash on a nipple nonresponsive to topical therapy should raise suspicion for Paget's disease of the breast. A skin biopsy is indicated.

What is Paget's disease of the breast?

Paget's disease of the breast occurs almost exclusively in women, rarely in men. It accounts for 1%–4% of new cases of female breast cancer diagnosed annually in the United States. For patients diagnosed with this, an underlying breast cancer (in situ or invasive) is present in 85%–88% of the cases.

What is the treatment plan?

Bilateral mammography is mandatory for patients with biopsy-proven Paget's disease of the breast. If any underlying mass or abnormality is detected, ultrasound can be used to evaluate and guide the core biopsy. The patient should then be referred to a breast cancer surgeon and oncologist for treatment.

This patient underwent a bilateral mammogram, which detected a 1.5-cm left retro-areolar mass. Ultrasound did not reveal any axillary lymphadenopathy. She underwent total mastectomy of the left breast, with histology showing Paget's disease of the breast with invasive ductal carcinoma (stage 1A); it stained positive for estrogen receptor. Her recovery was uneventful, and she has been well and is followed by the oncology department.

Case Summary

- **Complaint/History:** A 70-year-old female with chronic unilateral rash on left nipple.
- **Findings:** Eczematous thin plaque; no breast mass or axillary lymphadenopathy was palpated.
- **Test:** A skin biopsy was performed.

Diagnosis: Paget's disease of the breast.

- **Treatment:** The patient underwent a bilateral mammogram, which detected a left retro-areolar mass. She underwent total mastectomy of the left breast with histology showing Paget's disease of the breast with invasive ductal carcinoma.

BEYOND THE PEARLS

- The median duration of signs and symptoms prior to histologic diagnosis of Paget's disease of the breast is between 6 and 8 months.
- Between 84% and 91% of cases of Paget's disease of the breast overexpress HER2. HER2 is human epidermal growth factor receptor 2, which plays a role in breast cancer development. Overexpression of HER2 probably explains the poor prognosis reported for invasive breast cancer patients with Paget's disease.
- The differential diagnosis for Paget's disease of the breast can also include clear cell papulosis of the skin. This is common in children and rare in adults. It presents as scattered, white, flat-topped papules located on the lower abdomen and along the milk lines. Histology shows benign pagetoid cells in the basal cell of the epidermis that stain AE1 positive and CAM5.2 positive by immunohistochemical analysis.
- A KOH skin scraping can be performed for rapid in-office diagnosis of dermatophyte infection.
- In Paget's disease of the breast, a layer of basal cells often separates the Paget's cells from the basement membrane and can appear crushed beneath the nests of the Paget's cells. This histological feature helps to distinguish Paget's disease from pagetoid melanoma and squamous cell carcinoma in situ.

Bibliography

American Society of Clinical Oncology. Breast cancer guide. 2019. Available at: www.cancer.net/cancer-types/breast-cancer/introduction.

Chaudary, M. A., Millis, R. R., Lane, E. B., et al. (1986). Paget's disease of the nipple: A ten-year review including clinical, pathological and immunohistochemical findings. *Breast Cancer Research and Treatment*, *8*, 139.

Chen, C. Y., Sun, L. M., & Anderson, B. O. (2006). Paget disease of the breast: Changing patterns of incidence, clinical presentation, and treatment in the US. *Cancer*, *107*, 1448.

James, W. D., Berger, T. G., & Elston, D. M. (2006). *Andrews' diseases of the skin. Clinical dermatology.* (10th ed.). Canada: Saunders Elsevier.

Kothari, A. S., Beechey-Newman, N., Hamed, H., et al. (2002). Paget disease of the nipple: A multifocal manifestation of higher-risk disease. *Cancer*, *95*, 1.

Marshall, J. K., Griffith, K. A., Haffty, B. G., et al. (2003). Conservative management of Paget disease of the breast with radiotherapy: 10- and 15-year results. *Cancer*, *97*, 2142.

National Cancer Institute. Paget Disease of the Breast. 2012. Available at: https://www.cancer.gov/types/breast/paget-breast-fact-sheet#.

Rapini, R. P. (2005). *Practical dermatopathology*. China: Elsevier Mosby.

CASE 12

A 58-Year-Old Female With Progressive Facial Lesions

Brandon L. Adler ■ Binh Ngo

A 58-year-old Black female presents to the dermatology clinic with 5 years of skin lesions affecting her face, particularly her nose, that are slowly increasing in size and number. She denies associated pruritus, pain, or bleeding. On review of systems, she reports several years of bothersome sinus congestion. She denies any fevers, vision changes, cough, shortness of breath, palpitations, nausea, vomiting, diarrhea, or joint pain. Her medical history is significant for hypertension, hyperlipidemia, depression, and anxiety, for which she takes amlodipine, atorvastatin, and escitalopram. On physical examination, temperature is 37.0°C, blood pressure is 130/80 mmHg, pulse rate is 84/min, respiratory rate is 20/min, and oxygen saturation is 98% on room air. There are reddish-brown to violaceous papules and plaques with minimal overlying scale on the nose, upper lip, and cheeks (Fig. 12.1A). When a glass slide is pressed against the lesions to cause blanching, they appear to have an "apple jelly" color (Fig. 12.1B). The remainder of the examination is normal. Skin biopsy shows granulomas in the dermis (Fig. 12.2).

Why do granulomas form in the skin?

Granulomas are localized collections of macrophages and other inflammatory cells that function to limit inflammation, sequester pathogens, and protect nearby tissue. The differential diagnosis of granulomatous inflammation in the skin is wide but can be roughly divided into infectious and noninfectious etiologies (Table 12.1). Tuberculosis, Hansen's disease (leprosy), leishmaniasis, late syphilis, blastomycosis, coccidioidomycosis, and sporotrichosis are among the granulomatous infections of the skin. Noninfectious causes include sarcoidosis, granuloma annulare, necrobiosis lipoidica, rheumatoid nodules, cutaneous Crohn's disease, granulomatous rosacea, and reactions to foreign bodies and drugs.

On further histologic examination, the granulomas are noncaseating, with minimal surrounding inflammation.

Based on histologic features, cutaneous granulomas are divided into categories that help to narrow the differential diagnosis:

- *Sarcoidal granulomas* have sparse surrounding inflammation and, as the name implies, are strongly associated with sarcoidosis, although they are also found in foreign body reactions.
- *Tuberculoid granulomas* display a surrounding inflammatory infiltrate of lymphocytes and/or plasma cells and often have central caseation necrosis. Classically associated with tuberculosis, they can also be seen in other infections as well as inflammatory conditions. Thus, the presence of caseation necrosis signals the need to rule out an infectious process, but it is not pathognomonic for infection.
- *Palisading granulomas* surround a central focus of mucin, fibrin, or degenerated collagen, as found in granuloma annulare, rheumatoid nodules, and necrobiosis lipoidica, respectively.

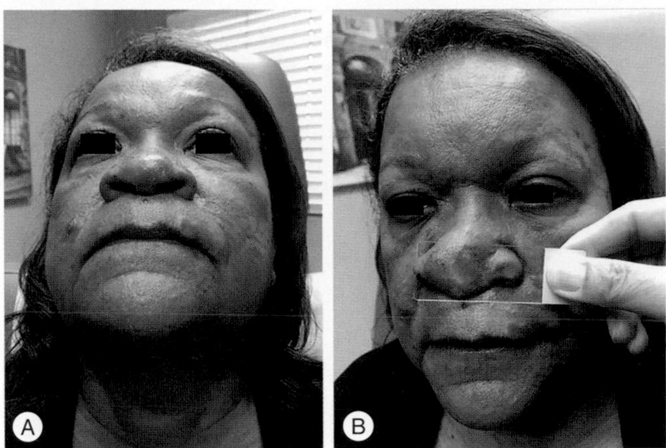

Fig. 12.1 (A) Violaceous papules and plaques on the nasal tip and alar rim, upper lip, and cheeks. (B) When a glass slide is pressed against the skin (diascopy), the lesions display a subtle "apple jelly" color.

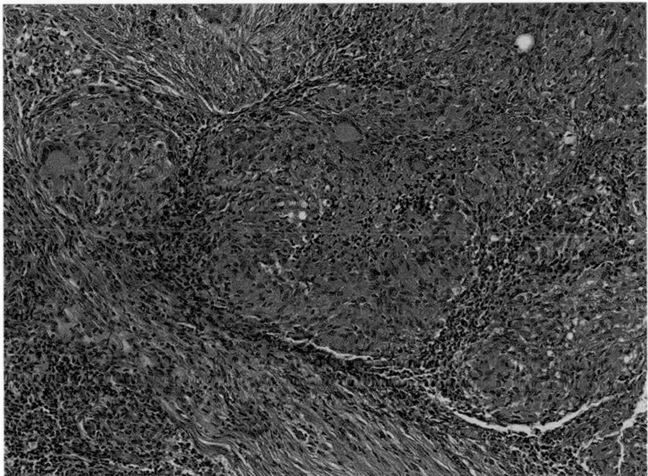

Fig. 12.2 Histologic examination reveals noncaseating granulomas with sparse surrounding inflammation in the dermis.

- *Suppurative granulomas* have a central collection of neutrophils and may be observed in various infections as well as ruptured cysts.
- *Foreign body granulomas* form as part of the immune response to exogenous (e.g., splinters, sutures, tattoo inks) and endogenous materials (most commonly keratin from ingrown hair or nails).

Clearly, there is overlap between the histologic subsets. Some uncommon disorders do not fit neatly into one category. Clinicopathologic correlation is essential to establish the correct diagnosis.

What is the pathogenesis of sarcoidosis?

Sarcoidosis is a chronic multisystem inflammatory disease of uncertain etiology in which an unchecked cell-mediated immune response drives the formation of noncaseating granulomas that can eventually damage tissues. It is thought to develop in genetically susceptible individuals as a

TABLE 12.1 ■ **Differential Diagnosis of Cutaneous Granulomas**

Infectious	Noninfectious
Mycobacterial	Sarcoidosis
Tuberculosis	Foreign body reactions
Hansen's disease (leprosy)	Granulomatous rosacea
Atypical mycobacterial infection	Perioral dermatitis
Fungal	Crohn's disease
Sporotrichosis	Granuloma annulare
Blastomycosis	Annular elastolytic giant cell granuloma
Coccidioidomycosis	Necrobiosis lipoidica
Paracoccidioidomycosis	Necrobiotic xanthogranuloma
Chromomycosis	Rheumatoid nodules
Pheohyphomycosis	Interstitial granulomatous dermatitis
Eumycotic mycetoma	Interstitial granulomatous drug eruption
Protozoal	Granulomatous mycosis fungoides
Leishmaniasis	Granulomatous cheilitis
Bacterial	
Syphilis (late)	
Actinomycosis	
Nocardiosis	
Blastomycosis-like pyoderma	
Cat-scratch disease	
Lymphogranuloma venereum	

reaction to one or more unidentified antigens, possibly autoimmune, environmental, or infectious in nature. Although it usually occurs sporadically, patients' first-degree relatives are at increased risk of developing sarcoidosis, implicating genetic factors in its development. Additionally, some medications can trigger cutaneous sarcoidosis or sarcoidosis-like reactions, including interferons, tumor necrosis factor (TNF)-α inhibitors, and cancer immunotherapies. Essential to granuloma formation is the differentiation of CD4+ T cells into T helper 1 (Th1) cells. Secretion of Th1 cytokines, including interleukin-2, interferon-γ, and TNF-α, promotes and supports ongoing granuloma formation.

BASIC SCIENCE PEARL **STEP 1**

Sarcoidosis is traditionally considered a Th1 cell-mediated immune process. More recent evidence suggests broader inflammatory pathways are at play, including the innate immune system and the Th17 pathway.

What is the epidemiology of sarcoidosis?

Sarcoidosis affects patients of all ages and racial/ethnic groups, with a slight female predominance. It most commonly presents in the third to fourth decades of life. Worldwide, sarcoidosis has its highest incidence in Scandinavia. In the United States, however, the incidence is approximately three times higher in Blacks compared with White Americans. Although epidemiologic data are limited, the incidence and prevalence of sarcoidosis appear to be lower in Asians and Hispanics than the White population.

CLINICAL PEARL **STEP 1/2/3**

In the United States, Black women have the highest incidence of sarcoidosis.

Cultures and special stains do not demonstrate infectious organisms or polarizable foreign material.

How is sarcoidosis diagnosed?

Sarcoidosis is a diagnosis of exclusion, without any definitive tests available to date. The diagnosis is made clinically with support from histology showing noncaseating granulomas (without infectious organisms or foreign substances) and compatible imaging findings. When feasible, a biopsy should be taken from the most accessible site of involvement, such as the skin, salivary glands, or peripheral lymph nodes.

CLINICAL PEARL **STEP 3**

Sarcoidosis is a diagnosis of exclusion; a biopsy demonstrating noncaseating granulomas is not sufficient to make the diagnosis. It is crucial to rule out infections and foreign body reactions and correlate with clinical and imaging findings.

Which organs are involved in sarcoidosis?

Sarcoidosis is a complex disease that can involve nearly any organ and display considerable phenotypic variability. Therefore, making the diagnosis often requires a multidisciplinary team approach. Most frequently, the lungs, thoracic lymph nodes, skin, and eyes are involved. Asymptomatic hilar lymphadenopathy is a very typical presentation. The most common ophthalmologic manifestation is chronic anterior uveitis, which can lead to blindness. Less often, neurologic (central or peripheral), hepatic, renal, cardiac, gastrointestinal, musculoskeletal, hematologic, endocrinologic, and upper respiratory tract/sinus sarcoidosis occur. Heerfordt syndrome (uveoparotid fever) comprises uveitis, parotitis, fever, and cranial nerve palsy (usually facial nerve). More generally, sarcoidosis negatively affects quality of life, with high prevalence of fatigue and psychological symptoms.

CLINICAL PEARL **STEP 2/3**

Sarcoidosis most often affects the lungs, lymph nodes, skin, and eyes, but can present in any organ.

How does sarcoidosis affect the skin?

As many as one-third of patients with sarcoidosis have cutaneous involvement. Skin variants are highly polymorphous; some are essentially pathognomonic and others are indistinct or even simulate more common conditions. There are two major divisions within cutaneous sarcoidosis: *specific lesions* that show granulomas on biopsy versus *nonspecific lesions* that represent reactive phenomena without granulomas. Specific lesions are typically reddish-brown to violaceous papules and plaques that favor the face, especially the nose and periocular and perioral areas (Fig. 12.3). Diascopy, in which a glass slide is pressed against skin lesions to induce blanching, produces a characteristic "apple jelly" color that heightens clinical suspicion. Lupus pernio is a term used to refer to a highly specific form of cutaneous sarcoidosis involving the central face, classically the alar rim of the nose. Sarcoidosis is well known to appear within scars and tattoos. Rarely, it presents as subcutaneous nodules (Darier-Roussy type), alopecia (hair loss, scarring [permanent] or nonscarring), erythroderma (generalized redness and scale involving greater than 80%–90% body surface area), or ichthyosis (extremely dry skin); it can also mimic psoriasis, lichen planus, or rosacea. Erythema nodosum, an inflammation of the subcutaneous fat, is the most common nonspecific lesion, presenting as tender, erythematous nodules on the shins. In addition to sarcoidosis,

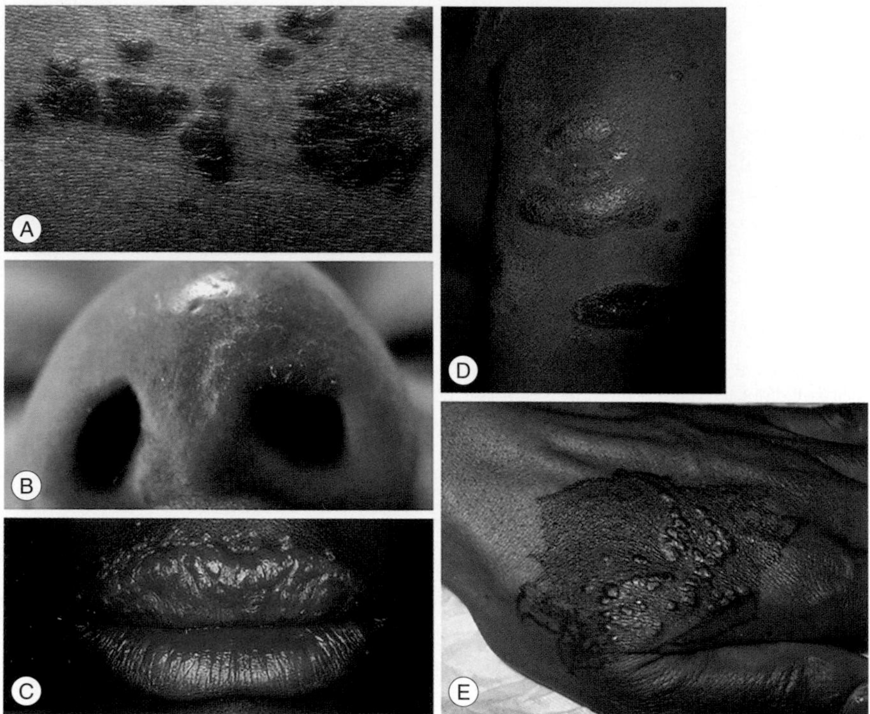

Fig. 12.3 Cutaneous sarcoidosis: papules and plaques. (A) Cutaneous sarcoidosis usually consists of papules and plaques with a typical reddish-brown to violet-brown color. (B, C) Lesions often favor the nose, lips, and perioral region. (D) Hyperpigmented plaques, some of which have scale. (E) Papules of cutaneous sarcoidosis arising within a tattoo; the differential diagnosis includes foreign body reaction. (From Bolognia, J. L., Schaffer, J. V., & Cerroni, L., eds. (2017). *Dermatology* (4th ed.). Philadelphia: Elsevier.)

erythema nodosum is seen in association with multiple infections, drugs, pregnancy, and inflammatory bowel disease, and is also frequently idiopathic.

CLINICAL PEARL **STEP 3**

Like syphilis, sarcoidosis is a great mimicker of many other dermatologic conditions. Although it sometimes shows classic or nearly pathognomonic findings on the skin, less common presentations may not be suspected prior to histopathologic examination.

Does the cutaneous presentation of sarcoidosis have clinical significance?

Classification of the cutaneous manifestations of sarcoidosis is not merely an academic exercise, because they can predict the degree of underlying systemic involvement. Erythema nodosum often occurs in Löfgren syndrome, an acute presentation that includes fever, arthritis, and bilateral hilar lymphadenopathy and portends a favorable prognosis, with most patients experiencing spontaneous resolution. On the other hand, as in the present case, lupus pernio is associated with chronic and refractory sarcoidosis with pulmonary, upper respiratory tract, and sometimes bone involvement, requiring intensive treatment. Since skin lesions may be the first sign of sarcoidosis, prompt recognition permits early diagnosis and timely initiation of treatment, thereby preventing or minimizing permanent organ damage.

CLINICAL PEARL **STEP 2/3**

Erythema nodosum is a positive prognostic factor in sarcoidosis, developing in cases that tend to resolve spontaneously.

What should be done during the initial workup of sarcoidosis?

All cases of suspected sarcoidosis require a comprehensive history (with a focus on exposures, and thorough review of systems), complete physical examination (including referral for ophthalmologic examination), and baseline laboratories, imaging, and functional testing, in order to delimit the extent of organ involvement (Table 12.2). With the exception of Löfgren syndrome's nonspecific skin lesions (erythema nodosum), a skin biopsy should be performed in all patients with cutaneous involvement. It is essential to rule out tuberculosis using a tuberculin skin test or interferon-γ release assay (IGRA). Without exception, the recommended examinations for all systems should be performed in all patients, regardless of symptoms, because of the risk of asymptomatic but clinically significant organ involvement. Silent cardiac sarcoidosis may present with sudden death.

BASIC SCIENCE/CLINICAL PEARL **STEP 1/2/3**

Macrophages in sarcoidal granulomas enzymatically convert 25-hydroxyvitamin D3 [25(OH)D_3] to its active metabolite, 1,25-dihydroxyvitamin D3 [1,25$(OH)_2D_3$] (calcitriol), causing hypercalcemia in around 10% of patients. Therefore, the level of 25(OH)D_3 may be low despite elevated 1,25$(OH)_2D_3$. In most clinical scenarios, only 25(OH)D_3 is routinely checked; in sarcoidosis, both levels should be assessed to avoid inappropriate vitamin D supplementation.

Laboratory tests are normal other than an elevated angiotensin-converting enzyme (ACE) level (101 nmol/ml/min; reference range, 9–67). IGRA is negative. A chest radiograph (CXR) shows bilateral hilar lymphadenopathy (Fig. 12.4). Pulmonary function testing shows mild airflow limitation. A whole-body positron emission tomography/computed tomography (PET/CT) scan highlights thickening of the bilateral maxillary sinuses; bilateral upper lobe reticulonodular and ground-glass opacities; and widespread cervical, mediastinal, abdominal, and pelvic lymphadenopathy.

TABLE 12.2 ■ **Initial Workup of Sarcoidosis**

History	• Occupational/environmental exposures (heavy metals, firefighters) • Family history • Complete review of systems
Examination	• Complete physical examination • Referral for ophthalmologic examination
Histopathology	• All patients except those with Löfgren syndrome (nonspecific findings) • Preferentially biopsy the most easily accessible tissue (e.g., skin, peripheral lymph node, lacrimal gland)
Laboratory testing	• Complete blood count with differential • Comprehensive metabolic panel • Urinalysis • Tuberculin skin test or interferon-γ release assay • Thyroid function testing • 25-hydroxyvitamin D and 1,25-dihydroxyvitamin D
Imaging and functional testing	• Chest radiograph • Pulmonary function testing (with diffusion lung capacity for carbon monoxide) • Electrocardiogram (possibly echocardiogram, Holter monitor)

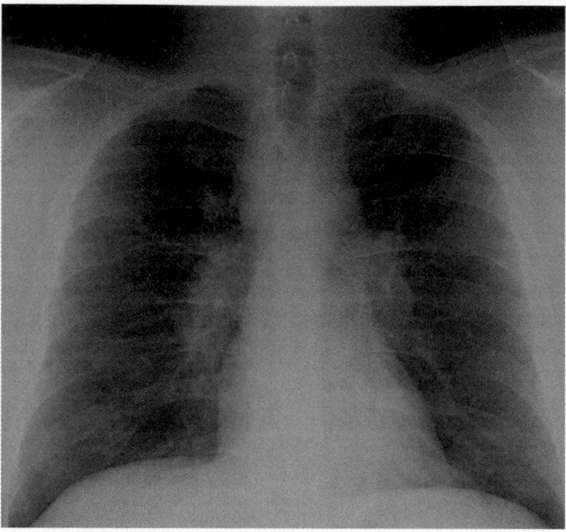

Fig. 12.4 Chest radiograph demonstrates bilateral hilar lymphadenopathy.

What is the significance of the serum ACE level in sarcoidosis?

The granulomas of sarcoidosis produce ACE, leading to increased serum levels in 60% of patients. Use of serum ACE as a diagnostic or therapeutic indicator is controversial, because it has been shown to lack sensitivity and specificity. A diagnosis of sarcoidosis is thought to be more likely when the ACE level is more than two or three times the upper limit of normal.

CLINICAL PEARL **STEP 2/3**

Serum ACE elevation is not limited to sarcoidosis. ACE may be increased in the setting of hyperthyroidism, diabetes mellitus, and osteoarthritis, as well as other granulomatous diseases. In patients with hypertension receiving ACE inhibitors, the ACE level may be falsely low.

The patient is started on prednisone 40 mg daily with a plan to taper over several months. Skin involvement is treated with pulse dye laser and a topical calcineurin inhibitor.

How is cutaneous sarcoidosis treated?

Because sarcoidosis is a disease of unknown etiology, there is no cure and it lacks a single, definitive therapy. At the outset, it is important to recognize that not every case of sarcoidosis requires treatment. Half of patients experience disease remission within 2 years. Accordingly, treatment of mild cases without evidence of organ damage must be balanced with potential side effects. The other half of patients have chronic disease, which may be stable or progressive.

Skin involvement, while not life threatening, is generally treated given its psychosocial effects and potential for disfigurement. Before proceeding, it is first vital to define the full extent of the disease because systemic therapy is dictated by the most severely compromised organ system. For instance, immunosuppressive treatment of cardiac sarcoidosis may be sufficient to control concomitant skin disease. If the skin does not improve during treatment of the most severely affected organ or if the skin itself is most impacted, treatment proceeds according to skin disease severity (Table 12.3). Notably, the US Food and Drug Administration has not approved any medications

TABLE 12.3 ■ **Cutaneous Sarcoidosis Treatment Ladder**

Disease Severity	Treatment Options
Mild	Topical glucocorticoids Intralesional glucocorticoids Topical calcineurin inhibitors Laser and light therapies
Moderate	Antimalarials (hydroxychloroquine, chloroquine) Tetracycline antibiotics (minocycline, doxycycline) Phosphodiesterase inhibitors (pentoxifylline, apremilast)
Severe	Systemic glucocorticoids Methotrexate Thalidomide Tumor necrosis factor-α inhibitors (infliximab, adalimumab)

for cutaneous sarcoidosis and there is a paucity of high-quality randomized controlled trials available to guide therapy. Local modalities (topical, intralesional, laser/light based) are preferred for mild cases because of their favorable safety profile. For deforming or quickly progressive skin disease, the first-line treatment is oral glucocorticoids (prednisone 0.5–1 mg/kg/day or equivalent), slowly tapered to the lowest dose able to control the disease. Otherwise, for moderate-to-severe disease, the therapeutic armamentarium includes a variety of steroid-sparing immunomodulatory and immunosuppressive agents, often used in combination. A well-established body of evidence supports the effectiveness of TNF-α inhibitors (specifically infliximab and adalimumab) for cutaneous sarcoidosis and emerging data suggest the utility of Janus kinase (JAK)–signal transducer and activator of transcription (STAT) pathway inhibitors.

Erythema nodosum resolves spontaneously within several weeks. Symptomatic treatment includes rest, elevation, and nonsteroidal antiinflammatory drugs.

BASIC SCIENCE/CLINICAL PEARL **STEP 1/2/3**

Several treatments used for sarcoidosis target the TNF-α pathway involved in granuloma induction and maintenance, including pentoxifylline, apremilast, thalidomide, and biologics.

Case Summary

- **Complaint/History:** A 58-year-old Black woman presents with 5 years of asymptomatic facial lesions, slowly increasing in size and number, as well as chronic sinus congestion.
- **Findings:** Vital signs are unremarkable. Violaceous papules and plaques are present on the nose, cheeks, and lips and exhibit an "apply jelly" color with diascopy. Other examinations are within normal limits.
- **Lab Results/Tests:** Skin biopsy reveals noncaseating granulomas with negative studies for infectious organisms and foreign materials; lab tests reveal elevated angiotensin-converting enzyme level and negative interferon-γ release assay; chest radiograph reveals bilateral hilar lymphadenopathy; pulmonary function testing reveals mild airflow limitation; positron emission tomography/computed tomography highlights thickening of the maxillary sinuses, bilateral pulmonary infiltrates, and multisite lymphadenopathy.

Diagnosis: Sarcoidosis.

- **Treatment:** The patient received prednisone 40 mg daily with a plan to taper over months. Her skin lesions were treated with pulse dye laser and a topical calcineurin inhibitor.

BEYOND THE PEARLS

- First responders to the September 11, 2001 World Trade Center terrorist attacks have a significantly increased incidence of sarcoidosis, possibly relating to exposure to triggering antigens or other inciting agents.
- Although it is essential to rule out foreign body reactions when working up sarcoidosis, as many as 25% of sarcoidosis biopsies contain tattoo ink or polarizable foreign material, possibly relating to prior unnoticed minor skin trauma. Careful clinicopathologic correlation is required in this scenario.
- PET/CT imaging is helpful in detecting occult foci of disease in sarcoidosis. In 12 patients initially presenting with cutaneous sarcoidosis, PET/CT showed asymptomatic myocardial involvement in four (33%), not found by electrocardiography or echocardiography. PET/CT is also useful to select a biopsy site in cases lacking easily accessible sites of involvement.
- TNF-α inhibitors are increasingly used to treat sarcoidosis because of the role played by this cytokine in granuloma formation and maintenance. Paradoxically, when used to treat other conditions such as rheumatoid arthritis and inflammatory bowel disease, TNF-α inhibitors can rarely induce sarcoidosis-like reactions in the skin and other organs. Recently, an increasing number of cases of sarcoidosis have been reported in patients on cancer immunotherapies, including ipilimumab, pembrolizumab, and vemurafenib, driven by mechanisms that remain to be elucidated.
- Fewer than 5% of patients die of sarcoidosis, usually from pulmonary, cardiac, or neurologic sequelae. In the United States, Black patients have higher mortality than other racial/ethnic groups.
- Several scoring systems have been devised to quantify cutaneous sarcoidosis activity, including the Sarcoidosis Activity and Severity Index (SASI) and the Cutaneous Sarcoidosis Activity and Morphology Instrument (CSAMI). The CSAMI demonstrated reliability and validity among dermatologists, pulmonologists, and rheumatologists, and also correlated with quality-of-life measures.
- Blau syndrome (familial juvenile systemic granulomatosis) is an autosomal dominant disease that is phenotypically similar to sarcoidosis, manifesting with early-onset granulomatous inflammation of the skin, eyes, and joints. It is caused by mutations in the nucleotide-binding oligomerization domain containing 2/caspase recruitment domain family, member 15 (NOD2/CARD15).

Bibliography

Adler, B. L., Wang, C. J., Bui, T. L., et al. (2019). Anti-tumor necrosis factor agents in sarcoidosis: A systematic review of efficacy and safety. *Seminars in Arthritis and Rheumatism*, *48*(6), 1093–1104.

Baughman, R. P., Field, S., Costabel, U., et al. (2016). Sarcoidosis in America. Analysis based on health care use. *Annals of the American Thoracic Society*, *13*(8), 1244–1252.

Grunewald, J., Grutters, J. C., Arkema, E. V., et al. (2019). Sarcoidosis. *Nature Reviews Disease Primers*, *5*(1), 45.

Iannuzzi, M. C., & Fontana, J. R. (2011). Sarcoidosis: Clinical presentation, immunopathogenesis, and therapeutics. *The Journal of the American Medical Association*, *305*(4), 391–399.

Iannuzzi, M. C., Rybicki, B. A., & Teirstein, A. S. (2007). Sarcoidosis. *The New England Journal of Medicine*, *357*(21), 2153–2165.

James, W. E., & Baughman, R. (2018). Treatment of sarcoidosis: Grading the evidence. *Expert Review of Clinical Pharmacology*, *11*(7), 677–687.

Johnson. R. B. (2016). Granulomatous Reaction Pattern. In R. B. Johnson (Ed.), *Weedon's skin pathology essentials* (2nd ed., pp. 133–161). London: Churchill Livingstone Elsevier.

Marcoval, J., Mana, J., Moreno, A., et al. (2001). Foreign bodies in granulomatous cutaneous lesions of patients with systemic sarcoidosis. *Archives of Dermatology*, *137*(4), 427–430.

Nakamura, S., Hashimoto, Y., Nishi, K., et al. (2014). High rate of cardiac sarcoidosis presenting with cutaneous plaque type sarcoidosis in 18F-fluorodeoxyglucose positron emission tomography-computed tomography: A case series. *Journal of Medical Case Reports*, *8*, 17.

Noe, M. H., & Rosenbach, M. (2017). Cutaneous sarcoidosis. *Current Opinion in Pulmonary Medicine*, *23*(5), 482–486.

Rosenbach. M. (2020). Janus kinase inhibitors offer promise for a new era of targeted treatment for granulomatous disorders. *Journal of the American Academy of Dermatology*, *82*(3), e91–e92.

Rosenbach, M. A., Wanat, K. A., Reisenauer, A., et al. (2017). Non-infectious granulomas. In J. L. Bolognia, J. V. Schaffer, & L. Cerroni (Eds.), *Dermatology* (4th ed., pp. 1644–1663). Philadelphia, PA: Elsevier.

Studdy, P. R., & Bird, R. (1989). Serum angiotensin converting enzyme in sarcoidosis—its value in present clinical practice. *Annals of Clinical Biochemistry*, *26*(Pt 1), 13–18.

Valeyre, D., Prasse, A., Nunes, H., et al. (2014). Sarcoidosis. *Lancet*, *383*(9923), 1155–1167.

Wanat, K. A., & Rosenbach, M. (2014). A practical approach to cutaneous sarcoidosis. *American Journal of Clinical Dermatology*, *15*(4), 283–297.

CASE 13

A 79-Year-Old Male With a Fungating Mass on the Left Lower Extremity

Maggie Chow ■ Binh Ngo

A 79-year-old male from Laos presents to the emergency department with nodules on his left lower extremity that have been slowly enlarging and spreading up his leg for 1 year. He reports weight loss and fatigue and denies any other systemic symptoms. He had just relocated from Laos to the United States. His medical history is generally unknown and he is not on any medications.

On examination, the left lower extremity has 3+ pitting edema. Over the plantar and dorsal feet, extending up to the knee, there are scattered fungating, friable, malodorous, tan hemorrhagic nodules (Fig. 13.1). No lymphadenopathy is palpated at the popliteal or inguinal regions.

What is the differential diagnosis of this patient's skin finding?
The differential diagnosis at this time is broad. It includes cutaneous neoplasms, infections, and inflammatory diseases. Table 13.1 shows a list of differential diagnoses.

CLINICAL PEARL **STEP 1/2/3**

The differential diagnosis for cutaneous nodular melanoma can be broad and include other cutaneous neoplasms, infections, and inflammatory diseases.

What is the appropriate next step in management?
Because of the broad list of differential diagnoses, we performed a skin biopsy for histopathology and also cultured for atypical mycobacteria, fungi, and aerobic and anaerobic bacteria.

All cultures came back negative and the patient's skin biopsy showed melanoma. Based on clinical and pathologic information, the patient was diagnosed with nodular melanoma.

What are the subtypes of melanoma?
The skin is made up of the epidermis, the dermis, and the subcutis. Melanoma is classified first by whether the disease is invasive into the dermis of the skin or whether the disease is circumscribed to the epidermis. Disease limited to the epidermis is designated as "melanoma in situ" or lentigo maligna if it clinically or histopathologically presents as a lentigo. Disease that invades the dermis of the skin is subclassified as superficial spreading melanoma, nodular melanoma, lentigo maligna melanoma, and acral lentiginous melanoma (if arising on acral surfaces). Other rare clinical and histologic variants of melanoma include amelanotic melanoma, spitzoid melanoma, desmoplastic melanoma, and pigment synthesizing melanoma. The depth at which the tumor invades directly correlates with the risk of metastasis and thus patient survival. Any location with melanocytes can

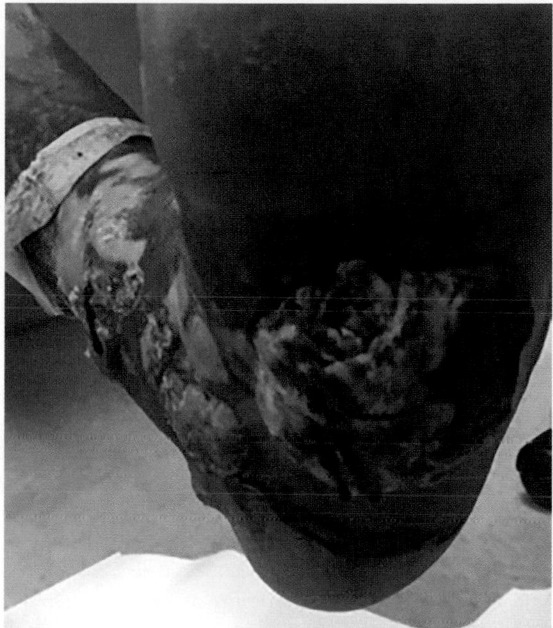

Fig. 13.1 Fungating nodule seen at presentation.

TABLE 13.1 ■ **Differential Diagnosis for Patient's Skin Findings**

Neoplasms	Infections	Inflammatory Diseases

• Squamous cell carcinoma
• Keratoacanthoma
• Pigmented basal cell carcinoma
• Melanoma
• Verrucous carcinoma
• Benign melanocytic neoplasms
  • Common nevus
  • Blue nevus
  • Lentigo
  • Spitz nevus
  • Dysplastic nevus
• Seborrheic keratosis
• Pyogenic granuloma
• Dermatofibroma
	• Cutaneous tuberculosis or atypical mycobacterial infection
	• Actinomycotic mycetoma
	• Eumycotic mycetoma
	• Deep fungal infections including blastomycosis, coccidioidomycosis, paracoccidioidomycosis
	• Verruca vulgaris
		• Hypertrophic lupus
		• Hypertrophic lichen planus

give rise to melanoma. Therefore, the locations can include the uvea of the eyes, vulva, mucous membranes, and intrathecal space.

CLINICAL PEARL **STEP 2/3**

The in situ forms of melanoma include melanoma in situ and lentigo maligna. The invasive forms of melanoma include nodular melanoma, superficial spreading melanoma, acral lentiginous melanoma, and lentigo maligna melanoma.

What are the reliable clinical clues that physicians can use to diagnose melanoma?

To aid in visual diagnosis of melanoma when evaluating a pigmented lesion, dermatologists rely on the ABCDEs of melanoma:

A. Asymmetry
B. Border irregularities
C. Color variegation
D. Diameter greater than or equal to 6 mm
E. Evolution: change in size, shape, color, or new development of a lesion

The more features present, the greater the likelihood that the lesion is a melanoma. Other criteria and checklists have been developed to help clinicians identify lesions suspicious for melanoma in special populations such as patients with skin of color and pediatric patients. Dermoscopy aids in the evaluation of pigmented lesions.

In patients with multiple nevi, dermatologists look for the "ugly duckling" sign. This sign is based on the observation that individuals with multiple nevi tend to have a unique nevus profile. Lesions that differ from this profile may deserve special attention. When comparing between experts, lesions that are different from signature nevi in a given patient are reliably identified.

Who is at risk of cutaneous melanoma?

Both genetic and environmental factors put patients at risk of developing cutaneous melanoma. Patients who have >100 congenital and acquired melanocytic nevi are at increased risk of developing melanoma. Individuals with a genetic susceptibility or a positive family history of melanoma are also at greater risk. There are a number of gene mutations that increase the risk for malignant melanoma. They include cyclin-dependent kinase inhibitor 2A (CDKN2A). This gene was identified as the first familial melanoma susceptibility gene more than 20 years ago and is responsible for the familial atypical malignant mole melanoma (FAMMM) syndrome. A few years later, cyclin-dependent kinase 4 (CDK4) was also identified as a melanoma susceptibility gene. Other genes identified as conferring increased risk of melanoma include: breast cancer 1 (BRCA1) associated protein 1 (BAP1), CXC genes, telomerase reverse transcriptase (TERT), protection of telomeres 1 (POT1), ACD, and TERF2IP, the latter four being involved in telomere maintenance. In addition, xeroderma pigmentosa, caused by several genetic mutations, has a markedly increased risk of melanoma.

Furthermore, variants in melanocortin 1 receptor (MC1R) and microphthalmia-associated transcription factor (MITF) are associated with a moderately increased risk. The MC1R gene is responsible for skin color phenotypes. Individuals with red hair, light eyes, and light complexion have a higher sensitivity to UV exposure.

Ultraviolet radiation (UV), and in particular the UVB spectrum, is the main environmental risk factor for developing melanoma. Patients with intense and intermittent sun exposure have a higher risk of melanoma than patients with chronic continuous sun exposure. Blistering sunburns and tanning bed use increase the risk of developing melanoma by two-fold and four-fold, respectively.

Patients who are immunosuppressed with medications for organ transplantation are at three-fold increased risk of developing melanoma compared with the general population. Patients who are on immunosuppressive drugs for their inflammatory bowel disease are also at high risk.

Is it possible for patients with skin of color to develop melanoma?

Although skin of color has a protective effect against development of skin cancer, there is a common misconception that skin cancer does not develop in dark-skinned individuals. That is not the case. Such misconception contributes to a delay in diagnosis and treatment. As a result, some studies suggest that patients with dark skin have poorer prognosis when they are diagnosed with skin cancer.

Across all ethnic groups, melanoma is the cutaneous tumor with the highest mortality. The incidence of cutaneous melanoma has been stable for the last several years according to the National Cancer Institute. However, rates of invasive melanoma in Hispanic individuals have been increasing in California since 1988. One study showed a 1.8% per year increase from 1988 to 2001 and 7.3% annual increase between 1996 and 2001. Five-year melanoma survival rates of Blacks and Hispanics are consistently lower than in White population. These statistics hold true even after adjusting for age, sex, stage, histology, site, socioeconomic status, and treatment. Although individuals with dark skin have a lower rate of skin cancer compared with White population, they experience significantly higher risk of mortality from skin cancer. Black in particular have the lowest 5-year survival rate for melanoma (72.2%), followed by Asians (80.2%) and Hispanics (81.1%). Comparatively, the survival rate is 89.6% for White population.

The differences in outcome between individuals with dark skin and White population may be due to multiple factors, including delays in correct diagnosis, inadequate access to healthcare, lack of education and awareness of skin cancer in patients with dark skin, and atypical presentation of skin cancer.

Atypical presentations of melanoma may contribute to a delay in the diagnosis in dark skin. The majority of melanoma in dark skin occurs in non-sun-exposed skin, including palmar and plantar surfaces, subungual surfaces, and mucous membranes. The plantar foot is the most commonly involved area in 30%–40% of cases; acral lentiginous melanoma is the most common type of melanoma in Black. At presentation, melanomas in Hispanics and Black tend to be thicker and are often at a later stage with regional and distant involvement than White population.

What are the prognostic factors for patients who have developed melanoma?

The most important prognostic feature for melanoma is the depth of the melanoma at biopsy, also known as the Breslow depth. Because of this, when dermatologists perform biopsies on lesions that we suspect may be melanoma, we aim to remove the entire lesion so that an accurate depth can be assessed.

The American Cancer Society has set up a complex staging system for melanoma (see Table 13.2). The most commonly used staging system is the AJCC staging. The key features are depth of invasion, ulceration, and spread to regional lymph nodes, as well as local and distant spread. Sentinel lymph node biopsy is performed to assess lymphatic spread.

TABLE 13.2 ■ **Staging System for Melanoma**

AJCC Stage	Melanoma Stage Description
0	The cancer is confined to the epidermis, the outermost skin layer (Tis). It has not spread to nearby lymph nodes (N0) or to distant parts of the body (M0). This stage is also known as melanoma in situ.
I	The tumor is no more than 2 mm (2/25 of an inch) thick and might or might not be ulcerated (T1 or T2a). The cancer has not spread to nearby lymph nodes (N0) or to distant parts of the body (M0).
II	The tumor is more than 1 mm thick (T2b or T3) and may be thicker than 4 mm (T4). It might or might not be ulcerated. The cancer has not spread to nearby lymph nodes (N0) or to distant parts of the body (M0).
IIIA	The tumor is no more than 2 mm thick and might or might not be ulcerated (T1 or T2a). The cancer has spread to one, two, or three nearby lymph nodes, but it is so small that it is only seen under the microscope (N1a or N2a). It has not spread to distant parts of the body (M0).

(Continued)

TABLE 13.2 ■ **Staging System for Melanoma** (Continued)

AJCC Stage	Melanoma Stage Description
IIIB	There is no sign of the primary tumor (T0) **AND:** • The cancer has spread to only one nearby lymph node (N1b) **OR** • It has spread to very small areas of nearby skin (satellite tumors) or to skin lymphatic channels around the tumor (without reaching the nearby lymph nodes) (N1c). It has not spread to distant parts of the body (M0). **OR** The tumor is no more than 4 mm thick and might or might not be ulcerated (T1, T2, or T3a) **AND:** • The cancer has spread to only one nearby lymph node (N1a or N1b) **OR** • It has spread to very small areas of nearby skin (satellite tumors) or to skin lymphatic channels around the tumor (without reaching the nearby lymph nodes) (N1c) **OR** • It has spread to two or three nearby lymph nodes (N2a or N2b). It has not spread to distant parts of the body (M0).
IIIC	There is no sign of the primary tumor (T0) **AND:** • The cancer has spread to two or more nearby lymph nodes, at least one of which could be seen or felt (N2b or N3b) **OR** • It has spread to very small areas of nearby skin (satellite tumors) or to skin lymphatic channels around the tumor, and it has reached the nearby lymph nodes (N2c or N3c) **OR** • It has spread to nearby lymph nodes that are clumped together (N3b or N3c). It has not spread to distant parts of the body (M0). **OR** The tumor is no more than 4 mm thick, and might or might not be ulcerated (T1, T2, or T3a) **AND:** • The cancer has spread to very small areas of nearby skin (satellite tumors) or to skin lymphatic channels around the tumor and it has reached nearby lymph nodes (N2c or N3c) **OR** • The cancer has spread to four or more nearby lymph nodes (N3a or N3b), or it has spread to nearby lymph nodes that are clumped together (N3b or N3c). It has not spread to distant parts of the body (M0). **OR** The tumor is more than 2 mm but no more than 4 mm thick and is ulcerated (T3b) **OR** it is thicker than 4 mm but is not ulcerated (T4a). The cancer has spread to one or more nearby lymph nodes **AND/OR** it has spread to very small areas of nearby skin (satellite tumors) or to skin lymphatic channels around the tumor (N1 or higher). It has not spread to distant parts of the body. **OR** The tumor is thicker than 4 mm and is ulcerated (T4b) **AND:** • The cancer has spread to one, two, or three nearby lymph nodes, which are not clumped together (N1a/b or N2a/b) **OR** • It has spread to very small areas of nearby skin (satellite tumors) or to skin lymphatic channels around the tumor, and it might (N2c) or might not (N1c) have reached one nearby lymph node). It has not spread to distant parts of the body (M0).
IIID	The tumor is thicker than 4 mm and is ulcerated (T4b) **AND:** • The cancer has spread to four or more nearby lymph nodes (N3a or N3b) **OR** • It has spread to nearby lymph nodes that are clumped together (N3b) • It has spread to very small areas of nearby skin (satellite tumors) or to skin lymphatic channels around the tumor, **AND** it has spread to at least two nearby lymph nodes, or to lymph nodes that are clumped together (N3c) **OR** It has not spread to distant parts of the body (M0).
IV	The tumor can be any thickness and might or might not be ulcerated (any T). The cancer might or might not have spread to nearby lymph nodes (any N). It has spread to distant lymph nodes or to organs such as the lungs, liver, or brain (M1).

The recent advent of gene expression analysis has added a new dimension to prognostic screening. There are strong correlations for certain gene expression patterns with risk of future recurrence and metastases.

Although the biopsy was transected at the base, it was estimated that our patient's Breslow depth was >4 mm, which confers poor prognosis. Additionally, PET/CT revealed metastasis to the left inguinal lymph nodes.

CLINICAL PEARL **STEP 2/3**

Depth of invasion is the most important prognostic factor in cutaneous melanoma.

How is melanoma treated?

When melanomas are diagnosed at an early stage, surgical excision is usually curative. The standard treatment for melanoma has always been surgical excision with wide margins. Typically, surgical margins of 5 mm or greater are recommended.

CLINICAL PEARL **STEP 2/3**

Early melanomas can be treated with surgery alone. Melanomas greater than Stage IB should be treated using a multidisciplinary approach with dermatology, surgical oncology, and medical oncology.

More recently, Mohs micrographic surgery (MMS) has been applied to treat melanomas in difficult locations and for superficial lesions that are large in diameter such as lentigo maligna and lentigo maligna melanomas. Although not yet standard of care, several series have shown encouraging results.

MMS is a specialized technique for locally invasive, high risk skin cancers with the goal of high cure rates and maximal preservation of normal unaffected tissue. MMS is usually performed under local anesthesia. The tumor is excised and the excised tissue is oriented, mapped, and processed such that the entire peripheral and deep margins can be evaluated by the surgeon, who also serves as the pathologist. Instead of the permanent vertical sectioning performed by standard laboratories, a frozen horizontal sectioning technique is performed. Residual tumor seen on the sections can be mapped to guide removal of additional tumor in subsequent stages, until all tumor has been removed. In difficult cases such as melanoma, immunostaining is often applied. Reconstruction is usually performed by the surgeon the same day.

A modification of MMS, namely staged excision with permanent horizontal sections, can also be applied for the treatment of melanoma. Using this technique, excision of the lesion is performed and the peripheral and deep margins are evaluated by a dermatopathologist with permanent horizontal sections.

CLINICAL PEARL **STEP 2/3**

MMS with rapid histologic stains and staged excision is currently in the process of being developed for the treatment of melanoma.

Because of the extent of our patient's disease, he was not a surgical candidate. Thus, he was started on systemic treatment with vemurafenib with stabilization and initial improvement of his disease.

How frequently should patients have their skin checked following the diagnosis of melanoma?

There are no standardized guidelines for follow-up with full body skin checks after the diagnosis of melanoma. At the University of Southern California, we perform skin checks every

3 months after diagnosis of melanoma for 2 years, followed by every 6 months for 2 years, then yearly after year 4.

At 2-year follow-up, the patient's melanoma continued to be stable on vemurafenib.

Case Summary

- **Complaint/History:** A 79-year-old male presents with an enlarging nodule on the left lower extremity.
- **Findings:** Over the left plantar and dorsal feet, extending up to his left knee, there are scattered fungating, hemorrhagic nodules.
- **Lab Results/Tests:** Skin biopsy was done as well as PET/CT scan.

Diagnosis: Melanoma with metastasis to left inguinal lymph nodes.

- **Treatment:** Patient was started on systemic treatment with vemurafenib with initial improvement and subsequent stablization of his disease.

BEYOND THE PEARLS

- All patients regardless of their skin color are at risk of cutaneous melanoma. Cutaneous melanoma is not just a disease affecting light-skinned individuals. A high index of suspicion is needed for early diagnosis and treatment of melanoma in darker-skinned individuals to prevent poor prognosis caused by diagnosis delay.
- For metastatic disease that cannot be surgically resected, immunotherapy is used. The current first-line treatment is to augment the immune response by removing checkpoint inhibition. The first successful agent was ipilimumab, an antibody to cytotoxic-T lymphocyte associated protein 4 (CTLA-4). This agent led to apparent cures in some patients with metastatic melanoma. Subsequently, inhibitors of the checkpoint protein for programmed cell death 1 (PD-1), namely pembrolizumab and nivolumab, have been even more successful in promoting long term survival in patients who had no hope in the past. Combinations of these therapies have also been applied (Mahoney et al., 2005).
- Targeted therapies have been developed more recently and are directed at oncogenes active in melanoma tumorigenesis. The MAP kinase pathway is important in the tumorigenesis of melanoma. Approximately 50% of cutaneous melanomas have the BRAF V600E mutation. Approximately 15%–20% of melanomas have a mutation in NRAS. These mutations contribute to BRAF activation of the MAPK pathway, which promotes tumorigenesis. For patients who harbor the BRAF V600E mutation, BRAF inhibitors vemurafenib or dabrafenib have been shown to improve disease-free progression. The addition of MEK inhibition downstream of the BRAF kinase in the MAPK pathway with trametinib or cobimetinib may prevent development of acquired BRAF resistance and also improve prognosis Eroglu et al. 2016.
- Fifteen percent of melanomas have mutations or amplification of the KIT tyrosine kinase proto-oncogene. However, treatment with KIT inhibitors such as imatinib have only shown clinically meaningful responses in patients with activating mutations in KIT. Other modalities such as radiation therapy and cytotoxic chemotherapy may be used for palliation.
- For melanoma that has reached stage IB and beyond without known metastases, adjuvant immunotherapy and targeted therapies postsurgical resection are now available with the checkpoint inhibitors and BRAF inhibitors.

Bibliography

Agbai, O. N., Buster, K., Sanchez, M., et al. (2014). Skin cancer and photoprotection in people of color: A review and recommendations for physicians and the public. *Journal of the American Academy of Dermatology*, *70*(4), 748–762.

Balch C, Houghton A, Sober A, Soong S, Atkins M, Thombpson J. *Cutaneous Melanoma.*; 1992.

Bradford. P. T. (2009). Skin cancer in skin of color. *Dermatology Nursing*, *21*(4). 170-177, 206; quiz 178.

Breslow. A. (1970). Thickness, cross-sectional areas and depth of invasion in the prognosis of cutaneous melanoma. *Annals of Surgery*, *172*(5), 902–908.

Byrd, K. M., Wilson, D. C., Hoyler, S. S., & Peck, G. L. (2004). Advanced presentation of melanoma in African Americans. *Journal of the American Academy of Dermatology*, *50*(1), 21–24.

Byrd-Miles, K., Toombs, E. L., & Peck, G. L. (2007). Skin cancer in individuals of African, Asian, Latin-American, and American-Indian descent: differences in incidence, clinical presentation, and survival compared to Caucasians. *Journal of drugs in dermatology: JDD*, *6*(1), 10–16.

Cockburn, M. G., Zadnick, J., & Deapen, D. (2006). Developing epidemic of melanoma in the hispanic population of California. *Cancer*, *106*(5), 1162–1168.

Coit, D. G., Andtbacka, R., Anker, C. J., et al. (2012). Melanoma. *Journal of the National Comprehensive Cancer Network: JNCCN*, *10*(3), 366–400.

Cormier, J. N., Xing, Y., Ding, M., et al. (2006). Ethnic differences among patients with cutaneous melanoma. *Archives of Internal Medicine*, *166*(17), 1907–1914.

Džambová, M., Sečníková, Z., Jiráková, A., et al. (2016). Malignant melanoma in organ transplant recipients: Incidence, outcomes, and management strategies: a review of literature. *Dermatologic Therapy*, *29*(1), 64–68.

Eroglu, Z., & Ribas, A. (2016). Combination therapy with BRAF and MEK inhibitors for melanoma: Latest evidence and place in therapy. *Therapeutic Advances in Medical Oncology*, *8*(1), 48–56.

Gandini, S., Sera, F., Cattaruzza, M. S., et al. (2005). Meta-analysis of risk factors for cutaneous melanoma: III. Family history, actinic damage and phenotypic factors. *European Journal of Cancer*, *41*(14), 2040–2059.

Gaudy-Marqueste, C., Wazaefi, Y., Bruneu, Y., et al. (2017). ugly duckling sign as a major factor of efficiency in melanoma detection. *JAMA Dermatology*, *153*(4), 279.

Gershenwald, J. E., Scolyer, R. A., Hess, K. R., et al. (2017). Melanoma staging: Evidence-based changes in the American Joint Committee on Cancer eighth edition cancer staging manual. *CA: a Cancer Journal for Clinicians*, *67*(6), 472–492.

Gloster, H. M., & Neal, K. (2006). Skin cancer in skin of color. *Journal of the American Academy of Dermatology*, *55*(5), 741–760.

Grob, J. J., & Bonerandi, J. J. (1998). The "ugly duckling" sign: Identification of the common characteristics of nevi in an individual as a basis for melanoma screening. *Archives of Dermatology*, *134*(1). 103-a-104.

Hu, S., Soza-Vento, R. M., Parker, D. F., & Kirsner, R. S. (2006). Comparison of stage at diagnosis of melanoma among Hispanic, black, and white patients in Miami-Dade County, Florida. *Archives of Dermatology*, *142*(6), 704–708.

Kim, G. K., Del Rosso, J. Q., & Bellew, S. (2009). Skin cancer in asians: part 1: Nonmelanoma skin cancer. *The Journal of Clinical and Aesthetic Dermatology*, *2*(8), 39–42.

Larkin, J., Chiarion-Sileni, V., Gonzalez, R., et al. (2015). Combined nivolumab and ipilimumab or monotherapy in untreated melanoma. *The New England Journal of Medicine*, *373*(1), 23–34.

Mahoney, M. -H., Joseph, M., & Temple, C. L. F. (2005). The perimeter technique for lentigo maligna: An alternative to Mohs micrographic surgery. *Journal of Surgical Oncology*, *91*(2), 120–125.

Pampena, R., Kyrgidis, A., Lallas, A., Moscarella, E., Argenziano, G., & Longo, C. (2017). A meta-analysis of nevus-associated melanoma: Prevalence and practical implications. *Journal of the American Academy of Dermatology*, *77*(5). 938-945.e4.

Rahman, Z., & Taylor, S. C. (2001). Malignant melanoma in African Americans. *Cutis*, *67*(5), 403–406. http://www.ncbi.nlm.nih.gov/pubmed/11381857.

Raziano, R. M., Clark, G. S., Cherpelis, B. S., et al. (2009). Staged margin control techniques for surgical excision of lentigo maligna. *Giornale Italiano Di Dermatologia E Venereologia*, *144*(3), 259–270.

Soura, E., Eliades, P. J., Shannon, K., Stratigos, A. J., & Tsao, H. (2016). Hereditary melanoma: Update on syndromes and management. *Journal of the American Academy of Dermatology*, *74*(3), 411–420.

Thomas, L., Tranchand, P., Berard, F., Secchi, T., Colin, C., & Moulin, G. (1998). Semiological value of ABCDE criteria in the diagnosis of cutaneous pigmented tumors. *Dermatology (Basel, Switzerland)*, *197*(1), 11–17.

WHO | Guidelines for the diagnosis, treatment and prevention of leprosy. *WHO*. 2019. https://www.who.int/lep/resources/9789290226383/en/.

Zell, J. a, Cinar, P., Mobasher, M., Ziogas, A., Meyskens, F. L., & Anton-Culver, H. (2008). Survival for patients with invasive cutaneous melanoma among ethnic groups: The effects of socioeconomic status and treatment. *Journal of Clinical Oncology*, *26*(1), 66–75.

CASE 14

A 38-Year-Old Female With a Diffuse Rash and Mucositis

Joan Leavens ■ Binh Ngo

A 38-year-old Asian female presents to the emergency department with a 3-day history of fever and rash. Her symptoms began with fevers, sore throat, and myalgias. The following day, she developed a diffuse rash that started on her trunk and spread to her extremities. By the third day, she noticed that her skin began to blister and slough off, her eyes became red, and she developed painful erosions in her mouth and vagina. Her medical history is significant for hypertension, hyperlipidemia, and a recent diagnosis of gout, for which she was started on allopurinol 10 days before her symptoms started.

On physical examination, her temperature is 38.6°C, blood pressure is 135/85 mmHg, heart rate is 125/min, respiratory rate is 22/min, and oxygen saturation is 98% on room air. There are diffuse erythematous to violaceous dusky-appearing macules, large erosions on the trunk and buttocks covering 15% of the body surface area, crusting of the vermilion lips, and erosions in the buccal mucosa and vagina. Placement of tangential digital pressure on the skin causes the epidermis to shear off and detach. A skin biopsy is performed. This is notable for full-thickness necrosis of the epidermis. (See Figs. 14.1–14.4.)

What is the difference between Stevens-Johnson syndrome and toxic epidermal necrolysis?

Stevens-Johnson syndrome (SJS) and toxic epidermal necrolysis (TEN) are thought of as the same disease on a spectrum and are generally referred to as SJS/TEN. SJS is characterized by detached and detachable skin that is less than 10% of the total body surface area (BSA). SJS-TEN overlap occurs when 10%–30% BSA is involved and TEN involves greater than 30% of the BSA. SJS can evolve into TEN.

CLINICAL PEARL **STEP 1/2/3**

SJS involves <10% of BSA. SJS-TEN overlap involves 10%–30% of BSA. TEN involves >30% of BSA. These are not separate diseases but rather the same disease on a spectrum.

What is the pathogenesis of SJS/TEN?

SJS/TEN is a severe adverse cutaneous reaction primarily involving the skin and mucous membranes that develops when genetically susceptible individuals are exposed to a culprit medication or, less commonly, another inciting event. Although the precise sequence of events leading to the development of SJS/TEN is not fully understood, research suggests that SJS/TEN is a result of the host's inability to detoxify the culprit drug and its metabolites. It has been proposed that the drug metabolite forms an antigenic complex with the host tissue that leads to a cell-mediated immune response. This immune response involves cytotoxic CD8+ helper T cells and

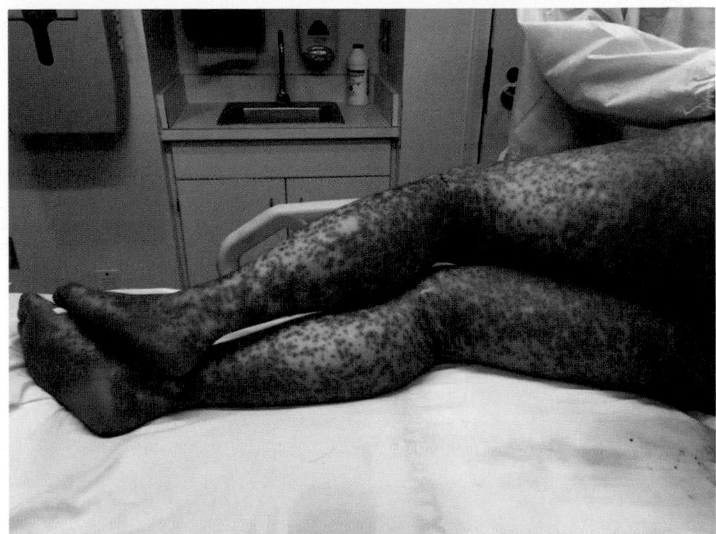

Fig. 14.1 Diffuse rash consisting of erythematous to violaceous dusky macules, demonstrated here on the lower extremities.

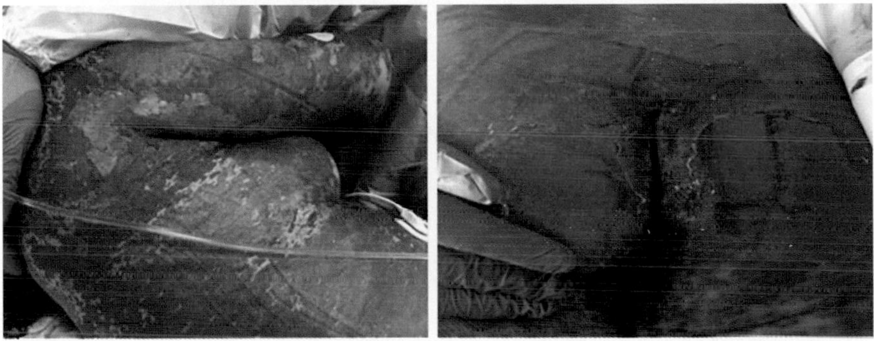

Fig. 14.2 Detachment of the necrotic epidermis from the dermis produces large erosions covering approximately 15% of the body surface area.

natural killer T cells, which secrete cytokines such as granulysin, perforin, and granzyme B. It is thought that these cytokines lead to necrosis of keratinocytes, which is the predominant cell type of the epidermis. Keratinocyte necrosis may also be mediated by the binding of Fas ligand (FasL) to Fas (also known as the death receptor). Necrosis of keratinocytes leads to the loss of cell adhesion in the epidermis and the loss of the attachment of the epidermis to the underlying dermis. This epidermal detachment produces the skin sloughing and erosions characteristic of SJS/TEN.

BASIC SCIENCE PEARL **STEP 1/2/3**

Keratinocyte necrosis in SJS/TEN is thought to be caused by drug metabolites that lead to a cell-mediated response involving cytotoxic CD8 T cells and natural killer T cells. Granulysin, perforin, granzyme B, and Fas-FasL are key players.

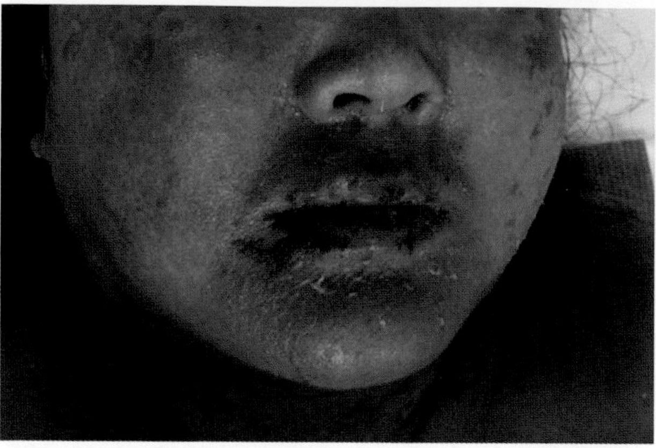

Fig. 14.3 Hemorrhagic crusting is present on the lips.

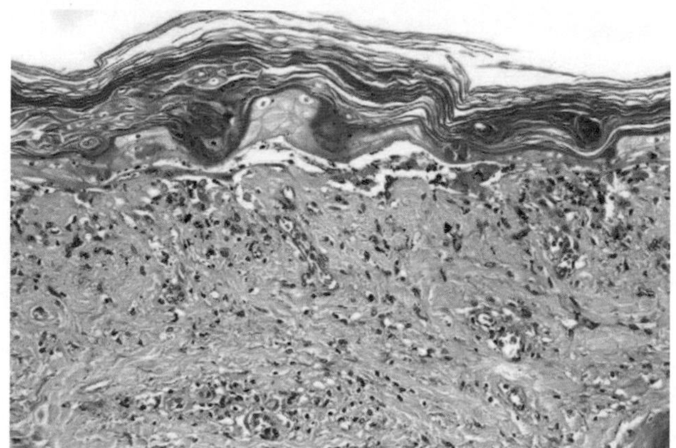

Fig. 14.4 Skin biopsy demonstrates subepidermal vesiculation, full-thickness necrosis of the epidermis, and a spare inflammatory infiltrate in the dermis.

Who is at risk of SJS/TEN?

SJS and TEN are rare diseases with an overall incidence of one or two cases per million. They can affect people of all ages and races, although they show a slight preponderance in women and in older age groups. In addition, certain patient groups are at higher risk of developing SJS/TEN. This includes patients who are immunocompromised (e.g., HIV positive) and those who metabolize drugs at a decreased rate (called slow acetylators). AIDS is associated with a 1000-fold increase in the risk of SJS/TEN. In addition, patients who have specific human leukocyte antigen (HLA) alleles are known to be genetically at a higher risk of developing SJS/TEN. Examples of high risk HLA types include Han Chinese with HLA-B*58:01 who are exposed to allopurinol and Asians and East Indians with HLA-B*15:02 exposed to carbamazepine. Sometimes HLA testing is required in these patient groups before administering higher risk medications.

Testing for HLAB*5801 is positive, which more definitely confirms allopurinol as the causative drug.

What are the most common drug culprits of SJS/TEN?

The majority of patients with SJS/TEN have a strong association between the ingestion of a drug and the development of the characteristic rash. The most frequently implicated medications include allopurinol, nonsteroidal antiinflammatory drugs (NSAIDs) such as piroxicam, antibiotics, anticonvulsants, and antiretrovirals, although more than 100 drugs have been found to be associated with SJS/TEN. Table 14.1 summarizes the common drug causes of SJS/TEN. Among the antibiotics, sulfonamides are the most strongly associated with the development of SJS/TEN; others include the penicillins, cephalosporins, fluoroquinolones, and tetracyclines. The risk of developing SJS/TEN is highest during the initial 1–3 weeks after the ingestion of the culprit medication. Less commonly SJS/TEN can develop as long as 8 weeks after the medication is started. Although rare, additional causes of SJS/TEN include immunizations and infections.

What is the differential diagnosis of SJS/TEN?

Although the diagnosis of SJS/TEN may be straightforward in the presence of the classic cutaneous eruption and a drug culprit, sometimes the patient lacks an obvious medication exposure or has been exposed to multiple medications, leading to diagnostic confusion. In addition, during the initial 1–2 days prior to the development of skin sloughing, the cutaneous eruption may be misdiagnosed as a simple morbilliform drug eruption. SJS may be difficult to distinguish from erythema multiforme (EM), especially EM major, which frequently demonstrates mucosal involvement. EM is classically characterized by targetoid lesions and tends to favor acral sites. Other diagnoses that may mimic SJS/TEN include generalized fixed drug eruption, autoimmune bullous diseases such as bullous pemphigoid and paraneoplastic pemphigus, Kawasaki disease, and more. Table 14.2 summarizes the differential diagnosis for SJS/TEN.

TABLE 14.1 ■ **Medications Most Frequently Associated With SJS/TEN**

Medication
Allopurinol
Aminopenicillins
Antiretroviral drugs, especially NNRTIs
Nevirapine
Efavirenz
Etravirine
Barbiturates
Carbamazepine
Cephalosporins
Checkpoint inhibitors
Ipilimumab
Nivolumab
Fluoroquinolones
Lamotrigine
Phenylbutazone
Phenytoin anticonvulsants
Piroxicam
Sulfonamide antibiotics
Sulfamethoxazole
Sulfadiazine
Sulfasalazine

NNRTIs, Nonnucleoside reverse transcriptase inhibitors.

TABLE 14.2 ■ **Differential Diagnosis of SJS/TEN**

Drug eruptions	Infectious
Morbilliform drug eruption Erythema multiforme major Generalized fixed drug eruption Acute generalized exanthematous pustulosis Drug-induced linear IgA bullous dermatosis Drug reaction with eosinophilic and systemic symptoms (DRESS) Toxic erythema of chemotherapy	Staphylococcal scalded skin syndrome Invasive fungal dermatitis
Autoimmune bullous disease	***Other***
Paraneoplastic pemphigus Bullous pemphigoid Cicatricial pemphigoid	Kawasaki disease Severe acute graft-versus-host disease Disseminated intravascular coagulation Purpura fulminans

What is the cutaneous clinical presentation of SJS/TEN?

SJS/TEN typically appears 1–3 weeks after exposure to the culprit medication but may occur as early as 4 days and as late as 4 weeks after ingestion of the drug. There is usually an initial nonspecific flu-like prodromal illness lasting 2 or 3 days that may include fevers, chills, malaise, fatigue, arthralgias, myalgias, rhinitis, sore throat, and irritation of the eyes and skin. When present, this typically precedes the cutaneous and mucosal eruption by 1 to 3 days. Cutaneous involvement usually begins as an eruption of erythematous, dusky red, or purpuric macules that tend to coalesce. These lesions tend to appear first on the trunk and then spread to the neck, face, and proximal upper extremities. The palms and soles may also be involved early on. This is in contrast to morbilliform drug eruptions, which tend to start on the proximal extremities, and erythema multiforme, which commonly begins on the palms and soles. As epidermal necrosis progresses, a fluid-filled space develops between the dermis and epidermis, leading to bulla formation. As the skin detaches, it reveals large areas of raw and bleeding dermis. This stage of the skin rash tends to be very painful. The Nikolsky sign is almost always present; this refers to detachment of the epidermis from the dermis when firm sliding pressure is applied by a finger to the skin. Although helpful, this sign is not specific for SJS/TEN and may be present in other blistering diseases.

CLINICAL PEARL **STEP 2/3**

SJS/TEN typically appears 1–3 weeks after initial exposure to the culprit medication.

Skin involvement starts as erythematous to dusky macules that progress to bullae and skin sloughing. A positive Nikolsky sign refers to when lateral digital pressure on the skin leads to detachment of the epidermis from the dermis.

The patient complains of eye redness and irritation. She has painful erosions inside her mouth, which makes talking, eating, and swallowing difficult. She also has painful vaginal erosions.

Besides the skin, which other areas and organ systems can SJS/TEN involve?

SJS/TEN always involves at least two mucosal surfaces, including the oral, ocular, and anogenital mucosa. Erythema and erosions of the buccal, ocular, and genital mucosa are present in more than 90% of patients and can be extremely painful. The vermilion (e.g., outer) lips can appear crusted and blackened and are often held slightly open. Oral mucosal involvement may make swallowing, eating, and talking difficult. The most common eye finding is conjunctivitis; however, ocular involvement may be severe and lead to ulceration, scarring, and ultimately blindness. Anogenital involvement is characterized by blisters and erosions, and urethral or vaginal bleeding may occur. Vaginal and anal stenosis may result.

Other organ systems that may be affected include the respiratory tract, which is involved in an estimated 25% of patients with TEN. Gastrointestinal (GI) involvement may also occur, leading to esophageal stenosis and gastrointestinal ulceration with bleeding and diarrhea. Other rare complications include hepatitis, urinary retention, nephritis, myocarditis, pneumothorax, and seizures.

CLINICAL PEARL **STEP 2/3**

SJS/TEN involves at least two mucosal surfaces, including the eyes, mouth, and anogenital area. Other organ systems that may be involved include the liver, GI tract, respiratory tract, kidneys, heart, and central nervous system.

What should be done during the initial workup of SJS/TEN?

The workup of SJS/TEN begins with a thorough history with a focus on medication exposures within the past 2 months and particularly the past 3 weeks, as well as a comprehensive review of systems. In addition, a complete physical examination and baseline laboratories and imaging to ascertain the complete extent of organ involvement should be performed. A chest X-ray should be obtained, particularly if the patient notes a history of respiratory symptoms. A skin biopsy is usually performed to confirm the diagnosis.

The patient's laboratory workup is remarkable for elevated erythrocyte sedimentation rate (ESR) to 85 mm/h (reference range, 0–29) and C-reactive protein (CRP) to 23 mg/dL (reference range, 0–0.8), complete blood count with leukocytosis to 13.8 × 10^9 cells/L (reference range, 3.5–9.5) with neutrophilia to 85% (normal, 40%–75%), and elevated aspartate aminotransferase (AST) to 90 U/L (reference range, 15–40) and alanine aminotransferase (ALT) to 139 (reference range, 9–50). Other laboratory tests were within normal limits, including the serum creatinine. Chest X-ray was unremarkable. A biopsy was performed for frozen section and permanent staining with hematoxylin and eosin (H&E). Histopathology demonstrated full-thickness necrosis of the epidermis.

How is SJS/TEN diagnosed?

SJS/TEN may be diagnosed clinically in the setting of the classic cutaneous eruption, involvement of at least two mucosal surfaces and the presence of an obvious drug trigger. However, a biopsy is usually performed for histopathologic analysis. Frequently, a frozen cryostat section is obtained because this enables immediate analysis of the biopsy specimen by the pathologist. This is useful for confirming the diagnosis on the same day of presentation so that treatment can be initiated. A frozen section is not usually performed alone, however, because permanent staining with H&E (which can take up to several days to prepare) yields a more accurate analysis of the tissue.

Early lesions of SJS show scattered apoptotic keratinocytes in the epidermis, while full-blown SJS/TEN classically demonstrates subepidermal blistering with overlying necrosis of the entire epidermis, as well as a spare lymphocytic perivascular infiltrate.

Laboratory abnormalities commonly seen in SJS/TEN include elevated inflammatory markers (ESR and CRP), leukocytosis with neutrophilia or less commonly eosinophilia, and low-grade elevations of AST and ALT. Leukopenia may also be seen and is a poor prognostic factor. Urinalysis may show proteinuria or hematuria.

CLINICAL PEARL **STEP 2/3**

Biopsy specimens in SJS/TEN classically show subepidermal blistering with full-thickness necrosis of the epidermis. Frozen sections are sometimes performed to allow for same-day tissue analysis.

How is SJS/TEN managed?

The management of SJS and TEN requires early diagnosis, immediate discontinuation of the causative drug, and ongoing supportive care. When cutaneous and/or systemic involvement is severe, patients are typically managed in tertiary care centers in the intensive care unit (ICU) or in specialized burn units when available. Care is aimed at limiting associated complications, which include hypovolemia, electrolyte imbalances, respiratory compromise from mucositis, renal insufficiency, and sepsis, because associated complications are the main cause of mortality in SJS/TEN. This is done through frequent laboratory monitoring and swabs from potentially infected areas, in addition to blood and urine cultures when clinically indicated. Antibiotics may be initiated when infection is suspected; however, the medical literature has not supported a role for prophylactic antibiotics.

Specialist consultations are mandatory and can include a dermatologist, an ophthalmologist, a gynecologist or urologist, and/or a burn or wound care specialist. Ophthalmology consultation is mandatory in patients with ocular involvement. If vaginal or urethral involvement is suspected, gynecology and/or urology should be consulted. Additionally, other consultants should be involved if organ involvement is suspected, including gastroenterology, pulmonology, cardiology, and so forth. If dermatology is not the primary team, a dermatologic consultation should be arranged.

Supportive care is similar to that performed for severe burns. Skin care should focus on the eyes, nose, mouth, face, anogenital region, and skin folds to help prevent scarring and infection. Intact areas of skin should not be manipulated to prevent further traumatization and epidermal detachment. Detached areas of skin should be kept covered using Vaseline gauze or other nonstick dressing until the epidermis has regenerated and the wound is closed.

Although milder forms of SJS may be treated with supportive care alone, more severe forms of SJS and TEN are treated with systemic agents. Because SJS/TEN is so rare, the literature on systemic medical therapies is mostly based on case reports and small case series, and no single specific therapy has a high level of evidence for its effectiveness. Treatments that have demonstrated some efficacy include TNF-α inhibitors (etanercept, infliximab), plasmapheresis, cyclosporine, cyclophosphamide, and high-dose intravenous immune globulin (IVIG). In a case series of 10 patients with TEN, a single 50 mg injection of etanercept led to a median healing time of 8.5 days. In comparison, in general it takes an average time of 3 weeks for the epidermis to regenerate and healing to occur in SJS/TEN survivors.

CLINICAL PEARL **STEP 3**

Management of SJS/TEN requires prompt discontinuation of the culprit drug, admission to an ICU or burn unit if involvement is severe, and specialty consultations when appropriate.

Associated complications are the main cause of mortality and include hypovolemia, electrolyte imbalances, renal insufficiency, respiratory compromise from mucositis, and sepsis.

The patient was admitted to the ICU. Allopurinol was discontinued. She was treated with a single 50 mg injection of subcutaneous etanercept and monitored closely for infection and end-organ damage. An ophthalmologist was consulted and serial eye exams were recommended with daily gentle cleansings and application of eye drops and antibiotic ointment. A gynecologist was consulted and recommended daily application of silver nitrate solution to the genital area.

The patient gradually improved with daily supportive wound care and, after 2 weeks, her erosions were mostly healed with overlying postinflammatory hyperpigmentation. She felt well and was discharged from the hospital.

TABLE 14.3 ■ **SCORTEN Criteria and Associated Mortality in SJS/TEN**

Prognostic factors	Points
Age >40 years	1
Heart rate >120 bpm	1
History of malignancy	1
BSA involved on day 1 >10%	1
Serum urea level (>10 mmol/L)	1
Serum bicarbonate level (<20 mmol/L)	1
Serum glucose level (>14 mmol/L)	1
SCORTEN	**Mortality (%)**
0–1	3.2
2	12.1
3	35.8
4	58.3
>5	90

What is the prognosis of SJS/TEN?

SJS and TEN are severe and life threatening. The average mortality is 1%–5% for SJS and 25%–35% for TEN. Risk factors that are related to a worse prognosis include the extent of skin involvement; older age; malignancy; number of medications; leukopenias; and elevated serum urea, glucose, and creatinine levels. An illness severity score called the SCORTEN has been developed to estimate mortality. SCORTEN accounts for the following factors: age, heart rate, history of malignancy, BSA, blood urea nitrogen (BUN), serum bicarbonate, and blood glucose. Table 14.3 shows the SCORTEN criteria.

More than 50% of patients who survive TEN suffer from long-term sequelae. Ocular sequelae may develop for as long as 8 years following SJS/TEN and include symblepharon, conjunctival synechiae, and entropion. Surviving patients may also experience irregular pigmentation, eruptive nevi, phimosis, nail dystrophy, and diffuse hair loss.

Case Summary

- **Complaint/History:** A 38-year-old Asian female presents with a 3-day history of fevers, sore throat, a rash consisting of dusky red macules progressing to bullae and skin sloughing, eye redness and blurry vision, and painful erosions of the oral and vaginal mucosa. Ten days earlier she had been started on allopurinol for gout.
- **Findings:** Vital signs are remarkable for fevers and tachycardia. Dusky red macules are present diffusely and large erosions are seen on the trunk and extremities involving 30% of the BSA. The exam is otherwise remarkable for conjunctival injection, hemorrhagic crusting of the lips, and mucositis of the oral and vaginal mucosa.
- **Lab Results/Tests:** Laboratory workup shows leukocytosis with neutrophilia, elevated ESR and CRP, and elevated AST/ALT. Skin biopsy shows subepidermal blistering with full-thickness necrosis of the epidermis.

Diagnosis: SJS/TEN.

- **Treatment:** The patient was admitted to the ICU. Allopurinol was discontinued. Consultations to ophthalmology, gynecology, dermatology, wound care, and dietician were arranged. She was treated with 50 mg etanercept once and gentle wound care was instituted. She was monitored closely for electrolyte imbalances, infection, and organ involvement.

BEYOND THE PEARLS

- SJS/TEN may rarely be caused by infections and vaccines. There are case reports of a number of vaccines, including hepatitis B, measles-mumps-rubella, smallpox, varicella, and more, leading to SJS/TEN. Rare infectious causes of SJS/TEN include herpes simplex virus.
- Rarely, SJS/TEN patients may present with involvement primarily in sun-exposed areas and report a history of recent significant sun exposure. This suggests that rarely SJS/TEN may be photoinduced or exacerbated.
- Survivors of SJS/TEN often suffer from chronic sequelae. The most common long-term complications are dermatologic and include postinflammatory dyspigmentation, scarring, eruptive nevi, and nail changes. Chronic ocular sequelae occur in up to 75% of survivors and are caused by scarring. Other long-term complications include oral and dental, pulmonary, urogenital/gynecological, gastrointestinal, renal, and psychological.
- SJS/TEN may be confused with EM major, which can also have mucosal involvement. The lesions in EM are classically targetoid, with three concentric zones of color, and SJS lesions are typically dusky macules with one or two zones of color. In addition, EM favors the extremities while SJS/TEN classically starts on the trunk (and may generalize subsequently). EM is usually precipitated by infections, such as herpes simplex virus and mycoplasma, rather than medications.
- Mycoplasma-induced rash and mucositis (MIRM) is another entity that may be difficult to distinguish from SJS/TEN. MIRM is more common in children and young adults. It is caused by mycoplasma pneumonia and typically presents as oral and ocular mucositis. Cutaneous involvement tends to be absent or milder than in SJS/TEN. Treatment for MIRM involves treating the underlying mycoplasma infection. In any patient with an SJS/TEN-like picture who complains of respiratory symptoms, a chest X-ray examination and mycoplasma serologies should be ordered. Sometimes it may not be possible to distinguish between MIRM and SJS, and some providers think these disorders are not mutually exclusive.
- Acute graft-versus-host disease (GVHD) may mimic SJS/TEN both clinically and histopathologically. The patient will have a history of bone marrow transplant in acute GVHD.

Bibliography

Bolognia, J., Jorizzo, J., & Schaffer, J. (2017). *Dermatology*. Philadelphia: Elsevier Saunders.

Canavan, T. N., Mathes, E. F., Frieden, I., & Shinkai, K. (2015). Mycoplasma pneumoniae-induced rash and mucositis as a syndrome distinct from Stevens-Johnson syndrome and erythema multiforme: A systematic review. *Journal of the American Academy of Dermatology*, *72*(2), 239–245.

Chahal, D., Aleshin, M., Turegano, M., Chiu, M., & Worswick, S. (2018). Vaccine-induced toxic epidermal necrolysis: a case and systematic review. *Dermatology Online Journal*, *24*(1): 3.

Guégan, S., Bastuji-Garin, S., Poszepczynska-Guigné, E., Roujeau, J. C., & Revuz, J. (2006). Performance of the SCORTEN during the first five days of hospitalization to predict the prognosis of epidermal necrolysis. *The Journal of Investigative Dermatology*, *126*(2), 272–276.

Harr, T., & French, L. E. (2010). Toxic epidermal necrolysis and Stevens-Johnson syndrome. *Orphanet Journal of Rare Diseases*, *5*, 39.

James, W., Berger, T., Elston, D., & Neuhaus, I. (2016). *Andrews' diseases of the skin: Clinical dermatology*. Philadelphia: Elsevier Saunders.

Lee, H. Y., Walsh, S. A., & Creamer, D. (2017). Long-term complications of Stevens-Johnson syndrome/toxic epidermal necrolysis (SJS/TEN): The spectrum of chronic problems in patients who survive an episode of SJS/TEN necessitates multidisciplinary follow-up. *The British Journal of Dermatology*, *177*(4), 924–935.

Paradisi, A., Abeni, D., Bergamo, F., et al. (2014). Etanercept therapy for toxic epidermal necrolysis. *Journal of the American Academy of Dermatology*, *71*(2), 278–283.

Wang, F., Ma, Z., Wu, X., & Liu, L. (2019). Allopurinol-induced toxic epidermal necrolysis featuring almost 60% skin detachment. *Medicine*, *98*(25), e16078.

Worswick, S., & Cotliar, J. (2011). Stevens-Johnson syndrome and toxic epidermal necrolysis: A review of treatment options. *Dermatologic Therapy*, *24*(2), 207–218.

Zimmermann, S., Sekula, P., Venhoff, M., et al. (2017). Systemic immunomodulating therapies for Stevens-Johnson syndrome and toxic epidermal necrolysis: A systematic review and meta-analysis. *JAMA Dermatologic*, *153*(6), 514–522.

CASE 15

A 62-Year-Old Woman With an 8-Year History of a Pruritic Rash

Michelle Walters ■ Meiling L. Fang Yuen

A 62-year-old woman presents to dermatology for evaluation of a rash, previously diagnosed as psoriasis. She has an 8-year history of a rash on her posterior legs and lower back and has tried medications for psoriasis, such as etanercept, without improvement. On review of systems she reports pruritus. Her medical history is significant for chronic obstructive pulmonary disease, congestive heart failure, and osteoporosis. She reports being recently hospitalized for a severe, intensely pruritic flare of this rash. On physical examination her temperature is 37°C, blood pressure is 110/55 mmHg, pulse rate is 97/min, respiratory rate is 18/min, and oxygen saturation is 97%. There are erythematous, lichenified, and poorly demarcated plaques with overlying excoriations covering >40% of her body surface area, including her upper back, gluteal cleft, posterior thighs, and extensor surfaces of both upper extremities (Fig. 15.1). A skin biopsy was consistent with atopic dermatitis. She was started on a high potency topical corticosteroid and counseled on bathing with mild cleansers and the frequent use of emollients.

CLINICAL PEARL **STEP 2/3**

Atopy is the predisposition to develop atopic dermatitis, allergic rhinitis, and asthma. These are known as the "atopic triad."

What is the epidemiology of atopic dermatitis?

In the United States, atopic dermatitis affects up to 25% of children and 7% of adults. In 50%–75% of cases, age of onset is 6 months or younger and a clearance rate of 60% is expected by the age of 16 years. A small percentage first develop symptoms as adults.

What is the pathogenesis of atopic dermatitis?

Atopic dermatitis (AD) is a chronic, inflammatory skin condition. The pathogenesis of atopic dermatitis is related to skin barrier dysfunction, immune system dysregulation, and alteration of the microbiome, resulting in skin that is characterized by severe dryness, inflammation, pruritus, and predisposition to infection. Filaggrin, a keratin protein, is a major structural component of the epidermis. In atopic dermatitis, mutations in the filaggrin (FLG) gene result in skin barrier dysfunction, causing dry skin through transepidermal water loss and allowing entry of irritants, allergens, and microorganisms, which trigger the release of inflammatory Th2 cytokines (IL-4, IL-10, and IL-13). Th2 cells also suppress macrophage activity, activate eosinophils, and downregulate the Th1 response and production of antimicrobial peptides, resulting in an increased susceptibility to infection.

BASIC SCIENCE PEARL **STEP 1**

Psoriasis is considered a Th1 cell-mediated immune process with resulting upregulation of antimicrobial peptides (defensins, cathelicidins). In contrast, atopic dermatitis is a Th2 cell-mediated immune process with downregulation of antimicrobial peptides. As a result, the lesions of atopic dermatitis are more susceptible to infection.

How is atopic dermatitis diagnosed?

The diagnosis of atopic dermatitis is often a clinical diagnosis. Atopic dermatitis is characterized by pruritic, poorly demarcated erythematous plaques with lichenification and scaling on the popliteal and antecubital fossae, as well as the neck, face, and extremities (Fig. 15.1). The differential diagnosis of atopic dermatitis is listed in Table 15.1.

Three criteria must be met for the diagnosis of atopic dermatitis: pruritus, a chronic or relapsing course, and a typical eczematous morphology and distribution pattern. Other features suggestive of atopic dermatitis include xerosis (dry skin), onset in early childhood, and a personal or family history of atopic disease, including allergic rhinitis or asthma. Skin biopsy may aid in diagnosis (see later section).

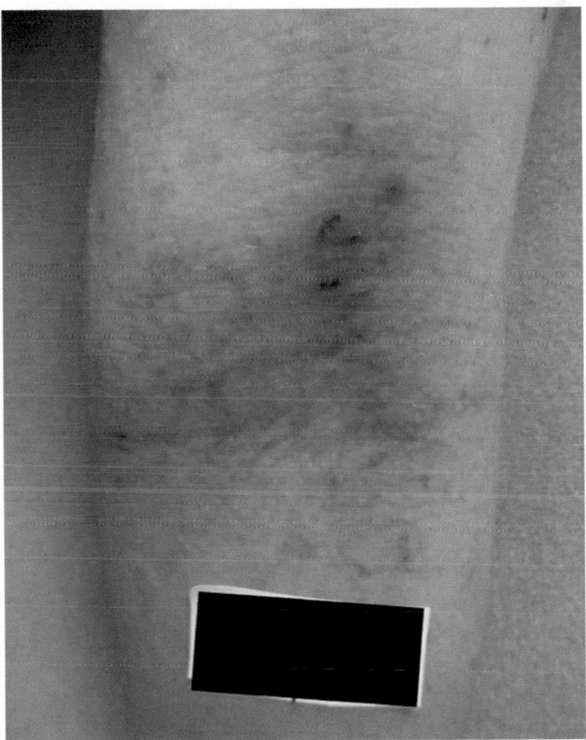

Fig. 15.1 Clinical photo of atopic dermatitis with poorly demarcated erythematous plaques with overlying excoriations. (From Bouthillette, M., Beccati, D., Akthakul, A., et al. (2020). A crosslinked polymer skin barrier film for moderate to severe atopic dermatitis: A pilot study in adults. *Journal of the American Academy of Dermatology, 82*(4), 895–901.)

TABLE 15.1 ■ **Differential Diagnosis of Atopic Dermatitis**

Atopic Dermatitis
Allergic or irritant contact dermatitis
Psoriasis
Nummular eczema
Asteatotic eczema
Lichen simplex chronicus
Mycoses fungoides
Sezary syndrome
Scabies
Dermatophytosis
Impetigo
Dermatitis herpetiformis
Keratosis pilaris
Eczematous drug eruptions
Langerhans cell histiocytosis
Wiskott-Aldrich syndrome

This patient was initially diagnosed with psoriasis because of the presence of thickened erythematous plaques on the skin. While atopic dermatitis presents with poorly demarcated erythematous plaques on the flexor surfaces, plaque psoriasis presents as sharply demarcated papules and plaques with overlying silvery scale that are symmetrically distributed and may be found on the elbows, knees, scalp, extremities, trunk, and intergluteal fold. If the two conditions cannot be distinguished clinically, they may be distinguished by skin biopsy.

CLINICAL PEARL **STEP 2/3**

Features associated with atopic dermatitis include increased prominence of the palmar creases, prominent horizontal folds beneath the lower lid (Dennie-Morgan lines), periorbital darkening, central facial pallor, thinning of the lateral eyebrows (Hertoghe sign), and follicular prominence (goose-bump-like appearance of the skin).

Further analysis of skin biopsy shows "spongiotic dermatitis and superficial perivascular dermatitis with eosinophils and without evidence of psoriasis, compatible with an eczematous dermatitis."

What are the histologic features of atopic dermatitis?

On histology, acute atopic dermatitis will show prominent spongiosis (intercellular edema), intraepidermal vesicles, and perivascular lymphohistiocytic inflammation with eosinophils. Subacute atopic dermatitis will show milder spongiosis with hyperkeratosis and increased acanthosis (proliferation of the epidermis), and chronic atopic dermatitis shows marked acanthosis with minimal to no spongiosis (Fig. 15.2).

What are variants of atopic dermatitis?

Hand eczema is common in adults with atopic dermatitis and dyshidrotic eczema occurs when the palms and sides of fingers develop vesicles. In nummular eczema, coin shaped erythematous scaly plaques appear on the trunk and extremities. Other regional variants of atopic dermatitis include nipple eczema, ear eczema in the retroauricular region, and eyelid eczema.

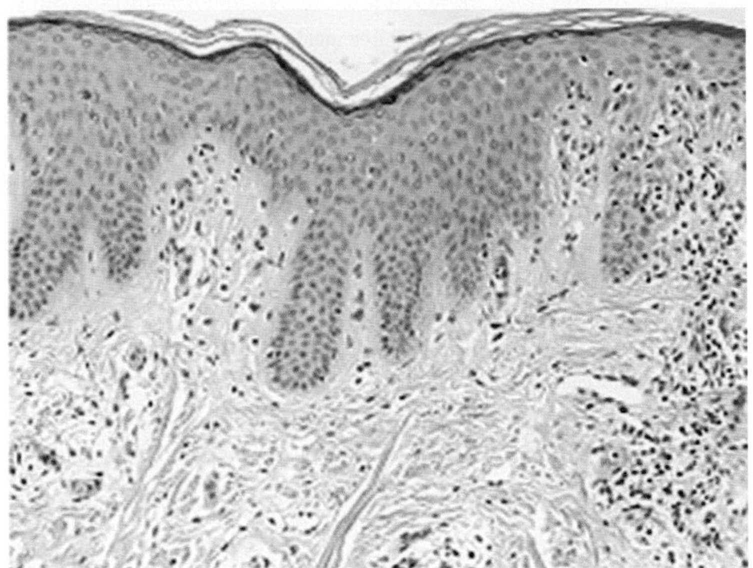

Fig. 15.2 Histology of chronic atopic dermatitis showing acanthosis of the epidermis, spongiosis, and a lymphohistiocytic infiltrate with few eosinophils. (From Hassan, A. S., Kaelin, U., Braathen, L. R., et al. (2007). Clinical and immunopathologic findings during treatment of recalcitrant atopic eczema with efalizumab. *Journal of the American Academy of Dermatology*, *56*(2), 217–221.)

How is atopic dermatitis treated?

Atopic dermatitis is a chronic, relapsing disease and its management requires treatment of active dermatitis, as well as maintenance of skin barrier function and avoidance of triggers.

Bathing with lukewarm water, using a mild cleanser, and the liberal use of emollients is recommended in order to maintain skin barrier function. For active lesions, topical corticosteroids are first-line therapy to control the inflammation. Topical calcineurin inhibitors (tacrolimus, pimecrolimus) may also be used, especially in areas that are susceptible to corticosteroid-induced skin atrophy, such as the face, axillae, and groin. Wet wrap therapy, in which moist occlusive dressings are used to improve the penetration of topical corticosteroids and increase skin hydration, is also beneficial.

Systemic antiinflammatory therapies and phototherapy with narrowband UVB, broadband UVB, psoralen plus UVA (PUVA), and UVA1 can be added for patients with moderate to severe atopic dermatitis that have not responded to topical corticosteroids. Systemic therapies effective in atopic dermatitis include methotrexate, mycophenolate mofetil, azathioprine, cyclosporine, and the IL-4/IL-13 inhibitor dupilumab. Sedating antihistamines (diphenhydramine, hydroxyzine) may be given at bedtime to control pruritus that disrupts sleep (Table 15.2).

The patient in this case improved with topical corticosteroids and diligent use of emollients.

BASIC SCIENCE/CLINICAL PEARL **STEP 1/2/3**

Methotrexate inhibits the enzyme dihydrofolate reductase, suppressing DNA synthesis, and is often concurrently administered with folic acid. It has the potential to cause bone marrow suppression and hepatotoxicity.

TABLE 15.2 ■ **Atopic Dermatitis Treatment Ladder**

Treatment Options
Moisturizers
Topical corticosteroids
Topical calcineurin inhibitors
Topical crisaborole
narrowband UVB, broadband UVB, psoralen plus UVA (PUVA), and UVA1
Dupilumab
Azathioprine
Mycophenolate mofetil
Methotrexate
Adjunctive Therapies
Sedating oral antihistamines (diphenhydramine, hydroxyzine)
Wet wraps
Dilute sodium hypochlorite (bleach) baths
Treatment of bacterial, viral, or fungal superinfection phototherapy

What are the complications of atopic dermatitis?

An impaired skin barrier and immune dysregulation make the lesions of atopic dermatitis susceptible to bacterial and viral infections. Impetiginization from *Staphylococcus aureus* and *Streptococcus pyogenes* infections may occur. Eczema herpeticum caused by herpes simplex virus infection presents as monomorphic "punched out" lesions over eczematous patches.

Case Summary

- **Complaint/History:** A 62-year-old woman presenting with 8 years of a pruritic rash previously diagnosed as psoriasis, for which she had recently been hospitalized, and which did not respond to the TNF-α inhibitor etanercept,
- **Findings:** Vital signs are unremarkable. Skin exam reveals erythematous, lichenified, and poorly demarcated plaques with overlying excoriations covering >40% of her body surface area, including the upper back, gluteal cleft, posterior thighs, and extensor surfaces of both upper extremities.
- **Lab Results/Tests:** Skin biopsy shows spongiotic dermatitis and superficial perivascular dermatitis with eosinophils and without evidence of psoriasis, consistent with atopic dermatitis.

Diagnosis: Atopic dermatitis.

- **Treatment:** Topical corticosteroids with counseling on the use of emollients for maintenance of the skin barrier.

BEYOND THE PEARLS

- Triggers for atopic dermatitis include extremes in temperature, wool and synthetic fabrics, detergents, environmental allergens such as dust mites and pollen, and skin infection with *Staphylococcus aureus*.
- More than 90% of individuals with atopic dermatitis have skin colonized with *Staphylococcus aureus*, compared with 5% of individuals without atopic dermatitis.
- Mutations in the filaggrin gene (FLG) are associated with earlier onset atopic dermatitis that is more likely to persist into adulthood.
- Filaggrin gene mutations also cause ichthyosis vulgaris, which presents with dry, scaling skin due to impaired formation of cornified keratinocytes.
- Keratosis pilaris, a condition that presents with keratotic follicular papules on the upper arms, thighs, face, and trunk, affects >40% of individuals with atopic dermatitis.
- Children and adolescents with atopic dermatitis may also be affected by pityriasis alba, which presents as hypopigmented macules and patches on the face with overlying fine scale.

Bibliography

Barrett, M., & Luu, M. (2017). Differential diagnosis of atopic dermatitis. *Immunology and Allergy Clinics of North America*, *37*(1), 11–34.

Bieber. T. (2008). Atopic dermatitis. *The New England Journal of Medicine*, *358*, 1483–1494.

Bouthillette, M., Beccati, D., Akthakul, A., et al. (2020). A crosslinked polymer skin barrier film for moderate to severe atopic dermatitis: A pilot study in adults. *Journal of the American Academy of Dermatology*, *82*(4), 895–901.

Eichenfield, L. F., Tom, W. L., Chamlin, S. L., et al. (2014). Guidelines of care for the management of atopic dermatitis: Section 1. Diagnosis and assessment of atopic dermatitis. *Journal of the American Academy of Dermatology*, *70*(2), 338–351.

Eichenfield, L. F., Tom, W. L., Berger, T. G., et al. (2014). Guidelines of care for the management of atopic dermatitis: Section 2. Management and treatment of atopic dermatitis with topical therapies. *Journal of the American Academy of Dermatology*, *71*(1), 116–132.

Hassan, A. S., Kaelin, U., Braathen, L. R., et al. (2007). Clinical and immunopathologic findings during treatment of recalcitrant atopic eczema with efalizumab. *Journal of the American Academy of Dermatology*, *56*(2), 217–221.

Irvine, A. D., McLean, W. H. I., & Leung, D. Y. M. (2011). Filaggrin mutations associated with skin and allergic diseases. *The New England Journal of Medicine*, *365*, 1315–1327.

MacAleer, M. A., O'Regan, G. M., & Irvine, A. D. (2017). Atopic Dermatitis. In J. L. Bolognia, J. V. Schaffer, & L. Cerroni (Eds.), *Dermatology* (4th ed., pp. 1644–1663). Philadelphia, PA: Elsevier.

Nestle, F. O., Kaplan, D. H., & Barker, J. (2009). Psoriasis. *The New England Journal of Medicine*, *361*, 496–509.

Sehra, S., Yao, Y., Howell, M. D., et al. (2010). IL-4 regulates skin homeostasis and the predisposition toward allergic skin inflammation. *Journal of Immunology*, *184*, 3186–3190.

Sidbury, R., Davis, D. M., Cohen, D. E., et al. (2014). American Academy of Dermatology. Guidelines of care for the management of atopic dermatitis: Section 3. Management and treatment with phototherapy and systemic agents. *Journal of the American Academy of Dermatology*, *71*(2), 327–349.

Van de Kerkhof, P. C. M., & Nestlé, (2017). Psoriasis. In J. L. Bolognia, J. V. Schaffer, & L. Cerroni (Eds.), *Dermatology* (4th ed., pp. 1644–1663). Philadelphia, PA: Elsevier.

SECTION 5

Neurology

CASE 16

A 28-Year-Old Male With Progressive Lower Back Pain, Paraplegia, and Urinary Incontinence

Colin M. McCrimmon ■ An H. Do

A 28-year-old male without significant medical history presents to the emergency department complaining of progressive lower back pain, inability to move the lower extremities, loss of lower extremity sensation, and urinary incontinence for 2 days. His back pain is constant, non- radiating, and 8 out of 10 in severity. He noticed decreased perianal sensation 2 days earlier and has lost bowel and bladder sensation. He denies recent history of trauma, infection, or IV drug abuse. On physical examination, the patient is not in acute distress but has soiled himself with urine and feces. His blood pressure is 119/74 mmHg, heart rate is 96/min, respiration rate is 16/min, and oxygen saturation is 96% on room air. His cranial nerve exam was normal, and the patient had normal strength and sensation in his upper extremities. His lower extremity strength is 0/5 bilaterally. When asked to sit up from a supine position, he is unable to and exhibits a positive Beevor's sign. The rectal exam reveals markedly reduced external sphincter tone. He exhibits diminished sensation to light touch and pinprick below the umbilicus with absent temperature and vibration sensation. His reflexes are absent in his lower extremities bilaterally with flexor plantar responses. He is unable to ambulate.

Fig. 16.1 provides a review of the neuroanatomical tracts that, when damaged, contribute to the above examination findings. Fig. 16.2 depicts a dermatomal map with the sensation in each segment corresponding to a specific spinal level.

BASIC SCIENCE/CLINICAL PEARL **STEP 2/3**

An injury to the spinal cord can result in:

- Weakness: Most spinal cord injuries affect bilateral corticospinal tracts and thus result in bilateral spastic paraparesis below the level of the injury (quadriparesis may occur if the injury involves the cervical spinal cord and paraparesis at the thoracic spinal cord or lower). In some cases where there is only injury to a unilateral corticospinal tract, ipsilesional spastic paresis will be seen below the level of the injury due to disruption in the ipsilesional corticospinal tract (upper motor neurons). At the level of the injury, or if nerve roots are involved, the lower motor neurons may also be affected causing flaccid paralysis. Spinal cord injuries can also lead to decreased anal tone as well as bowel and bladder incontinence.
- Sensory deficits: Most spinal cord injuries affect bilateral dorsal columns and spinothalamic tracts. This results in bilateral loss of touch, vibration, pain, and temperature sensation,

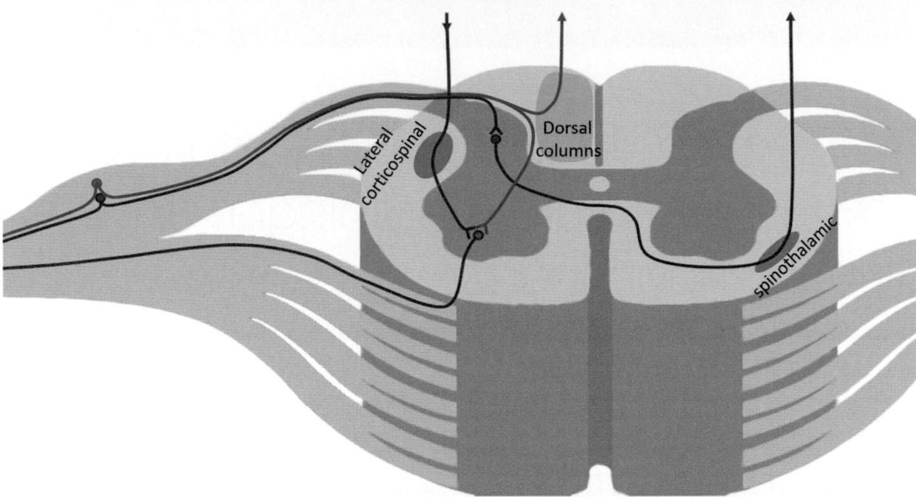

Fig. 16.1 Upper motor neurons descend primarily through the lateral aspect of the spinal cord—that is, the lateral corticospinal tract—to innervate corresponding lower motor neurons. This motor pathway is depicted in *red*. Note that another descending motor pathway, the anterior corticospinal tract, is not depicted. Neurons shown in *blue* are involved in the sensation of touch, vibration, and proprioception, and provide upgoing sensory input to the brain via the dorsal column-medial lemniscus pathway. Note that the cell bodies of these neurons lie in the dorsal root ganglia. Neurons shown in *purple* are involved in the sensation of pain and temperature and provide upgoing sensory input to the brain via the spinothalamic tract. The second-order neurons in this pathway appear to decussate near their cell bodies at the same spinal level in this figure. However, in reality, the second-order neurons may ascend a few spinal levels (typically 1–2) prior to their decussation and subsequent ascension through the spinothalamic tract.

as well as proprioception, below the level of the injury. In some cases where there is only injury to one side of the spinal cord, damage to the ipsilesional dorsal columns causes ipsilesional loss of touch and vibration sensation as well as proprioception at and below the level of the injury. Damage to the spinothalamic tract would cause contralateral loss of pain and temperature sensation one or two dermatomal segments below the level of the injury and ipsilesional loss of pain and temperature sensation at the level of injury.

- Abnormal reflexes: Damage to the lateral corticospinal tract results in ipsilateral hyperreflexia below the level of the injury. There can potentially be hyporeflexia at the level of the injury.

CLINICAL PEARL **STEP 2/3**

Note that in the acute phase of injury, flaccid rather than spastic paresis may predominate below the level of the injury. Similarly, in the acute phase of injury, hyporeflexia rather than hyperreflexia may predominate below the level of the injury.

CLINICAL PEARL **STEP 2/3**

The umbilicus corresponds to the 10th thoracic segment (T10) of the spinal cord. When there is a lesion in the spinal cord or nerve roots between T10–T12 or if there is weakness predominantly in the infraumbilical portion of the rectus abdominis muscle, the patient's umbilicus will migrate upwards when an attempt is made to sit up from a supine position. This is known as Beevor's sign. It is commonly seen with thoracic spinal cord lesions affecting T10–T12 but can also be seen in patients with myopathies, such as facioscapulohumeral muscular dystrophy, or other neuromuscular disorders.

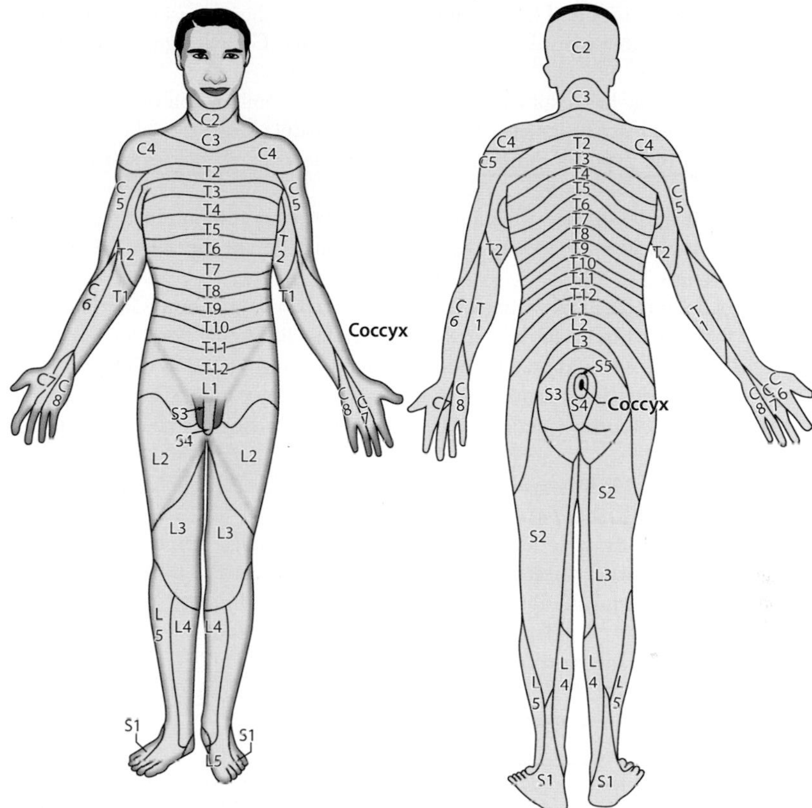

Fig. 16.2 Dermatomal map with the sensation in each segment corresponding to a specific spinal level. *C*, Cervical; *L*, lumbar; *S*, sacral; *T*, thoracic. (From Shankar N, Vaz M, Textbook of applied anatomy and applied physiology for nurses, ed 2. Delhi, Elsevier, 2022.)

What are some possible causes of motor weakness and loss of sensation in the lower extremities, together with loss of bowel and bladder control?

- Spinal cord lesions:
  The vast majority (>90%) of spinal cord injuries are traumatic/iatrogenic in etiology. Potential nontraumatic etiologies include transverse myelitis (e.g., multiple sclerosis, acute disseminated encephalomyelitis, infectious myelopathy, inflammatory disorders), compression (e.g., from epidural abscess, tumors, vertebral subluxation, severe and sudden disc herniation), vascular malformations, spinal cord infarction, metabolic diseases (e.g., vitamin B_{12} deficiency), and syringomyelia.
- Peripheral nerve disease:
  Examples include Guillain-Barré syndrome (GBS) and related variants (e.g., acute inflammatory demyelinating polyneuropathy, acute motor-sensory axonal neuropathy), infection (e.g., HIV, diphtheria, Lyme), and toxins (e.g., neurotoxic chemotherapeutic agents, organophosphates).
- Brain/brainstem:
  Certain brain lesions can produce some of the above array of signs and symptoms. For example, bilateral lower extremity weakness can be caused by bilateral anterior cerebral artery territory infarcts, parasagittal masses, and surgery involving the parasagittal region. However, overall, these causes are rare.

Given the patient's history and demographics, some of the above causes are more likely than others. For example, transverse myelitis, cord compression, and GBS are more typical of this age group and presentation.

The patient most likely has a spinal cord lesion, given the combination of paraplegia, incontinence, and bilateral lower-extremity sensory deficits with distinct sensory level (10th thoracic vertebrae, or T10, given the patient's diminished sensation below the umbilicus and the presence of Beevor's sign).

Acute peripheral nerve disease affecting motor, sensory, and autonomic systems is possible. However, it is less likely given the sharp delineation of sensation at the level T10 as well as the lack of recent infection.

Based on the somatotopic organization of the motor cortex, a brain lesion is less likely given that it must involve the parasagittal areas bilaterally. It is even less likely that both the left and internal capsule and thalamic areas would be affected. Although a brainstem lesion could produce motor, sensory, and autonomic deficits, it is unlikely in this case given the patient's lack of cranial deficits.

Due to the presence of sensory deficits, a disease process involving the neuromuscular junction can be ruled out.

What study should be done first as part of your workup?

Given the likelihood of a thoracic-level spinal cord injury, a thoracic-spine MRI should be performed to affirm the presence of any lesion and to narrow down the differential diagnosis. A lumbar-spine MRI may be justified to determine the extent of the lesion. Further imaging studies such as a brain MRI can be considered if previous spinal imaging is negative. If all neuroimaging studies were unremarkable, the next step would be to consider peripheral nerve disease. Serological testing, a lumbar puncture for cerebrospinal fluid (CSF) testing, and an electromyography/nerve-conduction study would be recommended in that case.

The patient underwent a thoracic- and lumbar-spine MRI (see Figs. 16.3 and 16.4) that revealed an intramedullary spinal lesion extending from T10 to L2. A brain MRI was also performed and was normal.

What is your differential diagnosis at this time?

Given the presence of an intramedullary enhancing lesion that involves both white and gray matter and extends through the thoracic and lumbar spine without any brain involvement, the patient probably has a primary or secondary malignancy.

Spinal cord tumors account for about 15% of all central nervous system tumors. These tumors can be classified based on their locations (Table 16.1).

What should your next steps in management be?

The tumor is most likely an ependymoma or astrocytoma. However, a biopsy must be performed first along with a neurosurgical consultation in order to make a definitive diagnosis.

The surgical biopsy of the spinal cord showed a WHO Grade IV, H3K27M, MGMT negative, mutated glioblastoma multiforme (GBM), a highly malignant type of infiltrative spinal cord astrocytoma.

CLINICAL PEARL **STEP 3**

Prognosis with primary spinal GBM is guarded, as overall mean survival has been estimated to be around 14 months. Mean survival is slightly improved for thoracic and thoracolumbar lesions compared with purely cervical and lumbar lesions.

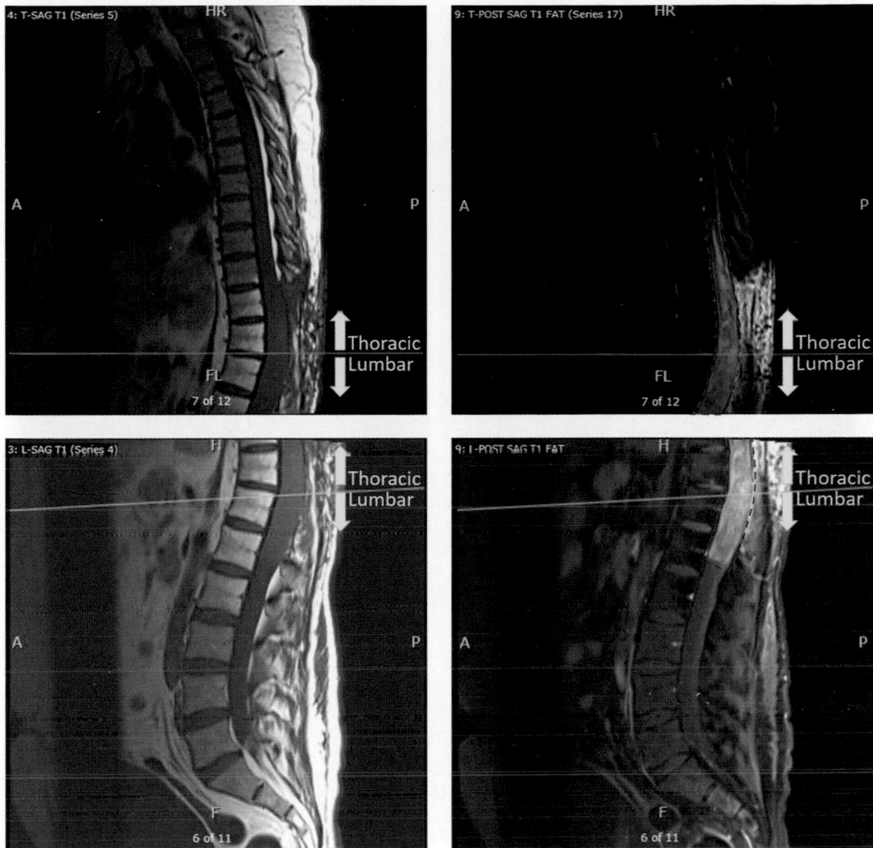

Fig. 16.3 Sagittal images from the precontrast thoracic *(top left)* and lumbar *(bottom left)* magnetic resonance imaging (MRI) and the fat-suppressed postcontrast thoracic *(top right)* and lumbar *(bottom right)* MRI. Note the presence of an intramedullary spinal cord lesion extending from T10 to L2 that is enhanced (bright) postcontrast (outlined in *red*). Note that the patient has lumbarization of S1.

How would you manage This patient's treatment?

Although surgical resection (gross or subtotal) may improve mean survival in patients with primary spinal GBM, resection may not always be feasible given the risk of further neurological injury. Thus, other modalities such radiation therapy, chemotherapy, and immunotherapy can be pursued. These therapies are typically coordinated by a neurooncology specialist.

While more definitive treatment is being pursued, temporizing measures to maximize preservation of neurological function can be administered. Such temporizing measures primarily include glucocorticosteroid administration, typically high-dose dexamethasone, to reduce perilesional vasogenic edema and temporarily preserve/improve neurological function.

For this patient, neurosurgery recommended no surgical intervention. He was treated with bevacizumab 10 mg/kg with a plan to start bevacizumab and panobinostat combination therapy three times weekly with radiation therapy. Initial high-dose dexamethasone therapy was also given to maximize preservation of neurological function. The patient is expected to remain paraplegic indefinitely and required supportive treatment that includes urinary catherization for neurogenic bladder and establishment of a daily bowel regimen.

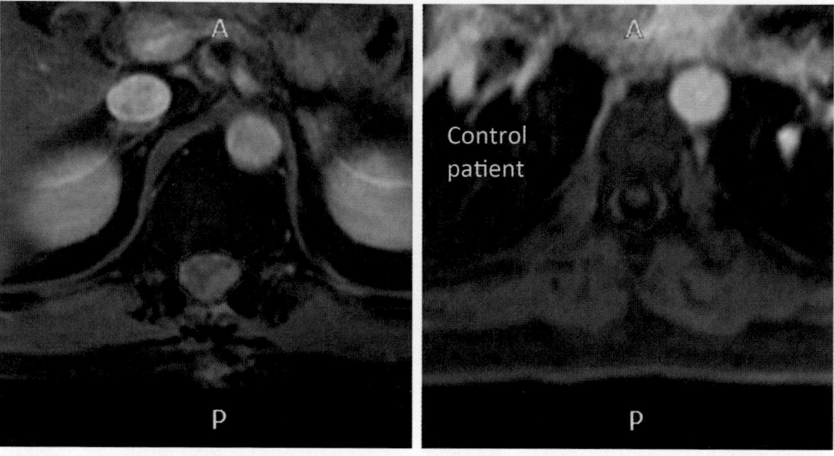

Fig. 16.4 On the *left* is an axial fat-suppressed postcontrast T1 magnetic resonance imaging (MRI) scan of the thoracic cord (around spinal level T12) showing an intramedullary mass with obliteration of the normal spinal cord architecture with no preferential sparing of the white or gray matter (outlined in *red*). Compare this with a fat-suppressed T1 MRI scan (on the *right*) of the thoracic cord of a normal control patient. (Image on right from Saeedan, M. S., Alabdulkarim, F. M., Aloufi, F.F., Alghofaily, K. A., Parkar, N., Ghosh S. (2020). Check the chest: review of chest findings on abdominal MRI. *Clinical Imaging, 59*(1), 68–77.)

TABLE 16.1 ■ **Tumors of the Spinal Cord**

- Intramedullary tumors occur inside the spinal cord parenchyma. Typical examples include ependymomas, astrocytomas, hemangioblastomas, and rare metastatic intramedullary tumors.
- Intradural–extramedullary tumors occur within the dura but outside the parenchyma. Typical examples include meningiomas and neurofibromas.
- Extradural tumors occur outside the dura. Typical examples include metastases from outside the spinal column.

Case Summary

- **Compaint/History:** A 28-year-old male with progressive lower back pain, inability to move the lower extremities, and urinary incontinence for 2 days.
- **Findings:** His lower extremity strength is 0/5 bilaterally with absent reflexes. Patient has markedly reduced external sphincter tone and exhibits diminished sensation to light touch and pinprinck below the umbilicus with absent temperature and vibration sensation.
- **Lab Results/ Tests:** A thoracic- and lumbar-spine MRI revealed an intramedullary spinal lesion extending from T10-L2. A biopsy was performed.

Diagnosis: glioblastoma multiforme

- **Treatment:** Patient was treated with high dose dexamethoasone and combination therapy with bevacizumab and panobinostat three times weekly with radiation therapy.

BEYOND THE PEARLS

- Intramedullary spinal tumors account for only 2%–5% of all spinal cord tumors. Gliomas comprise 80% of these and include ependymomas and astrocytomas.
- Ependymomas are typically found in middle-aged adults, and preferentially arise in the lumbosacral spinal cord. Gross total resection comprises the entirety of standard treatment, although adjuvant radiotherapy may have a role in myxopapillary and anaplastic subtypes (Welch, Schiff, & Gerszten, 2019).
- Astrocytomas are also typically found in middle-aged adults and arise most commonly in the thoracic level. The two subtypes, pilocytic and infiltrative, occur with similar frequency. For both subtypes, maximal resection is recommended, although complete resection is more difficult for infiltrative spinal cord astrocytomas due to the lack of clear tissue planes and risk of neurologic injury. Infiltrative astrocytomas are associated with poor prognosis and may be an indication for adjuvant radiotherapy. There may even be a role for chemotherapy and immunotherapy in the treatment of these tumors.
- Hemangioblastomas and metastatic intramedullary tumors are less common than gliomas. Metastatic intramedullary tumors typically originate from the lung or breasts but can also originate from the brain or colon. Other intramedullary tumors including lipomas, germ-cell tumors, gangliogliomas, germinomas, and lymphomas are extremely rarev.
- Spinal cord lesions can present with weakness and sensory deficits. Typically, both sides of the spinal cord are involved, yielding bilateral motor and sensory deficits (paraplegia or quadriplegia). However, unilateral lesions occasionally occur, causing ipsilesional motor impairment, ipsilesional proprioceptive and vibroceptive sensory loss, and contralesional pain and temperature sensory loss.
- If a spinal cord lesion is suspected, MR imaging should typically be performed.
- If a tumor is suspected in the spinal canal, a biopsy may be needed to make a definitive tissue diagnosis.
- The most common spinal cord tumors are meningiomas (extramedullary).
- The most common types of intramedullary spinal tumors are gliomas, such as ependymomas and astrocytomas.
- Management of spinal tumors with recent onset of weakness and sensory deficits includes temporizing measures, such as glucocorticosteroid administration, and surgical or chemotherapeutic treatment based on the biopsy results. Supportive measures such as urinary catheterization and establishment of a daily bowel regimen should always be considered. Rehabilitation will also be needed to maximize potential functional independence based on residual neurological functions.

Bibliography

Biller, J., Gruener, G., & Brazis, P.W. (2017). *DeMyer's the neurologic examination: A programmed text.* (7th ed). New York, NY: McGraw-Hill Education.

Blumenfeld, H. (2010). *Neuroanatomy through clinical cases.* (2nd ed). Sunderland, MA: Sinauer Associates.

Brazis, P. W., Masdeu, J. C., Biller, J. (2017). *Localization in Clinical Neurology.* (7th ed). Philadelphia, PA: Lippincott Williams & Wilkins/Wolters Kluwer.

Das, J. M., Hoang, S., Mesfin, F. B. (2020). *Intramedullary Spinal Cord Tumors. StatPearls.* Treasure Island, FL: StatPearls Publishing.

Shen, C.-X., Wu, J.-F., Zhao, W., Cai, Z.-W., Cai, R.-Z., & Chen, C.-M. (2017). Primary spinal glioblastoma multiforme. *Medicine*, 96(16), e6634.

CASE 17

A 23-Year-Old Male With Severe Headache Behind the Right Eye

Chelsea Stone ■ Esther Byun

A 23-year-old male presents to the emergency room with a severe 10/10 headache behind his right eye that started 30 minutes prior, peaking within minutes.

Which signs and symptoms must we ask about when a patient presents with this type of headache?
Red flag symptoms may suggest a secondary, serious etiology of headache. For example, in the setting of headache, fever, neck stiffness, and/or altered sensorium raises suspicion of meningitis or encephalitis. Thunderclap headache raises concern for subarachnoid hemorrhage. Worsening severe headache with focal neurological deficits is worrisome for cerebral venous sinus thrombosis. A recent head injury followed by headache raises the possibility of traumatic subdural hemorrhage.

The mnemonic "SNOOP" can be helpful:

- **S**ystemic symptoms (fever, neck stiffness, unstable vital signs, weight loss)
- **S**econdary risk factors (human immunodeficiency virus, malignancy, current/recent pregnancy)
- **N**eurological symptoms or signs (weakness, vision changes, papilledema, sensory changes, altered level of consciousness)
- **O**nset (sudden, severe)
- **O**lder (new, changed, or progressive headache in patient > 50 years of age)
- **P**rior headache history (is this the first headache or a different headache than usual?)

The patient reports he had three severe right-sided headaches in the past 5 days, similar in quality, lasting about 2 hours each. He was up late the night before with friends, drinking beer and smoking. The headache woke him from sleep but is not worsened by lying down. He denies nausea, vomiting, sensitivity to light or sound, neck pain, or trauma.

He was diagnosed with migraine headache after he suffered prior severe headaches; otherwise, he has no medical problems aside from seasonal allergies. He was prescribed oral sumatriptan for migraine headaches, and he did take this after headache onset with no benefit. He takes no other prescribed medications or supplements and has never used illicit drugs.

Temperature is 37°C (98.6°F), blood pressure is 155/85, pulse rate is 90/min, respiration rate is 20/min, and oxygen saturation is 99% on room air. He is a lean young man—at times sitting with his head in his hands, other times pacing the room in pain. He is upset, irritable, and sweating. There is redness, swelling, and tearing of the right eye. There is no papilledema. His neurologic exam is normal; there is no double vision, sensory loss in the face or body, motor weakness, or reflex asymmetry, and gait is normal. The emergency room performed a noncontrast CT of the head, which was normal.

What is your differential diagnosis for this patient?
Although the patient's headache is severe and sudden in onset, reassuringly he is young, has a prior history of similar headaches, and has no focal neurological deficits.

This patient complains of severe orbital pain and has trigeminal autonomic symptoms. The trigeminal autonomic cephalalgias (TACs) are a group of headaches involving a similar cranial distribution, varying in frequency, symptom duration, triggers, and treatments (Table 17.1). Top of the differential for this patient is cluster headache, one of the TACs.

- Cluster headaches last 15–180 minutes, occurring between one and eight times per day during certain times of the year.
- Paroxysmal hemicrania is similar to cluster headache, but attacks are less severe. Events are shorter (2–30 min) and more frequent.
- Short-acting unilateral neuralgiform headache attacks with conjunctival injection and tearing (SUNCT) and short-lasting unilateral neuralgiform headache attacks with cranial autonomic symptoms (SUNA) can last for a few seconds and can occur hundreds of times per day.
- Hemicrania continua is a constant aching headache in the trigeminal distribution with intermittent sharp, stabbing exacerbations throughout the day.

CLINICAL PEARL **STEP 1/2/3**

A good rule of thumb is the longer the name of the disorder, the shorter and more frequent the attacks.

TABLE 17.1 ■ **Typical Clinical Features of Trigeminal Autonomic Cephalalgias, Including Hemicrania Continua**

	Cluster headache	Paroxysmal hemicrania	Sunct syndrome	Hemicrania continua
Sex F:M	1:3.5–7	2.13–2.36:1	1:2.1	2.4:1
Pain:				
Type	Stabbing, boring	Throbbing, boring, stabbing	Burning, stabbing, sharp	Background dull ache, throbbing/stabbing exacerbations
Severity	Excruciating	Excruciating	Severe	Moderate background pain; severe exacerbations
Site	Orbit, temple	Orbit, temple	Periorbital	Orbit, temple
Attack frequency	1 every other day–8 daily	1–40/day	1/day–30/hr	Continuous
Duration of attack	15–180 min	2–45 min	5–250 sec	Continuous background pain; exacerbations quite variable and lasting minutes to days
Autonomic features	Yes	Yes	Yes (prominent conjunctival injection and lacrimation)	Yes—mainly with exacerbations; less prominent than with other TACs
Migrainous features*	Yes	Yes	Yes†	Yes—during exacerbations
Alcohol trigger	Yes	Occasional	No	Rare
Indomethacin effect	–	++	–	++
Abortive treatment	Sumatriptan injection or nasal spray Oxygen	Nil	Nil	Nil
Prophylactic treatment	Verapamil Methysergide Lithium Prednisolone	Indomethacin	Lamotrigine Topiramate Gabapentin	Indomethacin

TACs, trigeminal autonomic cephalalgias.
*Nausea, photophobia, or phonophobia.
†Photophobia homolateral to pain.
(From McMahon SB et al, Wall & Melzak's textbook of pain, ed 6. Philadelphia, Elsevier, 2013.)

Conjunctival injection, lacrimation, nasal congestion, and rhinorrhea can also be experienced in migraine disorders. Although there can be overlap between TACs and migraine, the description of this patient's headache is more consistent with a TAC—cluster headache in particular. Migraine is much more common than cluster headache, however; often there is a delay in diagnosis in cluster headache, as with this patient.

CLINICAL PEARL **STEP 1/2/3**

Migraine headaches tend to be less severe, last longer, and do not have the regularity/periodicity of cluster headache. Migraineurs often want to lie down in dark rooms during a headache, whereas patients with cluster headache often cannot sit still.

Trigeminal neuralgia also affects the trigeminal distribution, but pain is sudden and short, precipitated by touch, chewing, or wind. Trigeminal autonomic features are not typical. Temporal arteritis is unlikely in our young patient. The pain of temporal arteritis is typically continuous (although it may wax and wane); there may be jaw claudication, vision changes, and systemic symptoms such as fever and myalgia. Sedimentation rate and C-related peptide are often elevated.

Why is this pain syndrome called "cluster headache"?

Cluster headaches are known as the most painful of primary headache disorders, reportedly more painful than childbirth—leading to the name "suicide headache." They are called "cluster" because headache attacks cluster together, usually over a few weeks or months. Headaches may develop like clockwork at certain times of day, recurring every day during certain seasons of the year; then they might stop. The time between attacks is known as remission, lasting days to years. Most patients have episodic cluster headache (85%–90%), but some patients have continuous attacks without remission.

- Episodic cluster headache: at least two cluster periods lasting from 7 days to 1 year (untreated) separated by pain-free remission periods of ≥3 months.
- Chronic cluster headache: cluster periods occurring for 1 year or longer without remission or with remission periods lasting less than 3 months.

Most patients have a single cluster period in a year, but some have fewer and others have several bouts per year.

Which trigeminal autonomic symptoms should we ask about and seek out on examination when considering cluster headache?

In cluster headache, at least one of the following autonomic symptoms should be present ipsilateral to the headache (Fig. 17.1):

- Conjunctival injection and/or lacrimation
- Nasal congestion and/or rhinorrhea
- Eyelid edema
- Forehead and facial sweating
- Miosis and/or ptosis

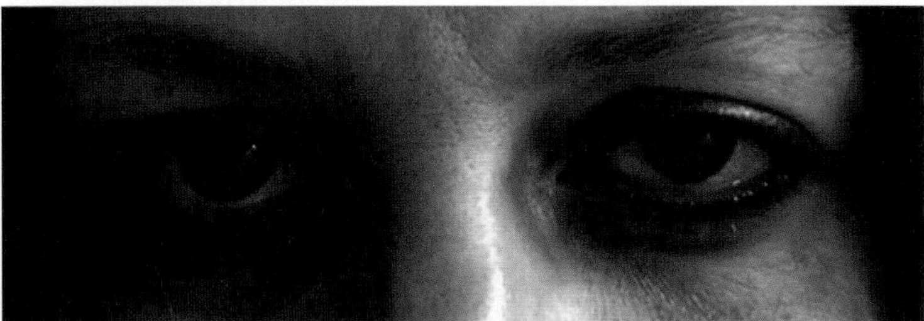

Fig. 17.1 Left-sided cluster headache with miosis, ptosis, increased lacrimation, and conjunctival injection. (From Hale, N. & Paauw, D. S. (2014). Diagnosis and treatment of headache in the ambulatory care setting. *Medical Clinics of North America*, *98*(3), 505–527.)

If there are no autonomic symptoms, patients must endorse restlessness and/or agitation to meet criteria for the disorder. Many patients will pace back and forth during an attack.

Which diagnostic tests should be performed?

Sometimes headaches secondary to a structural brain lesion can cause cluster headache–like symptoms, whether due to pituitary tumors or cavernous sinus disease. This patient's CT of the head is reassuring. An MRI of the brain can be pursued at some point, but not necessarily urgently in the ED. The clinical suspicion of cluster headache is high, given the presentation and history of similar headaches; therefore, lumbar puncture and angiography would typically not be pursued.

CLINICAL PEARL **STEP 2/3**

In a patient with longstanding headaches, a marked change in headache character or features would be indications for obtaining an MRI of the brain with contrast.

How should this patient's headache be treated?

Acute treatment options include 100% oxygen and triptan medications. High flow 100% oxygen has no side effects, is very effective for most patients, and is easily provided in the emergency room. Subcutaneous and intranasal triptan medications are also highly effective, but oral triptans are not. Alternative therapies include intranasal lidocaine, oral ergotamine, and intravenous dihydroergotamines. Noninvasive vagus nerve stimulation has also been FDA approved for the treatment of acute cluster attacks.

As with all headache sufferers, identification and avoidance of triggers is essential. Appropriate management can help minimize attack frequency and severity. Prophylactic therapy should be started immediately at the onset of a cluster period and can be weaned off after a cluster period has ended. Verapamil is the preventive treatment of choice. Because of concerns for cardiac conduction abnormalities with this medication, an electrocardiogram is often obtained at the onset of treatment and 10–14 days after dose changes. Glucocorticoids could be offered to this patient for short-term prophylaxis to reduce the frequency of headaches while the verapamil dose is increased. Second-line prophylactic medications are topiramate, lithium, and the calcitonin gene-related peptide antagonist, galcanezumab. Melatonin may be a useful adjuvant. Targeted interventions such as occipital nerve blocks and sphenopalatine ganglion blocks can be beneficial.

The patient received 100% oxygen and the pain improved within 5 minutes. For headache prevention, he received prescriptions for verapamil and a short course of glucocorticoids.

CLINICAL PEARL **STEP 2/3**

For migraine and cluster headache, patients should be offered both abortive therapy (treatments to stop the ongoing headache) and prophylactic treatment if the headaches are regular/recurrent (typically daily medications to prevent headache; in the case of migraine headache this could include monthly injectable medications or botulinum injections every 3 months). Sometimes patients and practitioners conflate the two and some patients inadvertently take their prophylactic medication on an as-needed basis (with little success).

What are some common triggers for this condition?

Alcohol, even in small quantities, can cause an attack in over half of patients during a cluster period. Nitroglycerin, histamine, and other vasodilators can also trigger cluster headache attacks. Patients report heat, exercise, strong smells (solvents and cigarette smoke), hypoxia, and high altitude can precipitate cluster headache during a cluster period.

Who develops cluster headaches?

Cluster headaches are the most common of the TACs, with a prevalence rate of about 1 in 1000. The typical patient is a 20- to 40-year-old man (3:1 male to female ratio). There is a high incidence of smoking in patients with cluster headaches.

Sometimes headaches are so severe that patients do not notice or think to mention their trigeminal autonomic symptoms. You should ask about them in all headache patients, especially if they are not experiencing the headache at the time of evaluation.

Case Summary

- **Complaint/History:** A 23-year-old man presents to the emergency room with a severe 10/10 headache behind his right eye that started 30 minutes prior, peaking within minutes. He has had three similar severe right-sided headaches in the past 5 days, similar in quality, lasting about 2 hours each.
- **Findings:** The patient is pacing the room in pain. There is redness, swelling, and tearing of the right eye. Neurologic exam is normal.
- **Lab Results/Tests:** None pursued. (MRI with contrast is ordered nonurgently and is ultimately normal; there are no structural brain lesions causing the trigeminal autonomic cephalalgia.)

Diagnosis: Cluster headache.

- **Treatment:** With high flow oxygen, the pain resolved. He was discharged from the emergency room with home oxygen. He received corticosteroids as cluster headache prophylaxis and his verapamil dose was increased.

BEYOND THE PEARLS

- Migraine and cluster headache can be confused. Migraine is far more common and cluster headache can be misdiagnosed as migraine headache. Cluster headache is a trigeminal autonomic cephalalgia that leads to bouts of severe pain with associated ipsilateral trigeminal symptoms. Usually patients are restless and agitated; in contrast, migraine patients often prefer to lie down in a dark room.
- Nausea, vomiting, photophobia, phonophobia, and aura can occur in cluster headache. They are not exclusively migraine headache accompaniments and their presence does not exclude the possibility of cluster headache.
- Although the severity of the headache is said to be more moderate in migraine headache compared with cluster, it is hard to use this to distinguish between the two conditions. Seldom do patients describe migraine headaches as moderate in severity. However, cluster headache is one of the most painful experiences a person can have.
- Paroxysmal hemicrania and hemicrania continua are exquisitely responsive to indomethacin. A trial of indomethacin is worthwhile in patients who are thought to have atypical migraine or cluster headache or are not responsive to typical therapies for these conditions.

Bibliography

Bahra, A., May, A., & Goadsby, P. J. (2002). Cluster headache: A prospective clinical study with diagnostic implications. *Neurology*, *58*(3), 354–361.

Burish. M. (2018). Cluster Headache and other trigeminal autonomic cephalalgias. *Continuum: Lifelong Learning in Neurology*, *24*(4), 1137–1156.

Do, T. P., Remmers, A., Schytz, H. W., Schankin, C., Nelson, S. E., Obermann, M., ... Schoonman, G. G. (2019). Red and orange flags for secondary headaches in clinical practice: SNNOOP10 list. *Neurology*, *92*(3), 134–144.

Dodick. D. W. (2003). Clinical clues and clinal rules: Primary vs secondary headache. *Advanced Studies in Medicine*, *3*, 87–92.

Dodick, D. W., & Campbell, J. K. (2008). Cluster headache: Diagnosis, management, and treatment: *Wolff's Headache and other head pain* (pp. 283–305) (7th ed.). New York, NY: Oxford University Press.

Headache Classification Committee of the International Headache Society (IHS). (2018). The international classification of headache disorders, 3rd edition. *Cephalalgia*, *38*(1), 1–211.

Nesbitt, A. D., & Goadsby, P. J. (2012). Cluster headache. *BMJ.*, *344*, e2407. Review.

CASE 18

A 61-Year-Old Female With Right-Hand Numbness

Nancy Baker ■ Esther Byun

A 61-year-old right-handed female presents to the emergency room with right-hand numbness that she noticed upon awakening. She is very concerned because her father had a stroke with right-arm numbness and weakness when he was 62 years old.

In the acute setting, what causes of hand numbness are most important to consider?
Acute stroke is important to recognize in a timely fashion. A thalamic stroke and a small cortical stroke can present with hand numbness. Hand numbness coincident with perioral numbness is a classic presentation of thalamic lacunar stroke (cheiro-oral syndrome). Embolic strokes affecting the sensory strip can also cause pure hand numbness, which can mimic a peripheral process such as median neuropathy (in these cases, vibratory sensation may be reduced; this is not affected in median neuropathy).

Other important causes of hand numbness to identify include disease of the cervical cord/nerves whether from structural cervical spine disease or myelopathy or radiculopathy from other causes.

On arrival in the emergency room, a computed tomography (CT) scan of the patient's head is performed and is unremarkable.

How does the CT result change your differential diagnosis?
A normal CT head scan excludes hemorrhage as a cause, e.g., hypertensive bleed into the thalamus. It does not change the differential diagnosis much, because many intracranial processes are not visible on a CT head scan. Importantly, we have not determined that this is even an intracranial process.

The causes of right-hand numbness can be broad, and it is important to determine whether an emergent workup is indicated at this time. The patient should be asked to describe the onset of her symptoms and whether they have occurred before. The patient should also be asked questions that help localize numbness and weakness (nerve, plexus, nerve root, cord, brainstem, cortex).

This is not the first time this patient has had numbness of her right hand. Over the last 6 months, she has awoken with pain and tingling in her right hand, but on the day of presentation symptoms were worse. Usually she can shake her hand out and symptoms improve, but today the numbness and tingling persisted. She has also noticed driving causes numbness and tingling of her hand. She thinks the entire right hand is affected. She has been dropping objects and has had difficulty opening jars. She is healthy, has never smoked, and has no other medical problems.

She denies weakness, numbness, or paresthesia of her left hand, face, or lower limbs. There is right-wrist pain that radiates up her arm. She does develop neck pain and tightness, especially when working long hours as an administrative assistant. Bowel/bladder function is normal. She denies additional medical history or surgeries. There have been no recent illnesses or injuries to her right hand, nor recent falls or traumatic injuries. Besides her father, no one in her extended family has had a stroke. There is no family history of unexplained recurrent blood clots or frequent miscarriages.

How does this new information affect our differential diagnosis?

Stroke now seems highly unlikely. Stuttering TIAs can cause recurrent symptoms, but not related to positioning or improved with shaking out the hand. Reassuringly, this patient has no risk factors for stroke.

CLINICAL PEARL **STEP 1/2/3**

Risk factors for stroke include hypertension, diabetes, hyperlipidemia, atrial fibrillation, or history of a hypercoagulable disorder or history of stroke in family members younger than 55 years old.

This is most likely a peripheral lesion. Top of the differential is carpal tunnel syndrome, the most common mononeuropathy, which is caused by compression of the median nerve at the wrist. Her description of symptoms is classic. Ulnar neuropathy, the second most common mononeuropathy, can present similarly, with paresthesia radiating up the arm (typically the ulnar aspect). Similar to median neuropathy, numbness/paresthesia that develops in ulnar neuropathy while sleeping and driving can improve with shaking out the arms. Patients with progressive polyneuropathy can also complain of hand numbness; however, in a length-dependent generalized polyneuropathy, both hands would be expected to be involved.

Cervical radiculopathy seems less likely given the provoking/alleviating factors, but this is a fairly common problem and remains on the differential. Lesions of the C6, C7, and C8 nerve roots can cause numbness or paresthesia of the hand. The presence of radiating neck pain, especially if provoked by specific head movements, is suggestive of cervical radiculopathy; however, patients may have no pain at all. In contrast, the presence of focal neck pain is very common and nonspecific.

CLINICAL PEARL **STEP 1/2/3**

In cervical radiculopathy, reflexes may be reduced (biceps/brachioradialis C5–6, triceps C7). There may be weakness in arm muscles (deltoid, biceps, brachioradialis C5–6, triceps C7, most hand muscles C8).

Brachial plexopathy seems unlikely. In brachial plexus lesions, the history is often most helpful. Patients may share a history of trauma, preceding median sternotomy, or severe shoulder pain (preventing sleep) that preceded weakness. If sensory changes are present in the forearm, brachial plexopathy is of higher concern; this would not be seen in median neuropathy at the wrist or ulnar neuropathy at the elbow.

In addition to stroke and TIA, central nervous system disorders that may present with right-hand symptoms include migraine and paresthesia associated with focal seizures. Finally, osteoarthritis and inflammatory arthropathies can present with wrist pain; this can be confused with conditions affecting the nervous system at times.

Neurological Examination Findings:

On examination, the patient's oral temperature is 37°C (98.6°F), pulse rate is 75/min, blood pressure is 118/78 mmHg, and respiration rate is 16/min. Examination showed slight wasting of the right thenar eminence compared with the left. Reflexes were normal. Thumb abduction was mildly weak on the right (Fig. 18.1). Sensation was reduced over the thumb, index, and middle fingers on both sides.

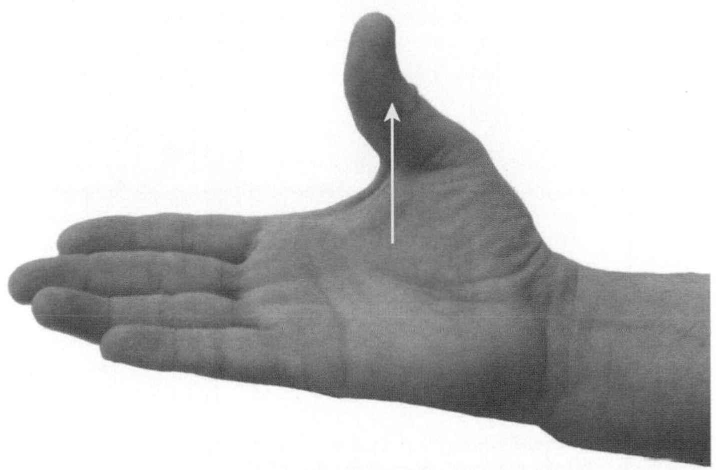

Fig. 18.1 How to test thumb abduction (abductor pollicis longus). (From Preston, D. C., & Shapiro, B. E. (2021). Medial neuropathy at the wrist. In *Electromyography and neuromuscular disorders: Clinical-electrophysiologic-ultrasound correlations* (4th ed.). Elsevier: Philadelphia.)

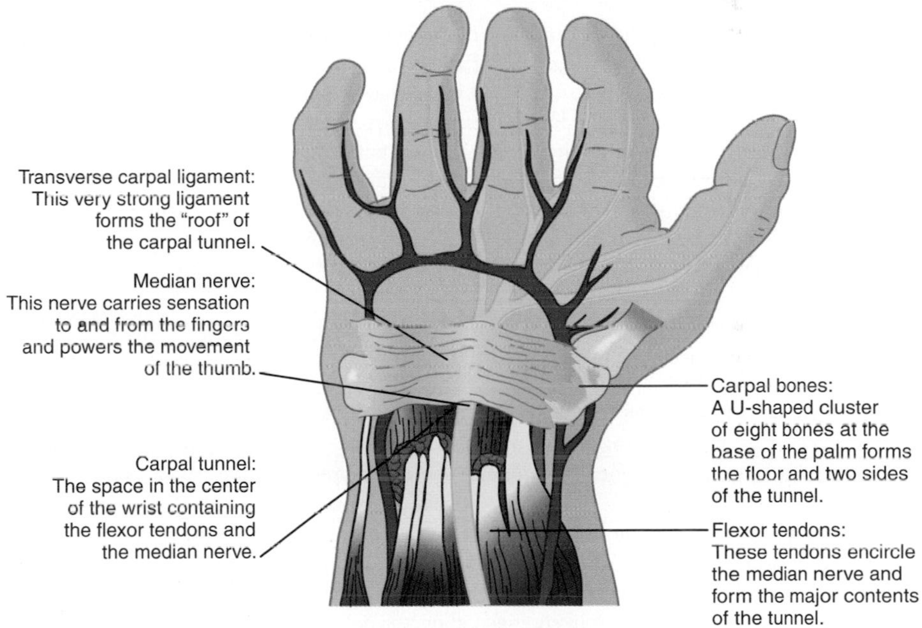
Transverse carpal ligament: This very strong ligament forms the "roof" of the carpal tunnel.
Median nerve: This nerve carries sensation to and from the fingers and powers the movement of the thumb.
Carpal tunnel: The space in the center of the wrist containing the flexor tendons and the median nerve.
Carpal bones: A U-shaped cluster of eight bones at the base of the palm forms the floor and two sides of the tunnel.
Flexor tendons: These tendons encircle the median nerve and form the major contents of the tunnel.

Fig. 18.2 The carpal tunnel is formed by carpal bones (floor, sides) and the transverse carpal ligament (roof). The median nerve travels in the carpal tunnel along with tendons. The ulnar nerve lies outside the carpal tunnel. (From Adams, J.G. (2014). Peripheral Nerve Disorders. In *Emergency medicine: Clinical essentials* (2nd ed.). Elsevier.)

What is the clinical diagnosis?

Carpal tunnel syndrome is the most likely diagnosis. This occurs when there is increased pressure on the median nerve in the carpal tunnel (Fig. 18.2). The distribution of numbness argues against an ulnar neuropathy.

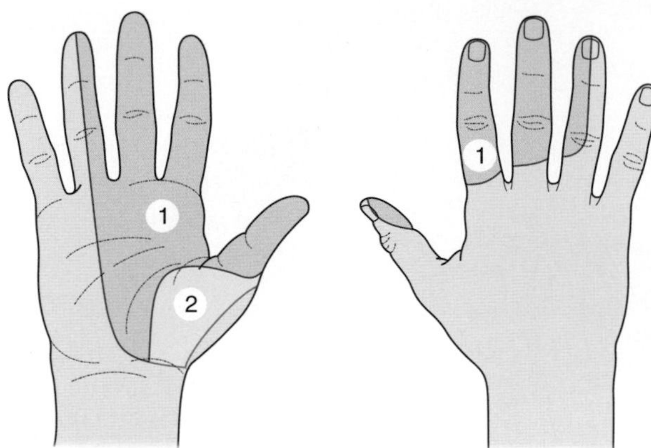

Fig. 18.3 Typical Median Sensory Territory. *(1)* The palmar digital sensory branch of the median nerve travels through the carpal tunnel; *(2)* the palmar cutaneous sensory branch of the median nerve does not and is unaffected in carpal tunnel syndrome. (From Preston, D. C., & Shapiro, B. E. (2021). Medial neuropathy at the wrist. In *Electromyography and neuromuscular disorders: Clinical-electrophysiologic-ultrasound correlations* (4th ed.). Elsevier: Philadelphia.)

The patient stated that her entire hand is numb, although the examination revealed the median distribution was primarily affected (Fig. 18.3). Patients with intermittent symptoms often cannot recall the exact location of sensory loss. If there is reduced sensation on examination, this can be very helpful. A normal examination does not exclude carpal tunnel syndrome, however, because symptoms and signs may be intermittent. Moreoever, patients may have full sensation to the modalities we test but nonetheless report something is qualitatively abnormal.

Sensory symptoms can be very difficult for patients to describe. In median neuropathy, patients often describe a feeling as if their hand fell asleep. Others mention a feeling of tightness or swelling. Sometimes these sensory disturbances are painful; other times they are not.

CLINICAL PEARL **STEP 1/2/3**

Tinel sign: pain/paresthesia in the median distribution elicited by percussion over the median nerve.
Phalen sign: pain or paresthesia on median distribution with full flexion of the wrists.

These signs are not very sensitive or specific for median neuropathy at the wrist, but their presence could support a diagnosis of carpal tunnel syndrome.

The normal vital signs argue further against stroke; normal blood pressure is not expected. High blood pressure is expected in most ischemic and hemorrhagic strokes, although sometimes with watershed strokes the blood pressure is low. A C5–6 radiculopathy leading to thumb, index, and middle finger numbness is not likely, given abductor pollicis brevis weakness (C8–T1 innervated) and symmetric reflexes. With cervical myelopathy, reflexes would be expected to be brisk.

What are the next steps for evaluation and treatment?

Practices vary. In this patient, there is atrophy of the abductor pollicis brevis—suggestive of axon loss and indicative of a more severe process; referral for carpal tunnel release is prudent to prevent further axon loss. Neutral wrist splints could be offered from the emergency room; this may relieve discomfort that develops when flexing the wrists, as often happens at night while sleeping. Increasingly, patients are referred for electrodiagnostic studies before surgery.

Electrodiagnostic testing (nerve conductions and electromyography) is completed in the outpatient setting. In this patient, there is electrophysiologic evidence of bilateral, moderately severe median neuropathies at the wrist (right worse than left).

Nerve conduction studies involve electrical stimulation of a standard set of sensory and motor nerves, recording along the nerve or muscle. Most laboratories have their specific norms, although national standards have been generated, which will hopefully improve comparisons between laboratories.

Carpal tunnel syndrome remains a clinical diagnosis. This clinical diagnosis can be supported by electrodiagnostic testing. Electrodiagnostic studies are valid and reproducible. They can confirm a clinical diagnosis of carpal tunnel syndrome; however, there can be false positives and false negatives. Electrodiagnostic testing can also be used to exclude other mononeuropathies, evaluate for a generalized polyneuropathy, and screen for radiculopathy. They are also used as a baseline for comparison in the future. Electrodiagnostic testing is recommended by the American Academy of Orthopedic Surgeons if surgery is being considered.

CLINICAL PEARL **STEP 2/3**

There may be little correlation between the degree or frequency of clinical signs or symptoms and the abnormalities seen on examination. A patient may report mild clinical symptoms but may have prominent physical examination findings, such as severe numbness and wasting of the thenar muscles.

Electrophysiologic severity may not correlate with severity of symptoms. Patients may have severe pain with electrophysiologically mild median neuropathy at the wrist. In contrast, even if patients have minimal symptoms, severe median neuropathy on nerve conductions suggests axon loss and patients should be offered carpal tunnel release.

What are treatments for carpal tunnel syndrome?

Injection of hydrocortisone into the carpal tunnel can be beneficial. Surgical division of the carpal tunnel ligament with decompression of the median nerve can be curative. This is typically an outpatient procedure and can be performed with local anesthesia.

The patient is not eager to pursue surgery because she would have to take time off work for the procedure. She is given a local corticosteroid injection and her symptoms improve.

However, symptoms return about 6 months later and are very bothersome. She undergoes right carpal tunnel release. Pain improves immediately. Numbness resolves more gradually over the following half year.

With carpal tunnel release, the majority of patients have improvement in symptoms and remain symptom free for years.

Case Summary

- **Complaint/History:** A 61-year-old woman with right-hand numbness that she noticed upon awakening. In the previous 6 months, pain and tingling in the right hand have repeatedly woken her from sleep. She drops objects unintentionally.
- **Findings:** There is slight wasting of the right thenar eminence with mild weakness of thumb abduction. Sensation is reduced over the thumb, index, and middle fingers.
- **Lab Results/Tests:** Electrophysiology can demonstrate median neuropathy at the wrist and support a clinical diagnosis of carpal tunnel syndrome.

Diagnosis: Carpal tunnel syndrome. This is a clinical diagnosis.

- **Treatment:** Neutral wrist splint, injection of corticosteroids, and surgical carpal tunnel release.

BEYOND THE PEARLS

- Carpal tunnel syndrome is a clinical diagnosis. Electrophysiology can support a diagnosis of median neuropathy and evaluate for mimics (ulnar neuropathy, generalized neuropathy, cervical radiculopathy).
- Numbness of the thumb, index, middle fingers, and half of the ring finger would be very suggestive of median neuropathy (as more proximal lesions do not typically produce such discrete borders) (Fig. 18.3). However, the distribution of numbness can vary in median neuropathy. Patients can present with numbness of just the thumb or the entire hand.
- Tinel and Phalen signs are not very sensitive or specific but are often performed. They can support a clinical diagnosis of carpal tunnel syndrome.
- Splinting and local corticosteroid injections can be beneficial in the short term. Surgical division of the carpal tunnel ligament with decompression of the median nerve can be curative.
- Clues that raise suspicion for a central cause of hand numbness include hyperreflexia and vague boundaries of sensory loss. Loss of vibration or joint position sense should also lead you to consider central causes of hand numbness (although vibratory sense loss is reportedly seen in median neuropathy at the wrist).

Bibliography

An, T. W., Evanoff, B. A., Boyer, M. I., & Osei, D. A. (2017). The prevalence of cubital tunnel syndrome: A cross-sectional study in a U.S. metropolitan cohort. *The Journal of Bone and Joint Surgery. American Volume, 99*(5), 408–416.

Colorado, B. S., & Osei, D. A. (2019). Prevalence of carpal tunnel syndrome presenting with symptoms in an ulnar nerve distribution: A prospective study. *Muscle & Nerve, 59*(1), 60–63.

Chen, S., Andary, M., Buschbacher, R., Del Toro, D., Smith, B., So, Y., ... Dillingham, T. R. (2016). Electrodiagnostic reference values for upper and lower limb nerve conduction studies in adult populations. *Muscle & Nerve, 54*(3), 371–377.

D'Arcy, C. A., & McGee, S. (2000). The rational clinical examination. Does this patient have carpal tunnel syndrome? *The Journal of the American Medical Association, 283*(23), 3110–3117. Review. Erratum in: JAMA 2000;284(11):1384.

Dawson DM, Hallet M, Wilbourn AJ. (1999). *Entrapment Neuropathies*, 3rd ed.

Keith, M. W., Masear, V., Chung, K. C., Amadio, P. C., Andary, M., Barth, R. W., ... American Academy of Orthopaedic Surgeons. (2010). American Academy of Orthopaedic Surgeons clinical practice guideline on the treatment of carpal tunnel syndrome. *The Journal of Bone and Joint Surgery. American Volume, 92*(1), 218–219.

Jablecki CK, Andary MT. Literature review of the usefulness of nerve conduction studies and electromyography for the evaluation of patients with carpal tunnel syndrome. *Muscle & Nerve* 16, 1392.

Louie, D. L., Earp, B. E., Collins, J. E., Losina, E., Katz, J. N., Black, E. M., ... Blazar, P. E. (2013). Outcomes of open carpal tunnel release at a minimum of ten years. *The Journal of Bone and Joint Surgery. American Volume, 95*(12), 1067–1073.

Preston DC, Shapiro BE. (2012). *Electromyography and Neuromuscular Disorders: Clinical-Electrophysiologic Correlations.* 3rd ed. Elsevier Saunders: Philadelphia.

Ropper R, Samuels M, Klein J, Prasad S. *Adam's and Victor's Principles of Neurology. Diseases of the peripheral nerves.* New York: McGraw Hill. Chapter 46, 1379–1384.

CASE 19

A 21-Year-Old Male With Sudden Onset of Right-Sided Hemiparesis and Aphasia

Anish R. Patel ■ Benjamin A. Emanuel

A 21-year-old male presents with sudden onset of aphasia, right facial droop, slurred speech, and weakness in his right arm and leg while he was eating breakfast with his family. He has no significant medical history. He takes no medications other than ibuprofen occasionally for headaches. The patient arrived 1 hour 15 minutes after onset of symptoms. According to his family there were no reports of headache, vomiting, or loss of consciousness. The patient is rapidly transported to the computed tomography (CT) department for advanced imaging. On physical examination, the patient is afebrile; his blood pressure is 175/105 mmHg, heart rate 76 beats/min, and respiratory rate 18 breaths/min. On auscultation, the patient has a persistently split S2 with a systolic ejection murmur in the upper left second intercostal area. Neurologic examination shows moderate expressive aphasia, moderate dysarthria, right facial palsy sparing the forehead, left gaze preference, and 2/5 right upper and lower limb weakness. National Institutes of Health Stroke Scale (NIHSS) score was 19.

What is the most important differential diagnosis to rule out with this patient's presenting symptoms? Given the sudden onset and severity of neurological symptoms, there should always be a high suspicion of the possibility of stroke. Timely response with rapid transport to a primary stroke center for imaging is essential to allow the patient the best chance of optimal intervention and treatment.

BASIC SCIENCE/CLINICAL PEARL **STEP 1/2/3**

Time is brain! An expedited yet thorough history is an absolutely critical first step toward making a diagnosis. A stroke should be high on the differential diagnosis for a patient presenting with sudden focal neurological deficits and/or altered level of consciousness. For each minute of a middle cerebral artery vessel occlusion, 1.9 million neurons, 14 billion synapses, and 7.5 miles of myelinated fibers are destroyed.

CLINICAL PEARL **STEP 2/3**

Neuroimaging is critical in the diagnosis of stroke. A noncontrast head CT should be performed in patients presenting with symptoms that suggest a stroke to assess the extent of ischemia and to exclude intracerebral hemorrhage. CT angiography should be performed to look for a treatable large vessel occlusion and a potential cause of the stroke. CT perfusion to can assess the metabolic state of a large vessel occlusion and whether there is a treatable ischemic penumbra.

A proper history and physical examination are essential and can provide valuable information about the likelihood of stroke, time of symptom onset, and potential treatment interventions. Utilizing the NIHSS is a quick and effective method of determining stroke possibility and severity.

BASIC SCIENCE/CLINICAL PEARL **STEP 1/2/3**

The NIHSS is the gold standard for stroke severity rating and stratifies patients based on:

- Level of consciousness
- Age of patient
- Ability to follow commands (blink eye and squeeze hands)
- Extraocular movements
- Visual fields
- Facial palsy
- Right/left arm motor drift
- Right/left leg motor drift
- Limb ataxia
- Sensation
- Language/aphasia
- Dysarthria
- Extinction/inattention

Which type of brain lesion do this patient's neurological deficits suggest?

The patient appears to have right-sided weakness, aphasia, and left gaze preference, suggesting a large cortical lesion to the left side of the brain. There are certain neurological symptoms that can be seen together that may help a clinician determine whether the stroke is small or large. The clinical and radiologic differences between these types of strokes are demonstrated in Table 19.1. Additionally, strokes that occur at specific locations in the brain present with certain patterns of neurological deficits. The deficits correlate to the specific cranial nerves and motor/sensory tracts that are compromised in the region of the brain injury.

Common acute ischemic stroke (AIS) syndromes are listed in Table 19.2. Familiarizing yourself with these stroke syndromes will allow you as a clinician to make a timely diagnosis and localize the region of the brain to look for an infarct/hemorrhage.

TABLE 19.1 ■ **Large Versus Small Vessel Infarct**

Type of Infarct	Clinical Features	Radiographic Features
Small vessel	• Lack of cortical signs • Pure motor • Pure sensory • Mixed motor/sensory deficits • Clumsy hand dysarthria • Ataxia-hemiparesis	• Occlusion of the small penetrating arteries that supply the deep cerebral structures (i.e., basal ganglia, thalamus, internal capsule, corona radiata, cerebellum) • Sometimes called lacunar infarcts • Most often caused by smaller thrombus that occurs in diseased vessels
Large vessel	• Cortical signs • Aphasia • Contralateral hemineglect • Ipsilateral gaze preference • Hemianopia	• Occlusion of the major blood vessels (i.e., ICA, MCA, ACA, PCA, basilar) • Occlusion is most often caused by emboli

ACA, Anterior cerebral artery; *ICA*, internal carotid artery; *MCA*, middle carotid artery; *PCA*, posterior carotid artery.

TABLE 19.2 ■ **CVA Syndromes and Associated Deficits**

Artery	Clinical Features
Anterior cerebral artery	Contralateral LE>UE weakness; urinary incontinence
Middle cerebral artery	Contralateral face/UE>LE; aphasia; neglect; ipsilateral gaze preference
Posterior cerebral artery	Weber's syndrome = contralateral hemiplegia + ipsilateral CN III palsy; homonymous hemianopsia
Deep/lacunar	Contralateral motor and/or sensory deficit without cortical signs
Basilar artery	Ipsilateral CN IV–VII palsy; ataxia; crossed deficits (ipsilateral face and contralateral body) or quadriplegia
Vertebral artery	Lower cranial nerve deficits (vertigo, nystagmus, dysphagia, dysarthria); diplopia; ataxia; crossed deficits (ipsilateral face and contralateral body)

LE, Lower extremity; *UE*, upper extremity.

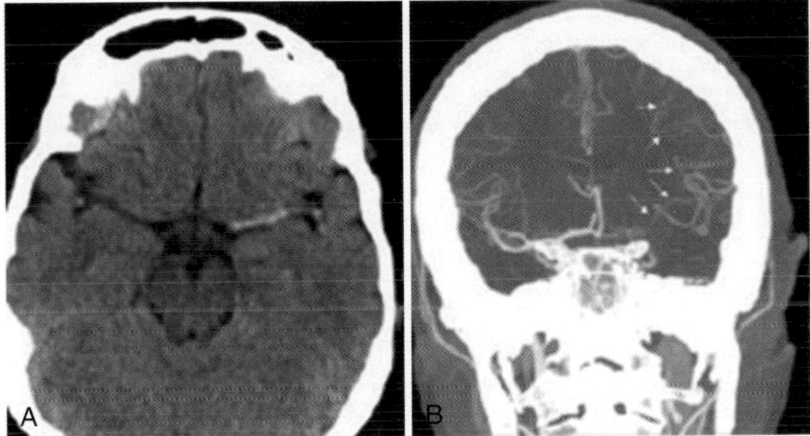

Fig. 19.1 (A) Noncontrast head CT scan with left MCA sign red *(arrow)* indicating thromboembolic clot in the left MCA artery. (B) CT angiogram with left MCA occlusion *(red arrow)* with robust collateral circulation *(white arrows)*. ((A) From Power, S., McEvoy, S. H., Cunningham, J., Ti, J. P., Looby, S., O'Hare, A., Williams, D., Brennan, P., & Thornton, J. (2015). Value of CT angiography in anterior circulation large vessel occlusive stroke: imaging findings, pearls, and pitfalls. *European Journal of Radiography*, *84*(7), 1333–1344; (B) from Jadhav, A. P., Desai, S. M., Liebeskind, D. S., & Wechsler, L. R. (2019). Neuroimaging of acute stroke. *Neurologic Clinics*, *38*(1), 185–199.)

The patient's noncontrast head CT showed no intracranial hemorrhage and (Fig. 19.1A) without early infarct changes. The Alberta Stroke Program Early Computed Tomography Score (ASPECTS) was 10 (Fig. 19.1).

Taking into consideration the severity of deficits, the patient's age and functional status, and the time of onset of symptoms, the possibility of IV alteplase administration was considered.

What are the major clinical considerations when deciding on administering IV alteplase for stroke?

Knowing which patients are IV alteplase candidates and applying the inclusion/exclusion criteria for using IV alteplase are both essential components of a physician's responsibility during an acute stroke evaluation. The inclusion and exclusion criteria for IV alteplase administration are given in Table 19.3. As you can see from these criteria, there are many components that require continuous measurement of vital signs along with an immediate set of lab test results.

TABLE 19.3 ■ **Inclusion and Exclusion Criteria for IV Thrombolysis**

Major Inclusion Criteria
- Age >18 years
- Severe or mild but disabling stroke symptoms with time since symptom onset <3 to 4.5 hours
- Blood pressure <185/110 mmHg
- Glucose >50 mg/dl

Major Exclusion Criteria
- Noncontrast head CT with extensive frank hypodensity of early infarction or with hemorrhage
- Ischemic stroke within 3 months
- Severe head trauma within 3 months
- Intracranial or spinal surgery within 3 months
- History of intracranial hemorrhage
- Signs and symptoms of subarachnoid hemorrhage
- Gastrointestinal malignancy or recent GI bleed within 21 days
- Platelets <100,000, INR >1.7, aPTT >40 seconds, PT >15 seconds
- Low-molecular-weight heparin given within 24 hours
- Dose of direct thrombin inhibitor or direct factor Xa inhibitor within 48 hours (unless aPTT, INR, thrombin time, and clotting time are normal)
- Infective endocarditis
- Aortic dissection
- Intra-axial intracranial neoplasm

Additional Exclusion Criteria in the 3–4.5 Hour Window
- Age >80 years
- NIHSS >25
- Patients taking warfarin regardless of INR
- Combined history of acute ischemic stroke and diabetes mellitus

The patient's vital signs remain stable. The initial laboratory workup including complete blood count, complete metabolic panel, blood glucose, partial thromboplastin time (PTT), and prothrombin time/international normalized ratio (PT/INR) are within normal limits. It was decided to treat the patient with intravenous alteplase with a door-to-needle time of 27 minutes.

Which major signs and symptoms should be monitored after administration of IV alteplase?

Treating patients with IV alteplase does not come without its consequences and it is therefore important to monitor the patient closely during and after IV alteplase administration. Patients are often taken to a critical care unit for continuous monitoring of vital signs and frequent neurological checks with the capability of a quick response to any potential complications. Strategies for monitoring and managing patients after IV alteplase administration are given in Table 19.4. Understanding the types of IV alteplase complications and rate of occurrence is another essential responsibility for clinicians using this medication.

A head CTA obtained at arrival showed a left middle cerebral artery (MCA) occlusion. CT perfusion demonstrated a large area of salvageable penumbra in the left MCA distribution (Fig. 19.2).

What type of infarct does this patient's stroke most likely suggest and what are the management strategies?

When one of the major arteries of the brain is blocked, it is considered a large vessel occlusion (LVO) or large vessel syndrome. Our patient appears to have an occlusion of the left middle

TABLE 19.4 ■ **Protocol for Postalteplase Management**

Monitor closely for:
• Severe headache
• Acute hypertension
• Nausea/vomiting
• Worsening neurological examination
Avoid nasogastric tube, urinary catheter, and lines for 24 hours (if possible)
Maintain BP below SBP 180 and DBP 105 (treatment: labetalol, nicardipine, clevidipine, hydralazine, enalapril)
Follow-up head CT or MRI 24 hours after treatment before starting antiplatelet and/or anticoagulant therapies
Management of Symptomatic Intracranial Bleeding Within 24 Hours of IV Alteplase
If you suspect a bleeding complication, stop alteplase infusion
CBC, PT/INR, aPTT, fibrinogen level, type and cross-match
Noncontrast head CT scan
Transfuse cryoprecipitate
Administer tranexamic acid or aminocaproic acid
Hematology and neurosurgery consultation
Supportive therapy to include BP management, temperature and glucose control
Management of Orolingual Angioedema Associated With IV Alteplase
Manage ABCs
Discontinue IV alteplase infusion and hold ACE inhibitors
Methylprednisolone 125 mg IV
Diphenhydramine 50 mg IV
Ranitidine 50 mg IV or famotidine 20 mg IV
For refractory cases, epinephrine subcutaneous or nebulized

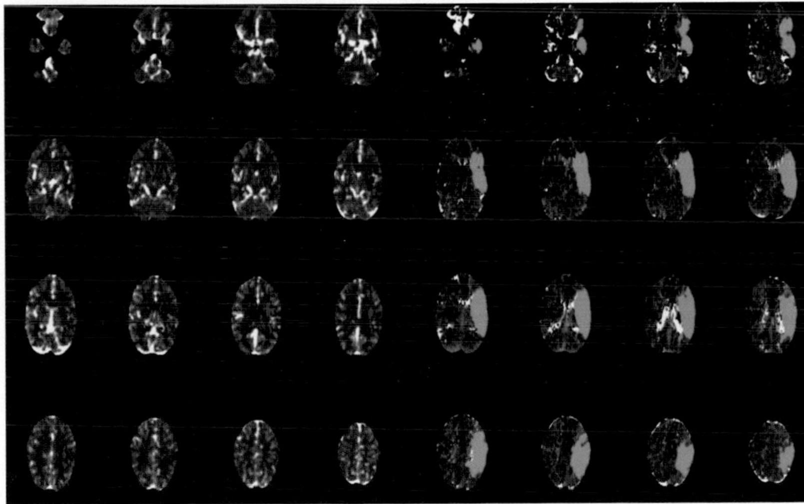

Fig. 19.2 CT perfusion imaging demonstrating large salvageable penumbra *(green)* with little irreversible core *(purple)*.

cerebral artery, which is considered to be one of the large cerebral vessels causing considerable deficits. This type of stroke tends to be more severe and warrants immediate intervention if possible. If the patient is within the time window for medical and/or surgical thrombectomy, should immediately be transported to a comprehensive stroke center capable of these treatment modalities.

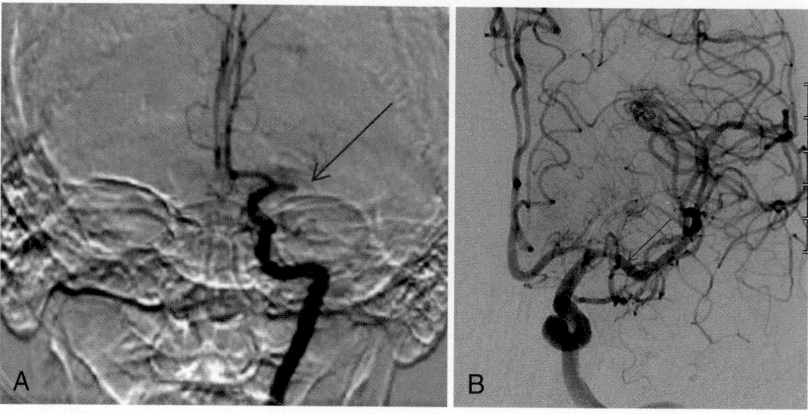

Fig. 19.3 (A) Cerebral angiogram with left middle cerebral artery occlusion *(red arrow)*. (B) Postthrombectomy angiogram with complete recanalization of left middle cerebral artery *(red arrow)*.

The patient is taken directly to the neurointerventional suite on arrival at the comprehensive stroke center. An MCA occlusion (Fig. 19.3A) is visualized. Thrombectomy achieved TICI III recanalization of the left MCA (Fig. 19.3).

The patient's post-IV alteplase and postthrombectomy neurological exam showed significant improvement with an NIHSS score of 19 that reduced to 6 within 24 hours.

What is the next step in managing this patient's condition?

The next step in this patient's workup should be to establish the actual cause of stroke. It is important to be familiar with the common risk factors that may contribute to a stroke.

BASIC SCIENCE PEARL **STEP 1**

Risk factors:

- Hypertension
- Diabetes
- Smoking
- Atrial fibrillation
- Mechanical valves
- Valvular abnormalities
- Patent foramen ovale
- Significant decreased ejection fraction
- Hypercoagulable state
- Family history
- Prior history of stroke
- Vascular disease

This patient is young with no significant medical history suggesting that the stroke event may not have been from a chronic comorbidity (e.g., hypertension, smoking, atrial fibrillation, diabetes mellitus) as commonly seen in the elderly. The workup of stroke in young patients with no history must include investigations into the atypical causes of stroke.

Full blood count and renal and liver function tests were normal, serum C reactive protein <2 mg/L, serum thyroid-stimulating hormone 1.25 mU/L, plasma glucose 93 mg/dL, plasma homocysteine 10.2 μmol/L, serum total cholesterol 75.6 mg/dL, serum triglyceride 36 mg/dL, serum high-density lipoprotein (HDL) cholesterol 18mg/dL, calculated low-density lipoprotein cholesterol

41.4 mg/dL, serum cholesterol/HDL ratio 4.2:1, anticardiolipin screen negative for IgG and IgM and IgA, antinuclear antibody negative, erythrocyte sedimentation rate 16 mm/h, total creatine kinase 75 U/L, lupus anticoagulant negative, antithrombin III activity normal, protein C activity normal, activated protein C (APC) resistance normal, prothrombin time normal, free protein S antigen normal, and factor V Leiden PCR negative.

Further investigation with transthoracic echocardiogram and transesophageal echocardiogram all indicate the presence of a grade 1 tunnel-shaped PFO with atrial septal aneurysm. No other cause for his stroke was found.

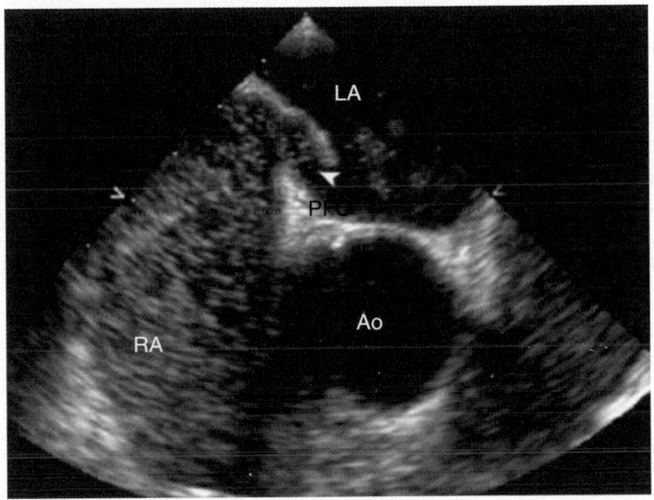

Fig. 19.4 Bubble study showing opacification of the right atrium with bubble and 2D echocardiography showing a patent foramen ovale *(arrowhead)* with some crossing of the bubble to the left atrium. *Ao*, Aortic valve; *LA*, left atrium.

BASIC SCIENCE/CLINICAL PEARL **STEP 1/2/3**

The sensitivity and specificity of transthoracic echocardiogram (TTE) for diagnosing patent foramen ovale (PFO) are 88% and 98%, respectively.

The presence of an atrial septal aneurysm has been shown to be independently associated with recurrent stroke.

CLINICAL PEARL **STEP 2/3**

PFO is a common congenital abnormality with a high prevalence of approximately 25% in the general population.

Two weeks after the stroke onset, the patient received transcatheter PFO closure. He continued to work with physical therapy as an outpatient. At his 3-month follow-up, he demonstrated complete resolution of symptoms and returned to college with no residual deficits.

CLINICAL PEARL **STEP 2/3**

Simply achieving "Life's Simple 7," a multifaceted approach to healthy living that includes no smoking, regular physical activity, healthy diet, maintaining normal weight, and controlling blood pressure, cholesterol, and blood glucose levels can reduce the long-term risk of dying after stroke.

Case Summary

- **Complaint/History:** Right Hemiparesis & Aphasia
- **Findings:** right-sided weakness, aphasia, and left gaze preference, suggesting a large cortical lesion to the left side of the brain.
- **Lab Results/Tests:** Normal Labs, No contraindications to tPA, No hypercoagulable predisposition, Transthoracic Echocardiogaphy with.

Diagnosis: Acute left middle cerebral artery ischemic stroke

- **Treatment:** IV alteplase and thrombectomy

BEYOND THE PEARLS

- Hemorrhagic complications from IV alteplase: 6%.
- Incidence of orolingual angioedema: 4%–5%.
- Unless the patient history suggests otherwise, given the extremely low risk of unsuspected abnormal platelet counts or coagulation studies in the general population, do not delay the administration of IV alteplase while waiting for hematologic or coagulation studies.
- Patients who are eligible for IV alteplase should receive IV alteplase even if mechanical thrombectomy is going to be performed.
- In patients with large vessel occlusion who receive IV alteplase, observation for a clinical response to IV alteplase should not delay mechanical thrombectomy.
- Recanalization rate with IV alteplase for ICA occlusions is 10% and for MCA occlusions is 30%.
- The Number Needed to Treat with IV alteplase to benefit one patient in each of the following windows:
  - 0–90 min = 3.6;
  - 91–180 min = 4.3;
  - 181–270 min = 5.9;
  - 271–360 min = 19.3;
- For every three patients that receive thrombectomy, one additional patient will achieve functional independence at 90 days.
- In patients who are at risk of stroke, 45% feel that a major stroke is a fate worse than death.
- Improvement in symptoms is not a contraindication to IV alteplase.

Bibliography

Hansen, C. K., Christensen, A., Ovesen, C., Havsteen, I., & Christensen, H. (2015). Stroke severity and incidence of acute large vessel occlusions in patients with hyper-acute cerebral ischemia: Results from a prospective cohort study based on CT-angiography (CTA). *International Journal of Stroke, 10*, 336–342.

Krishnamurthi, R. V., Moran, A. E., Feigin, V. L., Barker-Collo, S., Norrving, B., Mensah, G. A., et al. (2015). Stroke prevalence, mortality and disability-adjusted life years in adults aged 20-64 years in 1990–2013: Data from the global burden of disease 2013 study. *Neuroepidemiology, 45*, 190–202.

Lansberg, M., Schrooten, M., Bluhmki, E., Thijs, V., & Saver, J. (2009). Treatment time-specific number needed to treat estimates for tissue plasminogen activator therapy in acute stroke based on shifts over the entire range of the Modified Rankin Scale. *Stroke*, *40*(6), 2079–2084.

Lin, M. P., Ovbiagele, B., Markovic, D., & Towfighi, A. (2015). "Life's Simple 7" and long-term mortality after stroke. *Journal of the American Heart Association: Cardiovascular and Cerebrovascular Disease*, *4*, e001470.

Mozaffarian, D., Benjamin, E. J., Go, A. S., Arnett, D. K., Blaha, M. J., Cushman, M., et al. (2016). Heart disease and stroke statistics—2016 update: a report from the American Heart Association. *Circulation*, *133*, e38–e360.

Nogueira, R. G., Jadhav, A. P., Haussen, D. C., Bonafe, A., Budzik, R. F., Bhuva, P., … Jovin, T. G. (2018). Thrombectomy 6 to 24 hours after stroke with a mismatch between deficit and infarct for the DAWN Trial Investigators. *NEJM*, *378*, 11–21.

Palaskas N., & G.N. Levine. Cardiology Secrets, Chapter 7, 53–64.

Powers, W., Rabinstein, A., Ackerson, T., Adeoye, O., Bambakidis, N., et al. (2019). Guidelines for the early management of patients with acute ischemic stroke: 2019 update to the 2018 guidelines for the early management of acute ischemic stroke. *Stroke* e344–e41.8.

Ren, P., Xie, M., et al. (2012). Diagnostic accuracy of transthoracic echocardiography for patent foramen ovale: a systematic review and meta analysis. *Heart*, *98*, E304.

Saqqur, M., Ushin, K., Demchuk, A., Molina, C., et al. (2007). Site of arterial occlusion identified by transcranial Doppler predicts the response to intravenous thrombolysis for stroke. *Stroke*, *38*, 948–954.

Saver. J. L. (2006). Time is brain. *Stroke*, 263–266.

Turc, G., Lee, J. Y., Brochet, E., Kim, J. S., Song, J. K., & Masand, J. L. (2020). Atrial septal aneurysm, shunt size and recurrent stroke risk in patients with patent foramen ovale. *Journal of the American College of Cardiology*, *75*(18).

SECTION 6

Cardiology

CASE 20

A 62-Year-Old Female With Progressively Worsening Shortness of Breath, Fatigue, and Lower Extremity Edema

Neil Bhambi ■ Michael Fong

A 62-year-old female presents to the emergency department with progressively worsening shortness of breath, nonproductive cough, fatigue, and lower extremity edema over the past 3 weeks. She denies having fevers, hemoptysis, or chest pain. Her medical history is significant for nonis-chemic cardiomyopathy and hypertension. She had an implantable cardioverter-defibrillator (ICD) placed 4 years ago and is currently taking carvedilol, spironolactone, and furosemide. However, she has been inconsistently taking her medications and has been noncompliant with a low salt diet. On physical examination, temperature is 99°F, blood pressure is 84/53 mmHg, heart rate is 108 beats/min, respiration rate is 24 breaths/min, and oxygen saturation is 85% on room air. She has diffuse bilateral crackles on her lung examination. In addition, she has a laterally displaced precordial apical impulse, bilateral lower extremity edema, and jugular venous distention. Her skin is cool to the touch. She is placed on supplemental oxygen with improvement in her oxygen saturation to 92%. A chest radiograph is shown in Fig. 20.1.

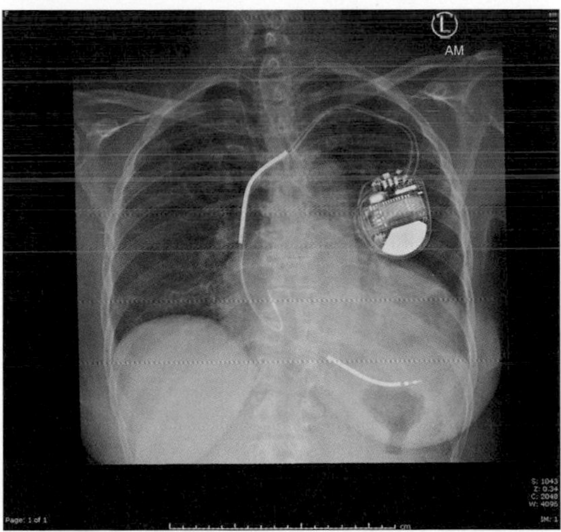

Fig. 20.1 Chest radiograph showing enlarged cardiac silhouette, interstitial edema, and dual-chamber implantable cardioverter-defibrillator.

What is your differential diagnosis for this patient with hypoxemic respiratory failure and hypotension?

The most likely etiology of this patient's presentation is an acute decompensated heart failure (ADHF) exacerbation. These patients present with worsening congestive symptoms, including dyspnea and peripheral edema. In severe cases, patients might present with hypotension and end-organ failure from severely reduced cardiac function, known as cardiogenic shock (CS). This patient has a history of dietary and medication noncompliance, which results in sodium and water retention. This increase in circulating volume worsens ventricular function and precipitates a heart failure (HF) exacerbation.

Other conditions to consider include septic shock and pulmonary embolism (PE). Patients with septic shock are hypotensive due to proinflammatory cytokines that cause systemic vasodilation. Hypoxemia is also common in infections, especially if pneumonia is suspected. However, the patient's nonproductive cough, lack of fever, and duration of symptoms favor a noninfectious etiology. Finally, a PE should be considered in patients with hypotension, hypoxemia, and tachycardia. Massive or submassive PE place significant strain on the right ventricle, causing reduced systolic function that results in decreased left ventricular preload and subsequently decreased stroke volume and hypotension. PE is less likely because this patient does not present with chest pain or syncope or have risk factors for venous thromboembolism.

What is the difference between hypotension and cardiogenic shock?

Hypotension is a state of low blood pressure (typically a systolic pressure <90 mmHg), which by itself is not pathologic. Many healthy people live with low blood pressure and are asymptomatic. Shock refers to a condition of circulatory failure marked by the inability to meet the metabolic needs of tissues and organs. Cardiogenic shock (CS) is a state of reduced cardiac function resulting in hypoperfusion and end-organ damage.

The primary insult in CS is reduced cardiac output (CO), which is the volume of blood ejected by the left ventricle per minute. It is equal to the product of the heart rate and stroke volume: $CO = HR \times SV$. CO is a key determinant of a patient's blood pressure (BP) and can be understood by applying a fundamental law of physics, Ohm's Law. This principle states that the change of voltage (ΔV) across a circuit is equal to the flow of electrical current (I) multiplied by the resistance (R) of the circuit: $\Delta V = I \times R$. Similarly, the change in BP across a circuit from the arterial to venous systems is the mean arterial pressure (MAP)-central venous pressure (CVP), and is equal to the flow of blood (cardiac output) multiplied by the systemic vascular resistance (SVR): $MAP - CVP = CO \times SVR$. Rearranged:

$$CO = (MAP - CVP)/SVR$$

From the above equation, MAP is directly proportional to CO. As CO decreases during CS, so does MAP and the patient becomes hypotensive. The body's primary objective is to preserve BP to maintain perfusion to critical organs, and it does so by increasing SVR. Although this compensatory mechanism can support BP in the short term, the increase in afterload further strains a weakened left ventricle because of its inverse relationship to CO. The result is a cycle of worsening CO, hypoperfusion, and clinical decompensation. The criteria used to help define shock are listed in Table 20.1.

CLINICAL PEARL **STEP 1/2**

MAP can be calculated as follows: MAP = 1/3 SBP + 2/3 DBP. A simple way to remember this is that more time is spent in diastole than systole.

TABLE 20.1 ■ **Criteria for Cardiogenic Shock**

- Clinical criteria: SBP<90 mmHg for ≥30 min OR support to maintain SBP ≥90 mm Hg AND end-organ hypoperfusion (UOP <30 mL/h, cool extremities, elevated lactate)
- Hemodynamic criteria: CI ≤2.2 L/min/m², PCWP ≥15 mmHg

CI, Cardiac index; *PCWP*, pulmonary capillary wedge pressure; *SBP*, systolic blood pressure; *UOP*, urine output.

What are some of the causes of cardiogenic shock?

The most common cause of CS is left ventricular failure following an acute ST-elevation myocardial infarction (STEMI). Nearly 80% of patients in CS have underlying acute coronary syndrome (ACS). ADHF exacerbations account for up to 30% of all cases. Additional causes including mechanical complications, valvular heart disease, and arrhythmias are listed in Table 20.2.

TABLE 20.2 ■ **Etiologies of Cardiogenic Shock**

Etiology	Examples
Myocardial	Myocardial infarction, ADHF, myocarditis, stress cardiomyopathy (Takotsubo), hypertrophic obstructive cardiomyopathy, myocardial contusion
Valvular	Valvular regurgitation, valvular stenosis
Arrhythmia	Supraventricular tachyarrhythmias, ventricular tachyarrhythmias, sinus node dysfunction, AV node dysfunction
Systemic	Hypothyroidism, toxidrome, myocardial depression caused by sepsis, hypothermia
Pharmacologic	Digoxin toxicity
Obstructive	Pulmonary embolism, cardiac tamponade

ADHF, Acute decompensated heart failure exacerbation.

What are the presenting symptoms and laboratory data of a patient in cardiogenic shock?

Patients can present with worsening signs and symptoms of congestive heart failure (CHF), including progressive dyspnea, orthopnea, and paroxysmal nocturnal dyspnea. They may also present with altered mental status resulting from poor cerebral perfusion. On physical examination, patients may be hypotensive and tachycardic, with evidence of hypervolemia such as pulmonary edema, elevated jugular venous pressure, peripheral edema, and ascites. Due to low CO, extremities will often feel cool and clammy.

The patient's presenting laboratory values are detailed in Table 20.3.

One of the hallmark laboratory findings seen in CS is an elevated lactic acid caused by hypoperfusion and tissue hypoxia. Troponin may be elevated due to acute ischemia, mismatch between myocardial oxygen supply and demand, or myocardial injury from myocardial inflammation. Patients will often have elevated serum creatinine and liver enzymes from hypoperfusion or venous congestion from right-sided HF.

How is cardiogenic shock diagnosed?

Although the patient's history, physical examination, and laboratory data support a diagnosis of CS, they are nonspecific findings. The diagnosis is ultimately established by confirming a state of

TABLE 20.3 ■ **Comprehensive Metabolic Panel and Initial Laboratory Values**

Sodium	137 mmol/L
Potassium	4.3 mmol/L
Chloride	102 mmol/L
Bicarbonate	22 mmol/L
Glucose	70 mg/dL
Calcium	9.0 mg/dL
Blood urea nitrogen	41 mg/dL
Creatinine	2.41 mg/dL
Albumin	3.6 g/dL
Total bilirubin	3.1 mg/dL
Aspartate aminotransferase	59 units/L
Alanine aminotransferase	66 units/L
Lactic acid	3.5 mmol/L
Troponin	0.12 ng/mL

low CO. Noninvasive testing with an electrocardiogram (ECG) and transthoracic echocardiogram (TTE) are useful initial steps. An ECG can help diagnose causes such as STEMI, arrhythmia, or PE. In addition, a TTE will help quantify the left ventricular function, characterize valvular pathology, and rule out cardiac tamponade.

However, there are complex cases when the diagnosis of CS remains unclear. For instance, a patient with a history of CHF may present with overlying sepsis, hypothyroidism, or acute liver failure causing hypoperfusion and hypotension. In these situations, further testing with a pulmonary artery (PA) catheterization is helpful to characterize a patient's CO and hemodynamic profile.

A pulmonary artery (PA) catheter (also known as a Swan-Ganz catheter) measures the CO and pressures in the right atrium (RA), right ventricle (RV), and pulmonary vasculature. During this procedure a catheter with an inflatable balloon tip is inserted into the vena cava and advanced into the right heart. It is floated into the PA with the balloon inflated until it reaches a distal pulmonary capillary. The balloon is wedged into the capillary, obstructing blood flow, and resulting in a characteristic dampening of the PA waveform. The pressure recorded at this point is referred to as the pulmonary capillary wedge pressure (PCWP) or pulmonary artery occlusion pressure (PAOP) and is an indirect measurement of the pressure in the left atrium, assuming that the absence of factors will alter the normal relationship such as pulmonary hypertension. Fig. 20.2 shows the characteristic waveforms of the PA catheter. Normal pressures in the cardiac chambers and PA are listed in Table 20.4.

CLINICAL PEARL **STEP 2/3**

A simple way to remember the normal pressures in the cardiac chambers and PA is by the mnemonic "nickel, quarter, dime, dollar." The pressure in the RA is around 5 mmHg, the systolic pressure in the RV (and therefore PA) is around 25 mmHg, the pressure in the left atrium is around 10 mmHg, and the systolic pressure in the LV is around 100 mmHg.

There are two methods in which CO is measured: thermodilution and Fick. With thermodilution, a known quantity and temperature of normal saline is injected in the RA at the proximal port of the PA catheter. The saline mixes with blood and passes through the RV and pulmonary circulation. At the distal end of the catheter in the PA is a thermal sensor that records the change in blood temperature from the RV. The integral of the area under the time–temperature curve generated after an injection is used to calculate blood flow and CO (Fig. 20.3).

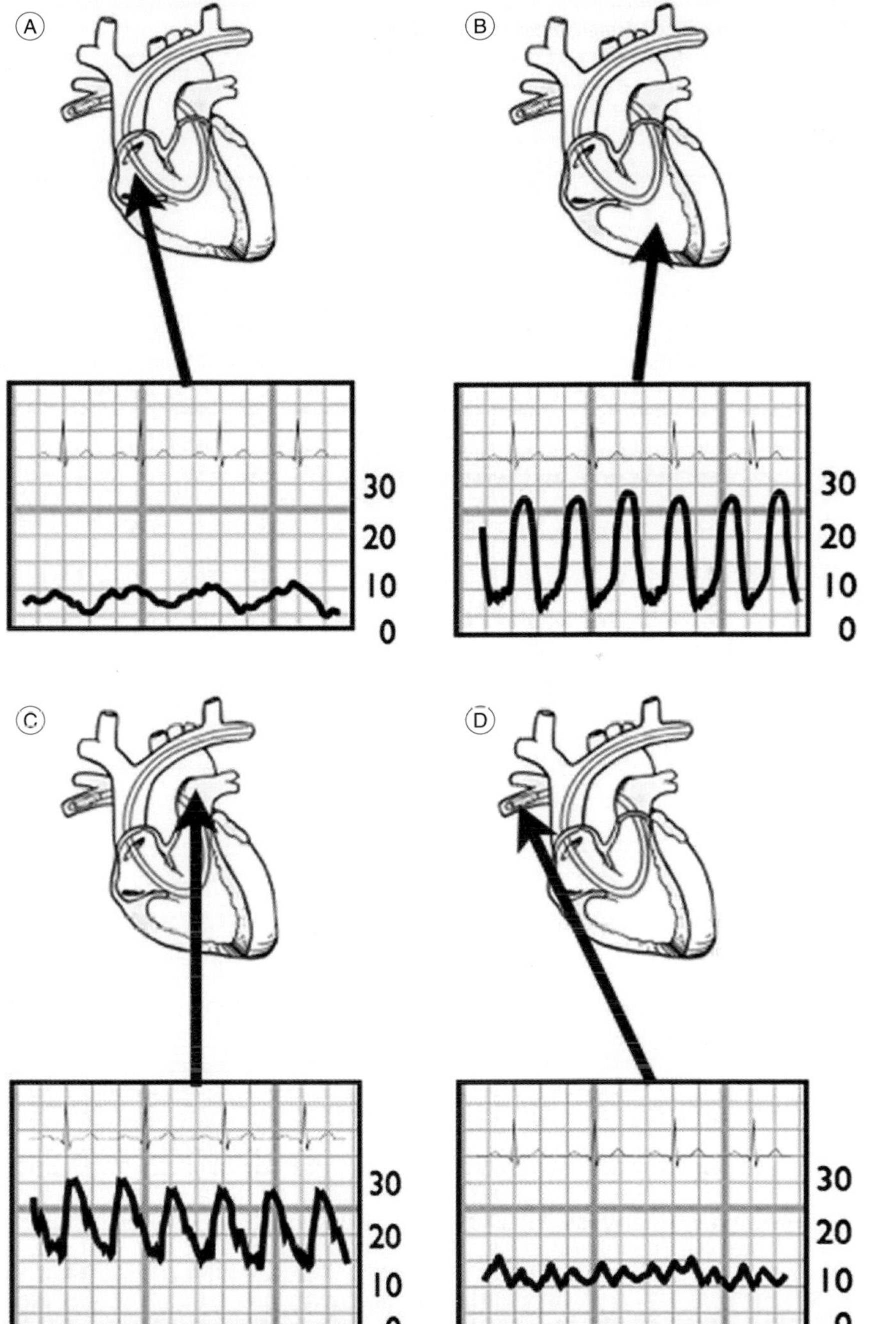

Fig. 20.2 Pulmonary artery catheterization waveforms. (A) Waveform seen when the catheter is in the right atrium. (B) Waveform of the right ventricle. (C) Waveform of the pulmonary artery. (D) Waveform of the pulmonary artery occlusion pressure. (From Hollenberg, S.M. (2013). Hemodynamic monitoring. *Chest, 143*(5), 1480–1488.)

TABLE 20.4 ■ **Simplified Normal Hemodynamic Values**

CVP/RA	0–5 mmHg
RV	25/5 mmHg
PA	25/10 mmHg (mean 15 mmHg)
PCWP/LA	8–12 mmHg
LV	120/10 mmHg
Ao	120/80 mmHg
SVR	800–1200 dynes/s/cm^5
CO	4.0–8.0 L/min
CI	2.5–4.0 L/min/m^2

Ao, Aorta; *CI*, cardiac index; *CO*, cardiac output; *CVP*, central venous pressure; *LA*, left atrium; *LV*, left ventricle; *PA*; pulmonary artery; *PCWP*, pulmonary capillary wedge pressure; *RA*, right atrium; *RV*, right ventricle; *SVR*, systemic vascular resistance.

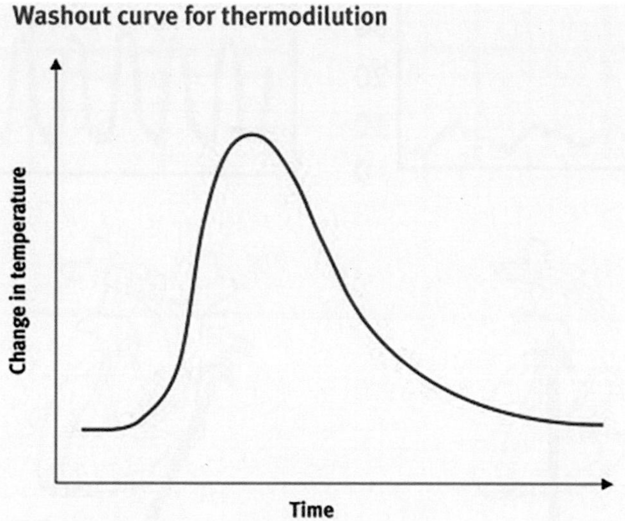

Fig. 20.3 Cardiac output measurement by thermodilution. (From Shah, A., & Oelofse, T. (2010). Advanced cardiovascular monitoring. *Surgery, 28*(4), 165–170.)

The second method used to calculate CO is known as the Fick principle. This principle states the uptake or release of a substance by an organ is equal to the product of blood flow to the organ and the arteriovenous concentration difference. Using oxygen as an example, oxygen consumption (VO_2) is equal to blood flow (CO) multiplied by the difference between arterial oxygen (CaO_2) and venous oxygen concentrations (CvO_2):

$$VO_2 = CO \times (CaO_2 - CvO_2)$$

CO can be measured by rearranging the formula and including the patient's hemoglobin (Hgb), the oxygen carrying capacity, and a correction factor:

$$CO = VO_2/[(CaO_2 - CvO_2) \times 1.34 \times Hgb]$$

CLINICAL PEARL **STEP 2/3**

CO measured according to thermodilution assumes that all blood from the proximal catheter reaches the distal sensor. Therefore, in conditions with retrograde flow or shunting (e.g., tricuspid regurgitation, ventricular septal defect, or atrial septal defect), thermodilution does not accurately reflect a patient's cardiac output.

CLINICAL PEARL **STEP 2/3**

CI is a measurement of cardiac function and can be calculated by dividing CO by patient's body surface area: CI = CO/BSA. CI is often used in clinical practice as it assesses cardiac function according to a patient's size. Normal values range from 2.6 to 4.0 L/min/m^2.

A PA catheter is placed in this patient with the results of her pressures and hemodynamics shown in Table 20.5.

TABLE 20.5 ■ **Patient's Pulmonary Artery Catheterization Values**

CVP	10 mmHg
PCWP	34 mmHg
CI	1.8 L/min/m^2
CO	3.5 L/min
SVR	1420 dynes/s/cm^5
PA	50/37 mmHg

CI, Cardiac index; *CO*, cardiac output; *CVP*, central venous pressure; *PA*; pulmonary artery; *PCWP*, pulmonary capillary wedge pressure; *SVR*, systemic vascular resistance.

How does PA catheterization help differentiate various forms of shock?

The PA catheter uses measurements of cardiac function and blood pressure to help determine the etiology of shock. In CS, left ventricular function and CO are reduced. This decrease in forward flow causes elevated pressure in the LA, pulmonary vasculature, and right heart. These patients will have increased PCWP, PA, and CVP measurements. In addition, SVR is elevated as a compensatory mechanism to maintain blood pressure. Another identifying feature of CS is a low venous oxygen concentration. As blood is pumped through the systemic circulation, peripheral tissues extract oxygen. In CS, blood flow is reduced, thereby allowing peripheral tissues more time to extract oxygen. The result is a low concentration of oxygen in the venous system.

Hypovolemic shock also has a low CI; however, this is not due to poor cardiac function but rather a result of low stroke volume. These patients will have decreased pulmonary and right heart pressures because of low intravascular volume.

In distributive shock (sepsis, anaphylaxis, liver disease), systemic vasodilation results in decreased SVR, but CO is preserved. Consequently, pulmonary and right heart pressures are normal because there is no left ventricular dysfunction. Table 20.6 summarizes the different types of shock.

The patient develops worsening dyspnea with increasing oxygen requirements. Her oxygen saturation is now 87% on 6 L of supplemental oxygen. A repeat chest radiograph shows worsening bilateral pulmonary edema. She is placed on BiPAP and treated with intravenous furosemide. However, she continues to be hypotensive.

TABLE 20.6 ■ **Differentiating Various Forms of Shock**

Type of Shock	CO/CI	SVR	PCWP	CVP	CvO_2
Cardiogenic	↓	↑	↑	↑	↓
Distributive	↑	↓	↓	↓	↑
Hypovolemia	↓	↑	↓	↓	↓

CI, Cardiac index; *CO*, cardiac output; *CvO_2*, venous oxygen concentration; *CVP*, central venous pressure; *PCWP*, pulmonary capillary wedge pressure; *SVR*, systemic vascular resistance.

How is cardiogenic shock treated?

The treatment of CS should be individualized to the specific patient and etiology of shock. In general, CS is managed through supportive care, pharmacologic treatment, revascularization if indicated, and sometimes mechanical circulatory support (MCS).

Many patients will have multiorgan failure as a result of decreased end-organ perfusion. In patients with acute renal failure, continuous renal replacement therapy (CRRT) is preferred to intermittent dialysis, because patients often do not tolerate large fluid shifts. In addition, patients who become oliguric or anuric will require renal replacement therapy (RRT) for removal of excess volume.

Hypoxemic respiratory failure from pulmonary edema is commonly seen in CS and there should be a low threshold for ventilatory support. Positive pressure ventilation with BiPAP or CPAP is especially useful in patients with ADHF, because the increased intrathoracic pressure reduces both preload and afterload.

However, the cornerstone of treatment for CS is pharmacologic therapy, using a combination of diuretics, inotropes, and vasopressors. Diuresis is essential for preload reduction and treatment of pulmonary edema. Many patients in renal failure may ultimately require RRT for volume removal. Inotropes and vasopressors are essential to maintain MAP by binding to sympathetic and dopaminergic receptors to increase cardiac contractility and, when necessary, vascular resistance. Table 20.7 provides a summary of the various catecholamines. There are limited data regarding the best vasopressor in CS; however, current guidelines suggest norepinephrine may be more favorable. In general, catecholamines should be started at the lowest doses and slowly uptitrated because they increase myocardial oxygen consumption and can precipitate arrhythmias. Negative inotropes should be avoided. Beta blockers are typically only prescribed once the patient's hemodynamics have improved.

TABLE 20.7 ■ **Affinity of Receptors for Vasopressors and Inotropes**

Medication	Receptor				
	α1	β1	β2	D1/D2	V1A
Dopamine (low dose)	0	+	0	++++	0
Dopamine (medium dose)	+	++	0	+++	0
Dopamine (high dose)	+++	++	0	+	0
Dobutamine	0	+++	++	0	0
Norepinephrine	++++	++	0	0	0
Epinephrine	+++	+++	++		
Phenylephrine	+++	0	0	0	0
Vasopressin	0	0	0	0	+++

BASIC SCIENCE/CLINICAL PEARL **STEP 1/2/3**

Milrinone is a phosphodiesterase (PDE) III inhibitor that works as an inodilator—increasing the heart's contractility and decreasing vascular resistance. By inhibiting PDE III, milrinone decreases the breakdown of cyclic adenosine monophosphate (cAMP). The subsequent increase in intracellular cAMP stimulates protein kinase activity that stimulates the release of calcium from the sarcoplasmic reticulum and the influx of calcium through L-type calcium channels, thus activating myocyte contraction.

In patients with suspected acute coronary syndrome, revascularization with percutaneous coronary intervention (PCI) or coronary artery bypass graft (CABG) should be performed as soon as possible. Clinical trials have demonstrated a significant mortality benefit with early revascularization compared with initial medical stabilization with delayed intervention in patients with an acute myocardial infarction complicated by CS.

Despite supportive care, vasoactive medications, and revascularization, some patients may still be unable to maintain adequate perfusion. In these cases, MCS is indicated. MCS includes temporary or permanent devices that are placed percutaneously or surgically and augment CO. The most widely used mechanical device is the intra-aortic balloon pump (IABP). The IABP is a device that is inserted percutaneously via the femoral (or sometimes axillary) artery and advanced into the descending aorta. The balloon inflates during diastole causing increased retrograde coronary perfusion and deflates during systole, thus decreasing afterload by creating a volume void. The IABP is therefore useful for afterload reduction and may have a modest impact on CO.

Mechanical support can be escalated further to ventricular assist devices (VADs), which reduce the workload of the heart by physically pumping blood for the ventricles. Left ventricular assist devices (LVADs) are predominantly used in CS, although some patients might also require right-sided support with a right ventricular assist device (RVAD). LVADs remove blood from the left ventricle through either continuous or pulsatile flow and return blood to the systemic arteries. LVADs can be placed either surgically or percutaneously. Surgically implanted LVADs remove blood through a tube at the apex of the left ventricle, which then pumps blood external to the heart before returning the blood to the ascending aorta. Percutaneous LVADs include the Impella and TandemHeart. The Impella device uses a catheter that is advanced into the left ventricle. Blood is aspirated from the left ventricle into the lumen of the catheter and ejected into the ascending aorta. On the contrary, TandemHeart provides external continuous flow. A catheter is advanced into the left atrium through transseptal puncture. Blood is drawn into a catheter in the left atrium and returned via an external pump to the femoral artery. VADs can provide hemodynamic support of 2.5–5.0 L/min but may cause vascular complications and hemolysis.

A final form of mechanical support is extracorporeal membrane oxygenation (ECMO), which is used in patients with cardiorespiratory failure despite mechanical ventilation. ECMO is a form of cardiopulmonary bypass where venous blood is pumped and oxygenated external to the body before being returned to the patient. Venovenous ECMO is used in isolated respiratory failure with preserved cardiac function—venous blood is removed, oxygenated, and returned to venous circulation. Venoarterial ECMO is used in cardiorespiratory failure and removes and oxygenates venous blood before returning blood to arterial circulation, thereby bypassing both the lungs and heart. Fig. 20.4 compares the various forms of MCS.

CLINICAL PEARL **STEP 3**

VADs are used in three clinical scenarios:

- In patients recovering from acute cardiogenic shock—"bridge to recovery"
- In patients waiting for cardiac transplant—"bridge to transplant"
- In patients as the final treatment—"destination therapy"

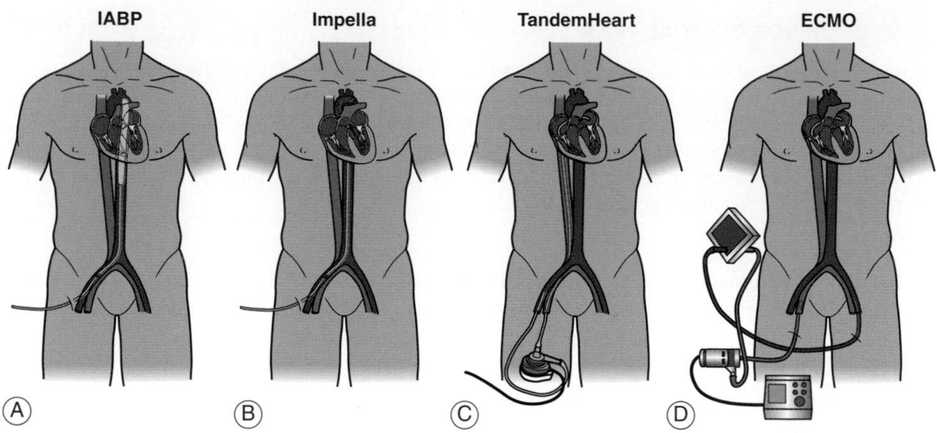

Fig. 20.4 Temporary mechanical circulatory support devices. (From Scheidt, S., Wilner, G., Mueller, H., Summers, D., Lesch, M., Wolff, G., Krakauer, J., Rubenfire, M., Fleming, P., Noon, G., Oldham, N., Killip, T., & Kantrowitz, A. (1973). Intra-aortic balloon counterpulsation in cardiogenic shock. *New England Journal of Medicine, 288*, 979.)

In addition to intravenous diuresis and BiPAP, the patient is treated with intravenous dobutamine for inotropic support. Her blood pressure begins to improve and over the following days she is weaned off BiPAP and back to room air. A repeat set of laboratory values are presented in Table 20.8.

The improvement in the patient's creatinine, liver enzymes, lactic acid, and troponin is a result of the increased contractility from dobutamine and decreased preload from furosemide. She is transitioned from intravenous to oral furosemide; however, she is unable to be weaned off dobutamine without becoming dyspneic and hypotensive. She is now dependent on inotropic support. A peripherally inserted central catheter (PICC) line is placed and the patient is discharged on dobutamine with plans for further evaluation for ventricular assist device therapy.

TABLE 20.8 ■ **Comprehensive Metabolic Panel and Laboratory Values**

Sodium	135 mmol/L
Potassium	3.9 mmol/L
Chloride	100 mmol/L
Bicarbonate	24 mmol/L
Glucose	82 mg/dL
Calcium	9.4 mg/dL
Blood urea nitrogen	28 mg/dL
Creatinine	1.31 mg/dL
Albumin	3.5 g/dL
Total bilirubin	2.1 mg/dL
Aspartate aminotransferase	44 units/L
Aspartate aminotransferase	46 units/L
Lactic acid	1.4 mmol/L
Troponin	0.04 ng/mL

Case Summary

- **Complaint/History:** A 62-year-old female presents with progressively worsening shortness of breath, nonproductive cough, fatigue, and lower extremity edema.
- **Findings:** Blood pressure is 84/53, and oxygen saturation is 85% on room air; lung exam reveals diffuse bilateral crackles; her skin is cool to the touch and she has bilateral lower extremity edema and jugular venous distention.
- **Lab Results/Tests:** Lab tests reveal elevated lactic acid, troponin, creatinine, and liver enzymes. A chest X-ray image shows an enlarged cardiac silhouette and interstitial edema. A pulmonary artery catheter shows low cardiac output, elevated pulmonary pressures, and increased SVR.

Diagnosis: Cardiogenic shock from acute decompensated heart failure exacerbation.

- **Treatment:** The patient received intravenous furosemide, intravenous dobutamine, and BiPAP. She was transitioned from intravenous to oral furosemide and weaned off BiPAP and supplemental oxygen. She was continued on intravenous dobutamine with future consideration of ventricular-assist device therapy.

BEYOND THE PEARLS

- Many patients with myocardial infarction–associated CS present with multivessel coronary artery disease, defined as stenoses in more than one coronary artery. A culprit lesion is defined as the lesion responsible for the myocardial infarct. Current guidelines from the American Heart Association recommend revascularization of the culprit lesion, in addition to hemodynamically significant nonculprit stenoses.
- Early revascularization of patients with myocardial infarction–associated CS confers a significant long-term mortality benefit at 6 months, 1 year, and 6 years when compared with initial medical stabilization.
- Norepinephrine is associated with fewer arrhythmias and lower mortality compared with dopamine in patients with shock.
- Pulmonary artery catheterization is an important tool for diagnosing and monitoring patients with cardiogenic shock. However, the use of PA catheters has not been associated with a mortality benefit. In addition, there is not a standard MAP target, because the ideal blood pressure varies from patient to patient. Instead, clinicians should use the hemodynamic parameters in conjunction with serum lactate, creatinine, liver enzymes, and the patient's urine output and mental status when determining treatment.
- Positive pressure ventilation offers several benefits. First, the increased positive end-expiratory pressure (PEEP) improves pulmonary edema by forcing fluid out of the alveoli and into the interstitium. Second, it can reduce pulmonary vascular constriction, which will further reduce pulmonary edema and can increase CO. Finally, elevated PEEP increases intrathoracic pressures and thereby decreases systemic venous return and RV preload.
- In patients refractory to a loop diuretic, a thiazide diuretic can be used as an adjunct therapy. Loop diuretics, such as furosemide, inhibit the sodium-potassium-chloride co-transporter in the thick ascending limb of the loop of Henle. Thiazide diuretics inhibit the sodium-chloride transporter in the distal convoluted tubule. The combination of a loop and thiazide diuretic provides sequential blockade in the nephron and may enhance diuresis.
- The IABP is the most widely used MCS device with about 50, 000 implanted per year. However, a randomized clinical trial of patients with acute myocardial infarction–associated CS found no difference in mortality, length of intensive care unit stay, or duration of catecholamine treatment among patients with IABP placement.
- Patient with single chamber or biventricular heart failure who are treated with MCS should be evaluated for cardiac transplant. Long-term durable MCS devices are often used in these patients as a bridge to transplant.

Bibliography

Diepen, S. V., et al. (2017). Contemporary management of cardiogenic shock: a scientific statement from the American Heart Association. *Circulation.*, *136*(16).

Hochman, J. S., Sleeper, L. A., Webb, J. G., Sanborn, T. A., White, H. D., Talley, J. D., Buller, C. E., Jacobs, A. K., Slater, J. N., Col, J., McKinlay, S. M., Picard, M. H., Menegus, M. A., Boland, J., Dzavik, V., Thompson, C. R., Wong, S. C., Steingart, R., Forman, R., Aylward, P. E., Godfrey, E., Desvigne-Nickens, P., LeJemtel, T. H. (1999). Early revascularization in acute myocardial infarction complicated by cardiogenic shock. *The New England Journal of Medicine*, *341*(9), 625–634.

Hollenberg, S. M. (2013). Hemodynamic monitoring. *Chest*, *143*(5), 1480–1488.

Reynolds, H. R., & Hochman, J. S. (2008). Cardiogenic shock. *Circulation.*, *117*(5), 686–697.

Shah, A., & Oelofse, T. (2010). Advanced cardiovascular monitoring. *Surgery*, *28*(4), 165–170.

Scheidt, S., Wilner, G., Mueller, H., Summers, D., Lesch, M., Wolff, G., Krakauer, J., Rubenfire, M., Fleming, P., Noon, G., Oldham, N., Killip, T., Kantrowitz, A. (1973). Intra-aortic balloon counterpulsation in cardiogenic shock. *New England Journal of Medicine*, *288*(19), 979–984.Thiele, Holger, Magnus Ohman, E., Desch, Steffen, Eitel, Ingo, & de Waha, Suzanne (2015). Management of cardiogenic shock. *European Heart Journal*, *36*(20), 1223–1230.

Thiele, H., Zeymer, U., Neumann, F. J., Ferenc, M., Olbrich, H. G., Hausleiter, J., Richardt, G., Hennersdorf, M., Empen, K., Fuernau, G., Desch, S., Eitel, I., Hambrecht, R., Fuhrmann, J., Böhm, M., Ebelt, H., Schneider, S., Schuler, G., Werdan. K., et al. (2012). Intraaortic balloon support for myocardial infarction with cardiogenic shock. *The New England Journal of Medicine*, *367*(14), 1287–1296.

CASE 21

A 77-Year-Old Female With Worsening Shortness of Breath and Leg Swelling

Shamili Allam ■ Michael Fong

A 77-year-old female presents to the emergency department with worsening shortness of breath and leg swelling. Her leg swelling first started about a year ago and has worsened gradually since that time. Over the past few months, she started noticing shortness of breath that is especially worse at nighttime when she is trying to sleep. Lately, she has been sleeping sitting up on several pillows. Her functional capacity has also decreased over the last few years, and she is now only able to walk short distances inside her house before becoming short of breath. Her only medical history is hypertension, for which she does not take medication. Her family history is significant for hypertension and diabetes in multiple individuals as well as a sister who had sarcoidosis.

On presentation, the patient's blood pressure is 163/75 mmHg, heart rate 95beats/min, and oxygen saturation 86% on room air. Physical examination is significant for jugular venous distension, crackles most prominent in the lung bases, and significant pitting edema in both lower extremities to her thighs. Chest radiograph (CXR, Fig. 21.1) shows pulmonary vascular congestion and bilateral pleural effusions.

What is the differential diagnosis for volume overload?

This patient is showing signs of both intravascular and extravascular volume overload. Jugular venous distension indicates intravascular overload. The presence of peripheral edema and pulmonary vascular congestion on CXR indicate extravascular overload. Although not seen in this patient, excess volume can also manifest as abdominal distension from ascites or generalized body swelling, known as anasarca.

Conditions that affect the heart, kidneys, and liver commonly lead to volume overload. Therefore, a close evaluation of these organs is indicated to look for diseases such as heart failure (HF), kidney disease, or liver failure. Although there are other etiologies that can be included to broaden our list of differential diagnoses (e.g., protein malnutrition, Cushing's syndrome, profound hypothyroidism), these are good places to start.

What should be part of the initial workup?

When such a patient presents to the emergency department, clinicians should start with basic lab work including a comprehensive metabolic panel and urinalysis to evaluate hepatic and renal function. To evaluate the heart, an electrocardiogram (ECG) should always be obtained as an initial diagnostic test given its low cost and broad availability. A transthoracic echocardiogram (TTE) with Doppler is the next step in evaluation and provides information about cardiac function. A B-type natriuretic peptide (BNP) level, a marker of cardiac stretch from volume overload, should also be obtained.

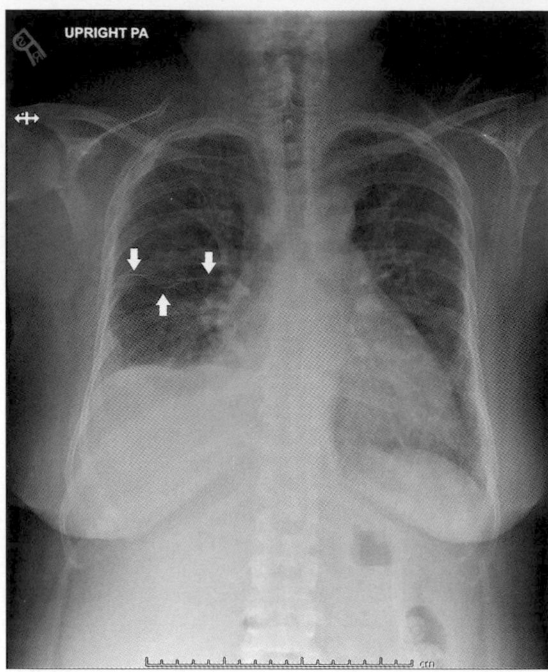

Fig. 21.1 This chest radiograph shows clear signs of volume overload. Notice that you can see prominent vessels and a prominent lateral fissure *(arrows)* suggestive of pulmonary venous congestion. There is also bilateral blunting of the costophrenic angles, indicative of pleural effusions.

CLINICAL PEARL **STEP 2/3**

An elevated BNP value is helpful in the diagnosis of HF but the value will probably not return to normal with treatment. BNP levels should be trended and a "baseline" value should be determined when the patient is at their dry weight. Note that a low BNP value (<25 pg/mL) makes HF less likely.

Basic lab results are shown in Table 21.1. Abdominal ultrasound shows trace ascites, kidneys that are normal in size, and a normal appearing liver. BNP is noted to be elevated. ECG (Fig. 21.2) shows left ventricular hypertrophy. TTE shows left ventricular basal septal and basal posterolateral wall thickness >1.1 cm, indicating hypertrophy. Grade III diastolic dysfunction is also noted, along with a left ventricular ejection fraction of 68%. The systolic pressure in the pulmonary arteries is estimated to be 59 mmHg, which is elevated.

CLINICAL PEARL **STEP 2/3**

An elevated pulmonary artery systolic pressure (>20–25 mmHg) is possibly an indication of pulmonary hypertension. Note that pulmonary hypertension is divided by the WHO into several groups. This patient probably has WHO Group II pulmonary hypertension, which is a result of left heart failure. The treatment for this is to treat the HF.

What is this patient's diagnosis?

This patient has heart failure with preserved ejection fraction (HFpEF). HF is a condition that is characterized by worsening functional status resulting from a decreased cardiac output. The lack of forward

TABLE 21.1 ■ **Laboratory Values**

Serum	
Sodium	141 mmol/L
Potassium	3.9 mmol/L
Chloride	103 mmol/L
Bicarbonate	24 mmol/L
Creatinine	1.23 mg/dL
Estimated GFR	49 mL/min
Albumin	3.1 g/dL
INR	1.1
Bilirubin (total)	0.5 mg/dL
BNP	250 pg/mL
Urine	
Protein	Negative
Casts	Hyaline casts present
Leukocytes	Negative
Nitrites	Negative
Blood	Negative

GFR, Glomerular filtration rate.

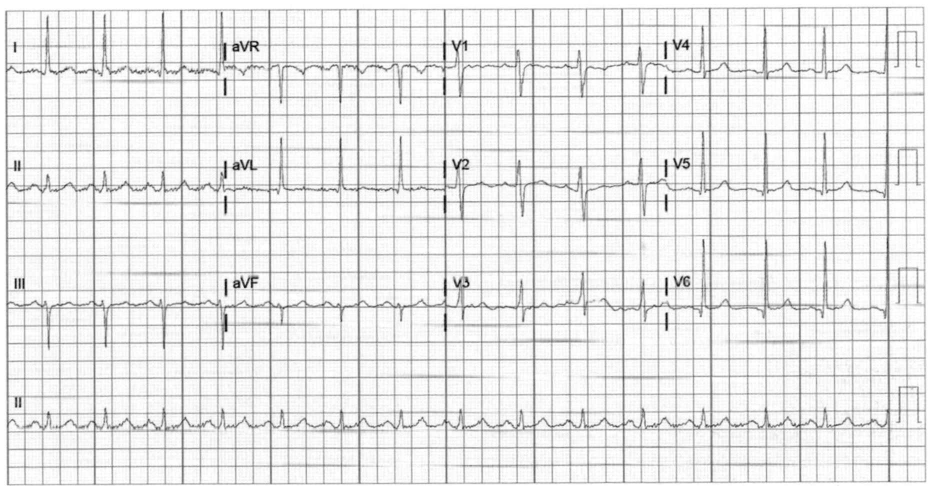

Fig. 21.2 This ECG shows left ventricular hypertrophy (note the R wave height in lead avL >11 mm).

flow through the heart often leads to a backup of fluid either in the pulmonary vasculature (causing pulmonary edema) or venous system (causing peripheral edema). HF describes a constellation of cardiac disorders, which can be further described as right or left sided. Left heart failure is further characterized as having a "reduced" ejection fraction (EF), <40%, termed heart failure with reduced ejection fraction (HFrEF), mildly reduced or mid-range EF, 40-49% (HFmrEF) or a "preserved" EF ≥50% (HFpEF).

Note that HF is a clinical diagnosis. It is defined by characteristic signs and symptoms caused by cardiac dysfunction. Diagnostic tests help support the diagnosis but are not strictly part of the diagnostic criteria. In this patient, worsening functional status and volume overload are suggestive of heart failure. Diastolic dysfunction is seen on the TTE and the BNP is elevated, both of which support the diagnosis. Prior to diagnosing HF, alternative diagnoses should be considered (e.g., pulmonary arterial hypertension, coronary artery disease).

It is important to ascertain the severity of HF. The two most commonly used systems are the New York Heart Association (NYHA) functional classification system, which ranges from I to IV, and the American College of Cardiology/American Heart Association (ACC/AHA) staging system, which ranges from A to D (see Table 21.2). Note that the NYHA class describes symptoms and a patient can go up or down between classes with interventions. The ACC/AHA stage describes the progression of the patient's disease. Patients go from A through D and cannot go backwards after a stage has been reached. At presentation, this patient would be classified as NYHA Class III, ACC/AHA Stage C. We hope that once optimized, she will be able to return to the NYHA Class I or II, but she will remain ACC/AHA Stage C.

What about this patient's kidneys and liver?

This patient's creatinine is elevated and her glomerular filtration rate (GFR) is decreased, which may be an indication of kidney disease. It is important to know that heart failure exacerbations can cause elevation in creatinine, a phenomenon known as cardiorenal syndrome. Poor heart function leads to a reduction in kidney perfusion. Clinically, it presents with bland urine sediment without cells, a lack of significant proteinuria, presence of hyaline casts, and a low fractional excretion of sodium.

The treatment is volume removal to decrease cardiac stretch, improve forward flow, and reduce renal venous hypertension, which further compromises renal perfusion. Cardiorenal syndrome can either be an acute phenomenon, where creatinine corrects with volume correction, or it can lead to chronic kidney disease.

You may be concerned about liver disease given this patient's decreased albumin. However, note that her INR (indicative of synthetic function of the liver) and bilirubin (indicative of secretory function) are normal. Also, the abdominal ultrasound, which is very sensitive for hepatic pathology, shows a normal-sized liver without mention of cirrhosis. Albumin is an "inverse" acute phase reactant, meaning that it decreases in patients who are ill, including with HF.

TABLE 21.2 ■ **Classification of Heart Failure**

NYHA Class		ACC/AHA Stage	
—		A	At high risk of HF but without structural heart disease or symptoms of HF.
I	No limitation of physical activity. Ordinary physical activity does not cause symptoms of HF.	B	Structural heart disease but without signs or symptoms of HF.
II	Slight limitation of physical activity. Comfortable at rest, but ordinary physical activity results in symptoms of HF.	C	Structural heart disease with prior or current symptoms of HF.
III[a]	Marked limitation of physical activity. Comfortable at rest, but less than ordinary activity causes symptoms of HF.	D	Refractory HF requiring specialized interventions.
IV	Unable to carry on any physical activity without symptoms of HF, or symptoms of HF at rest.		

[a]Sometimes, NYHA Class III is further divided into IIIa and IIIb without or with recent dyspnea at rest. Class IIIb is commonly used as a cutoff for "severe" heart failure and is encountered as an inclusion criteria for clinical trials and advanced heart failure therapies.

ACC/AHA, American College of Cardiology/American Heart Association; *HF*, heart failure; *NYHA*, New York Heart Association.

How is the volume removed?

The key to managing symptoms associated with HFpEF is to maintain euvolemia. This patient is volume overloaded; therefore, the volume must be removed either by aggressive diuresis or, if refractory, ultrafiltration. Loop diuretics are typically used, including furosemide, bumetanide, torsemide, and ethacrynic acid. While an inpatient, an intravenous loop diuretic is used (commonly furosemide or bumetanide), with transition to a lower oral dose to maintain euvolemia. The thiazide diuretics, such as metolazone or chlorothiazide, are sometimes used as adjunct agents to the loop diuretics to achieve a better diuretic response. While the patient is getting a high dose of diuretics, it is important to monitor closely for signs of electrolyte derangements (hyponatremia, hypokalemia, hypomagnesemia) and increasing BUN, creatinine, and CO_2 (indicative of contraction metabolic alkalosis).

CLINICAL PEARL **STEP 1**

Loop diuretics block the Na-K-2Cl cotransporters in the thick ascending limp of the loop of Henle. They are very efficient at removing sodium and thus volume. However, they also remove potassium, which can cause profound hypokalemia. The excretion of negative Cl-ions also promotes the excretion of positive Ca++ and Mg++ ions; therefore, these levels should also be monitored.

CLINICAL PEARL **STEP 2/3**

Bioavailability of the drug needs to be considered when transitioning from intravenous to oral formulations. Furosemide does not have good oral bioavailability, and most patients require twice the dose when given orally as compared with intravenously. Torsemide and bumetanide's oral formulations have closer to 100% bioavailability; therefore, oral formulations may be given in a 1:1 manner. Remember that gut wall edema in volume overloaded patients can reduce absorption regardless of bioavailability, necessitating the use of IV diuretics.

How would you manage the patient's hypertension?

Hypertension should be controlled with a goal systolic blood pressure <120 mmHg. There is increasing evidence to include an aldosterone inhibitor, such as spironolactone, as part of the regimen for patients with HFpEF. Spironolactone has been shown to decrease HF-related hospitalizations globally, and when tested in patients from North and South America, it was shown to have a mortality benefit. However, spironolactone is known as a "potassium sparing" diuretic and may cause hyperkalemia in some patients. Therefore, aldosterone inhibitors need to be used with caution in patients with chronic kidney disease who are already prone to hyperkalemia and all patients need close monitoring of serum potassium level. Ideally, most patients should receive a trial of spironolactone. Apart from that, the guidelines for medication choice do not differ significantly from management of other patients with hypertension. Although beta blockers, angiotensin converting enzyme inhibitors (ACE-I), and angiotensin receptor blockers (ARBs) have not been shown to have a survival benefit in HFpEF patients, they have been shown to decrease HF hospitalizations.

Your patient is admitted to the hospital for IV diuresis. Her symptoms of shortness of breath and peripheral edema are resolved with diuretics. Euvolemia is achieved prior to discharge and she is transitioned to oral torsemide. Her kidney function has returned to normal and spironolactone is initiated to help reach the blood pressure goal prior to hospital discharge.

How do you manage heart failure long term?

Apart from maintaining euvolemia and normotension, the etiology of heart failure should be determined and treated if indicated (see Table 21.3). Note that hypertensive heart disease is the

TABLE 21.3 ■ **Common Etiologies of Heart Failure With Preserved Ejection Fraction**

Hypertension	A very common cause of HFpEF, longstanding arterial hypertension causes concentric hypertrophy of the left ventricular wall, making the muscle stiff. This causes diastolic dysfunction. Controlling blood pressure early can prevent LV hypertrophy.
Coronary artery disease	Ongoing ischemia can cause impaired relaxation of the ventricular wall and eventually remodeling, leading to heart failure with either reduced or preserved EF.
Atrial fibrillation	The rapid ventricular rates associated with atrial fibrillation decrease diastolic filling time. This can cause left atrial pressure changes and volume backup.
Systemic inflammation	Patients with longstanding disorders (including chronic kidney disease, metabolic syndrome, hypertension, anemia, and diabetes mellitus) live in a state of chronic systemic inflammation. This causes cytokine release and the creation of reactive oxygen species, which can increase the resting tension of cardiac myocytes leading to heart failure.
Infiltrative disorders	Systemic infiltrative disease can cause infiltration of myocytes leading to ventricular hypertrophy and restriction. Such diseases include amyloidosis, sarcoidosis, and hemochromatosis.

EF, Ejection fraction; *HFpEF*, heart failure with preserved ejection fraction.

most common cause of HFpEF and your patient has a history of hypertension. However, all patients should undergo evaluation for coronary artery disease (either via coronary angiography or cardiac stress test). Many patients will additionally benefit from looking into alternate etiologies, including restrictive heart diseases. Positron emission tomography (PET) and cardiac magnetic resonance imaging (CMR) are useful tools to evaluate for these causes. Sodium glucose transport protein 2 (SGLT2) inhibitors are a class of medications initially developed for the treatment of diabetes, that have been shown to be effective in the treatment of HF regardless of the presence of diabetes. They are the first class of medications to demonstrate survival benefit in large clinical trials in HFpEF.

Given the patient's pertinent family history of sarcoidosis (which can present as an infiltrative cardiomyopathy causing restrictive disease), a PET scan was done as an outpatient. This showed an infiltrative process, which is possibly indicative of cardiac sarcoidosis (Fig. 21.3). The patient was referred for endocardial biopsy and rheumatologic evaluation for further workup of sarcoidosis.

How should you counsel your patient?

HFpEF is a chronic disease, and your patient should be counseled on its management prior to discharge. She should be told to maintain a low sodium diet (less than 3000 mg of sodium daily) to avoid volume overload. She should monitor her weight and symptoms at home closely, keeping a weight diary. If she notes an increase in her weight or worsening symptoms, she should take additional doses of diuretics or contact her providers. Additionally, she should be engaging in regular physical activity to improve her functional status.

Case Summary

- **Complaint/History:** A 77-year-old female with a history of hypertension complains of progressive shortness of breath and leg swelling as well as decreased functional capacity. She has a family history significant for sarcoidosis.
- **Findings:** Examination showed jugular venous distension, crackles in bilateral lung bases, and significant pitting edema in her thighs.

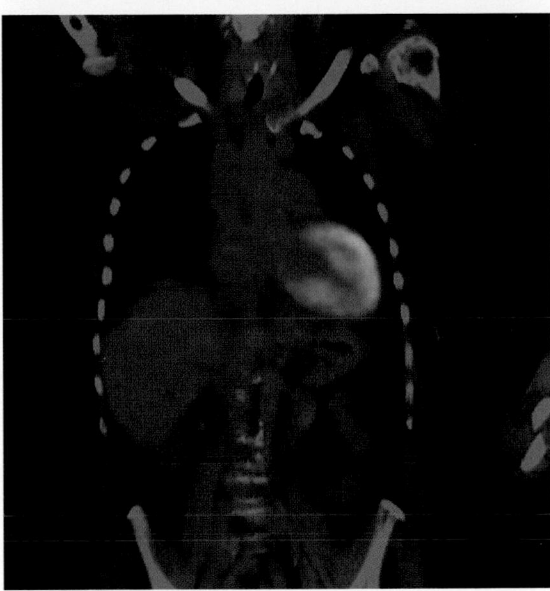

Fig. 21.3 This positron emission tomography scan shows increased uptake in the left ventricular myocardium, indicative of infiltrative disease.

- **Lab Results/Tests:** BNP was elevated to 250 pg/mL. TTE showed left ventricular hypertrophy and Grade III diastolic dysfunction. Left ventricular ejection fraction was 68%. Pulmonary artery systolic pressure was estimated at 59 mmHg.

Diagnosis: Presentation is consistent with heart failure with preserved ejection fraction complicated by volume overload.

- **Treatment:** The mainstays of treating HFpEF are diuretics to maintain euvolemia and control of hypertension.
- **Additional Workup:** Patients must be evaluated for etiology of HFpEF. In this patient's case, her PET CT was indicative of sarcoidosis and further evaluation and treatment were necessary.

BEYOND THE PEARLS

- HFpEF has been increasing in incidence. Some estimates show that it is more prevalent than HFrEF.
- The mortality of HFpEF is starting to approach that of HFrEF, although patients with HFpEF die more frequently from noncardiac causes.
- Consider HFpEF in your differential diagnosis when you have an elderly patient with hypertension and other systemic diseases who presents with classic heart failure symptoms.
- Unlike HFrEF, beta blockers and ACE-I/ARBs have not been shown to improve mortality.
- The EF cutoffs for diagnosing HFpEF have traditionally not been clearly defined. HFmrEF; EF between 40% and 49%) is a newly described entity, with management similar to HFrEF.
- HF, regardless of EF, necessitates treatment of its comorbidities. These include obesity, coronary artery disease, atrial fibrillation, and sleep apnea.

Bibliography

Anker SD, Butler J, Filippatos G, Ferreira JP, Bocchi E, Böhm M, et al. (2021). Empagliflozin in heart failure with a preserved ejection fraction. *The New England Journal of Medicine,* 14;385(16), 1451–1461. doi: 10.1056/NEJMoa2107038. PMID: 34449189.

Pitt, B., Pfeffer, M. A., Assmann, S. F., Boineau R, Anand IS, Claggett B, et al. (2014). Spironolactone for heart failure with preserved ejection fraction. *The New England Journal of Medicine, 370*(15), 1383–1392.

Ponikowski, P., Voors, A. A., Anker, S. D., Bueno H, Cleland JGF, Coats AJS, et al. (2016). 2016 ESC Guidelines for the diagnosis and treatment of acute and chronic heart failure: The Task Force for the diagnosis and treatment of acute and chronic heart failure of the European Society of Cardiology (ESC). Developed with the special contribution of the Heart Failure Association (HFA) of the ESC. *European Journal of Heart Failure, 18*(8), 891–975.

Redfield. M. M. (2016). Heart Failure with preserved ejection fraction. *The New England Journal of Medicine, 375*(19), 1868–1877.

Writing Committee Members, Yancy, C. W., Jessup, M., Bozkurt, B., Butler J, Casey DE Jr, Drazner MH, et al. (2013). 2013 ACCF/AHA guideline for the management of heart failure: a report of the American College of Cardiology Foundation/American Heart Association Task Force on practice guidelines. *Circulation, 128*(16), e240–327.

Yancy, C. W., Jessup, M., Bozkurt, B., Butler J, Casey DE Jr, Colvin MM, et al. (2017). 2017 ACC/AHA/HFSA focused update of the 2013 ACCF/AHA Guideline for the management of heart failure: A report of the American College of Cardiology/American Heart Association task force on clinical practice guidelines and the Heart Failure Society of America. *Circulation, 136*(6), e137–e161.

CASE 22

A 54-Year-Old Male With Bilateral Leg Pain

Ravi M. Rao ■ Prabhdeep S. Sethi

A 54-year-old male arrives at your clinic complaining of pain in both of his legs when he walks. This was first noted 2–3 years ago but has been gradually progressing. He states that it starts a few minutes after he starts to walk and then goes away if he rests. He describes the pain as achy and localized to his calves. He rates the pain at 8/10 at its worst. He denies any recent trauma or injuries. He denies leg swelling or skin changes. His medical history is significant for obesity (BMI 34), type 2 diabetes for which he takes metformin twice daily, and smoking 1 pack of cigarettes daily for the past 32 years. On physical examination, his pulse rate is 84 bpm, blood pressure is 137/84 mmHg, respiration rate is 18 breaths/min, and oxygen saturation is 94% on room air. He appears obese and his lower extremity pulses are weak. Upper extremity pulses are 2+. Reflexes are normal and there is no loss of sensation in any limb. There is no focal pain induced in his legs or hips with palpation over bony or muscular surfaces. Complete range of motion is preserved during passive movement. You also notice that his legs are somewhat shiny and that there is less leg hair than usual. Lab testing is unremarkable except for elevated low density lipoprotein (LDL) and total cholesterol levels and a hemoglobin A1c of 7.5%.

What is your differential diagnosis at this point?

There are many causes of lower extremity pain, which are summarized in Table 22.1. However, several key features of the history and physical examination will help to narrow our differential diagnosis. We note that this gentleman has pain in both of his calf muscles that is progressive, exertional, severe, and achy in quality. He has a history of obesity and type 2 diabetes, as well as a significant smoking history. The physical examination shows that he appears obese, has weak pulses in his legs, and has a reduced amount of leg hair. Based on these findings, we are more likely to consider a vascular cause of his leg pain rather than a neurogenic or musculoskeletal etiology.

CLINICAL PEARL **STEP 1/2/3**

True claudication and pseudoclaudication can be differentiated by history. True claudication worsens with exertion and improves with rest. Pseudoclaudication worsens when standing and improves with sitting or lying down.

Which tests would you order next to help narrow your diagnosis?

When the clinical indication of lower extremity atherosclerotic disease is high, we can order an arterial-brachial index (ABI) to assess the physiologic significance of reduced arterial blood flow and classify its severity. This test is performed by measuring blood pressures of the brachial arteries of both arms and the posterior tibial and dorsalis pedis arteries in both legs. To calculate the

TABLE 22.1 ■ **Differential Diagnosis of Bilateral Lower Extremity Pain**

	Neurogenic Causes aka "Pseudoclaudication"		
Vascular Causes	**Neurospinal**	**Neuropathic**	**Musculoskeletal Causes**
Progressive atherosclerotic disease	Degenerative disc disease	Diabetes	Hip/knee arthritis
Deep vein thrombosis	Spinal stenosis	Alcohol abuse	Leg muscle cramping
Arterial aneurysm	Tumor compression	Vitamin B_{12} deficiency	Iliotibial band syndrome
Arterial dissection		Medication-induced (e.g., chemotherapy)	Chronic exertional compartment syndrome
Embolism (blood, air, fat)			
Popliteal entrapment syndrome			
Adventitial cystic disease			
Thromboangiitis obliterans			

TABLE 22.2 ■ **Interpretation of Ankle-Brachial Index (ABI) Values**

ABI	Interpretation	Recommendation
>1.4	Stiffened blood vessels, calcification	Referral to vascular specialist
0.9–1.4	Normal	
0.8–0.9	Mild arterial disease	Treat reversible risk factors
0.5–0.8	Moderate arterial disease	Referral to vascular specialist
<0.5	Severe arterial disease	Referral to vascular specialist

ABI for one side, the highest systolic pressure from either artery of that leg should be divided by the highest systolic pressure from either brachial artery. An ABI less than 0.9 or greater than 1.4 is considered abnormal and prompts further workup, imaging, and treatment. If ABI is found to be between 0.9 and 1.4 and the patient still has concerning symptoms, a postexercise ABI can be measured and is considered abnormal if the ABI decreases by >20%. Table 22.2 elaborates more on the interpretation of the ABI test results (see Figs. 22.1 and 22.2).

CLINICAL PEARL **STEP 2/3**

An ABI cutoff of <0.9 has a sensitivity of 79%–95% and specificity of >95%, making it a good test to "rule in" the disease. [5]

Which risk factors does this patient have for developing peripheral arterial disease (PAD)?

Major risk factors for PAD include advanced age, male gender, Black Americans, a family history of atherosclerotic disease, known personal history of atherosclerotic disease at other sites, smoking history, hypertension, dyslipidemia, and diabetes. In regards to age, a patient older than 70 years is considered to have an increased risk of PAD, but patients aged 50–69 years of age are also considered higher risk if they smoke tobacco or have diabetes and patients aged 40–49 years of age are considered higher risk if they have diabetes and another risk factor for atherosclerosis.

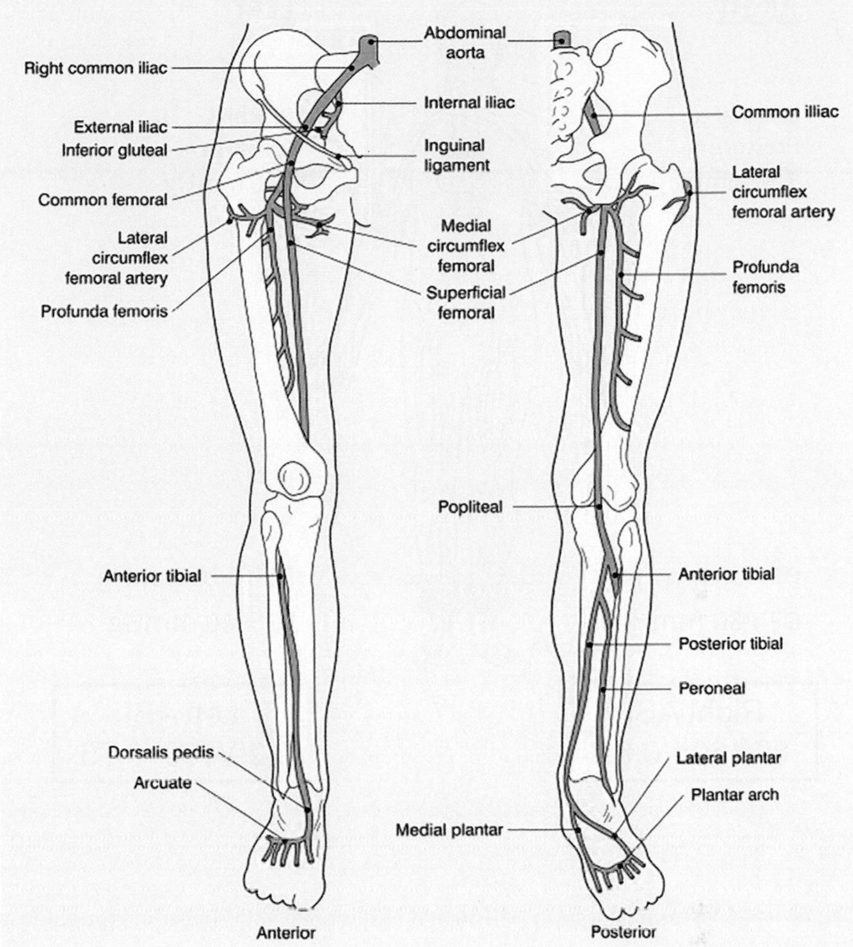

Fig. 22.1 Location of lower extremity arterial anatomy including aorta and peripheral arteries. Important arteries include internal and external iliac, superficial femoral, profunda femoris (deep femoral), popliteal, anterior tibial, posterior tibial, and dorsalis pedis.

Smoking is one of the strongest risk factors for peripheral arterial disease and is two or three times more strongly associated with the development of PAD compared with coronary heart disease.

Who should be screened for PAD?

Globally, there are approximately 200 million people with PAD and it is estimated that almost 20% of adults older than 55 years of age have PAD. However, patients do not always present with the typical symptoms of PAD such as exertional pain in the legs that is relieved with rest (claudication). It is estimated that approximately 20%–50% of patients with PAD are asymptomatic while 40%–50% present with atypical leg pain and only 10%–35% of patients present with typical leg claudication. Screening for PAD is not routinely indicated in asymptomatic patients. However, identification of the above risk factors in individuals can help to identify which asymptomatic patients are most likely to develop clinically significant PAD. If a patient with multiple

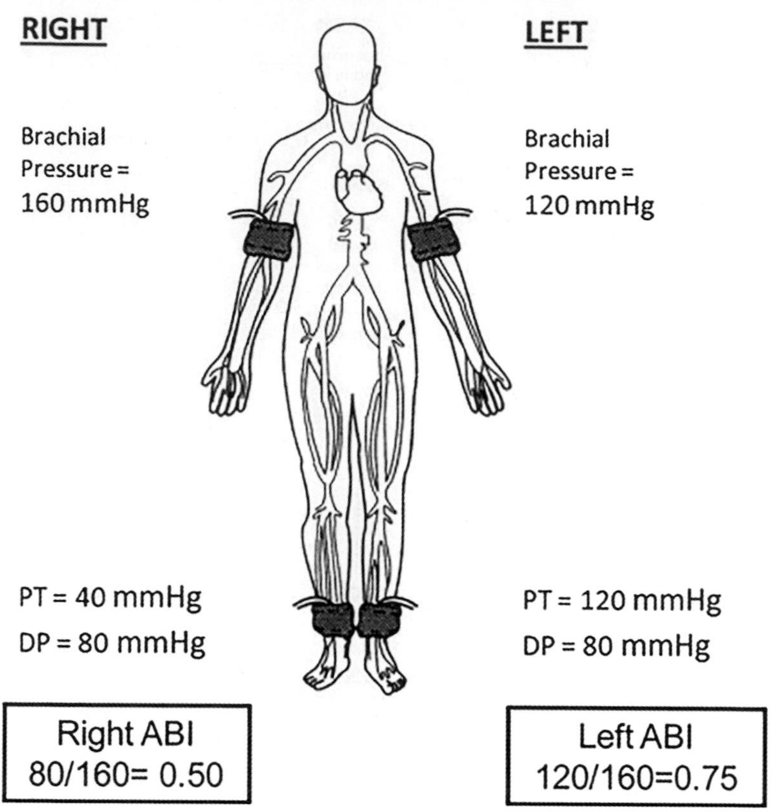

Fig. 22.2 Example of calculating ankle-brachial index (ABI) using brachial artery, dorsalis pedis artery (DP), and posterior tibial artery (PT) pressures.

risk factors desires a screening test, an ABI should be measured with similar interpretation as in a symptomatic patient.

Peripheral artery disease is a risk factor for the presence of arterial disease in other areas such as the coronary arteries. The presence of an abnormal ABI in an asymptomatic patient does not necessarily indicate a need for invasive evaluation of the PAD, but rather a thorough cardiovascular risk stratification of the patient and aggressive risk factor modification.

CLINICAL PEARL **STEP 2/3**

In patients with diabetes or end-stage renal disease, ABI values can be falsely elevated because of arterial calcifications. A toe-brachial index may be more reliable in these subsets of patients.

The gentleman in our case has a measured ABI of 0.75. What treatment would you offer at this time?
The treatment strategy for PAD aims to alleviate symptoms and prevent further progression of disease. Treatment choice is based on severity at time of presentation. Although several classification systems exist to categorize the severity of disease, based on this gentleman's ABI result of 0.75 and the absence of major complications (rest pain, nonhealing ulcers >2 weeks in duration, and gangrene), we can categorize his disease as mild to moderate. In such cases, we would

begin by recommending noninvasive management with risk factor modification and medication optimization.

The mainstays of medical therapy include antithrombotic pharmacologic treatment with aspirin or clopidogrel, lipid-lowering therapy with a statin medication, and other medications as needed to control comorbidities such as diabetes and hypertension. Risk factor modification is aimed to address daily exercise, maintaining a well-balanced diet, weight loss, and smoking cessation. A supervised weight-loss and exercise program is often utilized to increase compliance and monitor effectiveness. Follow-up should be conducted at regular 3-month intervals or more frequently as needed to assess improvement or lack of efficacy.

CLINICAL PEARL **STEP 3**

Although aspirin, clopidogrel, and statin medications have shown benefit in controlling progression of atherosclerotic disease and reduction in rates of myocardial infarction (MI) and cerebrovascular accidents (CVA), they have not consistently shown benefit in reducing symptoms of limb claudication.

We see the patient in the clinic 3 months later. At this time, he states that he has been compliant with all medications (aspirin, statin, and metformin). He also states that he has now quit smoking, is engaging in daily 30-minute walks with his wife, and has lost 10 pounds. His symptoms have improved slightly and he now can walk for longer distances before the onset of pain in his legs. You schedule a follow-up visit in 1 year.

What more do you want to know at this time?

At follow up visits for patients with PAD, it is important to ask certain questions to assess for improvement or worsening of the disease. First, we must ask detailed questions about existing symptoms and then assess for any new symptoms and/or signs of major complications. Key questions related to limb claudication include:

- How far can you walk before symptoms of leg pain occur?
- How severe is this pain?
- Does it cause you to stop walking and take a break?
- How long a break is required before you can resume walking?
- Does this pain come back after you resume walking for a similar distance?
- Is the limitation of walking getting worse over time?
- Is the limitation of walking having a significant effect on your overall lifestyle?

Key questions related to complications include:

- Do you experience pain in your limbs at rest?
- Do you experience pain in your limbs that causes you to wake from sleep?
- Do these symptoms improve if you hang the limb off the side of the bed?
- Have you noticed any ulcers or wounds on your limbs that are not healing? If so, how long have they been present?

The patient states that although his symptoms have gotten slightly better, the pain is still bothersome and is causing significant limitation to his lifestyle. He reports no nonhealing ulcers, wounds, or rest pain. He is curious about what more he could be doing.

What would you offer him at this time?

At this time, it would be reasonable to offer him pharmacologic therapy in the form of a medication called cilostazol, which is a phosphodiesterase-3 inhibitor that reduces platelet aggregation effects and is also an arterial vasodilator. It has shown to have a benefit in improving symptoms of limb claudication, as measured in walk distance, in patients with PAD. Beneficial effects can be noted as early as 4 weeks after initiation of treatment. Commonly reported side effects include headaches, gastrointestinal discomfort, and dizziness. It is also absolutely contraindicated in patients with any severity of heart failure with reduced ejection fraction.

At his 1-year follow-up visit, he states that his symptoms have unfortunately been slowly returning and are now worse than ever before. He reports no nonhealing ulcers, wounds, or rest pain. A repeat ABI done at this time results to 0.40.

What can you offer him at this time?

At this time, he would classify as having severe PAD and would warrant further workup with advanced imaging techniques including computed tomography (CT)/magnetic resonance (MR) angiography and/or digital subtraction angiography (DSA). CT angiography uses contrast dye injected into the vascular system to image the anatomy of arteries in peripheral limbs. MR angiography uses a similarly injected contrast dye to image peripheral anatomy but cannot easily be used in people with pacemakers, metal implants, or claustrophobia. DSA is considered the gold standard for arteriography and provides real-time imaging of peripheral vasculature by injecting contrast dye into the arterial system. It also provides vascular specialists the opportunity to perform simultaneous study and any necessary intervention in the same procedure. Depending on the location and size of any arterial narrowing or disease, different treatment modalities can be offered.

Disease involving the distal aorta and its iliac branches (aortoiliac disease) is called inflow disease and disease below the inguinal ligament in the femoropopliteal region is called outflow disease. In general, isolated arterial disease can be treated with angioplasty, stenting, or bypass surgery. If multilevel disease is identified, further angioplasty/stenting/bypass can be performed in this area. However, if long segments of arterial disease or severe calcific arterial disease are identified and the patient is a good surgical candidate (good surgical targets, medically fit, significant life expectancy to benefit from procedure), bypass surgery is preferred. Postprocedural medication choice is dependent on the procedure selected and the type of stent or graft used, if any. Follow-up should also be conducted on a regular basis to encourage compliance with lifestyle modification, ensure medication compliance, and monitoring of symptoms (see Figs. 22.3, 22.4, and 22.5).

The patient was found to have significant aortoiliac narrowing and elected to have an aortoiliac stent. He has recovered well from the procedure, continues to take his medications, exercises regularly, and no longer smokes. He now has near-complete resolution of his leg pain and enjoys an active lifestyle.

Case Summary

- **Complaint/History:** A 54-year-old male with type 2 diabetes mellitus, obesity, and smoking history presents with 2–3 years of gradually progressive bilateral leg pain that worsens with exertion.
- **Findings:** Weak lower extremity pulses, hair loss on legs.
- **Lab Results/Tests:** Lab results reveal elevated LDL level, elevated total cholesterol level, and hemoglobin A1c of 7.5%. Ankle-brachial index is 0.75.

Diagnosis: Peripheral arterial disease.

- **Treatment:** The patient received daily aspirin, statin medication, and metformin. He also quit smoking, exercised regularly, and lost 10 pounds. After 3 months, he saw a significant but incomplete improvement in his symptoms and cilostazol was added to his medications. One year later, his symptoms worsened and a repeat ABI was 0.40. He received a peripheral

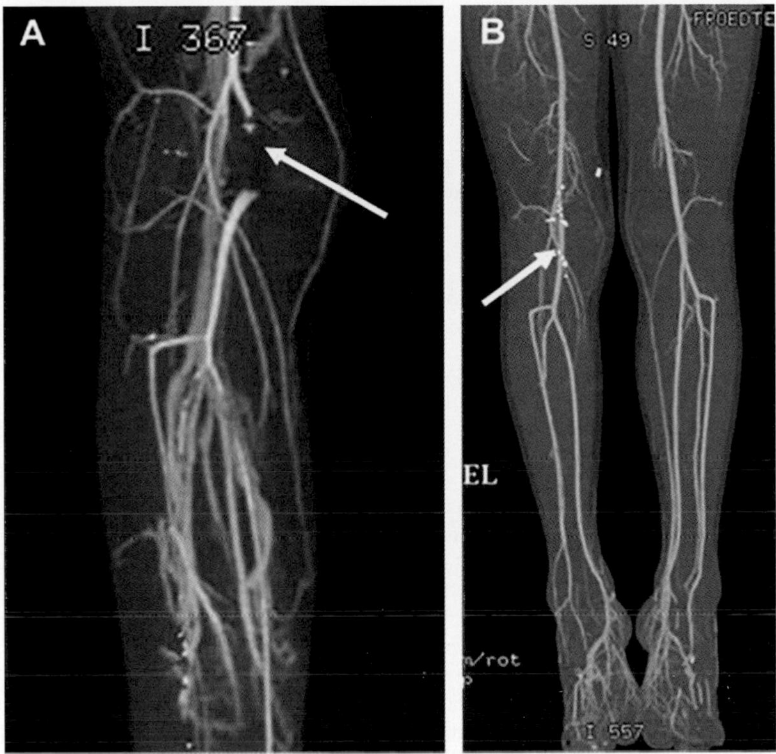

Fig. 22.3 CT Angiography. (A) Right-sided popliteal artery entrapment syndrome and (B) postoperative resolution of obstruction after placement of venous bypass graft.

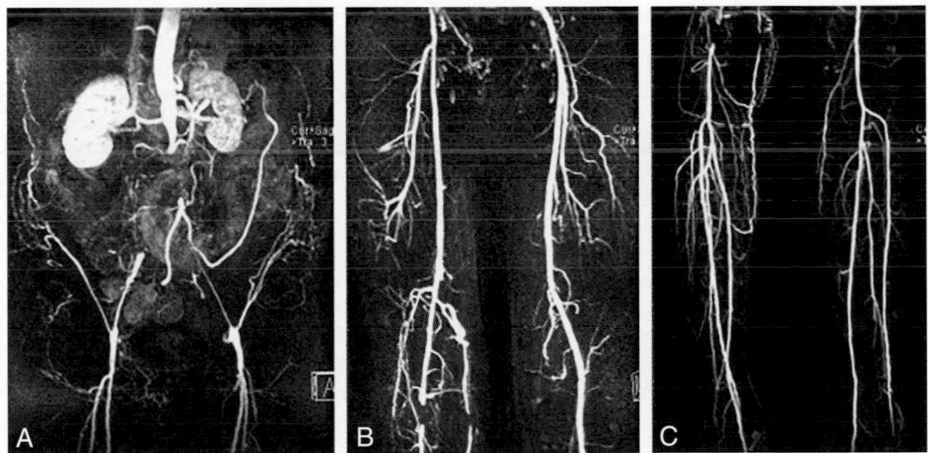

Fig. 22.4 MR Angiography. (A) Aortoiliac anatomy including significant narrowing and disease with collateral circulation; (B) femoropopliteal anatomy including a short segment of right-sided popliteal artery occlusion and disease with collateral circulation; (C) normal anatomy of further distal vessels bilaterally.

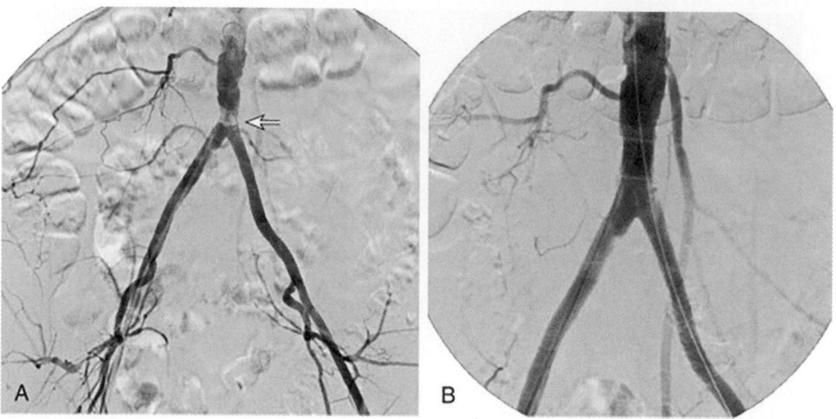

Fig. 22.5 Digital Subtraction Angiography. (A) Distal aortic disease and narrowing causing reduction in blood flow and (B) improved vascular blood flow after placement of aortic stent.

angiogram using digital subtraction angiography and was found to have significant aortoiliac narrowing. He chose to receive an aortoiliac stent with near-complete improvement in his symptoms.

BEYOND THE PEARLS

- Smoking cigarettes has a dose- and time-dependent relationship with the development of PAD. Studies have shown that smoking more than one pack per day is related to a higher likelihood of PAD compared with people who smoke less than one pack per day. The likelihood of developing PAD is also highest among current smokers, next highest in past smokers, and lowest in never smokers.
- Contrast induced nephropathy (CIN) is a possible complication of an angiography procedure. It is defined as an increase in serum creatinine levels (25% greater than baseline or more than 0.5 mg/dL) at 48–72 hours after exposure to a contrast agent. The population most at risk of developing CIN are people older than 75 years, diabetics, those with reduced kidney function at baseline, people with anemia, and people with congestive heart failure. The likelihood of developing this condition can be reduced by using N-acetylcysteine and limiting the amount of contrast used.
- Differentiating nonhealing arterial ulcers from venous ulcers is essential to arriving at the correct diagnosis. Arterial ulcers typically occur over the toes, heel, or bony prominences, have less exudative discharge, are more painful, and are treated with revascularization. Venous ulcers occur most commonly in the medial portion of the lower leg, have more exudative discharge, are less painful, and are treated with compression.
- The prevalence of abdominal aortic aneurysms has been reported in up to 10% of patients presenting with lower extremity claudication and should be considered in the differential diagnosis of this symptom. Additionally, 10%–20% of these patients will also have aneurysms in other vascular beds such as the popliteal artery and are more likely to present with claudication than those without popliteal artery aneurysms. A thorough and complete vascular exam is recommended for any patient presenting with typical claudication pain.
- Recent data from the COMPASS trial suggest that adding rivaroxaban 2.5 mg twice daily to aspirin 100 mg once daily in patients with stable coronary artery disease (27% of whom also had PAD) reduces rates of cardiovascular death, stroke, and myocardial infarction when compared with aspirin alone (4.1% versus 5.9%). However, there is no consensus yet on the addition of anticoagulants (vitamin K antagonist or direct oral anticoagulants) to antiplatelet agents for treatment of PAD alone.

Bibliography

Eikelboom, J. W., Connolly, S. J., Bosch, J., Dagenais, G. R., Hart, R. G., Shestakovska, O., ... COMPASS Investigators. (2017). Rivaroxaban with or without aspirin in stable cardiovascular disease. *The New England Journal of Medicine*, *377*(14), 1319–1330.

Fowkes, F. G., Rudan, D., Rudan, I., Aboyans, V., Denenberg, J. O., McDermott, M. M., ... Criqui, M. H. (2013). Comparison of global estimates of prevalence and risk factors for peripheral artery disease in 2000 and 2010: A systematic review and analysis. *Lancet*, *382*(9901), 1329–1340.

Giugliano, G., Laurenzano, E., Rengo, C., De Rosa, G., Brevetti, L., Sannino, A., ... Esposito, G. (2012). Abdominal aortic aneurysm in patients affected by intermittent claudication: Prevalence and clinical predictors. *BMC Surgery*, *12*(Suppl 1), S17.

Grey, J. E., Harding, K. G., & Enoch, S. (2006). Venous and arterial leg ulcers. *British Medical Journal*, *332*(7537), 347–350.

Hankey, G. J., Norman, P. E., & Eikelboom, J. W. (2006). Medical treatment of peripheral arterial disease. *The Journal of the American Medical Association*, *295*(5), 547–553.

Hirsch, A. T., Haskal, Z. J., Hertzer, N. R., Bakal, C. W., Creager, M. A., Halperin, J. L., ... Vascular Disease Foundation. (2006). ACC/AHA 2005 Practice Guidelines for the management of patients with peripheral arterial disease (lower extremity, renal, mesenteric, and abdominal aortic): A collaborative report from the American Association for Vascular Surgery/Society for Vascular Surgery, Society for Cardiovascular Angiography and Interventions, Society for Vascular Medicine and Biology, Society of Interventional Radiology, and the ACC/AHA Task Force on Practice Guidelines (Writing Committee to Develop Guidelines for the Management of Patients With Peripheral Arterial Disease): endorsed by the American Association of Cardiovascular and Pulmonary Rehabilitation; National Heart, Lung, and Blood Institute; Society for Vascular Nursing; TransAtlantic Inter-Society Consensus; and Vascular Disease Foundation. *Circulation*, *113*(11), e463–e654.

Price, J. F., Mowbray, P. I., Lee, A. J., Rumley, A., Lowe, G. D., & Fowkes, F. G. (1999). Relationship between smoking and cardiovascular risk factors in the development of peripheral arterial disease and coronary artery disease: Edinburgh Artery Study. *European Heart Journal*, *20*(5), 344–353.

Rooke, T. W., Hirsch, A. T., Misra, S., Sidawy, A. N., Beckman, J. A., Findeiss, L., ... American Heart Association Task Force. (2013). Management of patients with peripheral artery disease (compilation of 2005 and 2011 ACCF/AHA Guideline Recommendations): A report of the American College of Cardiology Foundation/American Heart Association task force on practice guidelines. *Journal of the American College of Cardiology*, *61*(14), 1555–1570.

Tuveson, V., Lofdahl, H. E., & Hultgren, R. (2016). Patients with abdominal aortic aneurysm have a high prevalence of popliteal artery aneurysms. *Vascular Medicine*, *21*(4), 369–375.

CASE 23

A 58-Year-Old Female With Recurrent Chest Pain With Exertion

Mateen Saffarian ■ Daniel Aldea ■ Shankar Chhetri ■ Sheila Sahni

A 58-year-old female with a history of smoking presents to the emergency department with several months of persistent left-sided chest pain on exertion. She describes her pain as a pressure sensation in the substernal region associated with diaphoresis. Pain is triggered after she walks briskly for over 20 minutes, which has remained unchanged over the previous 6 months. Symptoms improve upon rest. She currently has no chest pain, but she was brought into the emergency department by her daughter who was concerned about her symptoms. She has been smoking a half-pack of cigarettes daily for 20 years. On physical examination, blood pressure is 126/76 mmHg, pulse rate is 85/min, respiration rate is 16/min, and oxygen saturation is 98% on room air. The remainder of the examination is normal. Initial laboratory tests, including serial troponins, are normal. Chest radiography and serial electrocardiograms (ECGs) are also unremarkable. Acute coronary syndrome (ACS) is ruled out.

What are possible causes of chest pain?

The initial differential for chest pain is broad and includes respiratory, gastrointestinal, psychiatric, musculoskeletal, and cardiac etiologies. Potentially lethal diagnoses are often cardiovascular or respiratory in origin. A complete differential diagnosis is depicted in Table 23.1.

The initial workup of chest pain is guided by the history and laboratory evaluation for pulmonary embolism, pneumothorax, and acute coronary syndrome, as well as rarer entities such as esophageal rupture and aortic dissection that can be gleaned from a clinical scenario, if not by direct testing. Other etiologies such as pulmonary infection, musculoskeletal irritation or trauma, and gastrointestinal diseases including gastroesophageal reflux disease (GERD) or esophageal spasm can be successfully evaluated through careful history taking and examination of physical, radiographic, and laboratory evidence.

What is angina?

Ischemic heart disease manifesting as chest pain through myocyte tissue hypoperfusion caused by disrupted epicardial blood supply, defined formally as "angina," has certain characteristic features that can help distinguish it from competing entities as previously described.

Typical versus atypical anginal pain

Typical angina pain was formally defined by Diamond and Forrester as substernal chest pain of characteristic quality and duration (specified in Table 23.2) that is brought on by emotional or physical stress and is relieved by rest or nitrate medications. Atypical pain is defined as pain that possesses two of the three characteristic features. Noncardiac chest pain is defined as possessing one or none of these characteristic features.

TABLE 23.1 ■ **Differential Diagnosis for Chest Pain**

Nonischemic Cardiovascular	Pulmonary	Gastrointestinal	Chest Wall	Psychiatric
Aortic dissection	PE	Esophageal spasm	Costochondritis	Anxiety disorders
Pericarditis	Pneumonia			
	Pleuritis	Esophagitis	Fibrositis	Hyperventilation
		GERD	Rib fracture	Panic disorder
		Biliary colic		
		Cholecystitis	Sternoclavicular arthritis	Primary anxiety
		Choledocholithiasis		Affective disorders
		Cholangitis	Herpes zoster (prerash)	Somatoform disorders
		Peptic ulcer		Thought disorders
		Pancreatitis		

GERD, Gastroesophageal reflux disease; *PE*, pulmonary embolism.

TABLE 23.2 ■ **Typical Versus Atypical Chest Pain**

	Typical	Atypical
Duration	Minutes	Seconds or hours
Quality	Squeezing	Sharp
	Gripping	Pleuritic
	Suffocating	Localizable
	Heavy	Reproducible with palpation
	Levine sign	
	Gradually builds, gradually recedes	

While these descriptors are certainly helpful guides for clinicians, it is important to remember that the traditional features associated with angina may underestimate the prevalence of ischemic heart disease in a large subset of patients, most notably women. The Women's Ischemic Syndrome Evaluation (WISE) trial reported 65% of women presented with "atypical" chest pain. Numerous racial/ethnic groups are also historically underrepresented in medical research generally and specifically in the Framingham Heart Study, upon which a bulk of population assessment of cardiovascular disease is based.

Absence of these "characteristic" features does not sufficiently exclude ischemic heart disease, but their presence significantly elevates the statistical probability of a patient having coronary artery or ischemic heart disease.

What are the different types of angina?

Stable angina is a fixed response (chest pain) to a fixed stress (a certain distance traveled, activity performed, emotion experienced) that suggests that the degree of causative epicardial hypoperfusion is symmetrically stable in physiologic significance and low risk of sudden acceleration of cardiac injury leading to irreversible damage. Thus, there is no acute need for revascularization and further testing can be pursued to assess the necessity for angiography. Clinically, stable angina is defined as symptoms of at least 2 months' duration that have not worsened in severity or frequency as the result of consistent degrees of exertion or emotion.

Unstable angina, on the other hand, is defined as angina that is newly developed, occurring at lower levels of exertion than prior or occurring with increased frequency and severity. These symptoms are suggestive of an epicardial defect that is evolving rapidly and may merit urgent evaluation for revascularization to prevent further irreversible tissue injury and death.

Microvascular angina, historically known as *cardiac syndrome X*, is a type of anginal chest pain with signs associated with decreased blood flow to heart tissue but with normal epicardial coronary arteries on angiogram. It is more common in women and is believed to be related to hormones and other risk factors specifically unique to women.

What is your differential diagnosis?

The patient is a 58-year-old female with cardiovascular risk factors presenting with 2 months of *stable*, *typical* chest pain on exertion with stable vital signs and unremarkable physical, radiographic, and laboratory findings suggestive of underlying coronary artery disease (CAD).

The chronicity and pattern of symptoms in combination with an unremarkable physical examination and stable vital signs make other entities such as acute coronary syndrome (which was evaluated with serial cardiac biomarkers and electrocardiography), pneumothorax, clinically significant pulmonary embolism, and dissection unlikely and are indicative of anginal chest pain.

Is this patient experiencing stable or unstable angina?

Evaluating the stability of angina is crucial to facilitating adequate evaluation and therapy for the underlying disease process.

> This patient has consistent stress after 20 minutes of walking that provokes her likely anginal chest pain and thus merits evaluation for her *stable angina* in a way befitting the nonemergent nature of her condition via risk stratification for and evaluation of epicardial heart disease without immediately resorting to invasive testing.

What are the major risk factors for developing angina?

Major risk factors

- Age (≥45 years for men, ≥55 years for women)
- Smoking
- Diabetes mellitus
- Dyslipidemia
- Family history of premature cardiovascular disease (men <55 years, female <65 years old)
- Hypertension
- Kidney disease (microalbuminuria or GFR<60 mL/min)
- Obesity (BMI ≥30 kg/m^2)
- Sedentary lifestyle
- Prolonged psychosocial stress

What is the next step in making a diagnosis?

The first step in appropriately evaluating angina is estimating the pretest probability that a patient has CAD. Several studies have shown that a combination of patient age, nature of chest pain (typical versus atypical versus noncardiac), and gender can give a reasonable estimate of pretest probability of CAD. These data were aggregated in the 2002 Chronic Stable Angina American Heart Association (AHA) and American College of Cardiology (ACC) guidelines depicted in Table 23.3. Thus, by age, gender, and symptoms the patient falls into the "intermediate risk" category with a prerisk probability of 55%. For patients at intermediate risk (defined as pretest probability ranging from 25% to 75%), it is recommended that further evaluation be done with a stress test.

TABLE 23.3 ■ **Pretest Likelihood of Coronary Artery Disease in Symptomatic Patients According to Age and Sex**[a]

Pretest Likelihood of Coronary Artery Disease						
	Nonanginal Chest Pain		Atypical Angina		Typical Angina	
Age (years)	Men	Women	Men	Women	Men	Women
30–39	4	2	34	12	76	26
40–49	13	3	51	22	87	55
50–59	20	7	65	31	93	73
60–69	27	14	72	51	94	86

[a]Each value represents the percentage with significant coronary artery disease on catheterization.
Fihn, S. D., et al. for American College of Cardiology Foundation; American Heart Association Task Force on Practice Guidelines; American College of Physicians; American Association for Thoracic Surgery; Preventive Cardiovascular Nurses Association; Society for Cardiovascular Angiography and Interventions; Society of Thoracic Surgeons (2012). ACCF/AHA/ACP/AATS/PCNA/SCAI/STS guideline for the diagnosis and management of patients with stable ischemic heart disease. *Journal of the American College of Cardiology*, 60, 24, e44–e164.

Which stress modality should we order for this patient?

Choosing an appropriate stress test depends on a patient's ability to exercise and if they have an interpretable baseline ECG. For patients who are able to exercise and have a sufficiently normal baseline ECG, an exercise stress test with ECG is preferred because it can more closely mimic physiological stress and can better assess patients' symptom burden compared with pharmacologic stress testing. Exercise capacity itself is also one of the most useful predictors of major cardiac events; therefore, exercise ECG provides both *diagnostic* as well as *prognostic* information. The test is considered positive if there is a ≥1 mm horizontal or down sloping ST-segment depression at peak exercise on ECG. If patients cannot exercise, pharmacologically induced stress testing can be performed as a reasonable proxy for exertion. If patients have a baseline ECG that would complicate interpretation, either exercise echocardiography or nuclear stress test is recommended (Fig. 23.2).

CLINICAL PEARL **STEP 2/3**

Hold beta blockers and other antiischemic medications 24–48 hours prior to stress testing to avoid false negative findings. These medications can reduce heart rate and myocardial demand leading to a lack of ischemic ECG/imaging changes while a patient is undergoing a stress test.

The patient undergoes an exercise stress test with ECG and is found to have ≥2 mm of ST-segment depression at low workload (Fig. 23.1).

Does the patient warrant further workup?

Determining the utility of coronary artery catheterization is a complex decision that requires thoughtful shared decision making, assessment of candidacy for revascularization intervention, risk stratification of acuity and severity of symptoms, and disease response to appropriate pharmacological management. The goal of revascularization is to improve symptoms, improve survival, and decrease future CAD events. Patients with high-risk criteria and select patients with intermediate-risk criteria on noninvasive testing, regardless of symptom severity, should undergo catheterization for further evaluation. Additionally, patients who have persistent anginal

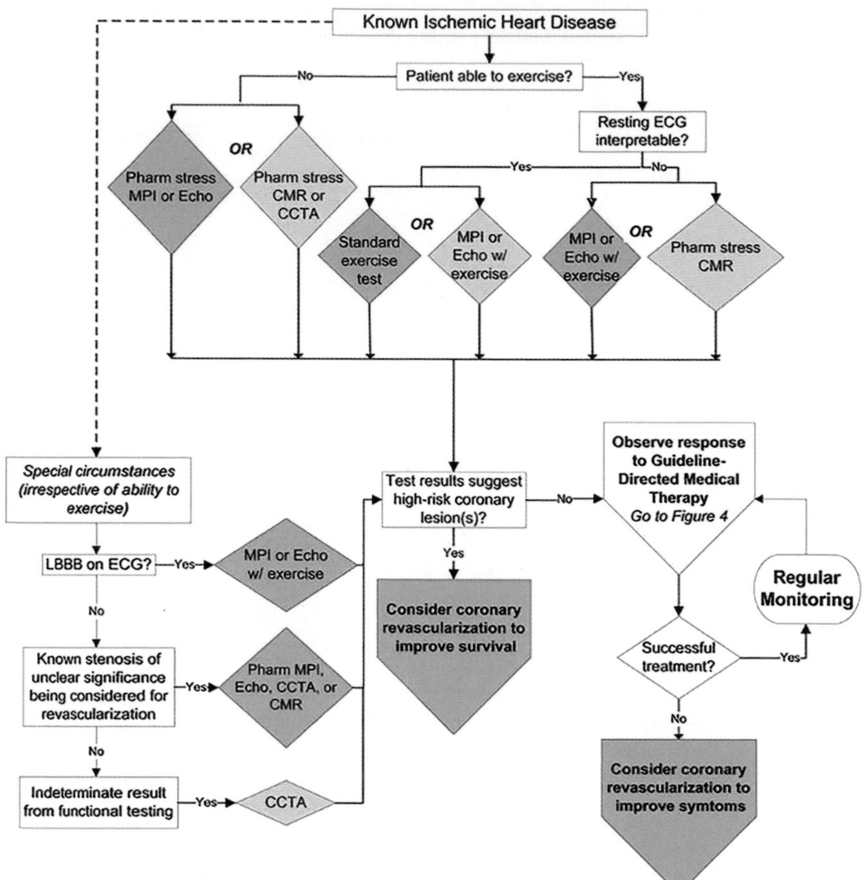

Fig. 23.1 Algorithm for diagnostic assessment of patients with stable ischemic heart disease. The algorithm does not represent a comprehensive list of recommendations (see text for all recommendations). *CCTA*, Coronary computed tomography angiography; *CMR*, cardiac magnetic resonance; *ECG*, electrocardiogram; *Echo*, echocardiography; *LBBB*, left bundle-branch block; *MPI*, myocardial perfusion imaging; *Pharm*, pharmacological. (From Fihn, S. D., et al. for American College of Cardiology Foundation; American Heart Association Task Force on Practice Guidelines; American College of Physicians; American Association for Thoracic Surgery; Preventive Cardiovascular Nurses Association; Society for Cardiovascular Angiography and Interventions; Society of Thoracic Surgeons (2012). ACCF/AHA/ACP/AATS/PCNA/SCAI/STS guideline for the diagnosis and management of patients with stable ischemic heart disease. *Journal of the American College of Cardiology, 60*, 24, e44–e164.)

symptoms despite maximal medical therapy or who are intolerant of medical therapy may also be candidates for catheterization and evaluation for revascularization. Patients who are found to have ≥2 mm of ST-segment depression at low workload meet high-risk criteria and have an estimated annual risk of myocardial infarction or death of >3%. Thus, this patient warrants further diagnostic evaluation with coronary artery catheterization.

This patient undergoes coronary artery catheterization and is found to have moderate diffuse coronary artery disease that is not amenable to revascularization.

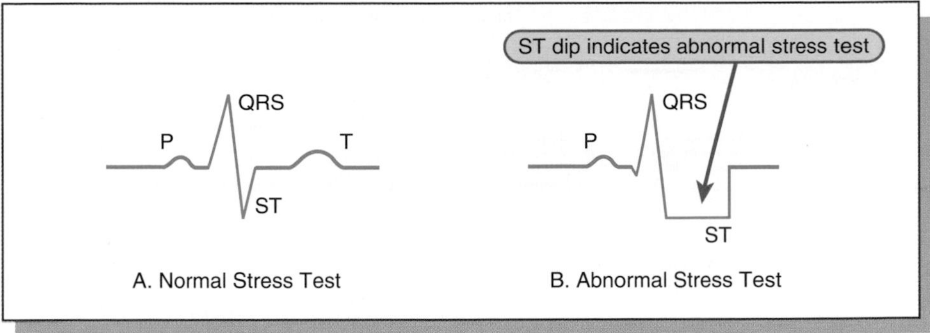

Fig. 23.2 Normal and Abnormal Stress ECG Comparison. *Left*, Normal exercise ECG complex. *Right*, A horizontal ST-segment depression of 2.0 mm as measured from the P–Q junction. (From Buck's step-by-step medical coding, 2021 edition. St. Louis, Elsevier, 2021.)

CLINICAL PEARL **STEP 2/3**

Generally, coronary artery bypass graft surgery (CABG) is preferred to percutaneous coronary intervention (PCI) in patients with extensive and complex CAD. CABG has been shown to improve survival and is superior to PCI or medical therapy in patients with left main disease or three-vessel CAD.

What are the next steps in patients with stable angina who have undergone diagnostic testing and are not currently candidates for revascularization?

Initial management of all patients with stable angina should include lifestyle modification to minimize or eliminate causes known to accelerate coronary artery disease. This often includes appropriate dietary changes, implementation of regular aerobic exercise, and smoking cessation as applicable. The goals of medication therapy in patients with stable angina are blood pressure control, risk reduction, and symptom mitigation. Patients with stable angina with a blood pressure of 140/99 mmHg or higher and refractory to lifestyle changes should be started on antihypertensives. Medication choice should be tailored to patients on a case-by-case basis depending on their specific comorbidities. Fig. 23.3 depicts a simple algorithm for guideline directed medical therapy.

CLINICAL PEARL **STEP 1**

Modifiable risk factors for atherosclerotic disease include smoking, hypertension, hyperlipidemia, and diabetes. Nonmodifiable risk factors include age, gender, and family history.

Which medications reduce mortality in patients with stable angina?

Two medications that should be started in all patients with stable angina are aspirin and a moderate- or high-dose statin. Unless contraindicated, all patients with stable angina and known coronary artery disease should be placed on aspirin indefinitely. A large metaanalysis illustrated that aspirin use was associated with 37% reduction in serious vascular events and 46% decrease in progression to unstable angina. Low-dose aspirin (75–163 mg/day) has been shown to be as effective as high-dose aspirin with lower bleeding risk. Clopidogrel can be used as a substitute if aspirin is contraindicated for any reason.

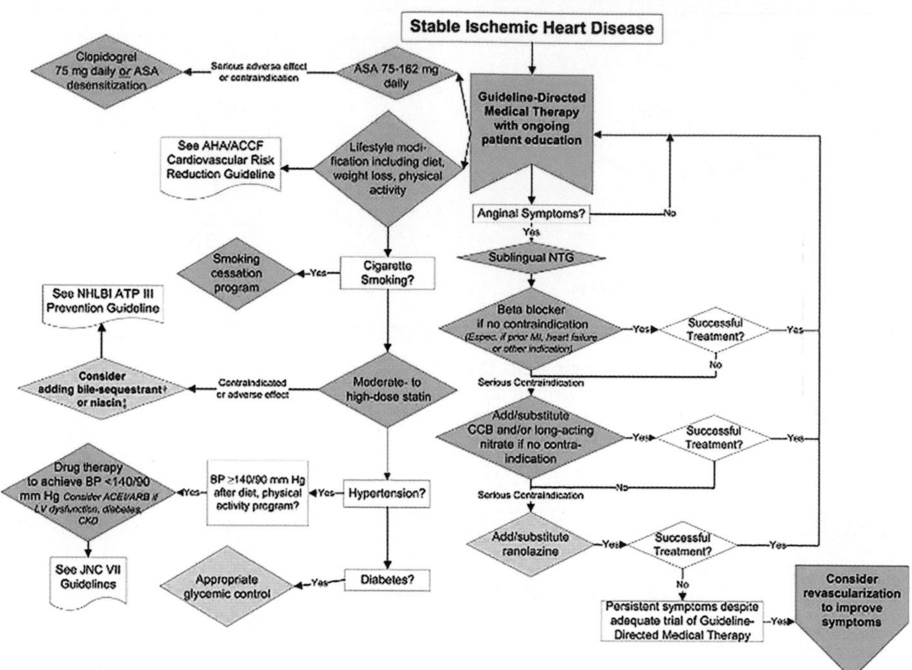

Fig. 23.3 Algorithm for guideline-directed medical therapy for patients with stable ischemic heart disease. The algorithm does not represent a comprehensive list of recommendations (see text for all recommendations). †The use of bile acid sequestrant is relatively contraindicated when triglycerides are ≥200 mg/dL and is contraindicated when triglycerides are ≥500 mg/dL. ‡Dietary supplement niacin must not be used as a substitute for prescription niacin. *ACCF*, American College of Cardiology Foundation; *ACEI*, angiotensin-converting enzyme inhibitor; *AHA*, American Heart Association; *ARB*, angiotensin-receptor blocker; *ASA*, aspirin; *ATP III*, Adult Treatment Panel 3; *BP*, blood pressure; *CCB*, calcium channel blocker; *CKD*, chronic kidney disease; *HDL-C*, high-density lipoprotein cholesterol; *JNC VII*, Seventh Report of the Joint National Committee on Prevention, Detection, Evaluation, and Treatment of High Blood Pressure; *LDL-C*, low-density lipoprotein cholesterol; *LV*, left ventricular; *MI*, myocardial infarction; *NHLBI*, National Heart, Lung, and Blood Institute; *NTG*, nitroglycerin. (From Fihn, S. D., et al. for American College of Cardiology Foundation; American Heart Association Task Force on Practice Guidelines; American College of Physicians; American Association for Thoracic Surgery; Preventive Cardiovascular Nurses Association; Society for Cardiovascular Angiography and Interventions; Society of Thoracic Surgeons (2012). ACCF/AHA/ACP/AATS/PCNA/SCAI/STS guideline for the diagnosis and management of patients with stable ischemic heart disease. *Journal of the American College of Cardiology, 60*, 24, e44–e164.)

In addition to aspirin, all patients with stable angina should be started on a moderate- or high-dose statin. Statins have been a staple of lipid lowering therapy for decades and have been shown to reduce the risk of cardiovascular events in patients with and without cardiovascular disease. Specifically, for patients with ischemic heart disease, the Heart Protection study showed that patients who were placed on simvastatin 40 mg daily had a 13% reduction in mortality and 8% reduction in coronary death rate compared with a placebo group. This improvement is probably driven in large part by statins' dose-dependent reduction of low-density lipoprotein (LDL) cholesterol levels. Several studies have shown that each reduction in LDL cholesterol of 40 mg/dL is associated with a 10% reduction in all-cause mortality and 20% reduction in coronary mortality.

Based on this, the patient should be started on aspirin 81 mg daily and atorvastatin 80 mg daily.

CLINICAL PEARL **STEP 2/3**

ACE inhibitor therapy is indicated in stable angina if the patient has concomitant diabetes, chronic kidney disease, heart failure with reduced ejection fraction, or a history of MI.

BASIC SCIENCE PEARL **STEP 1**

Statins are part of a class of medications known as HMG-CoA reductase inhibitors. They inhibit the conversion of HMG-CoA to mevalonate, which is a precursor of cholesterol.

Which medications help with symptoms of angina?

Beta blockers are generally recommended as first-line therapy to relieve symptoms in patients with stable angina. Beta blockers reduce myocardial oxygen demand by reducing heart rate, myocardial contractility, and afterload. There is no reported difference in efficacy among different beta blockers and dose titration is recommended to a target heart rate of 55–60 beats per minute at rest. Specific choice of a beta blocker will depend on the patient's comorbidities.

The patient is started on metoprolol tartrate 12.5 mg twice a day with the plan to uptitrate as tolerated if the patient has persistent stable angina symptoms upon follow-up visits.

CLINICAL PEARL **STEP 2/3**

Beta blockers should be used with caution in patients taking nondihydropyridine calcium channel blockers (verapamil and diltiazem) because of the combined negative inotropic and chronotropic effects.

Which additional therapies can be started if our patient continues to have anginal pain on maximum beta blocker therapy?

Calcium channel blockers can also be used in combination with beta blockers if symptom control with beta blockers is insufficient. Additionally, calcium channel blockers are the recommended second-line therapy for relief of angina if beta blockers are contraindicated or not tolerated. Calcium channel blockers decrease symptoms by both decreasing myocardial demand and increasing oxygen supply through negative inotropic effects and smooth muscle relaxation. All three classes of calcium channel blockers have been shown to be equally effective in treating angina symptoms. The specific choice of medication will depend on patient characteristics, potential adverse effects, and drug interactions. Adverse effects include headache, dizziness, palpitations, flushing, and peripheral edema.

If patients are unable to tolerate beta blockers or calcium channel blockers, or if symptoms remain uncontrolled despite maximal titration of these agents, long-acting nitrates are an additional therapy option. Nitrates cause vascular smooth muscle relaxation in both arteries and veins leading to improved collateral flow, improved flow at the site of coronary artery obstruction, and decreased preload. To minimize the occurrence of adverse effects, dosage should be titrated to the lowest dose needed for control of symptoms. Additionally, doses should be timed to give patients a nitrate-free period of around 12 hours daily to prevent development of nitrate tolerance. Adverse effects of nitrate medications include headache, flushing, and hypotension. Use with phosphodiesterase-5 inhibitors should be avoided because of the risk of severe hypotension.

Ranolazine is another therapy option that can be used for the treatment of chronic angina in combination with beta blockers, nitrates, or calcium channel blockers or as an alternative if patients cannot tolerate the aforementioned medications. Ranolazine improves ventricular diastolic tension and oxygen consumption with minimal changes in heart rate and blood pressure, making it an attractive option for patients who cannot tolerate other medications. It is generally well tolerated; however, it should not be prescribed in combination with inhibitors of enzyme CYP3A4 because they can significantly increase the serum levels of ranolazine.

The patient asks if there is anything that she can take to relieve her pain episodes acutely. What would you recommend?

For immediate relief of angina, all patients with stable angina should also be prescribed sublingual nitroglycerin tablets or nitroglycerin spray. Sublingual doses range from 0.3 to 0.6 mg for the sublingual formulation and 0.4 mg for the spray. They can be taken in 5-minute intervals for a maximum dose of ≤1.2 mg within 15 minutes. If symptoms do not improve in that time period, patients should seek immediate medical care.

Our patient is seen for follow-up 1 month after her initial presentation to the emergency department. Her symptoms have improved and the patient is now able to walk >40 minutes before chest pain returns. Her beta blocker is uptitrated and she is initiated on additional calcium channel blocker therapy.

Case Summary

- **Complaint/History:** A 58-year-old female with a significant smoking history presents with persistent typical angina that occurs when she walks for longer than 20 minutes. Symptoms have been stable over the previous 6 months.
- **Findings:** Blood pressure is 118/70 mmHg, pulse rate is 85/min, respiration rate is 16/min, and oxygen saturation is 97% on room air.
- **Lab Results/Tests:** Lab tests reveal negative serial troponins, serial ECGs are sinus rhythm with no concerning changes, and ACS is ruled out. Based on age, gender, and the typical nature of her angina, she is intermediate risk on CAD risk stratification warranting additional testing. Because the patient can exercise and has a normal baseline ECG, she undergoes an exercise stress with ECG. The stress test shows ≥2 mm of ST-segment depression at low workload, making it a markedly positive test with high risk features, which warrants coronary artery catheterization. Catheterization shows moderate diffuse CAD not amenable to revascularization. The diagnosis of stable angina and stable ischemic heart disease is confirmed.
- **Treatment:** The patient was started on aspirin 81 mg/day and atorvastatin 80 mg daily. For symptom control, our patient was started on beta blocker therapy with metoprolol tartrate 12.5 mg twice a day and was prescribed sublingual nitrate for immediate relief during anginal episodes. On follow-up, the patient's symptoms had improved although not completely resolved. The beta blocker was uptitrated and a calcium channel blocker was initiated.

BEYOND THE PEARLS

- Ischemic heart disease is the leading cause of death in the United States in both men and women despite marked advancements in diagnosis and therapy as well as a massively successful public health campaign to reduce smoking. Given the aging population of the United States generally, this number will probably continue to increase in coming years.
- ECG abnormalities affecting the ST segment, such as left ventricular hypertrophy, left bundle-branch block, ventricular-paced rhythm, or any resting ST-segment depression (≥0.5 mm) make it uninterpretable for use in a stress test. Patients with such findings should undergo an exercise echo stress or myocardial perfusion imaging.
- Generally, exercise stress tests start at 3.2 to 4.7 metabolic equivalents (METs) of work and increase by several METs every several minutes. Activities of daily living (ADLs) are

approximately 4 to 5 METs. Thus, evaluating a patient's ability to complete ADLs can help you quickly identify patients who will be able to complete an exercise stress test. Validated clinical calculators such as the Duke Activity Status Index can be used to estimate functional capacity.

- Findings from several individual studies and metaanalyses have shown that PCI does not demonstrate any survival benefit when compared with optimal medical therapy in patients with stable angina. However, it has been shown that PCI can reduce the severity of anginal symptoms.
- Smoking cessation reduces the risk of annual CAD mortality by 50% after 1 year of abstinence. After 5–15 years the annual coronary mortality risk reaches that of nonsmokers.
- Ivabradine, which reduces heart rate by inhibiting the sodium funny *(If)* channels in the SA node, has been shown to have additional anti-anginal and anti-ischemic effects in patients with stable angina who are already on standard therapy with beta-blockers.
- Current guidelines for dual anti platelet therapy in patients with stable ischemic heart disease who undergo percutaneous coronary intervention is 6 months for a drug eluting stent implantation and 1 month for bare metal stent implantation.

Bibliography

Antithrombotic Trialists' Collaboration Collaborative meta-analysis of randomised trials of antiplatelet therapy for prevention of death, myocardial infarction, and stroke in high risk patients. *BMJ.* 2002;324(7329):71–86.

Cholesterol Treatment Trialists' (CTT) Collaboration Efficacy and safety of more intensive lowering of LDL cholesterol: A meta-analysis of data from 170, 000 participants in 26 randomised trials. *Lancet.* 2010;376(9753):1670–1681.

Diamond GA, Forrester JS. Analysis of probability as an aid in the clinical diagnosis of coronary-artery disease. *The New England Journal of Medicine.* 1979;300(24):1350–8135.

Ellestad MH. *Stress testing: Principles and practice*: Oxford University Press; 2003.

Fihn SD, et al. 2012 ACCF/AHA/ACP/AATS/PCNA/SCAI/STS guideline for the diagnosis and management of patients with stable ischemic heart disease. *Journal of the American College of Cardiology.* 2012;60(24). e44–e164.

Goljan EF. *Rapid Review Pathology*: Elsevier; 2019.

Heart Protection Study Collaborative Group MRC/BHF heart protection study of cholesterol lowering with simvastatin in 20, 536 high-risk individuals: A randomised placebo-controlled trial. *Lancet.* 2002;360(9326):7–22.

Heidenreich PA, et al. Meta-analysis of trials comparing beta-blockers, calcium antagonists, and nitrates for stable angina. *JAMA.* 1999;281(20):1927–1936.

Levine, G. N., Bates, E. R., Bittl, J. A., Brindis, R. G., Fihn, S. D., Fleisher, L. A., . . . Smith, S. C. (2016). 2016 ACC/AHA guideline focused update on duration of dual antiplatelet therapy in patients with coronary artery disease: a report of the American College of Cardiology/American Heart Association Task Force on Clinical Practice Guidelines. *Journal of the American College of Cardiology*, *68*(10), 1082–1115.

Rousan TA, Thadani U. Stable angina medical therapy management guidelines: a critical review of guidelines from the European Society of Cardiology and National Institute for Health and Care Excellence. *European Cardiology.* 2019;14(1):18–22.

Tardif, J. C., Ponikowski, P., & Kahan, T. (2009). ASSOCIATE Study Investigators. Efficacy of the I(f) current inhibitor ivabradine in patients with chronic stable angina receiving beta-blocker therapy: a 4-month, randomized, placebo-controlled trial. *European Heart Journal*, *30*:540–548. https://doi.org/10.1093/eurheartj/ehn571.

CASE 24

A 59-Year-Old Male With Sudden, Burning Chest Pain

Christopher Bradley ■ Percy Genyk ■ Wilson Kwan ■ Antreas Hindoyan

A 59-year-old male presents to the emergency room complaining of chest pain. He reports having two episodes of chest pain earlier that day. Initially, he had acute onset, burning chest pain after dinner that lasted several minutes and did not improve with calcium carbonate tablets. Four hours later, he developed recurring chest pain, which prompted him to seek medical attention. He denies shortness of breath, diaphoresis, nausea, vomiting, leg swelling, or palpitations. His medical history is pertinent for hypertension and hyperlipidemia, for which he takes hydrochlorothiazide 25 mg daily and atorvastatin 20 mg daily. He denies prior history of tobacco or illicit drug use. On physical examination, blood pressure is 146/71 mmHg, pulse rate is 84/min, respiratory rate is 16/min, and oxygen saturation is 100% on room air. His heart rate is regular with normal heart sounds and no friction rub, gallop, or murmur. No jugular venous distension is noted. Lung sounds are clear bilaterally. The remainder of the examination is unremarkable. In the emergency room, the patient's pain resolves with aspirin, oral aluminum hydroxide/magnesium hydroxide, and lansoprazole.

Diagnostic workup

Initial evaluation of the patient's chest pain should include a complete blood count (CBC), complete metabolic panel (CMP), chest radiograph (CXR), electrocardiogram (ECG), and serum troponin-I or -T level. While awaiting the results for the laboratory tests, the ECG and CXR are completed (Figs. 24.1 and 24.2).

What is your differential diagnosis?

This is a 59-year-old male with a past medical history of hypertension and hyperlipidemia who presents to the emergency room with acute onset chest pain that resolves with aspirin, antacids, and a proton pump inhibitor (PPI).

What are some causes of chest pain?

The differential diagnosis of chest pain is broad. Common causes of chest pain are presented in Table 24.1.

Based on the features of this patient's chest pain, including burning sensation that occurred after a meal with resolution of symptoms upon administration of antacids and a PPI, gastrointestinal causes such as gastroesophageal reflux disease (GERD) or peptic ulcer disease (PUD) should be considered. However, it is important to consider serious, life-threatening causes of chest pain. Given this patient's age and comorbidities, acute coronary syndrome (ACS) should be high on the differential diagnosis.

In general, when should you consider ACS in a patient with chest pain?

ACS is defined as a group of signs and symptoms compatible with a state in which the heart is undergoing acute myocardial infarction or ischemia. The three types of ACS are unstable angina (UA), non-ST-elevated myocardial infarction (NSTEMI), and ST-elevated myocardial infarction

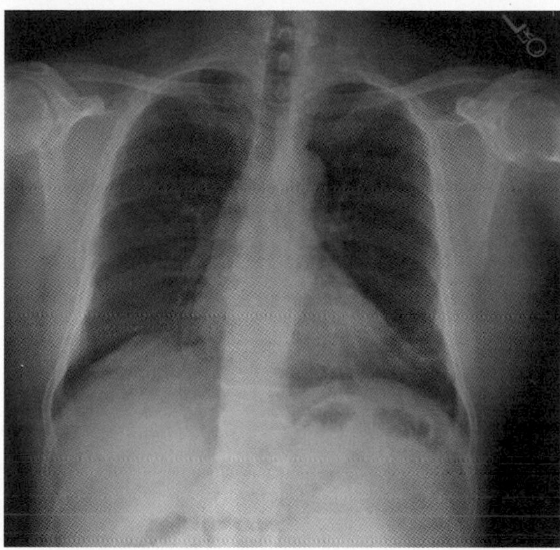

Fig. 24.1 Chest radiograph in the emergency department shows no acute processes.

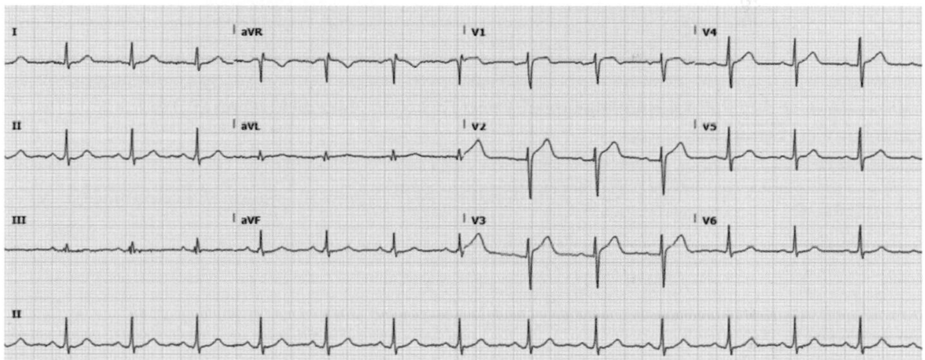

Fig. 24.2 Initial ECG shows normal sinus rhythm.

(STEMI) (see Table 24.2). Patients presenting with chest pain should be rapidly evaluated to determine whether their symptoms are suggestive of ACS. Ischemic chest pain, also known as typical angina, is characterized by sensations of squeezing, heaviness, pressure, burning, or tightness. The pain is classically located in the substernal area and may radiate to the left shoulder and arm, jaw, neck, or epigastrium. Duration of pain is variable, but 3–15 minutes is typical. Chest pain is often triggered by physical exertion or emotional stress and improves with rest or nitroglycerin. Patients who are elderly, female, or diabetic may experience atypical angina with ACS. Common atypical presentations include chest pain described as burning, pleuritic, or stabbing in nature (see next Clinical Pearl) and isolated symptoms of shortness of breath, nausea, or vomiting without pain.

CLINICAL PEARL **STEP 2/3**

Patients with a history of diabetes can present with silent myocardial infarction (without typical symptoms) as a result of diabetes-induced neuropathy.

TABLE 24.1 ■ **Differential for Chest Pain**

- Cardiac causes: acute coronary syndrome, aortic dissection, pericarditis and myopericarditis, uncontrolled hypertension
- Pulmonary causes: pneumothorax, pulmonary embolism, pneumonia, pleuritis, pulmonary hypertension
- Gastrointestinal causes: Boerhaave's syndrome, Mallory-Weiss tear, esophageal spasm, peptic ulcer disease, esophageal reflux, pancreatitis
- Miscellaneous causes: costochondritis, herpes zoster, anxiety

TABLE 24.2 ■ **Acute Coronary Syndrome**

	Unstable Angina	NSTEMI	STEMI
Coronary thrombosis	Subtotal occlusion	Subtotal occlusion	Total occlusion
ECG	ST-segment depression and/or T-wave inversion	ST-segment depression and/or T-wave inversion	ST-segment elevations
Troponin	Negative	Positive	Positive

NSTEMI, non-ST-elevated myocardial infarction; *STEMI*, ST-elevated myocardial infarction.

TABLE 24.3 ■ **Any Patient Fulfilling One of These Categories Should Have an ECG to Evaluate for Acute Coronary Syndrome**

Age	Symptoms
≥30 years old	Chest pain
≥50 years old	Dyspnea, encephalopathy, syncope, generalized weakness, upper extremity pain
≥80 years old	Abdominal pain, nausea, vomiting

In the original study, this ruleset had a sensitivity of 91.9% and negative predictive value of 99.98%.

When should you send a workup for ACS?

Because the presentation of ACS is variable and the workup is straightforward, evaluation for ACS is almost always conducted in patients who present to the emergency department (ED) with chest pain or discomfort. The initial workup for ACS includes an ECG and testing for the presence of biomarkers of cardiac injury (troponin T or I) in the serum. One study of over 3 million ED visits developed a set of rules for prioritizing patients at high risk of STEMI, including when to obtain an immediate ECG. The study recommendations are summarized in Table 24.3.

CLINICAL PEARL **STEP 2/3**

A positive troponin does not always indicate ACS. For example, patients with impaired renal function often have an elevated troponin at baseline, limiting its diagnostic utility. Other elevations in troponins include heart failure, severe sepsis, hypertension urgency/emergency, stroke, COVID-19, and so on. An elevated troponin suggests that the patient has increased morbidity from the underlying etiology.

Diagnostic workup continued

The results of laboratory testing and a repeat ECG are shown in Table 24.4 and Fig. 24.3, respectively. ACS is confirmed based on the elevated troponin level and ECG now showing dynamic changes (S–T segment abnormalities and new T-wave inversions in the precordial leads).

CLINICAL PEARL **STEP 2/3**

The initial ECG is often not diagnostic in ACS and troponin levels may only be detectable 3–4 hours after the onset of myocardial damage.

What are the differences between STEMI, NSTEMI, and UA?

Understanding the subtypes of ACS is important given their varying clinical management. The diagnosis of STEMI, NSTEMI, and UA depend on the ECG and serum troponin level.

STEMI is a condition in which a coronary artery (or arteries) have been totally occluded, leading to a transmural infarction and hallmark electrocardiographic findings secondary to abnormal conduction and repolarization. The diagnosis requires both an elevated troponin level and ECG findings of ST-segment elevation of 1 mm or more in two or more contiguous leads other than V2 and V3, where ST elevations must be greater than 2 mm in men or greater than 1.5 mm in women. The ST-segment elevation seen in contiguous leads is often paired with reciprocal changes or ST-segment depression in other leads (see Table 24.5). Other ECG changes considered STEMI equivalents include new

TABLE 24.4 ■ **Laboratory Tests**

Leukocyte count	7,900/
Hemoglobin	14.7 g/dL
Platelet count	171,000/μL
Serum sodium	140 mmol/L
Serum potassium	4.1 mml/L
Serum chloride	106 mmol/L
Serum CO_2	25 mmol/L
BUN	11 mg/dL
Serum creatinine	0.71 mg/dL
Troponin-T	0.45 ng/mL (normal <0.01 ng/mL)

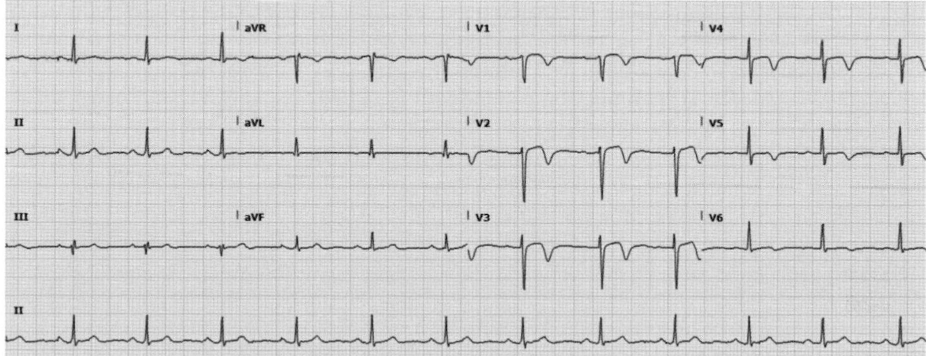

Fig. 24.3 Repeat ECG showing biphasic T-waves in leads V1–V4.

TABLE 24.5 ■ **ECG Changes in STEMI Can Often Show a Pattern That May Help Localize the Culprit Lesion in Myocardial Infarction**

Localization of Myocardial Infarction

Anatomic Area	ECG Leads with STE	ECG Leads with STD	Coronary Artery
Septal-anterior	V1–V4	—	LAD
Lateral	I, avL, V5–V6	II, III, avF	LCX or distal LAD
Inferior	II, III, avF	I, avL, V5–V6	RCA or LCX

LAD, Left anterior descending artery; *LCX*, left circumflex artery; *RCA*, right coronary artery; *STE*,; *STD*,; *STEMI*, ST-elevated myocardial infarction.

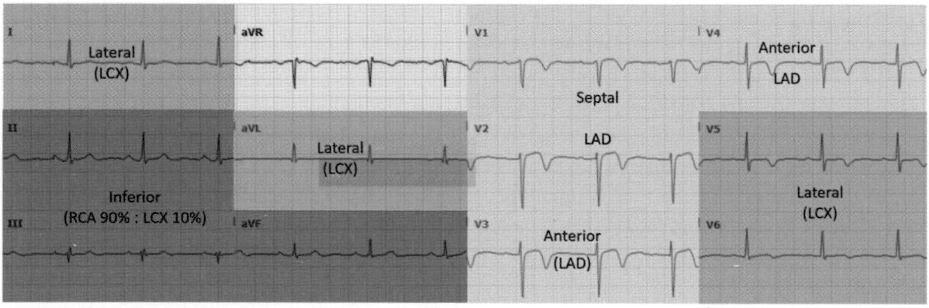

Fig. 24.4 Anatomic locations and supplying coronary arteries. *LAD*, Left anterior descending artery; *LCX*, left circumflex artery; *RCA*, right coronary artery.

left bundle branch block; tall, peaked T-waves in the precordial leads (DeWinter's T-waves); or ST-segment depression in V1 through V3 (posterior MI), among others (see next Clinical Pearl). Any suspicion of STEMI indicates urgent cardiology consultation (see Fig. 24.4).

CLINICAL PEARL **STEP 1/2/3**

Posterior MI presents with ST-segment depression in leads V1–V3. Reciprocal changes, in this case ST-segment elevation, can be identified by placing additional leads or V7–V9 on the patient's back.

NSTEMI is defined by an elevated troponin level with or without ECG changes that do not meet STEMI criteria. Once NSTEMI is identified, it is important to recognize patients at high risk of suffering an adverse cardiovascular event. High risk features include hemodynamic instability or cardiogenic shock, severe or new onset heart failure, recurrent or persistent angina at rest despite medical therapy, new or worsening mitral regurgitation or new ventricular septal defect, or sustained ventricular arrhythmia. If a patient with NSTEMI has any of these characteristics, cardiology should be consulted immediately to evaluate the patient for urgent intervention.

UA is characterized as new or worsening angina that occurs at rest, with or without ECG changes, and that is not accompanied by elevated troponin levels. This is distinguished from stable angina, which occurs with exertion but not at rest.

CLINICAL PEARL **STEP 1**

STEMI is indicative of a transmural infarct with the full thickness of the myocardial wall involved. NSTEMI indicates involvement of the subendocardium with the inner one-third of this region being especially vulnerable to ischemia.

Diagnosis

The ECG shown in Fig. 24.3 demonstrates sinus rhythm with biphasic T-waves in leads V1–V4 without ST elevation or depression, and an elevated serum troponin level.

Based upon the criteria, this patient is diagnosed with an NSTEMI. Cardiology is consulted and medical management for ACS is initiated with metoprolol tartrate 25 mg and atorvastatin 80 mg.

What if the troponin level is not elevated during workup for ACS?

If initial and serial troponin levels are not elevated, the primary diagnosis of ACS may need to be reconsidered. Nevertheless, these patients may require a stress test to ascertain the presence of inducible ischemia. Cardiology consultation may facilitate which, if any, additional investigations are warranted in these patients.

How is ACS managed in the early stages?

Patients suspected of having ACS are typically given high-dose aspirin (between 162 mg and 325 mg). If the patient has respiratory distress or an arterial saturation less than 90%, supplementation oxygen should be provided. Nitrates are administered sublingually at a dose of 0.4 mg every 2–5 minutes, up to three doses for active chest pain except when PDE-5 inhibitors have been recently used because of the potential to precipitate profound hypotension upon combining these drugs. Intravenous nitroglycerin may also be used if patients cannot tolerate sublingual or oral medications or in patients who have continued angina despite sublingual nitroglycerin. Intravenous nitroglycerin is started at an initial rate of 5–10 mcg/min and increased by 5–20 mcg/min every 10 minutes to achieve sufficient pain relief or reduce blood pressure by 10% or 25%–30% in normotensive and hypertensive patients, respectively. Caution should be exercised when the patient is preload sensitives (e.g., hypotension, aortic stenosis, right ventricular myocardial infarction). Although both sublingual and IV nitroglycerin provide symptom relief, they do not improve mortality in ACS. Beta blockers such as metoprolol tartrate are also administered to reduce myocardial oxygen demand provided that the patient is not significantly hypotensive. Notably, beta blockers are often contraindicated if the patient is markedly bradycardic or has second- or third-degree atrioventricular block or severe bronchospasm (see next Clinical Pearl). Cardioselective oral beta blockers such as metoprolol tartrate 25–50 mg every 6–12 hours or atenolol 25–50 mg twice daily are appropriate for treating ACS and generally preferred over intravenous beta blockers for their sustained effects. However, in the setting of ongoing ischemia or significant tachycardia, initial short-acting intravenous beta blockers may be appropriate because of their rapid onset of effect, with transition to oral medications when appropriate. Both oral and IV beta blockers have demonstrated improved mortality in ACS. Finally, a high-intensity statin such as atorvastatin 80 mg should be started as soon as possible, regardless of a patient's low-density lipoprotein levels.

CLINICAL PEARL **STEP 1**

Beta blockers are contraindicated in ACS caused by cocaine use because of the possibility of triggering coronary artery vasoconstriction and systemic hypertension resulting from unopposed alpha-adrenergic stimulation.

A second antiplatelet agent belonging to the P2Y12 inhibitor class is typically given in conjunction with aspirin at a loading dose at the discretion of the cardiologist (see Beyond the Pearls). Anticoagulant therapy should be initiated in most patients with suspected ACS except when significant bleeding is noted or suspected, particularly intracranial hemorrhage (ICH) or subdural hematoma (SDH). For this reason, many patients undergo a head CT examination prior to cardiac catheterization. Caution should be exercised in patients with hypertensive urgency or emergency because they are at higher risk of developing ICH while on anticoagulation. Anticoagulation should be continued for up to 24.48 hours from the time of diagnosis of ACS. Unfractionated heparin (UFH) is used more commonly than low molecular weight heparin (LMWH) in NSTEMI because of higher rates of bleeding with LMWH observed in some trials, although both are comparable in efficacy. UFH also has the advantage of a shorter half-life (in case of bleed) and is more easily titratable. In STEMI patients who will undergo percutaneous coronary intervention (PCI), there is some debate over the use of UFH or the direct thrombin inhibitor bivalirudin, although both are reasonable choices.

Upon examining the patient and the ECG results, the cardiology team orders a loading dose of clopidogrel 600 mg and unfractionated heparin drip and then activates a code STEMI, alerting the catheterization laboratory to prepare for urgent cardiac catheterization.

As the patient is being prepared for transport, the cardiologist explains that although the ECG and cardiac biomarkers are suggestive of NSTEMI, this patient's ECG demonstrates a concerning feature known as Wellen's syndrome.

Wellen's syndrome is frequently associated with high-grade stenosis of the left anterior descending coronary artery. Without intervention, Wellen's syndrome is very likely to progress to STEMI and should be treated urgently. Details on this ECG finding are discussed in Beyond the Pearls.

Images from the coronary angiogram are shown in Fig. 24.5. Fig. 24.5A shows 99% stenosis of the proximal left anterior descending artery. One drug-eluting stent (DES) is placed with return of flow distal to the lesion as shown in Fig. 24.5B.

What is the initial management when STEMI is recognized?

STEMI is typically caused by plaque rupture within a coronary artery resulting in acute obstruction of blood flow. The primary goal in acute management is to achieve reperfusion of blood flow, either through PCI or with thrombolytic agents such as alteplase. PCI is preferred, but if it is not available within 120 minutes of first medical contact, thrombolytic therapy is recommended. One-quarter to one-third of patients who receive thrombolytic therapy will fail to achieve reperfusion and all patients should be transferred to a PCI-capable hospital as soon as possible. Basic ACS treatment guidelines for STEMI are summarized in Table 24.6.

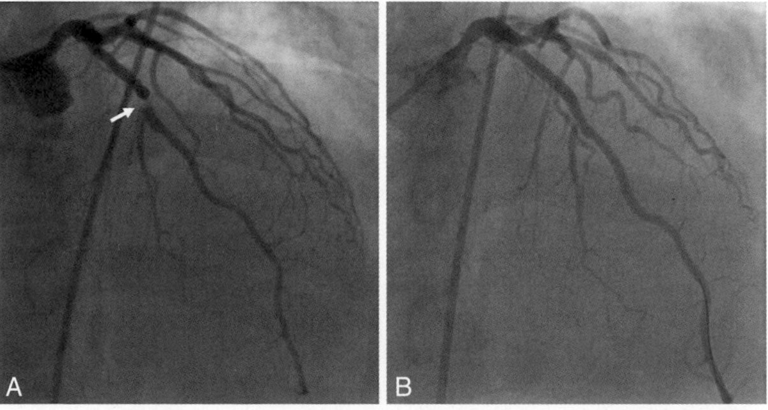

Fig. 24.5 Coronary angiogram before (A) and after (B) placement of one drug-eluting stent in the left anterior descending coronary artery.

TABLE 24.6 ■ **STEMI Management**

Initial Management
Mobilize all necessary resources for urgent cardiac catheterization
Administer loading doses of aspirin (325 mg) and clopidogrel (600 mg) unless contraindicated[a]
Initiate heparin drip to achieve therapeutic levels of anticoagulation (PTT goal 60–90 seconds)
Initiate beta blocker to reduce myocardial oxygen demand (blood pressure permitting)
Initiate high-intensity statin as soon as possible, preferably before PCI
Give morphine sulfate for persistent discomfort or anxiety related to myocardial ischemia
Post-PCI
Obtain post-PCI ECG and TTE
Continue dual antiplatelet therapy for 1 year and aspirin indefinitely
Continue beta blocker and statin
Perform risk-stratification with hemoglobin A1C, lipid panel
Consider additional medical therapy pending TTE results[a]

[a]See Beyond the Pearls for additional details.
ECG, Electrocardiogram; *PCI*, percutaneous coronary intervention; *PTT*, partial thromboplastin time; *STEMI*, ST-elevated myocardial infarction. *TTE*, transthoracic echocardiogram.

The patient is admitted to the coronary care unit to monitor for post-PCI complications. The patient is continued on dual antiplatelet therapy (DAPT) with aspirin 81 mg and clopidogrel 75 mg, as well as metoprolol and atorvastatin. A transthoracic echocardiogram (TTE) is ordered to assess for ischemic cardiomyopathy and ventricular dysfunction (see Beyond the Pearls). Post-PCI TTE shows a left ventricular ejection fraction of 60% and no wall motion abnormalities. After 72 hours of uneventful monitoring in the hospital, the patient is discharged with a plan to continue DAPT for 1 year followed by aspirin, atorvastatin, and metoprolol tartrate indefinitely.

Case Summary

- **Complaint/History:** A 59-year-old man presents with acute onset chest pain.
- **Findings:** Physical examination is unremarkable; initial CXR and ECG show no acute findings.
- **Lab Results/Tests:** Repeat ECG shows biphasic T-waves in leads V1–V4 and troponin-T is elevated.

Diagnosis: Wellen's syndrome.

- **Treatment:** The patient was given a loading dose of aspirin (325 mg) and clopidogrel (600 mg) and started on a heparin drip. Metoprolol tartrate was initiated and the patient was taken to the catheterization laboratory for PCI. One drug-eluting stent was placed in the LAD with successful reperfusion. The patient was monitored for post-MI complications and continued on dual antiplatelet therapy with aspirin and clopidogrel. After 1 year, discontinuation of the clopidogrel will be considered. The patient was also continued on a high-intensity statin and beta blocker indefinitely.

BEYOND THE PEARLS

- The ECG pattern demonstrated in this case is known as Wellen's syndrome and is associated with near or total occlusion of the proximal left anterior descending coronary artery. There are two subtypes of Wellen's syndrome: type A is characterized by biphasic T-waves in leads V2–V3 and type B is characterized by deep T-wave inversion in the same leads. In one of the initial studies describing this presentation, more than 75% of patients presenting with these ECG findings developed extensive anterior wall MI within weeks of presentation. Wellen's syndrome is considered a STEMI equivalent because of its high morbidity despite lacking typical features of STEMI and should be managed with early cardiac catheterization.

- Another commonly encountered clinical scenario is one in which a patient with a known left bundle branch block or ventricularly pacing pacemaker presents with chest pain or history indicating ACS. These conduction abnormalities impact ventricular depolarization and repolarization; standard STEMI ECG criteria do not apply in this situation. Instead, Sgarbossa's criteria may be used, which include: ST elevation ≥ 1 mm in a lead with concordant (upward) QRS complex; ST depression ≥ 1 mm in leads V1, V2, or V3; or ST elevation ≥ 5 mm in leads with a discordant (downward) QRS complex.
- ST-segment depression in leads V1–V3 should raise concern for posterior MI, particularly if they are accompanied by upright T-waves and/or a prominent R-wave. A posterior ECG should immediately be obtained to confirm diagnosis.
- Before initiating a P2Y12 inhibitor, the likelihood of multi-vessel CAD or other conditions which may require urgent surgical management should be considered. If a P2Y12 inhibitor is given but coronary angiography demonstrates lesions necessitating surgical revascularization via coronary artery bypass grafting, such an operation may be delayed by up to several days because of the prolonged effects of these medications and the increased risk of postoperative bleeding.
- Several studies have been conducted to assess the safety and efficacy of available oral P2Y12 inhibitors (clopidogrel, prasugrel, and ticagrelor). At this time, there is no consensus on a "best in class" agent, although practitioners should be aware that prasugrel is contraindicated in patients with any history of cerebrovascular accident or transient ischemic attack because of an increased risk of intracranial bleeding. Additional antiplatelet agents such as cangrelor (ATP analog that binds P2Y12 receptors) and abciximab (glycoprotein IIb/IIIa inhibitor) may also be given by a cardiologist in certain scenarios; their use and efficacy continues to be studied.
- Patients may often have significantly reduced left ventricular ejection fraction following their diagnosis with acute coronary syndrome. This may necessitate the initiation of goal-directed medical therapy for heart failure with reduced ejection fraction and possibly preventative measures for ventricular tachyarrhythmias prior to discharge.

Bibliography

de Zwaan C, Bär FWHM, Wellens HJJ. Characteristic electrocardiographic pattern indicating a critical stenosis high in left anterior descending coronary artery in patients admitted because of impending myocardial infarction. *American Heart Journal.* 1982;103:730–736.

Erlinge D, Omerovic E, Fröbert O, et al. Bivalirudin versus heparin monotherapy in myocardial infarction. *The New England Journal of Medicine.* 2017;377:1132–1142.

Ferguson JJ, Califf RM, Antman EM, et al. Enoxaparin vs unfractionated heparin in high-risk patients with non-ST-segment elevation acute coronary syndromes managed with an intended early invasive strategy: Primary results of the SYNERGY randomized trial. *The Journal of the American Medical Association.* 2004;292:45–54.

Fourth International Study of Infarct Survival Collaborative Group ISIS-4: a randomised factorial trial assessing early oral captopril, oral mononitrate, and intravenous magnesium sulphate in 58, 050 patients with suspected acute myocardial infarction. *Lancet.* 1995;345:669–685.

Glickman SW, Shofer FS, Wu MC, et al. Development and validation of a prioritization rule for obtaining an immediate 12-lead electrocardiogram in the emergency department to identify ST-elevation myocardial infarction. *American Heart Journal.* 2012;163:372–382.

Gruppo Italiano per lo Studio della Sopravvivenza nell'infarto Miocardico GISSI-3: effects of lisinopril and transdermal glyceryl trinitrate singly and together on 6-week mortality and ventricular function after acute myocardial infarction. *Lancet*. 1994;343:1115–1122.

Halkin A, Grines CL, Cox DA, et al. Impact of intravenous beta-blockade before primary angioplasty on survival in patients undergoing mechanical reperfusion therapy for acute myocardial infarction. *Journal of the American College of Cardiology*. 2004;43:1780–1787.

National Cardiovascular Data Registry. Outcomes in patients undergoing primary percutaneous coronary intervention for ST-segment elevation myocardial infarction via radial access anticoagulated with bivalirudin versus heparin: a report from the National Cardiovascular Data Registry - PubMed. Available at: https://pubmed-ncbi-nlm-nih-gov.libproxy2.usc.edu/28527778/.

Roberts R, Rogers WJ, Mueller HS, et al. Immediate versus deferred beta-blockade following thrombolytic therapy in patients with acute myocardial infarction. Results of the Thrombolysis in Myocardial Infarction (TIMI) II-B Study. *Circulation*. 1991;83:422–437.

Sgarbossa EB, Pinski SL, Barbagelata A, et al. Electrocardiographic diagnosis of evolving acute myocardial infarction in the presence of left bundle-branch block. GUSTO-1 (Global Utilization of Streptokinase and Tissue Plasminogen Activator for Occluded Coronary Arteries) Investigators. *The New England Journal of Medicine*. 1996;334:481–487.

Wallentin L, Becker RC, Budaj A, et al. Ticagrelor versus clopidogrel in patients with acute coronary syndromes. *The New England Journal of Medicine*. 2009;361:1045–1057.

Wiviott SD, Braunwald E, McCabe CH, et al. Prasugrel versus clopidogrel in patients with acute coronary syndromes. *The New England Journal of Medicine*. 2007;357:2001–2015.

CASE 25

A 55-Year-Old Female With Retrosternal Chest Pain

Shankar Chhetri ■ Sheila Sahni

A 55-year-old female presents to the emergency department with chest pain that started 25 minutes prior to her presentation. The pain initially started as a discomfort in the middle of the chest that gradually worsened and later radiated to the neck and jaws bilaterally. The pain is associated with palpitations, tooth pain, and presyncope, but she denies any nausea, vomiting, or diaphoresis. She also denies any recent illness, travel history, or sick contacts. She had a similar episode 3 months ago during which time cardiac catheterization was performed that showed nonocclusive coronary artery disease that was managed medically without any intervention. Past medical history is significant for hypertension for which she takes spironolactone and rheumatoid arthritis for which she takes hydroxychloroquine.

What is the differential diagnosis for a patient who presents with acute chest pain?

The differential diagnosis for women who present with acute chest pain is very broad and can be divided into cardiac and noncardiac causes (Table 25.1). Acute coronary syndrome (ACS) that includes ST-elevation myocardial infarction (STEMI), non-ST-elevation myocardial infarction (NSTEMI), and unstable angina (UA) are always high on the differential. The initial evaluation of any patient presenting with chest pain includes performing an electrocardiogram (ECG). Further imaging and laboratory tests can be obtained once the initial ECG is reassuring and the patient is hemodynamically stable.

What do you need to consider in women?

Although obstructive atherosclerotic disease of the epicardial coronary arteries remains the main cause of acute myocardial infarction (AMI) in both sexes, plaque characteristics have been observed to differ between men and women. Recent data suggest that women presenting with chest pain are more often found to have nonobstructive coronary artery dissection (CAD) even when presenting with ACS, particularly UA and NSTEMI. This has been attributed to more diffuse plaque erosion in women as opposed to acute plaque rupture with occlusion in men. Additionally, microvascular disease and dysfunction has been shown to play a role in the pathophysiology of coronary events among women. Spontaneous coronary artery dissection (SCAD) and stress (takotsubo) cardiomyopathy are two causes of ACS that are more common in women.

On initial physical examination, blood pressure is 172/87 mmHg, pulse rate is 92/min, temperature is 97.8°F, respiration rate is 26/min, and oxygen saturation is 97% on room air. She is in moderate distress but physical examination is otherwise unremarkable (Table 25.2).

ECG on presentation shows ST-segment elevation in leads III and aVF (Fig. 25.1).

TABLE 25.1 ■ **Causes of Chest Pain**

Cardiac Causes
- ACS (STEMI, NSTEMI, UA)
- Microvascular angina
- Myocarditis
- Pericarditis
- SCAD

Noncardiac Causes (including vascular causes)
- Aortic dissection
- Pulmonary embolism
- Pneumonia
- Tuberculosis
- Pneumothorax
- Costochondritis
- Rib fractures/trauma
- Peptic ulcer disease
- Esophageal tear/perforation
- Pancreatitis
- Panic attack

ACS, Acute coronary syndrome; *NSTEMI*, non-ST-elevation myocardial infarction; *SCAD*, spontaneous coronary artery dissection; *STEMI*, ST-elevation myocardial infarction; *UA*, unstable angina.

TABLE 25.2 ■ **Initial Laboratory Test Results**

Glucose	123 mg/dL
Hgb	15.6 gm/dL
Platelets	243 × 10^3/µL
BUN	15 mg/dL
Creatinine	0.8 mg/dL
Sodium	143 mmol/L
Potassium	4.3 mmol/L
Chloride	104 mmol/L
Calcium	10.1 mg/dL
Troponin I	<0.3 ng/mL

What is the differential diagnosis of ST-segment elevation in this patient?

There are various cardiac and noncardiac causes of ST-segment elevation in an ECG (Table 25.3). ACS with STEMI is the most common cause of ST-segment elevation of specific leads and is high on the differential diagnosis for any patient presenting with typical cardiac chest pain. Uncommon causes of ST-segment elevation of specific leads include Brugada syndrome (ST-segment elevation in leads V1–V3 with pseudo right bundle branch block) and SCAD. While ST-segment elevation is an alarming finding in a patient presenting with chest pain, it is always prudent to compare with prior ECG when possible.

The patient had a similar episode of chest pain 3 months ago (Fig. 25.2), which was more severe in intensity and also had elevated troponin I level of 15.73 ng/mL (reference range <0.3 ng/mL) at that time. She underwent emergent cardiac catheterization that did not reveal any flow-limiting coronary artery disease.

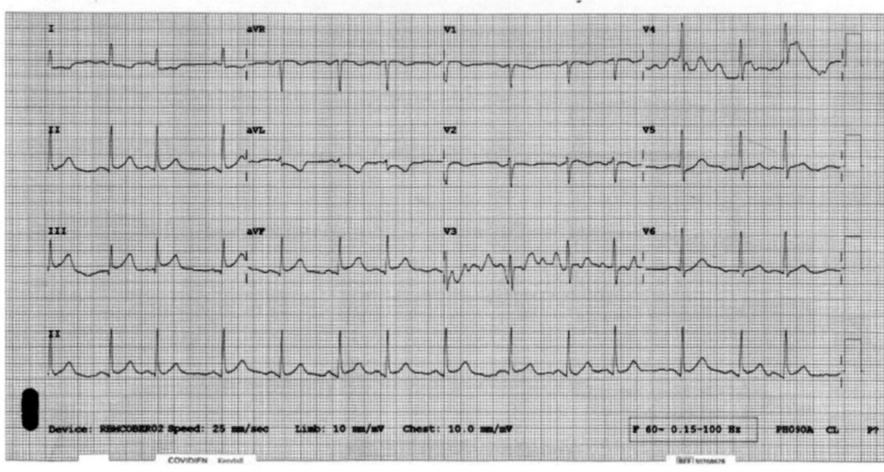

Fig. 25.1 Electrocardiogram on presentation to the emergency department.

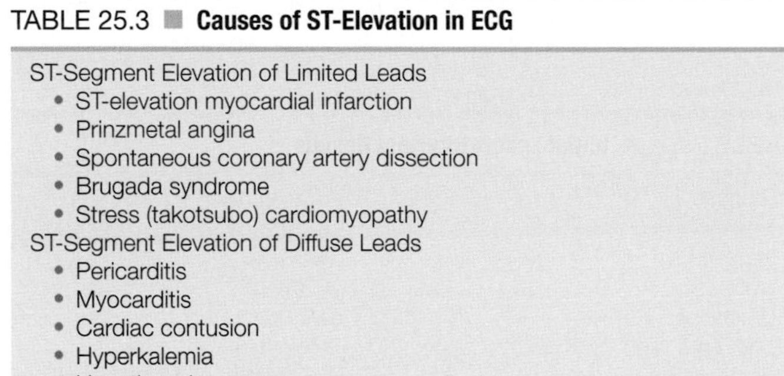

TABLE 25.3 ■ **Causes of ST-Elevation in ECG**

ST-Segment Elevation of Limited Leads
- ST-elevation myocardial infarction
- Prinzmetal angina
- Spontaneous coronary artery dissection
- Brugada syndrome
- Stress (takotsubo) cardiomyopathy

ST-Segment Elevation of Diffuse Leads
- Pericarditis
- Myocarditis
- Cardiac contusion
- Hyperkalemia
- Hypothermia

Approach to a patient with ST-segment elevation in ECG

About 38% of patients who present to the hospital with ACS have STEMI. In patients with myocardial infarction, time is critical. A common phrase for managing patients with STEMI is "time is muscle," meaning that delays in treating a myocardial infarction increases the likelihood and amount of cardiac muscle damaged as a result of localized hypoxia. Door-to-balloon time, which is the time between first medical contact and the insertion of guidewire into the culprit lesion, is 90 minutes in a primary percutaneous coronary intervention (PCI) center and 120 minutes in a non-PCI center. With the widespread availability of PCI and the benefits of PCI, patients with ST-segment elevation in ECG will almost always undergo cardiac catheterization for diagnostic cardiac catheterization with intervention as indicated. In patients who have no evidence of coronary artery occlusion upon cardiac catheterization, an alternative diagnosis should be considered depending on the findings of cardiac catheterization and presence of other risk factors.

What is your differential diagnosis?

This patient is a 55-year-old female who presents with retrosternal chest pain, ST-segment elevation in leads III and aVF and normal troponin I level (see Table 25.2).

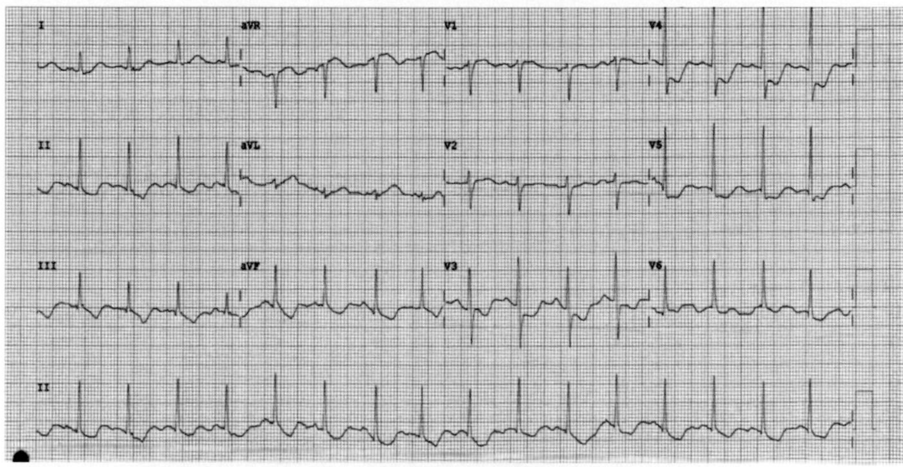

Fig. 25.2 Presenting electrocardiogram in the patient 3 months earlier.

CLINICAL PEARL/BASIC SCIENCE USMLE	STEP 1 AND 2
ST-segment elevation is not always caused by myocardial infarction.	

Given the nature of the patient's acute chest pain and ECG findings consistent with possible inferior acute STEMI, cardiac catheterization is performed. No focal lesion with 100% obstruction is found in the left coronary system. Upon selective injection of the right coronary artery, rupture of the vessel wall proximally is noted with contrast dye staining followed by a contrast filling defect (Fig. 25.3) in the distal vessel where the vessel tapered to a narrow caliber in a segment and then normalized. This is a finding inconsistent with obstruction of flow due to plaque. Further analysis of the angiogram reveals confirmed spontaneous dissection of the entire right coronary artery. Given that the patient reports no chest pain and has normal hemodynamics, the decision is made to manage the patient's condition with optimal medical treatment with no further intervention.

CLINICAL PEARL/BASIC SCIENCE PEARL USLME	STEP 1
The left anterior descending artery is the most frequently affected vessel and most patients have only one coronary artery involvement.	

What is spontaneous coronary artery dissection?

SCAD is a nonatherosclerotic, nontraumatic, and noniatrogenic separation of the coronary arterial wall and is an infrequent cause of acute myocardial infarction. The predominant mechanism of myocardial injury occurring as a result of SCAD is coronary artery obstruction caused by formation of an intramural hematoma or intimal disruption rather than atherosclerotic plaque disruption or intraluminal thrombus. This condition is more common in younger individuals and women.

BASIC SCIENCE/CLINICAL PEARL USMLE	STEP 1 AND 2
In SCAD, separation occurs in the outer third of the tunica media and development of an intramural hematoma occupying the dissection compresses the true lumen leading to coronary blood flow insufficiency and, ultimately, myocardial infarction.	

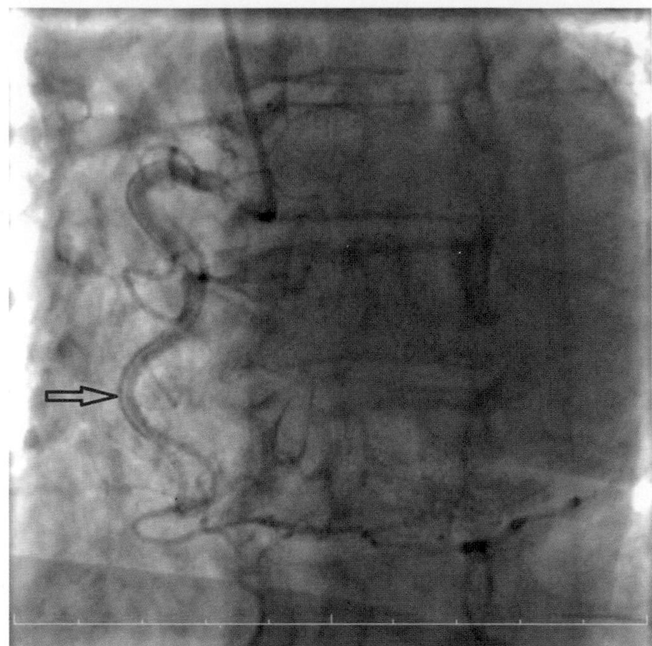

Fig. 25.3 Coronary angiogram showing tear of right coronary artery with contrast filling defect *(blue arrow)*.

When should a diagnosis of spontaneous coronary artery dissection be considered?

The diagnosis of SCAD should be considered in any young patients, particularly women, who present with ACS with or without ST-segment elevation in ECG and who do not have history of coronary artery disease or traditional cardiovascular risk factors. Fibromuscular dysplasia is a major risk factor for SCAD. In any patient with known fibromuscular dysplasia presenting with ACS, the diagnosis of SCAD must be high on the differential.

CLINICAL PEARL USMLE	**STEP 2**
Diagnosis of traumatic coronary artery dissection should be considered in patients who present with ACS following trauma.	

Epidemiology of SCAD

SCAD is the cause of 0.4%–1% of ACS in the general population. It is more prevalent among women, with approximately 85% of affected individuals being women compared with 15% being men. Men are slightly younger on presentation compared with women. Classically, SCAD was only thought to affect young women but now it is increasingly recognized in older and postmenopausal women. The mean age of women presenting with SCAD is between 44 and 53 years old.

Risk factors for SCAD

In most cases of SCAD, a predisposing arterial disease association or cause is identified; however, about 20% of cases are idiopathic. Potential risk factors (Table 25.4) include fibromuscular dysplasia (FMD), postpartum status, multiparity (≥4 births), connective tissue disorders, systemic inflammatory disorders, and hormonal therapy. The most common condition associated with SCAD is FMD, whereby almost 70% of affected patients have FMD of one or more areas.

BASIC SCIENCE/CLINICAL PEARL USMLE **STEP 1 AND 2**

In connective tissue disorders such as Marfan or Ehlers-Danlos syndrome, medial degeneration is believed to weaken the arterial wall and predispose to spontaneous dissection.

What are important historical questions to ask patients who present with SCAD or are suspected of having SCAD?

Patients with SCAD are at risk of having a missed diagnosis. Due to patients' relatively young age and absence of traditional atherosclerotic risk factors, provider awareness of this condition is extremely important. A careful history focused on SCAD-associated risk factors must be conducted in patients, particularly among young women, before reaching an alternative diagnosis. Early onset hypertension resistant to treatment can be a clue to fibromuscular dysplasia, whereas poor wound healing can be a sign of connective tissue disorder. Women should also be asked about hormonal contraceptives, supplements, and infertility treatment.

The only risk factor that can be associated with SCAD in this patient is rheumatoid arthritis which is well controlled with hydroxychloroquine. She lives in a two-story house with her family and admitted to doing a significant amount of laundry that day, which entailed multiple trips up and down the stairs earlier that morning. The patient also mentions that her father-in-law passed away recently and chaos during the funeral led to significant emotional distress.

TABLE 25.4 ■ **Conditions and Factors Associated With SCAD**

Associated Conditions

Fibromuscular dysplasia
Pregnancy/peripartum status
Multiparity (>4 births)
Connective tissue disorders

- Marfan syndrome, Ehlers-Danlos syndrome, polycystic kidney disease,
- α1-antitrypsin deficiency

Exogenous hormones

- Oral contraceptives, postmenopausal therapy, infertility treatments, testosterone, glucocorticoids

Systemic inflammatory diseases

- Systemic lupus erythematosus, inflammatory bowel disease, systemic vasculitis, rheumatoid arthritis, Kawasaki disease, celiac disease

Precipitating Factors

Intense exercise
Intense emotional stress
Intense Valsalva
Labor and delivery
Retching, vomiting, bowel movement, coughing, lifting heavy objects
Exogenous hormones/hormone modulators
Recreational drugs (cocaine, methamphetamines)
B-hCG (human chorionic gonadotropin) injections, glucocorticoid injections, clomiphene citrate

SCAD, Spontaneous coronary artery dissection.

Clinical manifestations

Patients with SCAD usually present with signs and symptoms of ACS. Chest pain is the most common symptom reported and is present in about 96% of patients. Other, less common symptoms include arm pain, neck pain, nausea or vomiting, diaphoresis, dyspnea, or back pain. ST-segment elevation is found in 25% to 50% of patients with the remaining patients presenting with non-ST-elevation myocardial infarction. However, about 1% of patients can present with no elevation of cardiac biomarkers. As many as 2% to 5% of patients present with cardiogenic shock (Lettieri et al., 2015) with ventricular arrhythmias or sudden cardiac death accounting for 3% to 11% of reported cases. About 30% of patients report physical exertion prior to the event and about 50% of patients report emotional stress.

Diagnosis

It is impossible to distinguish SCAD from ACS based on clinical features and laboratory test results alone, given similar presentations. The diagnosis of SCAD can be confirmed with cardiac catheterization, which may include the use of optical coherence tomography (OCT) or intravascular ultrasound (IVUS). It is critical to differentiate SCAD from ACS, particularly when patients present with ST-segment elevation, due to completely different management strategies. Even in patients who have preexisting conditions such as fibromuscular dysplasia that is strongly associated with SCAD, underlying coronary artery disease should be ruled out by cardiac catheterization. The typical treatment of patients who present with ST-segment elevation is to perform emergent coronary angiogram to treat completely obstructed coronary vessel(s) with percutaneous coronary intervention and salvage myocardial tissue. Upon proceeding with coronary angiogram as part of the STEMI algorithm, patients with SCAD are often found to have reduced coronary blood flow but not total occlusion. It is imperative to direct attention toward visualizing this difference in blood flow because proceeding with intervention is often riskier than conservative management in these patients. Based on angiographic findings, SCAD is classified into three types:

1. **Type 1:** Pathognomonic contrast dye staining of arterial wall with multiple radiolucent lumen, with or without the presence of dye hang-up or slow contrast clearing (Fig. 25.4)
2. **Type 2:** Diffuse long and smooth stenosis that can vary in severity from mild stenosis to complete occlusion (Fig. 25.5)
3. **Type 3:** Mimics atherosclerosis with focal or tubular stenosis and requiring optical coherence tomography (OCT) or intravascular ultrasound (IVUS) to differentiate the cause (Fig. 25.6)

In patients for whom the diagnosis is considered but not secured with coronary angiography, intracoronary imaging with OCT or IVUS may be helpful. Extreme technical detail is required to perform these imaging techniques in the laboratory to avoid propagation of the intramural hematoma. With these imaging modalities, SCAD diagnosis is made with the presence of an intramural hematoma and/or a double lumen (Fig. 25.7).

How do you approach treatment for SCAD?

The management goals of SCAD are twofold: to preserve myocardial function and maintain coronary myocardial perfusion (Fig. 25.8). In most cases, the primary treatment strategy is conservative management without intervention, unless there is evidence of ongoing ischemia, hemodynamic instability, or left main dissection. Patients with acute myocardial infarction who have symptoms of ongoing ischemia or hemodynamic compromise should be considered for revascularization with PCI or coronary artery bypass grafting. Observational studies have shown that PCI for the treatment of SCAD is associated with increased risk of complications and suboptimal outcome. Medical management with anticoagulation and antiplatelet agents lacks general consensus among practitioners in the absence of clear guidelines. Systemic anticoagulation is not preferred by most practitioners because of the risk of bleeding and/or extension of dissection. If systemic

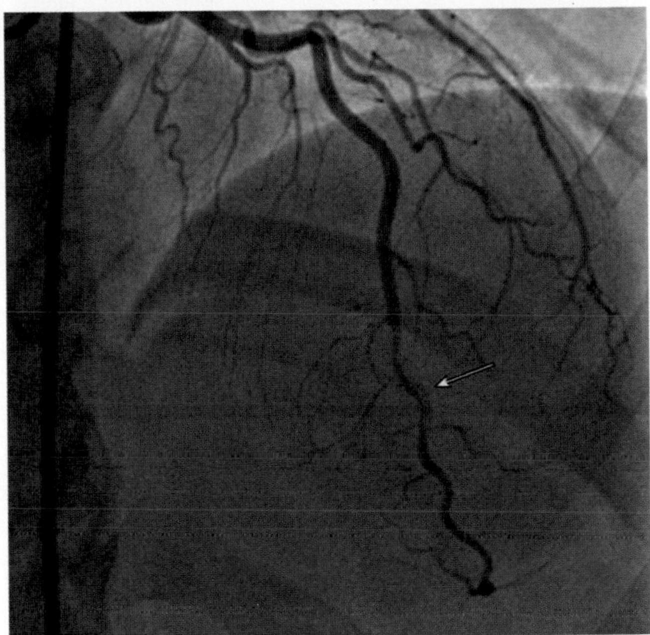

Fig. 25.4 Type 1 spontaneous coronary artery dissection *(yellow arrow)*. (From Saw, J. (2014). Coronary angiogram classification of spontaneous coronary artery dissection. *Catheterization and Cardiovascular Interventions*, *84*(7), 1115.)

anticoagulation is initiated on admission, it is prudent to consider discontinuation upon diagnosis of SCAD, unless there are other indications for systemic anticoagulation. Dual antiplatelet therapy has a theoretical benefit in preventing thrombus propagation but is infrequently used because of the potential for increasing bleeding risk. The routine use of beta blockers after SCAD is supported by a case series in which the use of beta blockers was protective, with a hazard ratio of 0.36 for recurrent SCAD in multivariable analysis. Retrospective studies have not demonstrated any clear benefit for routine use of statins after SCAD and statin therapy is reserved for patients meeting guideline-based indications for primary prevention of atherosclerosis or other guideline-based indications. The rarity of SCAD has resulted in limited clinical experience, dependence on registry data, and lack of randomized data. Thus, the optimal management of SCAD remains uncertain.

The patient denied chest pain, remained hemodynamic stability, and had no further changes in ECG. She also had no signs or symptoms of active ischemia. Therefore, no further invasive intervention was performed and she was managed conservatively with aspirin, atorvastatin, and metoprolol. She improved daily and was monitored in the hospital for a total of 4 days. She was discharged in a stable condition and referred to cardiac rehabilitation.

Prognosis

So far observational studies have demonstrated spontaneous healing of SCAD lesions in the majority of patients (70%–97%) with almost 90% of lesions healing within the first 35 days and most of the remaining cases healing after 35 days. Early complications of recurrent myocardial infarction may develop in 5%–10% of conservatively managed patients, mostly related to

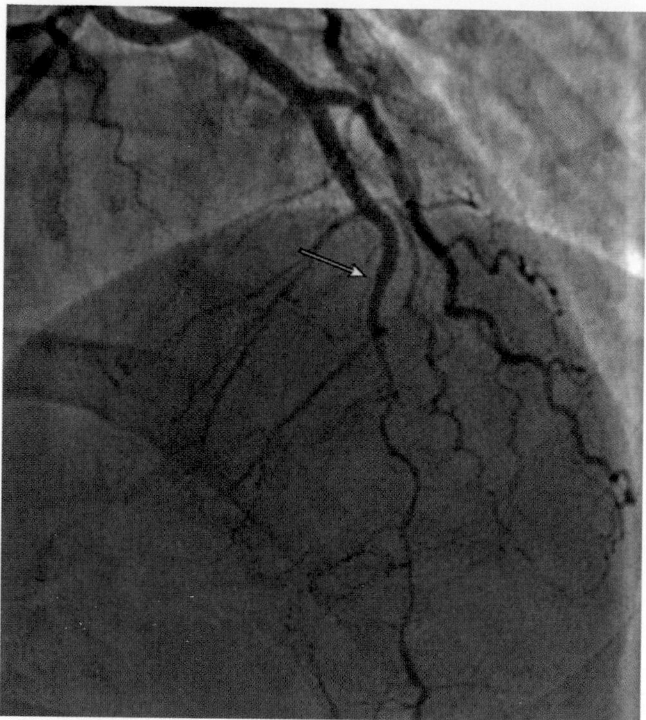

Fig. 25.5 Type 2 spontaneous coronary artery dissection *(yellow arrow)*. (From Saw, J. (2014). Coronary angiogram classification of spontaneous coronary artery dissection. *Catheterization and Cardiovascular Interventions*, *84*(7), 1115.)

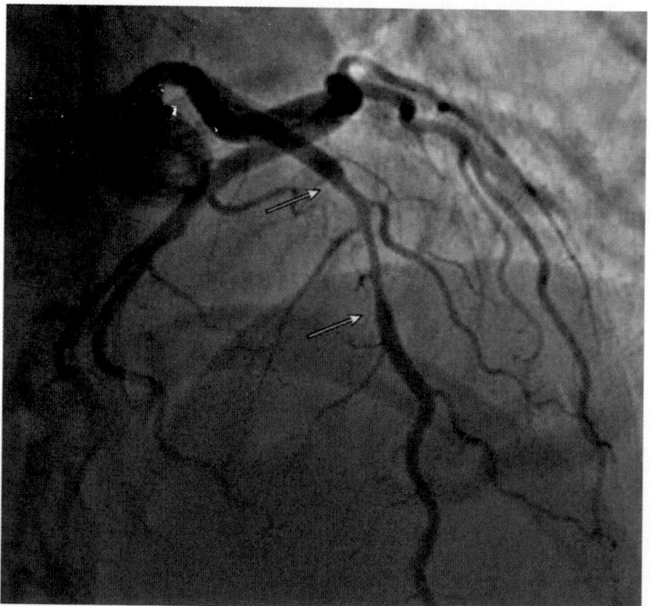

Fig. 25.6 Type 3 spontaneous coronary artery dissection *(yellow arrows)*. (From Saw, J. (2014). Coronary angiogram classification of spontaneous coronary artery dissection. *Catheterization and Cardiovascular Interventions*, *84*(7), 1115.)

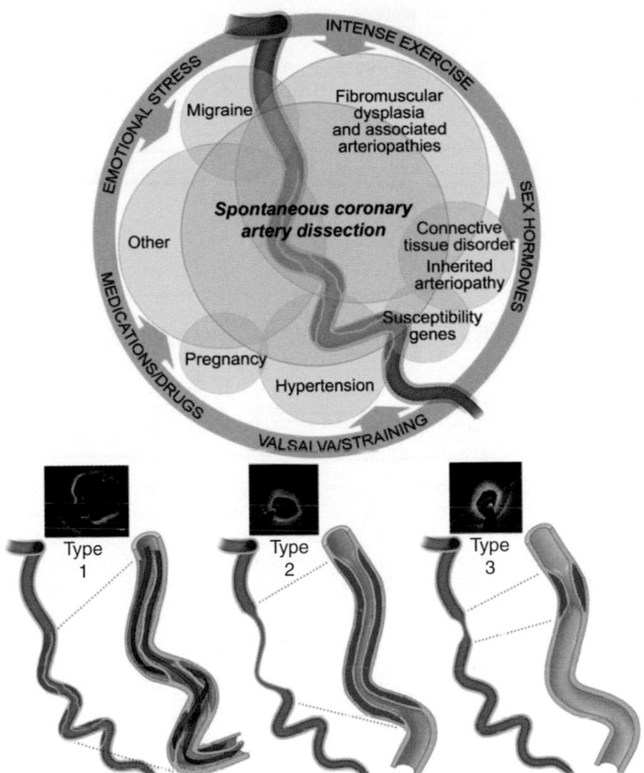

Fig. 25.7 Associated conditions, inciting factors, and angiographic diagnosis of spontaneous coronary artery dissection. (From Hayes, S. N., Tweet, M. S., Adlam, D., Kim, E. S. H., Gulati, R., Price, J. E., & Rose, C. H., (2020). Spontaneous coronary artery dissection. *Journal of the American College of Cardiology, 76*(8), 961–984.)

extension of dissection within the first 7 days after an acute episode (Saw et al., 2014) that may warrant inpatient monitoring for extended periods.

Case Summary

- **Complaint/History:** A 55-year-old female presents with chest pain FOR 25 minutes that initially started as a discomfort in the middle of the chest and gradually worsened with radiation to the neck and jaws bilaterally. The pain is associated with palpitations, tooth pain, and presyncope but without any nausea, vomiting, or diaphoresis.
- **Findings:** Blood pressure is 172/87 mmHg, pulse rate is 92/min, temperature is 97.8°F, respiration rate is 26/min, and oxygen saturation is 97% on room air. She is in moderate distress due to pain.
- **Lab Results/Tests:** Her labs are unremarkable and troponin I is <0.3ng/mL. EKG shows ST-segment elevation on leads III and aVF.

Diagnosis: On coronary angiogram, upon selective injection of the right coronary artery, rupture of the vessel wall proximally is noted with contrast dye staining followed by a contrast filling defect in the distal vessel where the vessel tapered to a narrow caliber in a segment and then normalized consistent with spontaneous dissection of the entire right coronary artery.

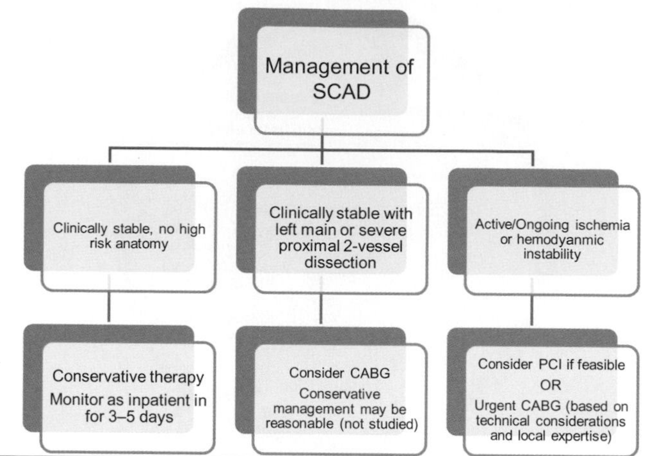

Fig. 25.8 Management of acute spontaneous coronary artery dissection. *CABG*, Coronary artery bypass graft surgery; *PCI*, percutaneous coronary intervention; *SCAD*, spontaneous coronary artery dissection. (From Hayes, S. N., Kim, E. S. H., Saw, J., et al. (2018). Spontaneous coronary artery dissection: current state of the science: a scientific statement from the American Heart Association. *Circulation*, *137*(19), e523–e557.; Hayes, S. N., Tweet, M. S., Adlam, D., et al. (2020). Spontaneous coronary artery dissection. *Journal of the American College of Cardiology, 76*(8), 961–984.)

- **Treatment:** Patient was managed conservatively with aspirin, atorvastatin, and metoprolol. She improved daily and was monitored in the hospital for a total of 4 days. She was discharged in a stable condition and referred to cardiac rehabilitation.

BEYOND THE PEARLS

- Women who present with UA and NSTEMI are more likely to have nonobstructive CAD when compared with men.
- SCAD is a clinically important diagnosis to make in women presenting with ACS and STEMI because of the distinct management strategy of conservative therapy as first-line treatment when possible. Decision-making is driven by proximal extension of the vessel involved, myocardial function, and electrical stability. Patients who only have chest pain can be managed conservatively but may require extended hospitalizations for observation.
- SCAD is an important diagnosis to consider in the setting of ACS because PCI can often lead to complications. Thus, a very high threshold should be utilized for proceeding with intervention, which is in stark contrast to the management of obstructive CAD in ACS.
- SCAD may be the first presentation of a systemic arteriopathy. Fibromuscular dysplasia has often been reported in patients with SCAD and has been associated with noncoronary related vascular abnormalities. Thus, it is an important condition to evaluate among patients presenting with SCAD.
- Clinical presentation could be precipitated by a number of factors, including pregnancy and extreme physical and emotional stress.

Bibliography

Alfonso, F., Paulo, M., Lennie, V., Dutary, J., Bernardo, E., Jiménez-Quevedo, P., Gonzalo, N., Escaned, J., Bañuelos, C., Pérez-Vizcayno, M. J., Hernańdez, R., Macaya, C., (2012). Spontaneous coronary artery dissection: Long-term follow-up of a large series of patients prospectively managed with a "conservative" therapeutic strategy. *JACC: Cardiovascular Interventions*, *5*(10), 1062–1070.

Hayes, S. N., Kim, E. S. H., Saw, J., Adlam, D., Arslanian-Engoren, C., Economy, K. E., Ganesh, S. K., Gulati, R., Lindsay, M. E., Mieres, J. H., Naderi, S., Shah, S., Thaler, D. Tweet, M. S. & Wood, M. J. (2018). Spontaneous coronary artery dissection: Current state of the science: a scientific statement from the American Heart Association. *Circulation, 137*(19), e523–e557.

Hayes, S. N., Tweet, M. S., Adlam, D., Kim, E. S. H., Gulati, R., Price, J. E., & Rose, C. H., (2020). Spontaneous coronary artery dissection. *Journal of the American College of Cardiology, 76*(8), 961–984.

Kolodgie, F. D., Burke, A. P., Farb, A., Gold, H. K., Yuan, J., Narula, J., Finn, A. V., Virmani, R. (2001). The thin-cap fibroatheroma: A type of vulnerable plaque: the major precursor lesion to acute coronary syndromes. *Current Opinion in Cardiology, 16*(5), 285–292.

Lettieri, C., Zavalloni, D., Rossini, R., Morici, N., Ettori, F., Leonzi, O., & Castiglioni, B. (2015). Management and long-term prognosis of spontaneous coronary artery dissection. *The American Journal of Cardiology, 116*, 66–73.

Luong, C., Starovoytov, A., Heydari, M., Sedlak, T., Aymong, E., & Saw, J. (2017). Clinical presentation of patients with spontaneous coronary artery dissection. *Catheterization and Cardiovascular Interventions, 89*, 1149–1154.

Mortensen, K. H., Thuesen, L., Kristensen, I. B., & Christiansen, E. H. (2009). Spontaneous coronary artery dissection: A Western Denmark Heart Registry study. *Catheterization and Cardiovascular Interventions, 74*, 710–717.

Mozaffarian, D., Benjamin, E. J., Go, A. S., Benjamin, E. J., Blaha, M. J., Chiuve, S. E., Cushman, M., Das, S. R., Deo, R., de Ferranti, S. D., Floyd, J., Fornage, M., Gillespie, C., Isasi, C. R., Jiménez, M. C., Jordan, L. C., Judd, S. E., Lackland, D., Lichtman, J. H., Lisabeth, L., Liu, S., Longenecker, C. T., ... Muntner, P. (2017). Heart disease and stroke statistics – 2017 update: A report from the American Heart Association. *Circulation, 135*, e146–e603.

Nishiguchi, T., Tanaka, A., Ozaki, Y., Taruya, A., Fukuda, S., Taguchi, H., Iwaguro, T., Ueno, S., Okumoto, Y., Akasaka, T. (2016). Prevalence of spontaneous coronary artery dissection in patients with acute coronary syndrome. *European Heart Journal. Acute Cardiovascular Care, 5*(3), 263–270.

Prakash, R., Starovoytov, A., Heydari, M., Mancini, G. B., & Saw, J. (2016). Catheter-induced iatrogenic coronary artery dissection in patients with spontaneous coronary artery dissection. *JACC: Cardiovascular Interventions, 9*, 1851–1853.

Saw. J. (2014). Coronary angiogram classification of spontaneous coronary artery dissection. *Catheterization and Cardiovascular Interventions, 84*(7), 1115.

Saw, J., Aymong, E., Sedlak, T., Buller, C. E., Starovoytov, A., Ricci, D., & Mancini, G. B. (2014). Spontaneous coronary artery dissection: Association with predisposing arteriopathies and precipitating stressors and cardiovascular outcomes. *Circulation: Cardiovascular Interventions, 7*, 645–655.

Saw, J., Humphries, K., Aymong, E., Sedlak, T., Prakash, R., Starovoytov, A., & Mancini, G. B. J. (2017). Spontaneous coronary artery dissection: Clinical outcomes and risk of recurrence. *Journal of the American College of Cardiology, 70*, 1148–1158.

Saw, J., Ricci, D., Starovoytov, A., Fox, R., & Buller, C. E. (2013). Spontaneous coronary artery dissection: Prevalence of predisposing conditions including fibromuscular dysplasia in a tertiary center cohort. *Circulation: Cardiovascular Interventions, 6*(1), 44–52.

Tweet, M. S., Eleid, M. F., Best, P. J., Lennon, R. J., Lerman, A., Rihal, C. S., & Gulati, R. (2014). Spontaneous coronary artery dissection: Revascularization versus conservative therapy. *Circulation: Cardiovascular Interventions, 7*, 777–786.

Yip, A., & Saw, J. (2015). Spontaneous coronary artery dissection: A review. *Cardiovascular Diagnosis and Therapy, 5*, 37–48.

CASE 26

A 48-Year-Old Male With Acute Shortness of Breath

James Onwuzurike ■ Katharine Yang ■ Shankar Chhetri ■ Sheila Sahni

A 48-year-old-male is brought to the emergency department for sudden-onset shortness of breath and diaphoresis for 4 days. He reports an episode of feeling faint 3 weeks previously while climbing three flights of stairs and intermittent episodes of dyspnea for the last 2 years. He has no fevers, chills, cough, or abdominal pain. The patient has no other medical problems and takes no medications. He had surgery for bilateral inguinal hernias at the age of 16 years. The patient does not use tobacco, alcohol, or illicit drugs. Blood pressure is 95/69 mmHg, pulse rate is 116/min and irregular, respirations are 28 breaths/min, and oxygen saturation is at 84%; he is immediately placed on 4 L nasal cannula, which brings his oxygen saturation to 94%. He is in marked respiratory distress. Pallor and diaphoresis are noted. His skin is velvety and has many atrophic scars. The apical impulse is hyperdynamic. Cardiac auscultation reveals a soft early-systolic decrescendo murmur at the cardiac apex. S1 is barely audible; S2 is normal. Lung examination reveals bibasilar crackles. Jugular venous distension (JVD) is present. His abdomen is soft, nontender, and nondistended. Neurologic examination shows no abnormalities.

What should be included in the differential diagnosis at this time?

Mr. Smith presents with acute on chronic dyspnea, with physical examination showing signs of hemodynamic instability, arrhythmia, and heart failure. The culprit organ system is most likely cardiac but could potentially be pulmonary as well. Differential diagnosis includes valvular disorders, especially given his systolic murmur, myocardial ischemia, and new onset heart failure. Lung processes to consider include acute pneumonia, exacerbation of a new diagnosis of rheumatological disorder, infiltrative process, autoimmune disease, or malignancy.

What are common causes for heart murmurs?

Heart murmurs are the direct result of blood flow turbulence. There are various causes of heart murmurs, which are summarized in Table 26.1. The most common cause of heart murmurs is valvular heart disease, which can include valvular stenosis or valvular regurgitation. Among the various types of valvular heart disease, aortic stenosis (AS), mitral regurgitation (MR), and tricuspid regurgitation (TR) are the most common valvular disorders in elderly adults.

What are common causes of valvular heart disease (VHD)?

The common causes of valvular heart disease are listed in Table 26.2.

The patient's lab tests return as follows: complete cell count revealed a WBC of 5.6 K/μL, Hgb of 13 g/dL, and platelet count of 334 × 10^9/dL. Basic metabolic panel (BMP) is notable for acute renal injury with blood urea nitrogen (BUN) and creatinine (Cr) of 45 mg/dL and 1.6 mg/dL, with baseline BUN and Cr of 13 mg/dL and 0.7 mg/dL. Troponin is 0.04 ng/mL. Pro-BNP was 3564 pg/mL. Two sets of blood cultures yielded no growth thus far.

TABLE 26.1 ■ **Differential Diagnosis: New Onset Murmur**

Cardiac	Acute coronary syndrome
	Atrial myxoma
	Congestive heart failure
	Hypertrophic cardiomyopathy
	Rheumatic heart disease
	Septal defect (atrial, ventricular)
	Valvular heart disease (stenosis, regurgitation)
Endocrine	Hyperthyroidism (thyrotoxicosis)
Pulmonary	Pulmonary embolism
Hematologic	Anemia
Infectious	Pericarditis
	Infective endocarditis
Vascular	Aortic dissection
	Aortopulmonary shunt
Benign	Growth in adolescence
	Pregnancy

TABLE 26.2 ■ **Common Causes of Valvular Heart Disease**

Endocarditis: infectious or rheumatological (Libman-Sacks endocarditis)
Papillary muscle rupture
Degenerative valve disease with chordal rupture and flail leaflet
Infiltrative diseases: sarcoidosis, hemochromatosis, amyloidosis
Rheumatic heart disease (often a result of untreated *Streptococcus pyogenes* in childhood)
Inherited genetic disorders: Turner's syndrome, Marfan syndrome, and other congenital defects
Chest radiation
Trauma causing mechanical changes to the valve
Cardiac tumors such as myxoma

How does this new information change your differential diagnosis?

The elevated pro-BNP and presence of pulmonary edema on chest X-ray (CXR) examination confirms our previous concern of signs of left-sided heart failure. Infectious endocarditis is less likely based on negative blood cultures and lack of known risk factors (e.g., intravenous drug use). A slight troponin elevation of 0.04 ng/dL without ischemic changes on electrocardiogram (ECG) would be atypical for an ischemic event, but it is important to continue to trend troponins and ECGs to monitor for ischemia. Given the acute symptoms of heart failure with a new apical systolic murmur, MR from a previous ischemic event or degeneration/rupture of papillary muscle and/or chordae tendineae should be considered.

How is valvular heart disease diagnosed?

Patients with valvular heart disease (VHD) may present with a heart murmur, symptoms, or incidental findings of valvular abnormalities on chest imaging or noninvasive testing. Given the range of presentations, all patients with known or suspected VHD should undergo a meticulous initial history and physical examination. Due to the slow, progressive nature of most valvular lesions, patients may not recognize symptoms because they may have gradually limited their daily activity levels without noticing changes. A detailed physical examination should be performed to diagnose and assess the severity of valve lesions based on a compilation of all findings made by inspection, palpation, and auscultation (see Table 26.3).

TABLE 26.3 ■ **Initial Testing in Valvular Heart Disease Workup**

Electrocardiogram (ECG)	Confirms present heart rhythm, assesses for bradycardia or conduction abnormalities. Important to note it is only a snapshot of the present rhythm.
Chest radiograph (CXR)	Assesses the presence or absence of pulmonary congestion, size of cardiac silhouette, as well as other lung pathology.
Transthoracic echocardiogram (TTE)	Key diagnostic test: Most commonly performed in two–dimensional imaging, TTE allows anatomic and functional data of cardiac chamber, cardiac valves, aortic root, great vessels, and other cardiac structures. Doppler interrogation allows physiologic assessment of blood flow across the valves to determine severity of pathologic lesions when present.

Depending on the findings from the initial diagnostic workup, additional testing may be performed. Transesophageal echocardiography (TEE) is an invasive ultrasound test performed by inserting a probe inside a patient's throat into the esophagus to allow high resolution images of cardiac structures. TEE is used to determine the extent of VHD conditions to guide management and treatment strategies. Other diagnostic testing may include computed tomography (CT), cardiac magnetic resonance (CMR) imaging, or exercise or pharmacological stress testing. Invasive hemodynamic or coronary angiography assessment are often performed, especially prior to surgical treatment or if the etiology of the valvular heart condition is ischemic in etiologies.

CLINICAL PEARL

Left atrial enlargement, left ventricle enlargement, and possible pulmonary congestion (most often normal) are common findings on CXR that may suggest valvular dysfunction (Lam, 2019).

Mr. Smith's ECG shows sinus tachycardia with occasional premature ventricular complexes (PVCs). Posteroanterior CXR reveals borderline cardiomegaly with pulmonary edema (see Fig. 26.1).

How important is follow-up for patients with suspected VHD?

Follow-up of these patients is important and should consist of an annual history and physical examination in most stable patients. An evaluation of the patient may be necessary sooner than annually if there is a change in the patient's symptoms. In some valve lesions, there may be unpredictable adverse consequences on the left ventricle in the absence of symptoms necessitating more frequent follow-up. The frequency of repeat testing, such as echocardiography, will depend on the severity of the valve lesion and its effect on the left or right ventricle, coupled with the known natural history of the valve lesion.

Case Recap: Mr. Smith is a 48-year-old man who was to the emergency department suffering from sudden-onset shortness of breath and diaphoresis and found to have oxygen desaturations, soft early-systolic decrescendo murmur at the cardiac apex, JVD, bibasilar lung crackles on physical examination, sinus tachycardia with PVCs on ECG, and severe pulmonary edema on CXR.

What remains on the differential diagnosis at this point?

Valvular heart disease is high on the differential diagnosis at this point given the patient's clinical symptoms of shortness of breath and diaphoresis, in conjunction with a newly found early-systolic decrescendo murmur at the cardiac apex. Table 26.1 summarizes other conditions that should be considered in a patient who presents with these symptoms. JVD and bibasilar lung crackles on physical

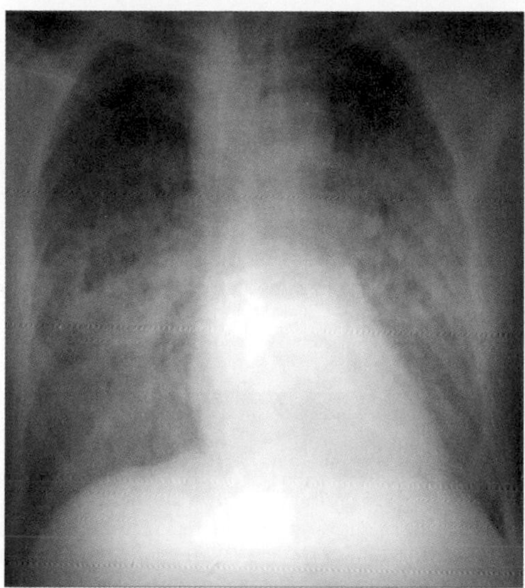

Fig. 26.1 Chest X-ray shows borderline cardiomegaly with severe pulmonary edema *(arrow)*. (From Thomas, J., *Rosen's emergency medicine: concepts and clinical practice*, (pp. 891–928).e4.)

examination suggest decompensated heart failure that may result from acute valvular dysfunction, including acute mitral stenosis (MS), mitral regurgitation(MR), aortic regurgitation (AR), or aortic stenosis (AS). Given that systolic murmur is heard best at the cardiac apex, involvement of the mitral valve is suspected. In some patients with acute MR, presentation can be dramatic given less time for adaptation of the left heart compared with chronic MR, resulting in sudden-onset hypotension (as seen in our patient), which can rapidly progress to cardiogenic shock with poor tissue perfusion and peripheral vasoconstriction. Cardiac examination reveals a hyperdynamic precordium and decrescendo holosystolic murmur at the cardiac apex. Patients with acute, severe MR have early equalization of left atrial and left ventricular pressures and up to 50% (especially with ischemic MR) may have no audible murmur (silent MR). The diagnosis is typically confirmed by rapid bedside echocardiography.

Papillary muscle rupture with acute, severe MR can occur as a life-threatening mechanical complication of acute MI, typically 3–5 days after the infarct. The patient's presenting and ECG findings do not show evidence of ischemia or recent MI. Spontaneous papillary muscle rupture in young patients without any symptoms suggestive of recent MI is uncommon.

Infective endocarditis involving the mitral valve can lead to acute MR as a result of inadequate leaflet coaptation, leaflet perforation, or papillary muscle involvement. This patient's absence of preceding fever combined with his velvety skin with scar formation and previous bilateral hernias (suggestive of underlying connective tissue disease) make chordae tendineae rupture from the mitral valve more likely.

Massive, acute pulmonary embolism can cause sudden-onset dyspnea, hypotension, right heart failure, and syncope. However, patients do not typically develop acute pulmonary edema.

CLINICAL PEARL

Patients with underlying connective tissue disease (e.g., Marfan syndrome, Ehlers-Danlos syndrome) are at risk of mitral chordae tendineae rupture, leading to a flail leaflet and acute MR.

How do you establish a diagnosis of VHD?

Major advances in cardiac surgery have resulted in the prompt and accurate diagnosis of valvular heart disease, which can affect the consideration of surgical treatment in elderly patients who previously may not have been surgical candidates. Among patients who survive the surgery and perioperative period, the quality of life and, in some studies, survival, are the same as in a general population of age-matched subjects. Echocardiography remains the gold standard for diagnosis and periodic assessment of patients with valvular heart disease.

CLINICAL PEARL

Normal left ventricle function and elevations of brain natriuretic peptide (BNP) >105 pg/mL have an independent and additive prognostic value that may identify high-risk patients and aid in the selection of patients for early surgery in patients with severe asymptomatic MR (Lam, 2019).

A transthoracic echocardiogram with Doppler was obtained on Mr. Smith, showing the presence of a prominent flail mitral valve leaflet caused by ruptured chordae resulting in MR (Fig. 26.1). A transesophageal echocardiogram was obtained for further definition revealing the vena contracta (VC) width of 0.7 cm with a 50% central regurgitant jet cover of the left atrium, and a systolic flow reversal in the pulmonary veins. (The quantitative parameters include an effective regurgitant orifice area (ERO) >40 cm^2, a regurgitate volume (RV) >60 mL, and a regurgitant fraction (RF) >50%.) No vegetations were seen on mitral, aortic, tricuspid, or pulmonic valves.

Still frames of transthoracic echocardiogram (TTE) are shown in Figs. 26.2 and 26.3. Left ventricular ejection fraction was 60% with no wall motion abnormalities and no diastolic dysfunction.

CLINICAL PEARL

Left ventricle systolic performance, estimated right ventricular (RV) systolic pressure vena contracta width >0.7 cm, regurgitant volume >60 mL, regurgitant orifice area >0.40 cm^2 by proximal isovelocity surface area (PISA), and systolic pulmonary vein flow reversal are all echocardiographic criteria of severe MR (Lam, 2019).

Based on clinical history, examination, and echocardiographic findings, we established a diagnosis of acute on chronic MR in Mr. Smith, secondary to long-standing connective tissue disease, that in the moments before presenting to the emergency room led to chordae rupture, causing acute MR and flash pulmonary edema.

Diagnosis: Chordae tendineae rupture leading to acute regurgitation, superimposed on chronic MR from connective tissue disease.

How is MR treated?

Management of MR requires the assessment of a number of factors to help elucidate the urgency as well as the modality of treatment that will be most effective in addressing the underlying cause. We must determine: (1) the level of hemodynamic compromise at time of presentation, (2) acute versus chronic presentation, and (3) the etiology of mitral regurgitation (Watanabe, 2019) (see Fig. 26.4).

CLINICAL PEARL

When evaluating for the management of mitral regurgitation, determine (1) the level of hemodynamic compromise, (2) the acuity of presentation, and (3) the etiology of mitral regurgitation.

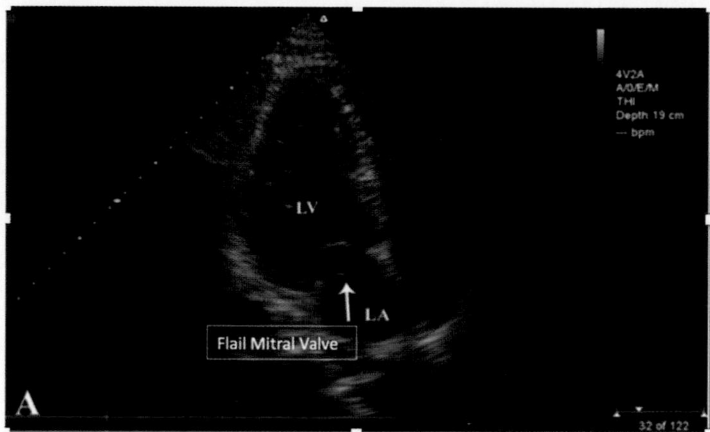

Fig. 26.2 Echocardiography revealed mitral chordae tendineae rupture *(arrow)* and the leaflet of the mitral valve turnover into left atrium during systole. (From Lijun, C., Ya, S., Liju, H., Zhao, L., Xianghong, M., Changyu, Z., Guangping, L. (2015). Ruptured mitral chordae tendinae induced by acute inferior myocardial infarction. *International Journal of Cardiology, 181*, 216–217.)

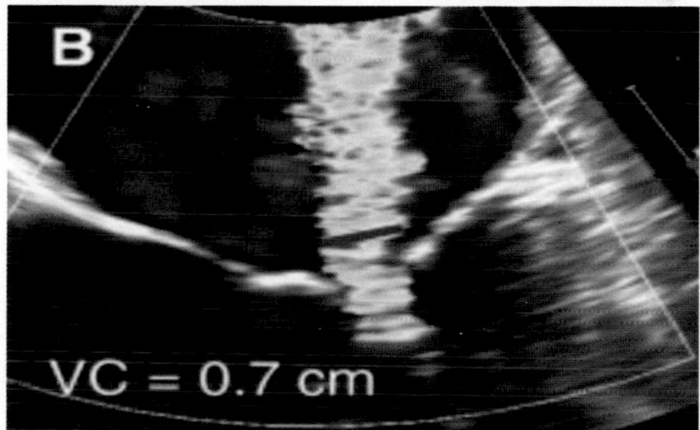

Fig. 26.3 Transesophageal echocardiography four-chamber view measuring vena contracta (VC) width at 0.7 cm, confirming severe MR. (From Omran, A. S., Arifi, A. A., Mohamed, A. A. (2011). Echocardiographic atlas of the mitral regurgitation. *Journal of the Saudi Heart Association, 23*(3), 163–170.)

How does hemodynamic compromise affect management?

If the level of hemodynamic compromise is severe enough for the patient to require ICU level of care, vasopressors, and continuous intravenous diuretic therapy, and presentation is secondary to acute mitral regurgitation, urgent surgical intervention is warranted. However, if hemodynamic compromise is the result of another issue such as sepsis (as can be seen in infective endocarditis), optimization with antimicrobial therapy to optimize surgical mortality may be beneficial.

Why is it important to distinguish between acute and chronic presentations?

The acuity of presentation goes hand-in-hand with hemodynamic compromise. Acute presentations of MR will often present with sudden onset of shortness of breath, orthopnea, and hemodynamic compromise, and early consultation with cardiology and cardiothoracic surgery is critical for appropriate timing of surgical intervention.

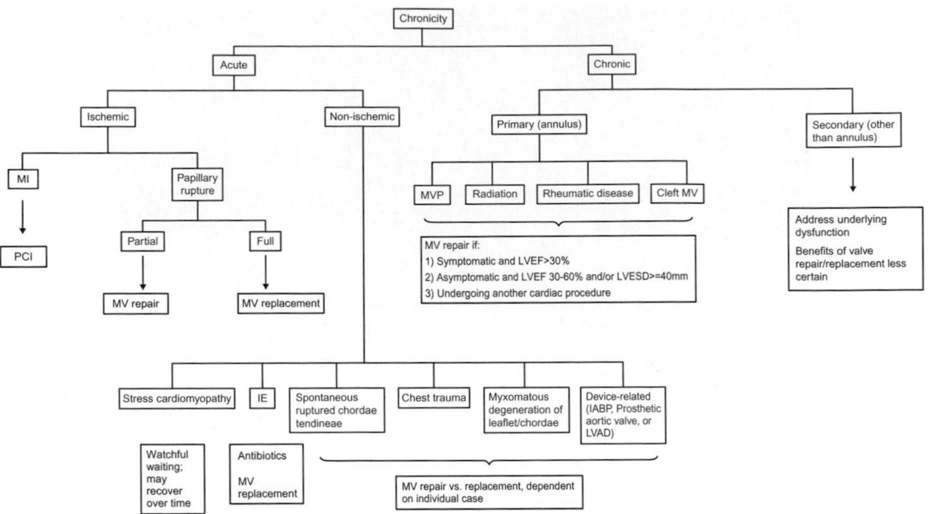

Fig. 26.4 Algorithm for classifying mitral regurgitation for management. *IABP*, Intraaortic balloon pump; *IE*, infective endocarditis; *LVAD*: left ventricular assist device; *LVEF*, left ventricular ejection fraction; *LVESD*, left ventricular end-systolic diameter; *MI*, myocardial infarction; *MV*, mitral valve; *MVP*, mitral valve prolapse; *PCI*, percutaneous coronary intervention.

How is etiology determined?

Once MR has been classified as acute with hemodynamic instability requiring hospital admission, as seen in Mr. Smith's case, it is crucial to identify the etiology to address proper management of the patient. Certain imaging characteristics on TTE can provide useful information regarding presence of vegetations, papillary muscle rupture, structural prolapse, tear, or mass to help guide the determination of etiology. Etiology is important because it guides treatment. In the case of ischemic MR, there can be a spectrum of etiologies for the MR. One scenario is that ischemic MR occurs as a result of shutdown of blood flow to the muscle supplying the mitral valve. On TTE imaging, this appears as a wall motion abnormality that prevents the mitral valve leaflets from closing properly, thus causing regurgitation. Treatment for this form of ischemic MR involves revascularization of the affected coronary vessel supplying the heart muscle associated with the mitral valve. This differs, however, for papillary muscle rupture, which is an extreme form of ischemic MR where the muscle that attaches the mitral valve to the ventricle is acutely damaged as a result of blood flow loss. Papillary muscle rupture is more often associated with inferior myocardial infarction as a result of the posterior descending artery being the single blood supply to the posteromedial papillary muscle. Surgical mitral valve replacement is recommended emergently with possible bridge with mitral valve repair if complete replacement is not possible (Watanabe, 2019).

Possible nonischemic causes of MR include: (1) infective endocarditis, (2) spontaneous ruptured chordae tendineae, (3) myxomatous degeneration of leaflet or chordae, (4) spontaneous rupture of chordae tendineae, (5) systemic inflammatory disease (e.g., lupus), (6) chest trauma, (7) device-induced from intraaortic balloon pump (IABP), prosthetic aortic valve, and left ventricular assist device (LVAD) (Watanable, 2019). In infective endocarditis, because an infection was the underlying cause, appropriate medical management for septic shock with antibiotics, fluids, vasopressors, and volume overload with diuresis will be crucial for optimization prior to surgery. For the other listed conditions, because the root problem is anatomical, surgical or transcatheter mitral repair/replacement will be necessary.

Chronic MR can further be split into primary (a problem with the mitral annulus) or secondary (a problem outside the mitral annulus). Given its chronic nature and more gradual onset of symptoms, there is less urgency for surgical intervention. However, appropriate management is still crucial (see Fig. 6) (Alguire, 2018). If it is a primary (or annulus) problem, potential etiologies include MVP, weakened valve from radiation therapy, rheumatic heart disease, or cleft mitral valve. In these cases, surgical mitral repair should be pursued if (1) the patient is symptomatic and left ventricular ejection fraction (LVEF) > 30%, (2) the patient is asymptomatic and LVEF 30%–60% and/or left ventricular end-systolic diameters (LVESD) ≥ 40 mm, or (3) the patient is undergoing another cardiac procedure (Alguire, 2018).

Chronic secondary MR is most often secondary to heart failure with reduced left ventricular function, and this is managed with goal-directed medical therapy and implantable cardioverter-defibrillator, if indicated. Utility of repairing or replacing the mitral valve in chronic secondary MR is not clear and requires more investigation.

When should transcatheter mitral repair be considered?

If patients are elderly and/or have other comorbidities that lead to a high operative mortality and require an intervention to ameliorate an acute decompensation of mitral regurgitation, cardiologists may offer a transcatheter mitral repair such as the FDA-approved mitral clip, which is lower risk but may improve quality of life for a period of time (Alguire, 2018).

What is the role of pharmacological and mechanical circulatory support device in mitral regurgitation?

The principles for pharmacological and device therapy in MR include:

- Afterload reduction with vasodilatory therapy (such as nitroprusside) that will allow for more forward flow into the aorta
- Diuresis to offload pulmonary edema that can lead to respiratory compromise
- Mechanical circulatory support such as IABP, extracorporeal membrane oxygenation (ECMO), and VAD to improve systemic and coronary perfusion to bridge the patient to definitive surgical mitral repair/replacement (Alguire, 2018; Watanabe, 2019).

Our patient's underlying connective tissue disorder manifested as bilateral inguinal hernias and velvety skin. It is also likely reshaping his mitral valve. His gradual onset of symptoms over the past few years were compounded by an acute event several hours prior to his presentation, which led to a rupture of his chordae tendineae. This event led to acute MR with flash pulmonary edema. Thus, we would classify this case as an acute on chronic mitral regurgitation.

The patient was admitted to the Medical Intensive Care Unit and placed on IV diuresis and, IV nitroprusside, and cardiology and cardiothoracic surgery teams were consulted promptly. Once transthoracic echocardiogram confirmed the ruptured chordae tendineae, the patient was transferred to the Cardiac Critical Care Unit and he was subsequently taken for a surgical mitral valve replacement with the cardiothoracic surgery team.

CLINICAL PEARL

Approximately 50% of those with acute moderate to severe ischemic MR do NOT have an audible murmur, also known as silent MR (Watanabe). Especially in cases of respiratory distress, which can accompany the acute pulmonary edema experienced by someone in acute MR, a soft murmur is even less audible.

Case Summary

- **Complaint/History:** Mr. Smith is a 48-year-old-male with no known past medical history who presents to the ED with sudden-onset shortness of breath for 4 days, superimposed on a gradual worsening dyspnea for the previous 2 years. He had surgery for bilateral inguinal hernias at the age of 16 years and is currently not taking any medications.
- **Findings:** Blood pressure is 95/69 mmHg, pulse rate is 116/min and regular, and respirations are 28/min. He is in marked respiratory distress. Pallor and diaphoresis are noted. His skin is velvety and has many atrophic scars. The apical impulse is hyperdynamic. Cardiac auscultation reveals a soft early-systolic decrescendo murmur at the cardiac apex. S1 is barely audible; S2 is normal. Lung examination reveals diffuse crackles bilaterally. Jugular venous distension (JVD) to the jaw is present. ECG shows sinus tachycardia with occasional premature ventricular complexes (PVCs). CXR reveals borderline cardiomegaly, but severe pulmonary edema.
- **Lab Results/Tests:** Complete cell count revealed a WBC of 5.6 K/μL, Hgb of 13 g/dL, and platelet count of 334 × 10^9/dL. BMP was notable for acute renal injury with BUN and Cr of 45 mg/dL and 1.6 mg/dL, with baseline BUN and Cr of 13 mg/dL and 0.7 mg/dL. Pro-BNP was 3564 pg/mL. Two sets of blood cultures yielded no growth.
  - A transthoracic echocardiogram with Doppler was obtained on Mr. Smith, showing the presence of a prominent flail mitral valve leaflet and ruptured chordae and a vena contracta (VC) width of >0.7 cm with a central regurgitant jet cover >40% of the left atrium, and a systolic flow reversal in the pulmonary veins in Fig. 2. (The quantitative parameters include an ERO >40 cm^2, an RV >60 mL, and an RF >50%.)

Diagnosis: With the confirmed echocardiographic findings of a flail mitral valve leaflet and ruptured chordae, without evidence of infective endocarditis, the diagnosis of acute severe MR was established. This acute MR is secondary to ruptured chordae tendineae, superimposed on a chronic regurgitation caused by underlying undiagnosed connective tissue disease in Mr. Smith. This acute rupture then led to hemodynamic compromise and pulmonary edema.

- **Treatment:** He was admitted to the Medical Intensive Care Unit and placed on IV diuresis and, IV nitroprusside, and cardiology and cardiothoracic surgery teams were consulted promptly. Once transthoracic and transesophageal ECG confirmed the ruptured chordae tendineae, the patient was transferred to the Cardiac Critical Care Unit and he was taken subsequently for a surgical mitral valve replacement with the cardiothoracic surgery team.
- **Complaint/History:** A 59-year-old man presents with acute onset chest pain.
- **Findings:** Physical examination is unremarkable; initial CXR and ECG show no acute findings.
- **Lab Results/Tests:** Repeat ECG shows biphasic T-waves in leads V1–V4 and troponin-T is elevated.

Diagnosis: Wellen's syndrome.

- **Treatment:** The patient was given a loading dose of aspirin (325 mg) and clopidogrel (600 mg) and started on a heparin drip. Metoprolol tartrate was initiated and the patient was taken to the catheterization laboratory for PCI. One drug-eluting stent was placed in the LAD with successful reperfusion. The patient was monitored for post-MI complications and continued on dual antiplatelet therapy with aspirin and clopidogrel. After 1 year, discontinuation of the clopidogrel will be considered. The patient was also continued on a high-intensity statin and beta blocker indefinitely.

- **Complaint/History:** A 54-year-old female presents with difficulty swallowing solids and liquids over the past four years.
- **Findings:** Temperature is 98.5; Physical exam was unrevealing.
- **Lab Results/Tests:** Labs reveal ____. Chest x-ray shows a retrocardiac air-fluid level in the mediastinum at the level of the aortic arch. Upper endoscopy showed no signs of obstruction or inflamation in the esophagus, although it was difficutl for the ednoscopist to pass the endscope from the esophagus to the stomach which was normal in appearance. Manometry showed multiple areas of the esophagus with increased pressure readings simultaneously as the patient swallowed.

Diagnosis: Type III Achalasia

- **Treatment:** The patient was started on Nifedipine 10mg before meals and a liquid diet for symptomatic management. She was scheduled for definitive treatment wiht peroral endoscopic myotomy (POEM).

Bibliography

Lam, U. T. (2019). Mitral regurgitation. In F. F. Ferri (Ed.), *Ferri's clinical advisor 2020: 5 books in 1.* Philadelphia, PA: Elsevier.

Lijun, C., Ya, S., Liju, H., Zhao, L., Xianghong, M., Changyu, Z., & Guangping, L. (2015). Ruptured mitral chordae tendinae induced by acute inferior myocardial infarction. *International Journal of Cardiology, 181,* 216–217.

Alguire. P. C. (2018). *MKSAP, 18: Medical Knowledge Self-Assessment Program, Cardiovascular Medicine.* Philadelphia: American College of Physicians.

Omran, A. S., Arifi, A. A., & Mohamed, A. A. (2011). Echocardiographic atlas of the mitral regurgitation. *J Saudi Heart Assoc, 23*(3), 163–170.

Thomas, J. J., Rosen's emergency medicine: concepts and clinical practice, Chapter 68, 891–928.e4.

Watanabe, N. (2019). Acute mitral regurgitation. *Heart, 105*(9), 671–677. https://doi.org/10.1136/heartjnl-2018-313373.

SECTION 7

Rheumatology

CASE 27

A 32-Year-Old Female With Right Lower Extremity Edema

Arezoo Haghshenas ■ Vaneet K. Sandhu

A 32-year-old female with a known history of systemic lupus erythematosus (SLE) presents to the emergency department with acute onset right lower extremity pain and swelling with associated shortness of breath for 4 days. She also suffers chest pain, described as sharp, 9/10 in intensity, intermittent, and worse with deep breathing. Upon further questioning, she mentions two episodes of deep vein thrombosis in the past 2 years for which she took oral warfarin for 6 consecutive months and stopped 3 months ago after being evaluted by her primary care doctor and determined to be asymptomatic.

On physical examination, her blood pressure is 100/50 mmHg, pulse is 110 beats/min, respiratory rate is 20 breaths/min, and oxygen saturation is 90% on room air. Tenderness is noted on palpation of the right calf muscle, which also demonstrates overlying erythema. There is point tenderness on palpation of the upper right side of the chest. No murmur or gallop is noted on heart exam, lungs are clear to auscultation, the abdomen is not tender or distended, and there is no swelling in her joints.

What are common causes of acute shortness of breath?

Acute shortness of breath has an extensive differential diagnosis (Fig. 27.1). Some include:

- Respiratory: asthma, chronic obstructive pulmonary disease, pulmonary edema, pulmonary hypertension, pulmonary fibrosis, infections (including tuberculosis), lung cancer, and pulmonary embolism.
- Cardiac: arrhythmias, heart failure, pleuritis, and pericarditis.
- Other factors: anemia, anxiety, musculoskeletal disease (i.e., costochondritis, rib fracture).

What are common causes of unilateral peripheral edema?

Peripheral edema can be pitting or nonpitting. The approach to peripheral edema is dependent on its laterality. Acute onset unilateral lower extremity edema is concerning for deep vein thrombosis (DVT). Local involvement such as cellulitis or trauma should also be considered. Alternatively, bilateral lower extremity edema may be caused by heart failure, pulmonary hypertension, renal disease, medications, or other systemic processes.

The patient denies any history of trauma to the right leg or surgeries. She denies any fever, chills, night sweats, or weight loss. She denies a family history of stroke or blood clots. She denies smoking, drinking alcohol, or using illicit drugs. She has no history of surgeries. She is not taking any oral contraceptives nor is she allergic to any medications. She later says that she has a history of two miscarriages, one at 12 weeks and one at 14 weeks of gestation.

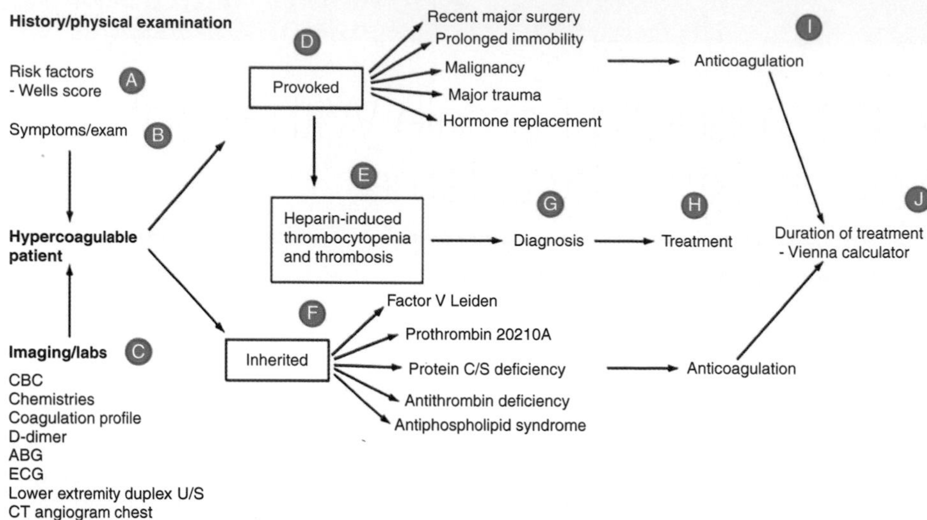

Fig. 27.1 Differential diagnosis and management of the hypercoagulable patient. *ABG*, Arterial blood gases; *CBC*, complete blood count; *EKG*, electrocardiogram; *U/S*, ultrasound. (From Ehlert, B.A. (2020). Hypercoagulable patient. In R. C. McIntyre & R. Schulick (Eds.), *Surgical decision making* (6th ed.) (pp. 14–15). Elsevier.)

Considering the patient's risk factors, including history of miscarriages, what are your differential diagnoses for this patient?

Alternative causes of thrombosis such as inherited or acquired thrombophilia, heparin-induced thrombocytopenia, and alternative causes of pregnancy complications such as chromosomal or anatomical abnormalities or hypothyroidism.

CLINICAL PEARL **STEP 1/2/3**

Risk factors for multiple DVTs include:

- Age greater than 40 years
- Immobilization
- Obesity
- Genetics
- Malignancy
- Bone fractures
- Smoking
- Recent surgeries
- Antiphospholipid syndrome

What are the inherited causes of a hypercoagulable state that should be considered in this case?

There are several inherited defects associated with a hypercoagulable state, including factor V Leiden deficiency, antithrombin III deficiency, prothrombin 20210 A mutation, protein C deficiency, protein S deficiency, antiphospholipid syndrome, and homocysteinemia.

CLINICAL PEARL **STEP 2/3**

Factor V Leiden is the most common inherited defect, occurring in 2% to 7% of European ancestry and found in 10% of individuals with DVT. It accelerates the conversion of prothrombin to thrombin. A homozygous mutation is associated with greater risk of thrombosis compared with heterozygous mutation. Clinical presentation is typically venous thrombosis at unusual sites such as retinal veins, splenic veins, renal veins, or upper extremity veins.

Which laboratory tests should be ordered for this patient?

- Prothrombin time (PT), partial thromboplastin time (PTT), and mixing study to evaluate for the presence of antibodies versus factor deficiency
- Antithrombin III activity
- Protein C activity
- Protein S activity
- Factor VIII, IX, XI levels
- Factor V Leiden mutation
- Factor II 20210 A mutation
- Homocysteine levels
- Antiphospholipid antibodies (lupus anticoagulant, beta-2-glycoprotein IgG/IgM, and anticardiolipin IgG/IgM)

CLINICAL PEARL **STEP 1/2/3**

In a young patient without a family history of diabetes or blood clots, screening should focus on thrombotic risk factors. In patients without a family history of a hypercoagulable state, testing for antiphospholipid antibodies and age-appropriate cancer screening should also be prioritized (see Fig. 27.2).

Which imaging studies should be ordered for further evaluation?

Chest X-ray image is the initial modality of choice for individuals with shortness of breath. If the image is normal, screening for a pulmonary embolism (PE) can be done with pulmonary angiogram, which is the imaging modality of choice but is limited by contrast exposure and its invasive nature. Computed tomography pulmonary angiography (CTPA) is a noninvasive alternative but

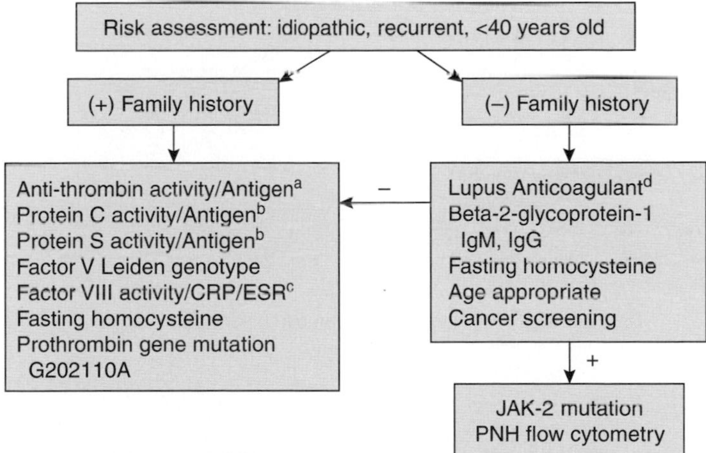

Fig. 27.2 Evaluation and laboratory testing for hypercoagulability in patients with venous thromboembolism.

is also limited by the use of intravenous (IV) contrast. If the patient has contraindications for CTPA, a ventilation/perfusion mismatch scan can be used to screen for PE.

CLINICAL PEARL **STEP 1**

Hemostasis is a series of actions that starts with platelet adhesion and the formation of a platelet plug and extends to activation of coagulation proteins, resulting in thrombin formation. Thrombin then triggers platelet aggregation and promotes fibrin clot formation by activation of fibrinogen.

The activated thrombin activates factor XI, then activation of factors IX and VIII. Factors VIII, IX, and X together form a complex that activates thrombin, which then promotes fibrin formation from fibrinogen (see Fig. 27.3).

When should antiphospholipid syndrome (APS) be considered?

There are two scenarios indicating APS:

- Adverse outcomes of pregnancy such as premature birth secondary to preeclampsia, any fetal death beyond 10 weeks' gestation, or multiple miscarriages prior to 10 weeks gestation.
- Unexplained venous or arterial thrombosis particularly in young patients with unexplained stroke, myocardial infarction, DVT, or PE, or in individuals with known autoimmune disease (especially SLE), valvular heart disease, or neurologic impairments such as cognitive deficits who present with unexplained stroke, myocardial infarction, DVT, or PE.

CLINICAL PEARL **STEP 2/3**

APS is an autoimmune hypercoagulable disorder that occurs with venous or arterial thrombosis and/or pregnancy-related complications such as preterm labor, preeclampsia, or miscarriages in the setting of positive antiphospholipid. The definitive diagnosis requires two positive antibodies 3 months apart and one clinical complication related to either thrombosis or pregnancy.

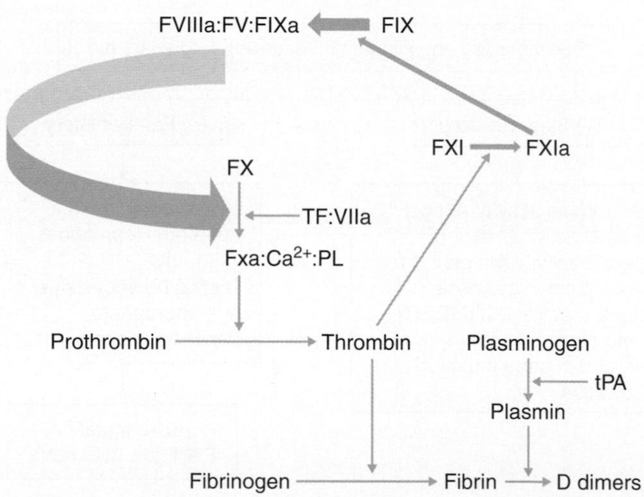

Fig. 27.3 Secondary hemostasis. Exposed tissue factor binds factor VII, producing an initial small amount of thrombin that triggers an amplifying cascade, resulting in a thrombin burst that converts enough fibrinogen to fibrin to form a stable clot. *PL*, Phospholipid; *TF*, tissue factor; *tPA*, tissue plasminogen activator.

What are the clinical manifestations of APS?

The most common features of APS are:

- Thrombosis: more commonly venous than arterial. Lower extremity veins are more prone to thrombosis; however, it can also be seen in renal, pulmonary, subclavian, cerebral, or pelvic veins. Venous thrombosis usually occurs at a single site, with the tendency to recur in the same site. Arterial thrombosis occurs anywhere in the vascular tree from the aorta to the small capillaries. Strokes or transient ischemic attacks are common in APS patients and are the most common presentation of arterial thrombosis. The risk of recurrence in patients who have arterial thrombosis is higher than venous thrombosis. Stroke in a young patient with no other risk factors such as atherosclerosis should be concerning for APS.
- Pulmonary embolism.
- Superficial thrombophlebitis.
- Thrombocytopenia is more common in SLE-related APS than in primary APS. It occurs in 16% to 46% of patients with APS. The pathogenesis is unclear but is suspected to be a result of binding of antiphospholipid antibodies (aPLs) to platelet membranes. Coombs positive hemolytic anemia is noted in up to 10%–20% of APS patients and is referred to as Evans syndrome.
- Cutaneous manifestations include ulcers, livedo reticularis, splinter hemorrhages, necrosis, and gangrene of the digits.
- Cardiac disease may be a result of thrombosis or valvular involvement, which is typically left sided. Although valvular lesions maybe hemodynamically insignificant, 25% of these patients have reported mitral regurgitation.
- Pulmonary hypertension.
- Cognitive dysfunction varies from minor findings to permanent loss of function that is typically associated with white matter lesions.
- Renal disease is not a common manifestation. When present, however, thrombotic microangiopathy is the clinicopathologic presentation, manifesting the triad of hypertension, proteinuria, and renal failure.
- Pregnancy complications include miscarriage, fetal loss, and preterm birth. Other less common complications are HELLP (hemolysis, elevated liver enzymes, low platelets) syndrome, intrauterine growth restriction, and placental insufficiency. Individuals are deemed high risk if they demonstrate triple positive aPLs (positive lupus anticoagulant, cardiolipin and beta-2-glycoprotein-1 antibodies), prior pregnancy complications, or a history of thrombosis.
- Ocular involvement is typically of vascular ischemia or thrombosis, typically of the retinal arteries and/or veins.

See Figs. 27.4–27.6.

All the requested workup has been performed. The patient is found to have positive cardiolipin antibody, lupus anticoagulant, and beta-2-glycoprotein. The rest of the tests including PT/INR/PTT are normal.

The patient has a positive compression ultrasonography on her right lower extremity. She underwent CTPA, which was positive for pulmonary embolism.

What are positive laboratory findings of APS?

Three major antiphospholipid antibodies (aPLs) are indicative of APS:

- Beta-2-glycoprotein-I antibodies IgG/IgM (anti-β_2-GPI) is relatively specific for APS associated with thrombosis and pregnancy loss.
- Lupus anticoagulant (LA) represents a less sensitive but more specific test. It presents an inhibitor of coagulation, which inhibits phospholipid-dependent coagulation reactions.

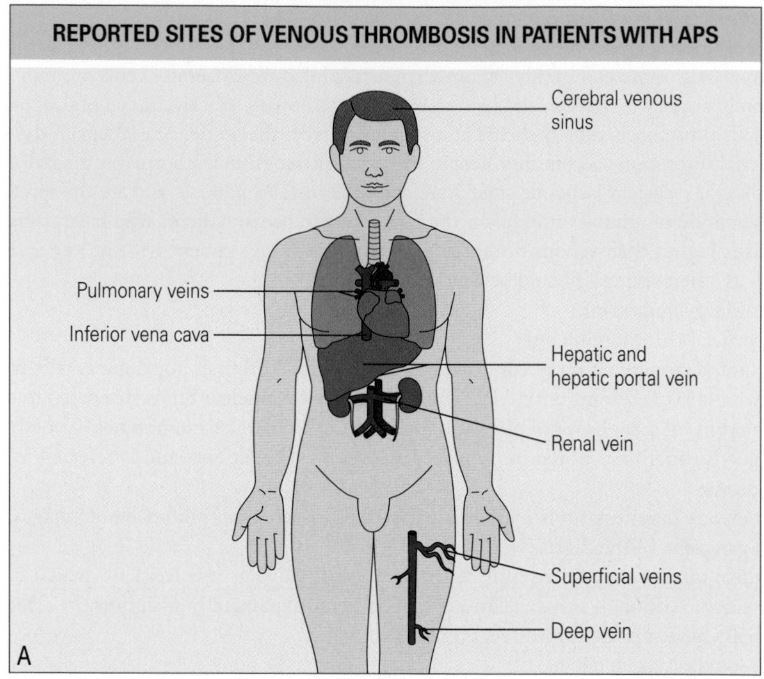

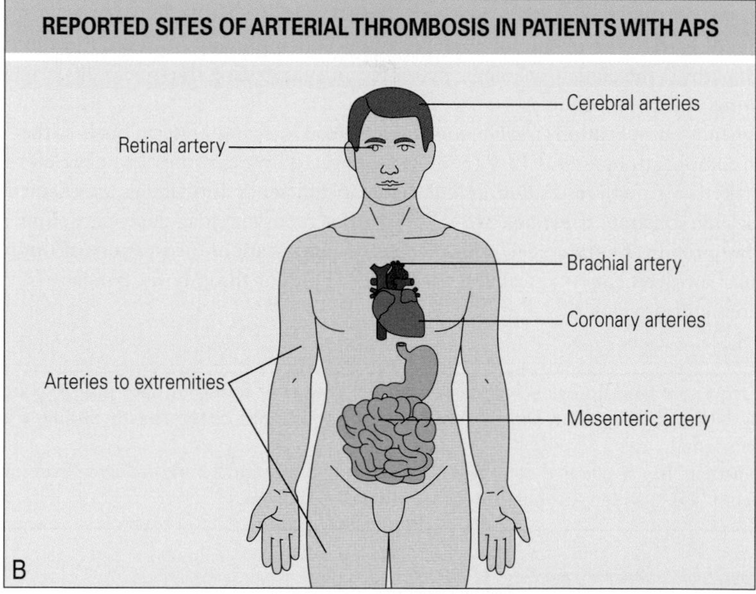

Fig. 27.4 Sites of potential thrombotic events in antiphospholipid syndrome. (From Amigo, M. C., & Khamashta, M. A. (2019). Antiphospholipid syndrome: pathogenesis, diagnosis, and management. In M. C. Hochberg, E. M. Gravallese, A. J. Silman, J. S. Smolen, M. E. Weinblatt, & M. H. Weisman, (Eds.), *Rheumatology* (7th ed.). Philadelphia: Elsevier.)

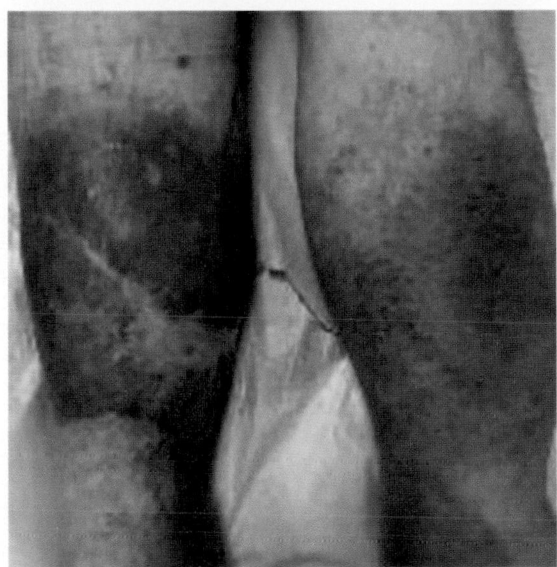

Fig. 27.5 Livedoid vasculitis with atrophie blanche in a patient with antiphospholipid syndrome. (From Lally, L., & Sammaritano, L.R. (2015). Vasculitis in antiphospholipid syndrome. *Rheumatic Disease Clinics of North America*, *41*(1), 109–123.)

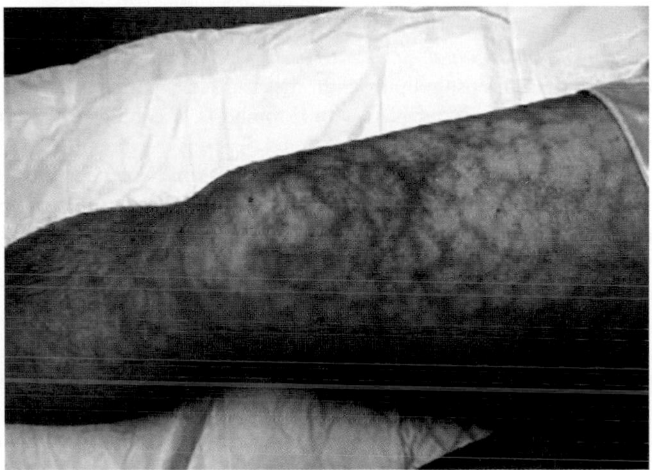

Fig. 27.6 Livedo reticularis caused by antiphospholipid syndrome. (From Ruiz-Irastorza, G., Crowther, M, Branch, W., & Khamashta, M.A. (2010). Antiphospholipid syndrome. *The Lancet*, *376*(9751), 1498–1509.)

- Cardiolipin antibodies (aCLs) IgG and/or IgM: aCL titer of more than 40 GPL is associated with increased risk of thrombosis.
- **Seronegative APS:** In daily practice, there are scenarios in which patients have clinical signs of APS, with persistently negative APS lab results. In these patients, providers may pursue newer immunoassays or start treatment based on clinical judgment.

In addition to the aPLs, there are other common laboratory findings such as prolonged PTT, thrombocytopenia, hemolytic anemia, and low complements.

How can APS be diagnosed?

The diagnosis is a combination of a complete and thorough history and physical examination with laboratory findings.

CLINICAL PEARL **STEP 2/3**

In patients suspected of having APS, the history should be focused on thrombotic events such as DVTs, PEs, or any strokes; the nature of the thrombotic event; and whether it was provoked by any risk factors such as contraceptive use, immobility, cancer, or recent surgeries. Other important parts of the history to take into account are the outcomes of pregnancies, history of thrombocytopenia, and review of systems for autoimmune disease such as SLE.

Physical examination has the same importance as the diagnosis of APS. Findings such as livedo reticularis, digital gangrene, heart murmurs, and neurologic findings consistent with strokes are important.

What are the causes of false-positive aPLs?

Infections: Bacteremia, Lyme disease, syphilis, leprosy, tuberculosis, infective endocarditis, and viral infections such as HIV, HTLV-I, mumps, rubella, zoster virus, and hepatitis A, B, and C.

Medications: Some medications have been associated with aPL including hydralazine, procainamide, quinine, amoxicillin, oral contraceptives, and propranolol.

Malignancy: Malignancies, especially solid tumors such as lung and colon cancers, and lymphomas such as Hodgkin and non-Hodgkin have been associated with aPLs.

What is the management of individuals with antiphospholipid antibodies?

The primary treatment of antiphospholipid syndrome is anticoagulation or antiplatelet therapy.

Patients with positive aPL without history of thrombosis: Treating these patients with anticoagulation or antiplatelet therapy is controversial and depends on variables such as existing risk factors. These variables include circulating aPLs, hypertension, hypercholesterolemia, smoking, or underlying autoimmune disease. Some studies support low-dose aspirin to prevent the first thrombosis. However, the effectiveness of aspirin monotherapy has not been significant in randomized clinical trials. Some studies have demonstrated benefit in using aspirin in addition to low-dose warfarin.

In patients with SLE and aPL with or without thrombosis, hydroxychloroquine has also demonstrated protection from thrombosis.

Patients with positive aPL is correct (can unbold text for consistency) with acute thromboembolism: Anticoagulation with heparin bridging for long-term warfarin, which should be followed by warfarin indefinitely secondary to the high risk of recurrent thrombosis. The preferred anticoagulation in this case will be warfarin rather than a direct oral anticoagulant (such as apixaban, rivaroxaban, or dabigatran). In pregnant patients warfarin is contraindicated and low-molecular-weight heparin will therefore be the drug of choice.

CLINICAL PEARL **STEP 2/3**

Patients with venous or arterial thrombosis in the setting of APS warrant lifelong anticoagulation with warfarin. If the patient has arterial thrombosis, low-dose aspirin may also be added.

The goal international normalized ratio (INR) in this population should be in the range of 2–3.

If the patient becomes pregnant, the anticoagulation method should be switched from warfarin to low-molecular-weight heparin to avoid the teratogenicity of warfarin.

Can you stop the anticoagulation in this population? No. Lifelong anticoagulation is recommended.

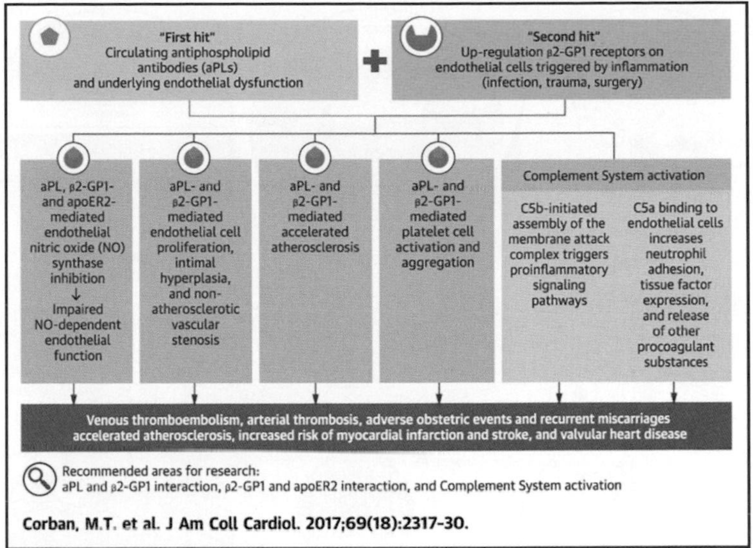

Fig. 27.7 Pathogenesis of antiphospholipid syndrome: "first hit" circulating antiphospholipid antibodies (aPLs) and underlying endothelial dysfunction and "second hit" inflammatory insult result in impaired nitric oxide (NO) dependent endothelial function, accelerated atherosclerosis, nonatherosclerotic vasculopathy, platelet activation and aggregation, and complement system activation. (From Corban, M.T., Duarte-Garcia, A., McBane, R. D., Matteson, E. L., Lerman, L. O., & Lerman, A. (2017). Antiphospholipid syndrome: Role of vascular endothelial cells and implications for risk stratification and targeted therapeutics. Journal of the American College of Cardiology, 69(18), 2317–2330.)

CLINICAL PEARL **STEP 1**

What is the pathophysiology of APS?

Endothelial cells and the circulating aPLs have crucial roles in APS pathophysiology, and they have been considered the initial necessary strike for thrombosis (first hit). However, the thrombotic events cannot be initiated without additional triggers such as inflammation (second hit). Endothelial cell dysfunction facilitates the binding of aPLs to the endothelial cell B2-GP1 receptors and increases the risk of thrombosis, atherosclerosis, stroke, and myocardial infarction. Any inflammatory insult such as surgery or trauma can increase the B2-GP1 receptors on the endothelial surface. Endothelial nitric oxide (NO) is produced by endothelial cells and is one of the key factors for endothelial function. In patients with APS, reduced NO production results in impaired endothelial vascular response and, hence, enhanced platelet aggregation and thrombosis (see Figs. 27.7 and 27.8).

How is APS in pregnancy managed?

To reduce the chance of fetal and maternal complications, preconception counseling is of utmost importance in women with APS. Despite close monitoring and complying with treatment recommendations, patients with APS are at a greater risk of miscarriage, fetal death, preeclampsia, and preterm birth.

All pregnant patients with APS need very close observation for maternal complications during the second and third trimesters with arterial Doppler ultrasound for umbilical artery Doppler flow and placental insufficiency. Preconception aspirin is recommended in this group of patients with continuation of aspirin during the pregnancy. Apart from warfarin, which is contraindicated in pregnancy, treatment of APS in pregnancy is the same as with nonpregnant patients.

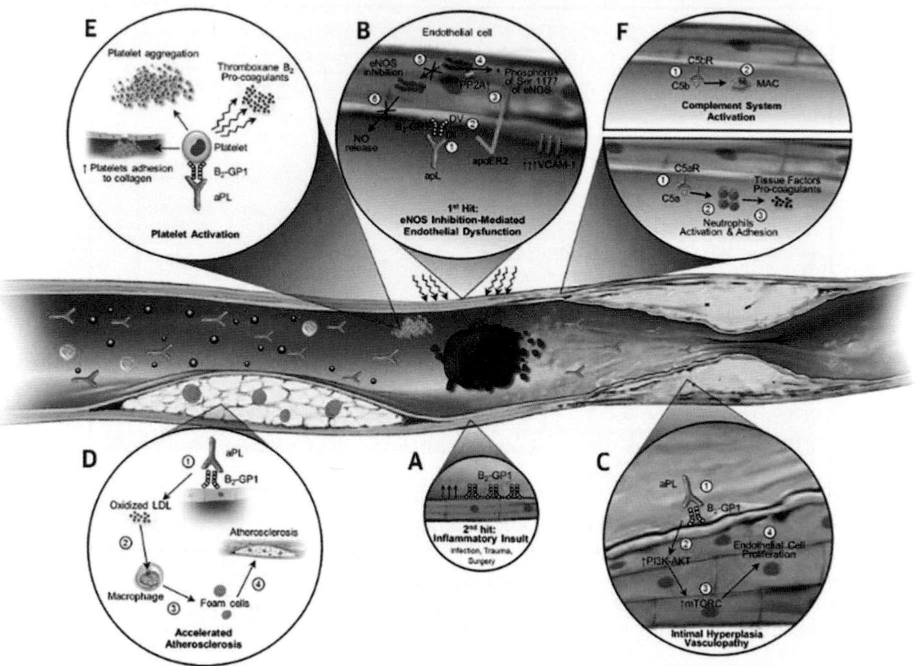

Fig. 27.8 (A) Up-regulation of beta-2-glycoprotein 1 *(β_2-GP1)* receptors on endothelial cells following a "second hit" inflammatory insult. (B) Antiphospholipid antibody *(aPL)*–mediated endothelial nitric oxide synthase *(eNOS)* inhibition, impaired nitric oxide *(NO)* production and release, and endothelial dysfunction. (C) "First hit" aPL-mediated endothelial cell proliferation, intimal hyperplasia, and nonatherosclerotic vascular stenosis. (D) Antiphospholipid syndrome (APS)–associated accelerated atherosclerosis. (E) aPL-mediated platelet cell activation, aggregation, and thrombosis. (F) Complement system activation and thrombosis. *apoER2*, Apolipoprotein E receptor 2; *C5a*, complement component 5a fragment; *C5aR*, complement component 5a fragment receptor; *C5b*, complement component 5b fragment; *C5bR*, complement component 5b fragment receptor; *DI*, domain I of β_2-GP1 receptor; *DV*, domain V of β_2-GP1 receptor; *LDL*, low-density lipoprotein; *MAC*, membrane attack complex; *mTORC*, mammalian target of rapamycin complex; *PI3K-AKT*, phosphatidylinositol 3-kinase–AKT pathway; *PP2A*, protein phosphatase 2A; *VCAM*, vascular cell adhesion molecule. (From Corban, M.T., Duarte-Garcia, A., McBane, R. D., Matteson, E. L., Lerman, L. O., & Lerman, A. (2017). Antiphospholipid syndrome: role of vascular endothelial cells and implications for risk stratification and targeted therapeutics. *Journal of the American College of Cardiology, 69*(18), 2317–2330.)

Case Summary

- **Complaint/History:** A 32-year-old female with SLE presents with acute onset of right lower extremity pain and edema and shortness of breath.
- **Findings:** There is edema and tenderness of the right lower extremity, tachypnea, tachycardia, pleuritic chest pain, and tenderness.
- **Lab Results/Tests:** Patient has a normal chest X-ray image. Duplex ultrasound of the right lower extremity demonstrates thrombosis of the femoral vein. CTPA is positive for pulmonary embolism. Serum hypercoagulable workup is significant for a positive lupus anticoagulant, beta-2-glycoprotein-I (β_2) antibody, cardiolipin antibody.

Diagnosis: Pulmonary embolism and DVT in the setting of antiphospholipid syndrome.

- **Treatment:** Start heparin with warfarin, which should be followed by warfarin indefinitely because of the high risk of recurrent thrombosis.

Bibliography

Alarcón-Segovia D, Boffa MC, Branch W, Cervera R, Gharavi A, Khamashta M, Shoenfeld Y, Wilson W,… Roubey R. (2003). Prophylaxis of the antiphospholipid syndrome: a consensus report. *Lupus*, 2003.

Amigo, M. C., & Khamashta, M. A. (2019). Antiphospholipid syndrome: Pathogenesis, diagnosis, and management. *Rheumatology*

Avčin, T., & O'Neil, K. M. (2016). Petty Laxer Lindsley (Eds.), *Antiphospholipid syndrome. Textbook of pediatric rheumatology* (7th ed., pp. 318–335). Wedderburn: Elsevier. e10.

Corban, M. T., Duarte-Garcia, A., McBane, R. D., Matteson, E. L., Lerman, L. O., & Lerman, A. (2017). Role of vascular endothelial cells and implications for risk stratification and targeted therapeutics. *JACC*

Ehlert. B. A. (2020). Hypercoagulable patient. In C. Robert, R. C. McIntyre, & Richard Schulick (Eds.), *Surgical decision making* (6th ed., pp. 14–15). Elsevier.

Erkan, D., Merrill, J. T., Yazici, Y., Sammaritano, L., Buyon, J. P., & Lockshin. (2001). High thrombosis rate after fetal loss in antiphospholipid syndrome: effective prophylaxis with aspirin. *Arthritis and Rheumatism*

Farzamnia, H., Rabiei, K., Sadeghi, M., & Roghani, F. (2011). The predictive factors of recurrent deep vein thrombosis. *ARYA Atherosclerosis*

Holbrook A, Schulman S, Witt DM, Vandvik PO, Fish J, Kovacs MJ, … Guyatt GH. (2012). Evidence-based management of anticoagulant therapy: Antithrombotic Therapy and Prevention of Thrombosis, 9th ed: *American College of Chest Physicians Evidence-Based Clinical Practice Guidelines.*

Keeling, D., Mackie, I., Moore, G. W., Greer, I. A., & Greaves, M. (2012). Guidelines on the investigation and management of antiphospholipid syndrome. *British Journal of Haematology*

Lallly, L., & Sammaritano, L. R. (2015). Vasculitis in antiphospholipid syndrome. *Rheum Dis Clinics Nor Amer*, *41*(1), 109–123.

Liebman, H. A., & Weitz, I. C. (2018). Hypercoagulable states. In Anton N. Sidawy & Bruce A. Perler (Eds.), *Rutherford's vascular surgery and endovascular therapy*. Elsevier. Chapter 38.

Mary Mathias, R Liesner. Understanding haemostasis, Symposium: Haematology.

Ruiz-Irastorza, G., Crowther, M., Branch, W., & Khamashta, M. A. (2010). Antiphospholipid syndrome 2010.. *The Lancet*, *376*(9751), 1498–1509.

Ruiz-Irastorza, G., Cuadrado, M. J., Ruiz-Arruza, I., Brey, R., Crowther, M., Derksen, R., … Khamashta, M. (2011). Evidence-based recommendations for the prevention and long-term management of thrombosis in antiphospholipid antibody-positive patients: Report of a task force at the 13th International Congress on antiphospholipid antibodies. *Lupus*

Wahl, D. G., Bounameaux, H., de Moerloose, P., & Sarasin, F. P. (2000). Prophylactic antithrombotic therapy for patients with systemic lupus erythematosus with or without antiphospholipid antibodies: do the benefits outweigh the risks? A decision analysis. *Archives of Internal Medicine*

Yachoui, R., Sehgal, R., Amlani, B., & Goldberg, J. W. (2015). Antiphospholipid antibodies-associated diffuse alveolar hemorrhage. *Seminars in Arthritis and Rheumatism*, *44*(6), 652–657.

CASE 28

A 35-Year-Old Female With Dry Eyes and Dry Mouth

Micah Yu ■ Kevin Kaplowitz ■ Sophia Li

A 35-year-old female is evaluated for a 1-year history of progressive dry eyes and dry mouth with proximal interphalangeal phalangeal (PIP) joint pain involving bilateral hands. She states that she has been chewing gum to relieve the dry mouth and has been using over-the-counter lubricating eye drops. Her joint pain is worse in the morning, associated with 20 minutes of morning stiffness, and is relieved with activity. In addition, her PIP joints occasionally become swollen. She does not take any medications, smoke, drink alcohol, or use any recreational drugs and is employed as a teacher.

How does the history help to narrow your differential diagnosis?

Keratoconjunctivitis sicca (dry eyes) and xerostomia (dry mouth) are known as sicca syndrome. There are many causes of sicca syndrome, including medications, infections, and systemic processes. A detailed review of a patient's current medications list is important in identifying any culprit agents. Infections such as hepatitis C and HIV can cause dry eyes and dry mouth. Finally, a comprehensive review of symptoms is important to identify any associated symptoms that might point to a systemic process such as malignancy or an autoimmune process. Sicca symptoms occur in almost all patients with Sjögren's syndrome, but not all patients with sicca symptoms have Sjögren's.

A differential diagnosis for dry eyes and dry mouth is listed in Tables 28.1 and 28.2.

Which symptoms do patients with oral dryness report?

Symptoms include difficulty speaking continuously, difficulty swallowing dry food, burning sensation in the mouth, and a change in taste. Oral examination may reveal a decreased sublingual salivary pool, dry fissured or atrophic tongue, angular stomatitis, and dental caries.

On physical examination, vital signs are normal and her body mass index (BMI) is 28 kg/m^2. Examination of her oral mucosa shows a decreased sublingual salivary pool and poor dentition with multiple cavities. Palpation of her neck reveals slightly enlarged bilateral parotid glands. There is swelling of her second and third PIP joints bilaterally. Her other joints are nontender to palpation without evidence of synovitis. Her strength is 5/5 throughout her upper and lower extremities (see Fig. 28.1).

Sjögren's syndrome is suspected. Which laboratory studies would you order?

There are several laboratory tests that can be helpful in diagnosing Sjögren's. Antinuclear antibody (ANA) is nonspecific but positive in up to 90% of patients with Sjögren's. Anti-Ro/SSA and/or anti-La/SSB are present in 60% to 80% of patients with Sjögren's. Isolated anti-La/SSB antibody is uncommon and these patients do not exhibit the typical Sjögren's phenotype. Rheumatoid factor

TABLE 28.1 ■ **Differential Diagnosis for Dry Eyes**

Drugs	Antihistamines Beta blockers Antispasmodics Diuretics
Infectious disease	Human immunodeficiency virus Hepatitis C
Rheumatic disease	Sjögren's syndrome Sarcoidosis IgG4 disease
Oncologic disease	Lymphoma
Endocrine disease	Diabetes mellitus
Miscellaneous	Aging Blepharitis Vitamin A deficiency Contact lens irritation Allergic conjunctivitis Graft versus host disease

TABLE 28.2 ■ **Differential Diagnosis for Dry Mouth**

Drugs	Antihistamines Antihypertensives Anticholinergics Tricyclic antidepressants Diuretics
Infectious disease	Human immunodeficiency virus Hepatitis C
Inflammatory disease	Sjögren's syndrome Sarcoidosis IgG4 disease
Oncologic disease	Lymphoma
Endocrine	Diabetes mellitus
Amyloidosis	
Cystic fibrosis	
Miscellaneous	Mouth breathing Dehydration Psychological factors Head and neck irradiation Head and neck surgery Graft versus host disease

is another common autoantibody present in 40% to 50% of patients with Sjögren's. Erythrocyte sedimentation rate (ESR) is often elevated secondary to elevated globulins but is not specific nor high in all cases.

The results of the patient's laboratory studies are listed in Table 28.3.

In addition to laboratory studies, which other tests can be done when evaluating a patient for Sjögren's?

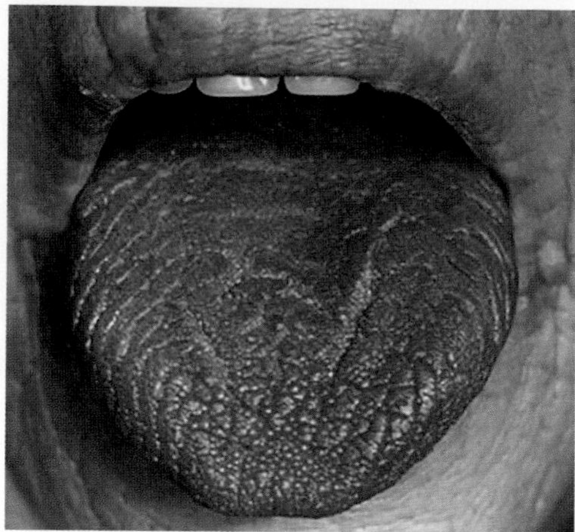

Fig. 28.1 Dry, fissured tongue in Sjögren's syndrome.

TABLE 28.3 ■ **Laboratory Values**

Leukocyte count	8100/μL (8 × 10^9/L)
Hematocrit	37%
Platelet count	450,000/μL (450 × 10^9/L)
Serum creatinine	0.9 mg/dL
Urinalysis	Normal
Erythrocyte sedimentation rate	40 mm/h
C-reactive protein	5 mg/L
Rheumatoid factor (RF)	Negative
Anticitrullinated protein (anti-CCP) antibody	Negative
Antinuclear antibody (ANA)	1:160 speckled
Anti-Ro/SSA	Positive
Anti-La/SSB	Positive

A Schirmer test can be performed as an objective measure of ocular dryness. A standard strip of filter paper is placed at the junction of the middle and lateral thirds of the inferior conjunctival sac for 5 minutes. A positive test is ≤5 mm of wetting (see Fig. 28.2).

Corneal staining patterns can be another tool in evaluating dry eyes. Dyes such as fluorescein bind to degenerated cells to highlight sites of corneal and conjunctival epithelial disease. Unlike fluorescein or lissamine green, rose bengal can also bind to healthy cells. In a healthy eye it is probably blocked from doing so by tear components such as mucin. Therefore, it also highlights areas where the tear film is disturbed. The dye can be toxic to corneal epithelial cells and stinging upon instillation can be severe; therefore, it may not be the dye of choice.

Because lissamine green does not stain healthy cells, it is less toxic. However, it is probably just as sensitive as rose bengal. As with rose bengal, a 1% drop is applied to the inferior conjunctival sac and the staining pattern is assessed under white light. In aqueous tear deficiency, the staining pattern (often punctate keratitis) may start in the interpalpebral nasal conjunctiva and move temporally. When the cornea becomes involved, staining may start inferiorly. Besides the general pattern of staining, quantitative grading can be tracked by recording the intensity (van Bijsterveld Score) or number (Ocular Staining Score) of punctate stains.

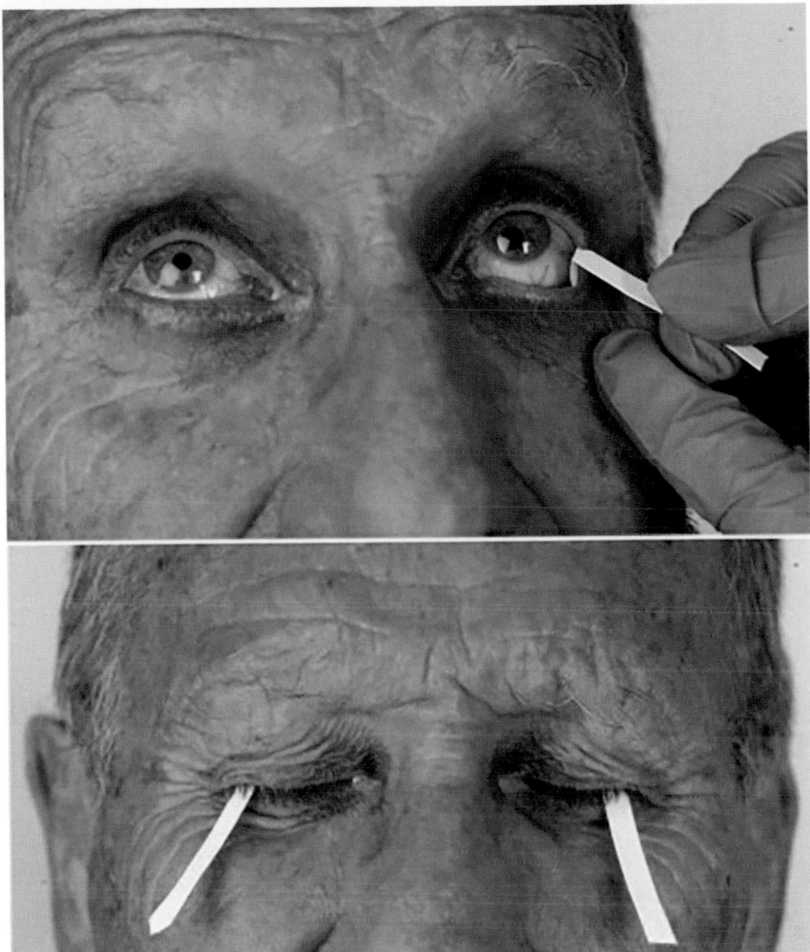

Fig. 28.2 Schirmer test.

A minor salivary gland biopsy is a more invasive test that remains an important diagnostic procedure for Sjögren's. A positive biopsy will show periductal lymphocytic infiltration. Pathologists report a focus score, which is the number of mononuclear cell infiltrates containing at least 50 inflammatory cells in a 4-mm^2 glandular section. A focus score of ≥1 is considered positive (see Figs. 28.3 and 28.4).

BASIC SCIENCE PEARL **STEP 1/2/3**

Genetic predisposition to Sjögren's syndrome can be attributed to alleles within the MHC class II gene region, in particular HLA-DR and HLA-DQ alleles.

The results of the Schirmer test is 4 mm on the left eye and 4 mm on the right eye. A biopsy of the salivary gland is obtained with a focus score of 2.

Diagnosis: Sjögren's syndrome.

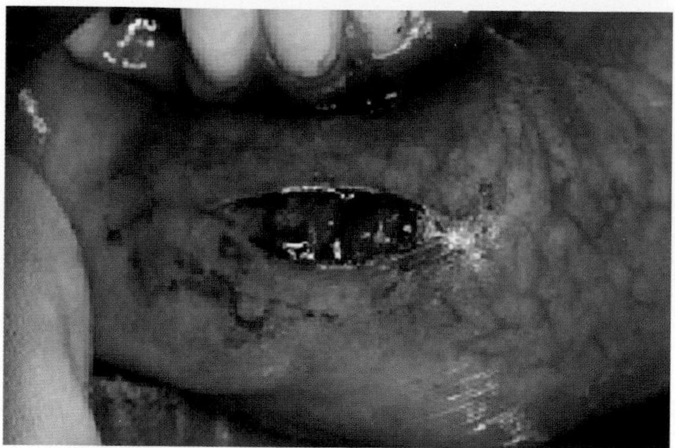

Fig. 28.3 Lip biopsy with salivary glands exposed.

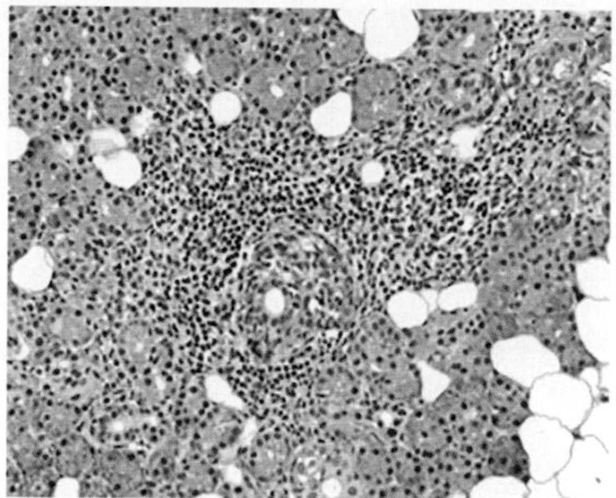

Fig. 28.4 Focal lymphocytic infiltration of salivary gland seen in Sjögren's.

TABLE 28.4 ■ **American College of Rheumatology (ACR)/European League Against Rheumatism (EULAR) 2016 Classification Criteria**

Item	Weight/Score
Labial salivary gland with focal lymphocytic sialadenitis and focus score ≥1	3
Anti-SSA(Ro)+	3
Ocular Staining Score ≥5 (or van Bijsterveld score ≥4) on at least one eye	1
Schirmer ≤5/5 min on at least one eye	1
Unstimulated whole saliva flow rate ≤0.1 ml/min	1

What are the 2016 ACR/EULAR classification criteria of Sjögren's syndrome?

Sjögren's syndrome is characterized by lymphocytic infiltration of the exocrine glands. The classification criteria are met when the sum of the total points is ≥4 (see Table 28.4).

CLINICAL PEARL **STEP 2/3**

Fatigue is often the most prominent and disabling symptom of Sjögren's.

Exclusion criteria:
Prior diagnosis of the following conditions would exclude a diagnosis of Sjögren's syndrome:

- History of head and neck radiation treatment
- Active hepatitis C infection (with positive PCR)
- Acquired immunodeficiency syndrome
- Sarcoidosis
- Amyloidosis
- Graft versus host disease
- IgG4-related disease

What is the initial treatment strategy for Sjögren's syndrome?

Treatment for Sjögren's syndrome is organ specific. The goal of treating keratoconjunctivitis sicca is to restore a healthy tear film, beginning with lifestyle modification such as avoiding a desiccating environment, eliminating offending medications, and attention to activities that limit blinking such as reading. First-line treatment includes artificial tears to reinstate the tear film. If four times daily is insufficient, more frequent dosing requires preservative free formulations. For the evaporative component of dry eyes, which often overlaps with tear deficiency, eyelid hygiene with attention to warm compresses can be started as well. In more severe cases, short courses of topical antibiotics and/or low-dose topical steroids are sometimes used. Cyclosporine drops have also been used and punctal plugs can increase tear retention.

Xerostomia is treated with muscarinic agonists such as pilocarpine hydrochloride and cevimeline hydrochloride. Systemic symptoms such as fatigue and arthritis are treated with activity modification, and depending on severity, immunosuppressants such as hydroxychloroquine or methotrexate can be used. For severe systemic complications, azathioprine, mycophenolate, and cyclophosphamide can be efficacious.

CLINICAL PEARL **STEP 1/2/3**

The main side effect of muscarinic agonists such as pilocarpine and cevimeline is sweating.

The patient receives pilocarpine hydrochloride for her dry mouth and lubricating eye drops for her dry eyes. She is also started on hydroxychloroquine 200 mg daily for her joint pain. The patient follows up with you in 3 months and states that she feels much better. Her mouth and eyes are no longer dry. Her arthritis has also improved.

What noninvasive tests can be done to determine salivary gland involvement?

Three noninvasive tests performed to determine salivary gland involvement include sialometry, scintigraphy, and ultrasonography.

1. Sialometry (sensitivity 56%, specificity 81%): This test is a measure of saliva flow, either unstimulated (primarily from the sublingual and submandibular glands) or stimulated saliva production (primarily from the parotid glands) for a period of 5–15 minutes. An unstimulated whole salivary flow rate of ≤0.1 mL/min indicates abnormal salivary function.
2. Scintigraphy (sensitivity 75%, specificity 78%): In this nuclear medicine procedure, an intravenous injection of a radioactive tracer, technetium 99, is taken up and secreted during a 60-minute period to determine salivary flow rates. It is best used to differentiate an inflammatory process from a neoplasm in the salivary glands.
3. Ultrasonography (sensitivity 63%, specificity 99%): This is another technique that can help determine involvement of the salivary gland. Ultrasound can detect typical structural salivary gland abnormalities characteristically seen in Sjögren's (see Fig. 28.5).

What are the systemic manifestations of Sjogren syndrome?
See Table 28.5.

CLINICAL PEARL **STEP 1/2/3**

Distal renal tubular acidosis presenting as severe hypokalemia can occur in 5% to 23% of patients with Sjögren's syndrome.

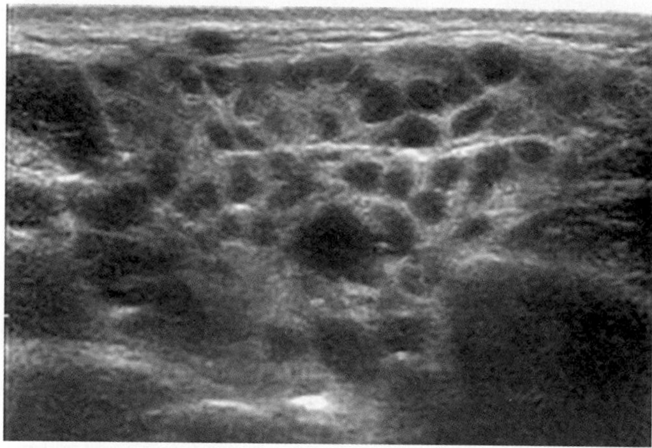

Fig. 28.5 Ultrasound of a parotid gland. There is parenchymal inhomogeneity with many rounded hypoechoic areas surrounded by hyperechogenicity.

TABLE 28.5 ■ **Systemic Manifestations of Sjögren's Syndrome**

Constitutional	Fatigue
Musculoskeletal	Arthralgia
	Arthritis
	Myositis
Pulmonary	Interstitial pneumonitis
	Interstitial lung disease
Renal	Tubulointerstitial nephritis
	Glomerulonephritis
Neurologic	Peripheral neuropathy
	Neuromyelitis optica
Cutaneous	Vasculitis
	Subacute cutaneous lupus
	Annular erythema
Systemic vasculitis	Necrotizing vasculitis of medium-sized arteries
Hematologic	Leukopenia
	Anemia
	Thrombocytopenia
	Hypergammaglobulinemia
	Cryoglobulinemia
	Monoclonal gammopathy

How do you differentiate the arthritis in Sjögren's from other forms of arthritis?
The arthritis in Sjögren's can be similar to rheumatoid arthritis with symmetric joint involvement of the metacarpophalangeal (MCP) joints, PIP joints, and wrists. Morning stiffness for

>30 minutes is common just as in rheumatoid arthritis. In contrast to rheumatoid arthritis, however, the arthritis in Sjögren's is nonerosive and not deforming.

What is the difference between primary and secondary Sjögren's syndrome?

Primary Sjögren's is diagnosed in patients with keratoconjunctivitis sicca and xerostomia in the absence of an underlying autoimmune disease. Anti-Ro/SSA and anti-La/SSB are typically elevated. Secondary Sjögren's is diagnosed in patients who present with sicca syndrome alongside another autoimmune disorder such as systemic lupus erythematosus, scleroderma, or rheumatoid arthritis. Clinical manifestations in primary and secondary Sjögren's are similar.

Which malignancy are Sjögren's patients at risk of developing?

Sjögren's syndrome patients are at risk of developing non-Hodgkin's B cell lymphoma at a rate of 6 to 20 times greater than the general population. The overall lifetime risk is 5% to 10%. The most common is marginal zone B cell subtype. Persistent mass of a salivary or lacrimal gland should raise concern for malignancy. Therefore, it is important to ask patients about constitutional symptoms including fevers, chills, weight loss, and night sweats. Initial evaluation should begin with a fine-needle aspiration.

CLINICAL PEARL **STEP 1/2/3**

It is important to obtain a biopsy if the etiology of the parotid gland enlargement is unclear given the increased risk of lymphoma in patients with Sjögren's.

Case Summary

- **Complaint/History:** A 35-year-old female presents with 1 year of progressive dry eyes, dry mouth, and joint pain.
- **Findings:** Patient has poor dentition with decreased salivary pool. Her second and third PIP joints are swollen.
- **Lab Results/Tests:** Lab tests reveal an elevated ESR of 40. She is also found to have positive anti-Ro/SSA, anti-LA/SSB and ANA. Schirmer test is positive and her lip biopsy reveals a focus score of 2.

Diagnosis: Sjögren's syndrome.

- **Treatment:** The patient was treated with lubricating eye drops and pilocarpine. Her arthritis was treated with hydroxychloroquine with clinical improvement.

BEYOND THE PEARLS

- Patients with Sjögren's syndrome can present with interstitial lung disease, typically lymphocytic interstitial pneumonitis. Consider Sjögren's syndrome in a patient with unexplained lung disease and a positive ANA.
- Complement levels (C4) are commonly low in Sjögren's.
- Pregnant women with positive SSA antibodies are at risk of having babies with neonatal lupus syndrome, which can cause a congenital heart block.
- Patient's with Sjögren's can be checked for dry eyes by looking for punctate staining with fluorescein or lissamine green dye.
- A thorough history is needed to find risk factors for dry eye such as high air-flow masks, dry environments, polyunsaturated fatty acid deficiency, medications, contact lens use, or prior eye surgery.
- Consider screening your dry eye patients for xerostomia by asking whether they can eat dry foods such as a cracker without drinking fluids.

Bibliography

Cornec, D., Saraux, A., Jousse-Joulin, S., Pers, J., Boisrame-Gastrin, S., Renaudineau, Y., Gauvin, Y., Roguedas-Contios, A., Genestet, S., Chastaing, M., Cochener, B., & Devauchelle-Pensec, V. (2015). The differential diagnosis of dry eyes, dry mouth, and parotidomegaly: a comprehensive review. *Clinical Reviews in Allergy & Immunology*, *49*(3), 278–287.

Hochberg, M. C. (2019). *Rheumatology*. Philadelphia, PA: Elsevier.

Mariette, X., & Criswell, L. A. (2018). Primary Sjögren's syndrome. *New England Journal of Medicine*, *378*(10), 931–939.

Segerberg-Konttinen, M., Konttinen, Y. T., & Bergroth, V. (1986). Focus score in the diagnosis of Sjögren's syndrome. *Scandinavian Journal of Rheumatology. Supplement*, *61*, 47–51.

Shiboski, C. H., Shiboski, S., Seror, R., Criswell, L., Labetoulle, M., Lietman, T., Rasumussen, A., Scofield, H., Vitali, C., Bowman, S., & Mariette, X. (2017). 2016 ACR-EULAR classification criteria for primary Sjögren's syndrome: a consensus and data-driven methodology involving three international patient cohorts. *Arthritis & Rheumatology (Hoboken, N.J.)*, *69*(1), 35–45.

Nair, J., & Singh, T. (2017). Sjögren's syndrome: review of the aetiology, pathophysiology & potential therapeutic interventions. *Journal of Clinical and Experimental Dentistry*, *9*(4), e584–e589.

Vivino, F. (2017). Sjögren's syndrome: Clinical aspects. *Clinical Immunology*, *182*, 48–54.

Thorne, I., & Sutcliffe, N. (2017). Sjögren's syndrome. *British journal of Hospital Medicine*, *78*(8), 438–442.

Baer, A., DeMarco, M., Shiboski, S., Lam, M., Challacombe, S., Daniels, T., Dong, Y., Greenspan, J., Kirkham, B., Lanfranchi, H., Schiodt, M., Srinivasan, M., Umehara, H., Vivino, F., Vollenweider, C., Zhao, Y., Criswell, L., & Shiboski, C. (2015). for the Sjögren's International Collaborative Clinical Alliance (SICCA) Research Groups: The SSB positive/SSA negative antibody profile is not associated with key phenotypic features of Sjögren's syndrome. *Annals of the Rheumatic Diseases*, *74*, 1557–1561.

CASE 29

A 36-Year-Old Male With 3 Years of Worsening Joint Pain

Anna Lafian ■ Nasim Daoud

A 36-year-old male with no significant medical history presents to his primary care provider with 3 years of worsening joint pain. He reports pain in his hands with occasional swelling of his fingers and toes, right elbow, and low back that wakes him up around 4–5 a.m. with 2 hours of morning stiffness. Symptoms are improved by taking ibuprofen. Patient always felt he was too young to have "serious arthritis" and did not seek medical care earlier. Given his clinical features, the patient is referred to rheumatology.

What can we discern from knowing the duration of this patient's symptoms?

Acute and chronic polyarthritis have different etiologies. When presented with a case of acute arthritis (symptoms ongoing for a few days or less), differentials to consider are septic arthritis and crystal-induced arthritis (gout or pseudogout). When dealing with chronic polyarthritis (symptoms ongoing for >6 weeks), the differential is broad and includes two categories: inflammatory and noninflammatory.

Inflammatory arthritides have the following features: morning stiffness >1 hour, improvement of joint symptoms with activity, no improvement with rest, pain at night, improvement with corticosteroids or nonsteroidal antiinflammatory drugs (NSAIDs), and fatigue.

The list of differentials for inflammatory polyarthritis is broad and includes rheumatoid arthritis, systemic lupus erythematosus, polyarticular gout, psoriatic arthritis, spondyloarthropathy, juvenile idiopathic arthritis, systemic sclerosis, polymyalgia rheumatica, vasculitis, reactive arthritis, enteropathic or inflammatory bowel disease associated arthritis, sarcoid arthritis, and chronic calcium pyrophosphate disease (CPPD).

The list of differentials for noninflammatory polyarthritis includes osteoarthritis, chronic CPPD, fibromyalgia, hemochromatosis, and hypermobility syndrome.

What is the definition of inflammatory back pain?

According to the Assessment of Spondyloarthritis International Society (ASAS),

1. Age at onset younger than 40 years
2. Insidious onset
3. Improvement with exercise
4. No improvement with rest
5. Pain at night (with improvement on getting up)

If four out of five parameters are present, there is a sensitivity of 77% and specificity of 91.7%. Sensitivity and specificity refer to the presence of inflammatory back pain, not to a specific diagnosis.

Upon physical examination, vital signs are normal. Body mass index (BMI) is 31 kg/m^2. The right second and fourth distal interphalangeal (DIP) joints are swollen and tender as well as the left second and fifth DIP joints. He has pitting of multiple nails and has pain upon palpation of the right elbow and sacroiliac (SI) joint. While examining his elbows, it is noted that he has small silvery scales on the extensor surfaces of bilateral elbows as well as bilateral knees. He mentions that he has had these lesions as well as flaking of his scalp for 8 years but did not mention them to his doctor as he felt they were unrelated and due to "eczema and dandruff." You highly suspect psoriatic arthritis and want to order some lab tests and imaging for further evaluation.

What are some differentials of inflammatory back pain?

Spondylarthropathies including psoriatic arthritis, enteropathic arthritis, and reactive arthritis.

How does the distribution of arthritis in this patient's presentation help narrow the diagnosis?

Most patients with psoriatic arthritis have peripheral joint disease (synovitis, dactylitis, enthesitis). A small percentage of patients have axial spine involvement alone.

Joint involvement in psoriatic arthritis varies and patients can have more than one subtype of disease manifestation.

- Asymmetric oligoarticular disease occurs in 15%–20% of patients and involves distal interphalangeal (DIP) joints, proximal interphalangeal (PIP) joints, metacarpal phalangeal (MCP) joints, metatarsal phalangeal (MTP) joints, knees, ankles and hips.
- Predominant DIP involvement occurs in 2%–5% of patients and involves DIPs.
- Arthritis mutilans occurs in 5% of patients and involves DIPs and PIPs.
- Polyarthritis occurs in 50%–60% of patients and involves MCPs, PIPs, and wrists (and resembles rheumatoid arthritis).
- Isolated axial involvement occurs in 2%–5% of patients and involves the vertebrae and SI joints.

As a quick review, refer to Table 29.1 for distribution of joint involvement in various arthritides.

What is the importance of nail changes/pitting in this clinical scenario?

Nail involvement is a strong predictor for development of psoriatic arthritis. Skin disease may precede symptoms of arthritis by 7–10 years, but nail changes occur only 1–2 years before onset of arthropathy.

The nail is closely related to the distal phalanx and the involvement of nails in psoriatic arthritis typically denotes the presence of DIP arthritis. In other words, patients with DIP joint involvement also have more severe nail changes. In fact, when there is a flare of DIP joints or worsening of nail disease, a flare of skin and arthritis can be expected.

Which nail changes can occur in this clinical scenario?

The various nail changes that can occur are pitting, ridging, hyperkeratosis, and onycholysis (see Figs. 29.1–29.3).

What is enthesitis?

Inflammation and swelling at the insertion of tendon into bone, which is postulated to be the key pathogenic process in all forms of spondyloarthritis. This occurs in 20%–40% of patients with psoriatic arthritis.

A comprehensive list of anatomical sites for assessment of enthesitis is given in Fig. 29.4. The most common sites of enthesitis include the Achilles tendon, the plantar fascia insertion into the calcaneus, and the ligamentous insertions into the pelvic bones (Fig. 29.5).

TABLE 29.1 ■ **Typical Distribution of Joint Involvement in Some Commonly Encountered Forms of Polyarthritis**

	Rheumatoid Arthritis	Osteoarthritis	Psoriatic Arthritis	Gout/Pseudogout
Large weight-bearing joints	Knees and ankles, usually symmetric; hips only rarely	Hips, knees, ankles	Knees and ankles, usually asymmetric	Knees and ankles; wrists in pseudogout
Small joints	MCP and PIP joints in the hands; MTP joints in the feet	DIP, PIP, and first CMC joints in the hands; first MTP joint in the feet	Frequently DIP joints along with nail involvement; other small joints	Small joints of the feet; MCP joints in pseudogout
Spine	Cervical spine	Cervical spine and LS spine	LS spine and SI joints	No

CMC, Carpometacarpal; *DIP*, distal interphalangeal; *LS*, lumbosacral; *MCP*, metacarpophalangeal; *MTP*, metatarsophalangeal; *PIP*, proximal interphalangeal; *SI*, sacroiliac.

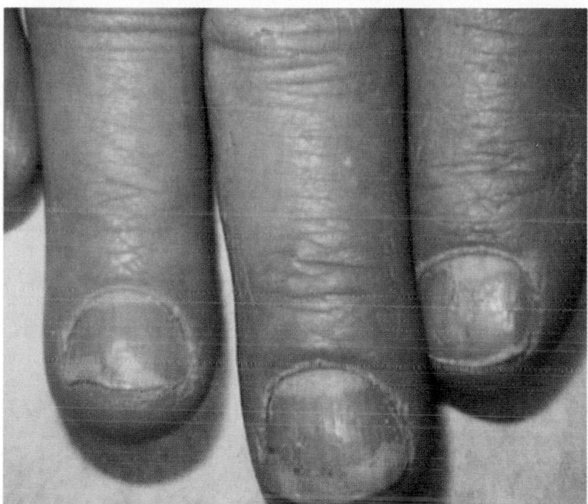

Fig. 29.1 Psoriasis affecting nails (onycholysis and pitting). (From Zitelli, B.J., Nowalk, A.J., & McIntire, S.C. (2018). *Zitelli and Davis' atlas of pediatric physical diagnosis* (7th ed.). Elsevier.)

CLINICAL PEARL **STEP 2/3**

Symptoms include asymmetric joint involvement (often DIP, spine can be involved) associated with joint pain and stiffness. Physical examination identifies swelling in affected joints, dactylitis ("sausage digits"), psoriatic lesions (pink plaques with silvery scales), and nail changes (pitting, ridging, onycholysis). Sacroiliitis and uveitis can also be present.

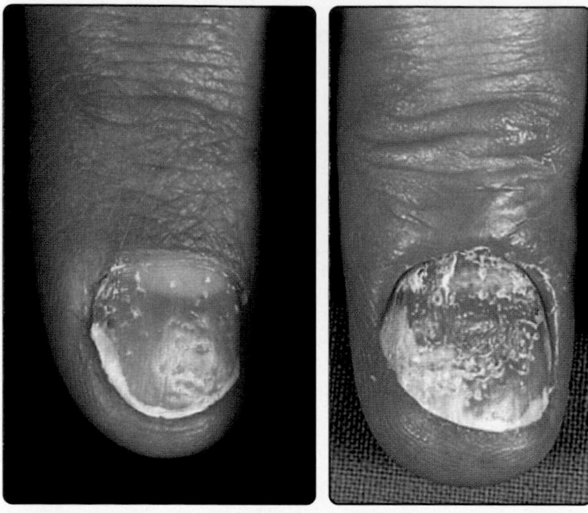

Fig. 29.2 Nail involvement in psoriasis: pitting *(left)* and subungual hyperkeratosis with onycholysis *(right)*. (From Ardern-Jones, M. R. & Gawkrodger, D. J. (2021). *Dermatology: an illustrated colour text* (7th ed.). Elsevier.)

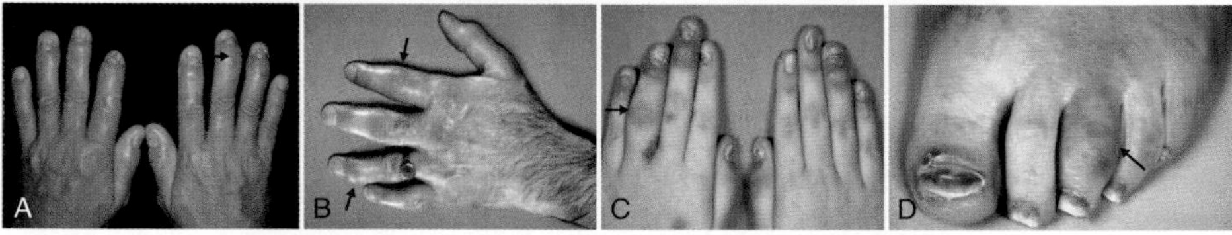

Fig. 29.3 Psoriatic arthritis: joint inflammation. (A) Distal interphalangeal synovitis. (B) Proximal interphalangeal and distal oligoarthritis synovitis. (C) Asymmetrical oligoarthritis. (D) Dactylitis with nail changes. (From Scott, W.N. (2018). *Insall & Scott surgery of the knee* (6th ed.). Elsevier.)

Lab tests obtained show ESR 64 and CRP 12.9 (both elevated). Rheumatoid factor (RF) and anticitrullinated peptide antibodies (anti-CCP) are normal. Complete blood count (CBC) is normal except for elevated platelet count. Complete metabolic panel (CMP) and uric acid levels are normal. HLA-B27 is positive.

X-ray of bilateral hands/wrists shows erosive changes at the DIP and proximal interphalangeal (PIP) joints with no involvement of the metacarpophalangeal (MCP) joints or wrists.

What is the significance of HLA-B27?

Psoriatic arthritis is a polygenic disorder. In genome-wide association studies, the following genes have been identified as possibly being involved in psoriatic arthritis: HLA-Cw6, HLA-B38, HLA-B39, and HLA-B27.

HLA-B27 and HLA-B39 are associated with sacroiliitis and spondylitis. Of patients with psoriatic sacroiliitis, 50% are HLA-B27 positive.

How do this patient's lab tests help us with the diagnosis?

Psoriatic arthritis is considered a "seronegative" arthritis and therefore a negative rheumatoid factor is telling. However, in up to 10% of patients, there can be a low titer positive RF, which can

Anatomic region	Enthesitis exam
Foot and ankle	Achilles tendon insertion to calcaneus Plantar fascia insertion to calcaneus Plantar fascia insertion to metatarsal heads Plantar fascia insertion to base of fifth metatarsal
Knee	Quadriceps tendon insertion to patella (2 and 10 o'clock) Infrapatellar ligament insertion to patella (6 o'clock) and tibial tuberosity
Pelvis	Hip extensor insertion at greater trochanter of femur Sartorius insertion at anterior superior iliac spine Posterior superior iliac spine Abdominal muscle insertions to iliac crest Gracilis and adduction insertion to pubis symphysis Hamstring insertion to ischial tuberosity
Spine	5th lumbar spinous process
Upper extremity	Common flexor insertion at medial epicondyle of humerus Common extensor insertion at lateral epicondyle of humerus Supraspinatus insertion into greater tuberosity of humerus
Chest	Costosternal junctions (1st and 7th)

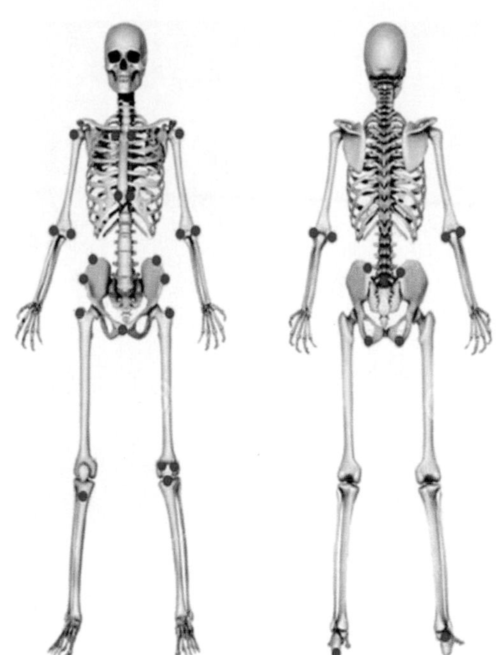

Fig. 29.4 Anatomical sites for assessment of enthesitis in enthesitis-related arthritis and juvenile ankylosing spondylitis. (From Petty, R. E., Lindsley, C. B., Laxer, R. M., Mellins, E. D., Wedderburn, L. R., & Fuhlbrigge, R. C. (2021). *Textbook of pediatric rheumatology* (8th ed.). Elsevier.)

confuse the clinical picture. What helps confirm the diagnosis are the DIP involvement, enthesitis, and dactylitis. Inflammatory markers can be elevated but are nonspecific and portend a worse prognosis and correlate with polyarticular involvement.

CLINICAL PEARL **STEP 2/3**

These patients usually have a negative rheumatoid factor (seronegative spondyloarthritis) and can have a positive HLA-B27.

What are common X-ray findings in this disease process?

See Fig. 29.6.

CLINICAL PEARL **STEP 2/3**

X-ray findings include bone proliferation, bone resorption, "pencil-in-cup deformity" of DIP joints, and erosive changes.

Diagnosis: Psoriatic arthritis.

What treatments are available in psoriatic arthritis?

Conservatively, patients must be counseled on weight loss. This may reduce disease activity.

Medically, patients should be started on NSAIDs, which is first-line treatment for mild joint symptoms. There is also evidence that NSAIDs are effective in treating spinal pain in axial psoriatic arthritis.

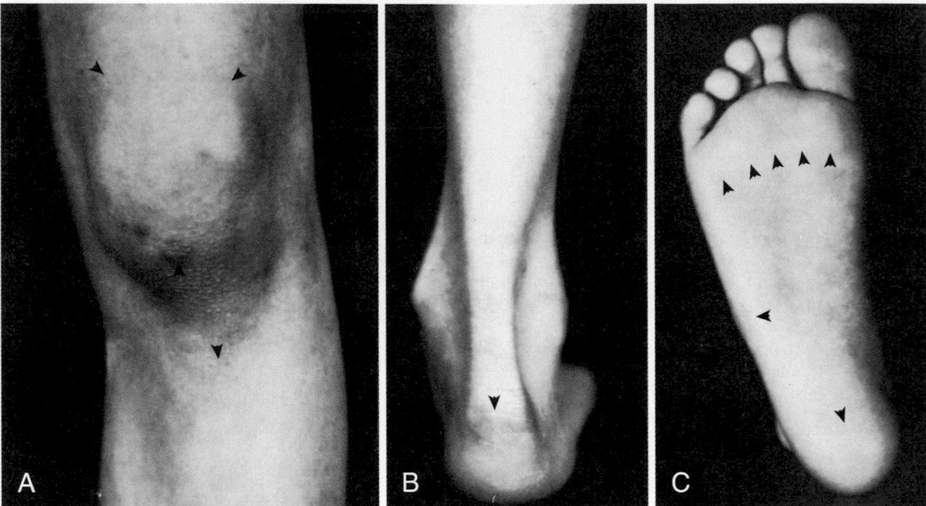

Fig. 29.5 (A) *Arrowheads* indicate the most common sites of tenderness associated with enthesitis at the insertions of the quadriceps muscles into the patella and the attachments of the patellar ligament to the patella and tibial tuberosity. (B) *Arrowhead* indicates the site of tenderness at the insertion of the Achilles tendon into the calcaneus. (C) *Arrowheads* indicate the most common sites of tenderness associated with enthesitis at the insertion of the plantar fascia into the calcaneus, base of fifth metatarsal, and heads of the first through fifth metatarsals. (From Petty, R. E., Lindsley, C. B., Laxer, R. M., Mellins, E. D., Wedderburn, L. R., Fuhlbrigge, R. C. (2021). *Textbook of pediatric rheumatology* (8th ed.). Elsevier.)

In mild situations or when few joints are affected, glucocorticoid therapy (intraarticular injections) is also effective. If symptoms persist, more joints are involved (>5), or there are elevated inflammatory markers, disease-modifying antirheumatic drugs (DMARDs) should be considered. The following DMARDs can be used: methotrexate, sulfasalazine, leflunomide, cyclosporine, and apremilast. However, these DMARDs do not prevent progression of radiographic changes and none is effective for nail disease or axial involvement. In this case, biologics should be attempted:

- Tumor necrosis factor-alpha inhibitors (etanercept, infliximab, adalimumab, golimumab, certolizumab)
- Monoclonal antibody against IL-12/23 (ustekinumab)
- Monoclonal antibody against IL-23 (guselkumab)
- Selective costimulation modulator: inhibits T-cell activation (abatacept)
- Monoclonal antibody against IL-17A (secukinumab, ixekizumab)
- Janus kinase inhibitor (tofacitinib)

Patient presents for follow-up. NSAIDs improved the patient's pain slightly, but he continues to have multiple tender and swollen joints as well as inflammatory back pain. Methotrexate is started, which helps with his peripheral joint pain, but his SI joint pain persists. He is agreeable to adalimumab in addition to methotrexate and, upon initiation, reports significant improvement in all symptoms with normalization of his inflammatory markers.

BASIC SCIENCE PEARL **STEP 1**

Increase in interferon (IFN)-alpha precipitates psoriasis. IFN-alpha promotes differentiation to Th1 and Th17 into skin and joints. Th1 releases tumor necrosis factor (TNF) and IFN-gamma. Th17 produces IL-17, TNF, IL-1, and IL-22. There is also stimulation in IL-6 production.

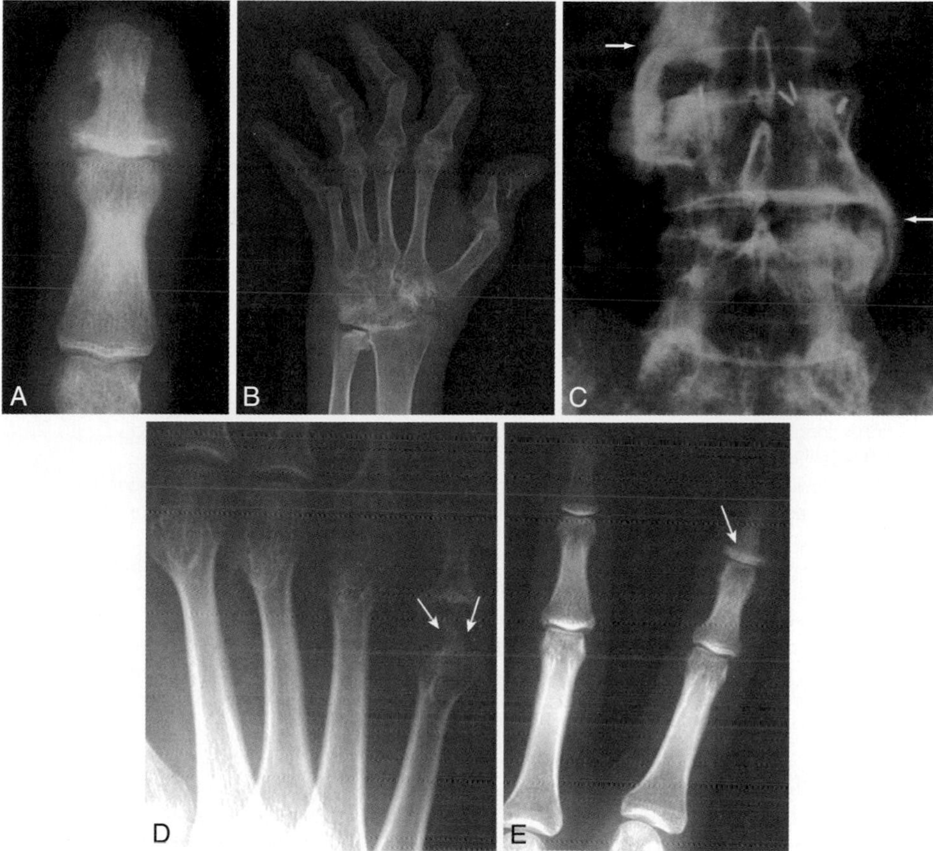

Fig. 29.6 Psoriatic arthritis (radiography). (A) DIP with soft tissue swelling, bone erosions with accompanying bone proliferation, and lack of osteoporosis. (B) Arthritis mutilans resulting from psoriatic arthritis with destructive change and joint deformity of the hand and pancompartmental ankyloses of the wrist. (C) Psoriatic spondylitis. Thick asymmetric paravertebral ossifications *(arrows)*, which are characteristic of psoriatic spondylitis. (D) Radiograph of the foot shows erosive changes at the distal end of the fifth metatarsal, with "pencil-in-cup" appearance at the metacarpal-phalangeal joint *(arrows)*. (E) Radiograph of the hand shows bony proliferation at the base of the distal phalanx *(arrow)*. (A–C from Koretzky, G.A., et al. (2021). *Firestein & Kelley's textbook of rheumatology* (11th ed.). Elsevier; and Resnick, D., & Niwayama, G. (1988). *Diagnosis of bone and joint disorders*. Philadelphia: W.B. Saunders; D, E from Coley, B.D. (2019). *Caffey's pediatric diagnostic imaging* (13th ed.). Elsevier.)

What if this patient presented with all of the same symptoms but developed these symptoms over the past 2 weeks?

Concurrent HIV infection should be considered with sudden onset psoriasis or psoriatic arthritis.

Case Summary

- **Complaint/History:** A 36-year-old male presents with inflammatory back pain, joint pain, skin lesions, and nail abnormalities.
- **Findings:** Exam demonstrates scattered DIP tenderness and swelling, nail pitting and psoriatic lesions on extensor surfaces of elbows and on knees. Enthesitis of right elbow and tenderness of SI joint is also noted.

- **Lab Results/Tests:** Lab results show elevated inflammatory markers, negative RF and CCP, and positive HLA-B27.

Diagnosis: Psoriatic arthritis.

- **Treatment:** The patient received NSAIDs with mild improvement in symptoms. He was then started on methotrexate with improvement in peripheral arthritis but ongoing inflammatory back pain. After adding adalimumab to his therapy, his symptoms significantly improved.

BEYOND THE PEARLS

- Other extraarticular manifestations in psoriatic arthritis include eye disease (iritis), oral ulcers, urethritis, nonspecific colitis, and aortic insufficiency (caused by dilatation of the aortic arch).
- Dermatologic conditions associated with psoriatic arthritis are palmoplantar pustulosis, acne conglobata, acne fulminans, psoriatic onycho-pachydermo periostitis, and hidradenitis suppurativa.
- Musculoskeletal ultrasound features of enthesitis are entheseal thickening, hypoechoic change, increased vascularity on power Doppler, tenosynovitis, bony erosion, or enthesophyte formation.
- Magnetic resonance imaging in psoriatic arthritis patients can demonstrate entheseal-related bone marrow edema, which is why it is suggested that psoriatic arthritis is an entheseal-based disease.
- Common comorbidities in psoriatic arthritis patients include increased risk of myocardial infarction, ischemic heart disease, diabetes, dyslipidemia, and metabolic syndrome.
- Anticitrullinated peptide antibodies are found in about 5% of patients with psoriatic arthritis.

Bibliography

Arthur, M., Schwarz, D. A., & Paul, B. (2019). Chapter 136, Arthritis and differential inflammatory joint disorders. In B. Coley (Ed.), *Caffey's pediatric diagnostic imaging* (13th ed.). Philadelphia: Elsevier. 1323–1348.e5.

Bruce, I., & Ho, P. (2015). Chapter 120, Clinical features of psoriatic arthritis. In M. C. Hochberg, A. J. Silman, J. S. Smolen, M. E. Weinblatt, M. H. Weisman, & E. Gravallese (Eds.), *Rheumatology* (6th ed., pp. 989–997). Philadelphia: Elsevier.

Christopher, R., & Dennis, M. (2015). Chapter 121, Etiology and pathogenesis of psoriatic arthritis. In M. C. Hochberg, A. J. Silman, J. S. Smolen, M. E. Weinblatt, M. H. Weisman, & E. Gravallese (Eds.), *Rheumatology* (6th ed., pp. 998–1005). Philadelphia: Elsevier.

FitzGerald, O., & Elmamoun, M. (2017). Chapter 77, Psoriatic arthritis: *Kelley & Firestein's textbook of rheumatology* (pp. 1285–1308) (10th ed.). Philadelphia: Elsevier.

Mikkel, O., Robert, L., Ho, J., & Walter, G. (2017). Chapter 58, Imaging in rheumatic diseases: *Kelley & Firestein's textbook of rheumatology* (10th ed.). Philadelphia: Elsevier. 858–907.e8.

Shalini. N. (2013). Dermatological history and examination. *Medicine*, *41*(6), 321–326.

Thomas. H. (2015). Chapter 8, Psoriasis and other papulosquamous diseases: *Clinical dermatology* (pp. 263–328) (6th ed.). Philadelphia: Elsevier.

Vollenhoven. R. (2017). Chapter 42, Evaluation and differential diagnosis of polyarthritis: *Kelley & Firestein's textbook of rheumatology* (pp. 615–624) (10th ed.). Philadelphia: Elsevier.

Weisman. M. (2012). Inflammatory back pain. *Rheumatic Disease Clinics of North America*, *38*(3), 501–512.

CASE 30

A 55-Year-Old Female With Muscle Weakness

Howard Yang

A 55-year-old Black-American female presents for evaluation of bilateral shoulder and hip weakness. She is a yoga instructor and noticed the weakness has significantly limited her ability to teach her classes as well as perform simple tasks like washing her hair. She has a history of hypothyroidism, type 2 diabetes mellitus, and hypercholesterolemia. Her medications include levothyroxine, metformin, and atorvastatin.

What are important questions to ask when a patient complains of weakness?

The causes of weakness are broad; therefore, a proper history is extremely important. First, try to isolate the location of weakness. Is the weakness diffuse or focal? Proximal or distal? Ascending or descending? Endocrine and electrolyte disturbance typically present with generalized weakness, whereas strokes commonly present with focal weakness. Inflammatory myopathies present with proximal > distal weakness, but some can present with isolated distal weakness. Neuromuscular disorders such as Guillain-Barré syndrome are characterized by ascending weakness with absent or depressed deep tendon reflexes.

The duration of symptoms is another important question to ask in order to help narrow the differential diagnosis. Acute focal weakness suggests infectious myopathies, medication-related myopathies, toxin-related myopathies, or neurologic causes.

Third, it is important to ask for any constitutional symptoms such as fever, unintentional weight loss, and night sweats that can point toward an underlying systemic process or malignancy.

She states the weakness has been getting progressively worse for the past 8 months and is associated with fatigue, subjective fever, and 13-pound unintentional weight loss. She denies any rashes or discoloration of her skin. There are no recent changes to her medications. She denies any recent travel or animal exposures.

What are some alarming symptoms to be aware of in someone with weakness?

Shortness of breath can result from diaphragm impairment as a result of inflammatory myopathies or neuromuscular disorders. When severe, patients can require mechanical ventilation and there should be a low clinical threshold for airway management for inpatient admission. Another alarming symptom is difficulty swallowing. Dysphagia can be related to oropharyngeal muscle weakness and increases the risk of aspiration.

Patient denies shortness of breath or trouble swallowing. On physical examination, her temperature is 36.1°C (97.5°F), blood pressure is 120/72 mmHg, pulse rate is 65/min, respiratory rate is 16/min, and oxygen saturation is 96% on room air. She is able to speak in full sentences without distress. Lung exam is clear bilaterally. No rashes are seen. She has bilateral proximal upper and lower extremity weakness, which is more pronounced in the upper extremities. She has trouble raising her arms above her head. Distal muscle strength is fully intact. Initial lab tests are shown in Table 30.1.

CLINICAL PEARL **STEP 2/3**

Serum aspartate aminotransferase (AST) and alanine aminotransferase (ALT) are often referred to as "poor man's" muscle enzymes that can be elevated in patients with myositis.

What is the difference between myalgia, myopathy, myositis, and myonecrosis?

Myalgia: muscle discomfort with normal creatine kinase (CK) level.

Myopathy: muscle weakness not attributed to pain with or without elevated CK level.

Myositis: muscle inflammation.

Myonecrosis: muscle enzyme elevation.

What is the differential diagnosis?

The differential diagnosis for weakness is listed in Table 30.2.

Inflammatory myositis, in particular polymyositis (PM), is at the top of the differential diagnosis. The mean age of onset for PM is between ages 50 and 60 years with female to male ratio 2–3:1. In the United States, Black Americans are more affected than White American with a ratio of 3–4:1. Dermatomyositis (DM) is another type of inflammatory myositis but typically presents with characteristic skin findings, including Gottron papules (erythematous rash over the extensor aspect of metacarpophalangeal and/or interphalangeal joints) or heliotrope rash (reddish purple rash around the eyelids), which are absent in our patient. It is possible to develop DM without skin findings but this is rare. Inclusion body myositis (IBM) typically presents with asymmetrical, proximal, and distal weakness, which is different from our patient who only has proximal weakness. Necrotizing myopathies will also present with symmetrical proximal weakness, but serum enzymes are typically higher (see Table 30.3).

Inflammatory myositis may also be associated with other connective tissues diseases such as systematic lupus erythematosus (SLE), mixed connective tissue disease (MCTD), scleroderma, and vasculitis.

TABLE 30.1 ■ **Laboratory Tests**

Complete blood count	Within normal limits
Erythrocyte sedimentation rate	75 mm/h
C-reactive protein	4.2 mg/dL
Creatine kinase	2300 units/L
Aldolase	21 units/L
Serum creatinine	0.8 mg/dL
Aspartate aminotransferase	380 units/L
Alanine aminotransferase	218 units/L
Thyroid-stimulating hormone	1.4 mIU/mL

TABLE 30.2 ■ **Differential Diagnosis for Weakness**

Drugs and toxins	Statins, alcohol, cocaine, zidovudine, D-penicillamine, antifungals, antimalarials, colchicine, amiodarone, steroids, and anti-TNF inhibitors
Endocrine	Hyperthyroidism, hypothyroidism, Addison's disease, Cushing's disease, acromegaly, diabetic amyotrophy, and diabetic muscle infarction
Infectious	Bacterial (*Staphylococcus, Streptococcus, Borrelia burgdorferi*) Viral (e.g., influenza, human immunodeficiency virus (HIV)) Parasitic (e.g., toxoplasma, trichinella)
Neuromuscular	Muscular dystrophies (e.g., Becker's, Duchenne's) Neuromuscular junction disorders (e.g., myasthenia gravis, Eaton-Lambert syndrome) Denervation disorders (e.g., amyotrophic lateral sclerosis)
Metabolic	Abnormal lipid metabolism (e.g., carnitine deficiency, carnitine palmitoyl transferase deficiency) Glycogen storage disease (e.g., McArdle's, acid maltase deficiency) Mitochondrial disorders Nutritional (e.g., vitamin D deficiency, malabsorption) Electrolyte (e.g., hypercalcemia, hypocalcemia, hypokalemia, hypophosphatemia)
Rheumatological	Dermatomyositis, polymyositis, inclusion body myositis, myositis associated with connective tissue disorders (systemic lupus erythematosus (SLE), rheumatoid arthritis, vasculitis), sarcoidosis
Genetic	Limb-girdle muscular dystrophy, dysferlinopathy, facioscapulohumeral muscular dystrophy, sarcoglycanopathy
Oncological	Paraneoplastic syndrome secondary to malignancy

TABLE 30.3 ■ **Inflammatory Muscle Diseases**

	Polymyositis	Dermatomyositis	Inclusion Body Myositis	Necrotizing Myopathy
Age	Adults	Children and adults	Adults >50 years	Adults
Sex	Female	Female	Male	Female
Onset	Months	Months	Years	Months
Weakness	Proximal	Proximal	Proximal and distal	Proximal
Symmetry	Symmetric	Symmetric	Asymmetric	Symmetric
Skin finding	No	Yes	No	No
Serum enzymes (CK, aldolase)	Normal to high	Normal to high	Normal to high	High
Associated with systemic autoimmune disease	Yes	Yes	Yes	No

CK, Creatine kinase.

Malignancy should be of concern because of the patient's age, subjective fever, and unintentional weight loss. Of patients with PM/DM, 10% to 20% are reported to have an underlying malignancy and the risk is highest within the first 3 years of diagnosis. Cancers associated with PM/DM include breast, lung, colon, stomach, pancreas, ovaries, and lymphoma. It is strongly recommended that patients with inflammatory muscle diseases (particularly PM and DM) undergo age-appropriate malignancy screening.

CLINICAL PEARL **STEP 2/3**

Malignancy should be considered in any patient with symptoms of fever, night sweats, and weight loss, particularly Hodgkin's lymphoma and non-Hodgkin's lymphoma.

TABLE 30.4 ■ **Difference Between Inflammatory Myopathy, Hyperthyroid Myopathy, and Hypothyroid Myopathy**

	TSH	T4	CK	Weakness
Inflammatory myopathy	Normal	Normal	↑	Mild to severe
Hyperthyroidism	↓	↑	Normal	Mild
Hypothyroidism	↑	↓	↑	Mild

CK, Creatine kinase; *TSH*, thyroid-stimulating hormone; *T4*, thyroxine

Medications or toxin-induced myopathies can also present with weakness. Alcohol, cocaine, statins, steroids, colchicine, amiodarone, antiretrovirals like zidovudine, antifungals, and antimalarials are known culprits. Statins are commonly used for treatment of hypercholesterolemia by inhibiting 3-hydroxy-3-methylglutaryl-coenzyme A reductase (HMGCR). Up to 20% of patients will develop statin-related myalgia but rarely myopathy or myonecrosis. Anti-HMGCR autoantibodies have been discovered in patients with immune-mediated necrotizing myopathy with the majority of patients having been exposed to statins.

The most common endocrine abnormality that leads to muscle weakness is thyroid disorders. Both hyperthyroidism and hypothyroidism can present with muscle weakness, but it is far more common to see elevated CK with hypothyroidism (see Table 30.4).

Infectious etiologies are low on the differential because of the chronicity of symptoms, but human immunodeficiency virus (HIV) infection should be ruled out. It would be extremely rare for inherited metabolic disorders or genetic disorders to present at the age of 55 years.

Which diagnostic workup should be performed?

First, it is important to assess the patient's safety. Is the patient in danger of choking on food? Does the patient have trouble breathing because of muscle weakness? Is the patient a fall risk?

Obtaining a muscle biopsy is the most important diagnostic test to confirm the diagnosis. Histopathological findings help differentiate various type of myopathies. Electromyography (EMG) and magnetic resonance imaging (MRI) are often used as a roadmap to help guide the location of the muscle biopsy. EMG can also aid in differentiating inflammatory myositis from neuropathic disorders, such as myasthenia gravis. MRI is another important diagnostic tool and would demonstrate increased signal on T2-weighted images with fat suppression (short tau inversion recovery (STIR) images) but not on T1-weighted images.

CLINICAL PEARL **STEP 2/3**

Do not perform an EMG and MRI on the same extremity. An EMG can cause muscle irritation and lead to an abnormal MRI finding.

CLINICAL PEARL **STEP 2/3**

Do not biopsy any muscle that has undergone recent EMG (<2 to 4 weeks) to avoid an erroneous result.

Atorvastatin is held. An EMG of the right upper extremity is obtained and shows early recruitment, variable fibrillations, small amplitude, and short duration suggestive of myopathy. An MRI of the left upper extremity shows patchy signal on T2-weighted images with fat suppression of the left deltoid muscle consistent with inflammatory myositis. She undergoes a left deltoid muscle biopsy which reveals focal endomysial infiltrates with predominant CD8+ cytotoxic T cells without vasculopathy or immune complex deposition.

Diagnosis: Polymyositis.

Serologic workup for the patient shows a positive antinuclear antibody (ANA) by indirect immunofluorescence assay (IFA) with a titer of 1:1280 homogeneous pattern, but negative double antidouble-stranded DNA (anti-DsDNA) antibody, anti-Smith antibody, and antiribonucleoprotein (anti-RNP) antibody. Myositis specific antibodies are positive for antinuclear matrix protein 2 (NXP2). She undergoes chest, abdomen, and pelvis CT scans to screen for malignancy in addition to a transvaginal ultrasound.

What is the significance of these autoantibodies?

Autoantibodies are often intimidating and confusing to interpret. A key concept is that autoantibodies alone are not diagnostic and rarely correlate with disease activity. Autoantibodies can also precede development of symptoms. Certain autoantibodies can be associated with a specific clinical phenotype. For example, our patient is positive for anti-NXP2 antibody, which is associated with malignancy. Therefore, a CT scan and an ultrasound were ordered to rule out an underlying malignancy (see Table 30.5).

CLINICAL PEARL **STEP 2/3**

Never order an ANA ELISA test that only gives a positive or negative result. ANA should always be ordered by IFA testing with a corresponding titer.

Chest, abdomen, and pelvis CT scans and vaginal ultrasound scan are unremarkable. The patient is started on oral prednisone 60 mg daily with sulfamethoxazole/trimethoprim for *Pneumocystis jirovecii* pneumonia (PJP) prophylaxis.

What is the initial treatment for polymyositis?

The focus of the therapy is to stop muscle inflammation and improve muscle strength. The initial treatment for polymyositis is systemic glucocorticoids. There is no standardized dosing for glucocorticoids, but the general rule is high dose glucocorticoids during the initial onset of disease with gradual tapering over 6 to 12 months. High dose glucocorticoids are typically defined as 1 mg/kg/day. However, in a critically ill patient with severe respiratory distress, a pulse-dose-steroid of methylprednisolone 1000 mg daily for 3 days is reasonable.

TABLE 30.5 ■ **Myositis Specific Antibodies**

Antibody	Clinical Significance
Aminoacyl tRNA synthetases: Jo-1, PL7, PL12, EJ, OJ, KS	Antisynthetase syndrome (fever, severe myositis, ILD, Raynaud's phenomenon, polyarthritis, and mechanic hands)
SRP	Aggressive necrotizing myopathy
Mi2	Typical dermatomyositis skin lesion with mild myositis
MDA5	Rapidly progressive ILD
NXP2	Malignancy associated

ILD, Interstitial lung disease.

What is the long-term treatment for polymyositis?

Long-term treatment focuses on safely reducing systemic glucocorticoids while monitoring for disease flare and any related complications. Immunosuppressive agents are used early on to help reduce glucocorticoid use as steroid-sparing agents can often take several months to take effect. Methotrexate and azathioprine are two of the commonly used steroid-sparing agents in polymyositis. In patients who are unable to tolerate methotrexate or azathioprine, cyclophosphamide and rituximab have also been used. Monthly infusions of intravenous immunoglobulin (IVIG) are often used for acute flares. Physical therapy is an important part of the treatment plan in order to regain and maintain muscle strength.

The patient sees her outpatient rheumatologist and reports that she is feeling great and able to get through her yoga classes without any problem. Methotrexate 15 mg weekly is chosen as the steroid-sparing agent with folic acid daily. She will continue to follow her rheumatologist with plans to taper off glucocorticoids in 6 months.

Case Summary

- **Complaint/History:** A 55-year-old African American female presents with an 8-month history of progressive weakness, subjective fever, and unintentional weight loss.
- **Findings:** Proximal muscle weakness.
- **Lab Results/Tests:** Lab tests reveal elevated aspartate aminotransferase (AST), alanine aminotransferase (ALT), creatine kinase (CK), aldolase, antinuclear antibody (ANA) with titer of 1:1280 homogeneous pattern, and antinuclear matrix protein-2 (NXP2) antibodies. Electromyography shows early recruitment, variable fibrillations, small amplitude, and short duration. Magnetic resonance imaging shows deltoid muscle with patchy signal on T2-weighted images with fat suppression. Muscle biopsy shows focal endomysial infiltrates with predominant CD8+ cytotoxic T cells without vasculopathy or immune complex deposition.

Diagnosis: Polymyositis.

- **Treatment:** Prednisone 1 mg/kg daily with methotrexate 15 mg weekly as steroid-sparing agent with a plan to taper off the steroids in 6 months.

BEYOND THE PEARLS

- It is important for inflammatory myositis patients to be up-to-date with age-appropriate malignancy screening. The peak incidence of cancer diagnosis is 3 years before or after the diagnosis of inflammatory myositis.
- Repeating myositis specific autoantibodies is unnecessary because it does not correlate with disease activity.
- Normal muscle enzymes do not always rule out a disease flare of myositis. Patients with advance disease might have significant muscle atrophy in which muscle enzymes would not be elevated.
- Creatine kinase (CK) and aldolase are not muscle specific. CK is found in muscle, heart, and brain tissues, and aldolase is found in muscle, liver, and brain tissues.
- Chronic steroid use can lead to steroid-induced myopathy, which also presents with proximal weakness and muscle wasting. Clinicians should have a high index of suspicion for anyone who is on chronic steroids and develops weakness.
- Anti-HMGCR–associated myopathy is related to statin exposure, but statin exposure is not a requirement for anti-HMGCR–associated myopathy. Patients who have never been exposed to statin therapy can still develop anti-HMGCR–associated myopathy.
- Inclusion body myositis should be considered in any patient over the age of 50 years who is resistant to steroid and immunosuppressive therapy.

Bibliography

Satoh, M., Tanaka, S., Ceribelli, A., Calise, S.J., Chan E. et al. (2017). A comprehensive overview on myositis-specific antibodies: new and old biomarkers in idiopathic inflammatory myopathy. *Clinical Reviews in Allergy & Immunology*, *52*(1), 1–19.

Rosenson. R. S., Baker, S.K., Jacobson, T.A., Kopecky, S.L., Parker B.A. et al. (2014). An assessment by the statin muscle safety task force: 2014 update. *Journal of Clinical Lipidology*, *8*, S58–71. https://doi.org/10.1016/j.jacl.2014.03.004.

West. S. G. (2014). *Rheumatology secrets* (Third Edition). Mosby: Elsevier.

Mohassel, P., & Mammen, A. L. (2018). Anti-HMGCCR myopathy. *Journal of Neuromuscular Diseases*, *5*(1), 11–20.

CASE 31

A 46-Year-Old Female With Purpura and Arthralgia

Kristal Choi ■ Talha Khawar

A 46-year-old female presents to the emergency department with 4 months of worsening fatigue, weakness, and arthralgia. In the previous 2 weeks, she had developed a raised purpuric rash on the legs. She denies any hemoptysis, headaches, chest pain, urinary symptoms, and neuropathy. Her past medical history is significant for hepatitis C, for which she has never received treatment. On physical examination, her blood pressure is 124/78 mmHg, pulse rate is 95/min, respiration rate is 18/min, and oxygen saturation is 95% on room air. There are purpuric macules and papules on the bilateral lower extremities (Fig. 31.1). Symmetric joint tenderness of the metacarpophalangeal joints, shoulders, and knees is noted without joint swelling. The remainder of the examination is normal.

What is the differential diagnosis for purpura?

Purpura is caused by the extravasation of red blood cells into the skin, causing a nonblanchable rash. Purpura can be further divided into nonpalpable and palpable purpura. Nonpalpable purpura is caused by bleeding into the skin without vascular inflammation and is more often caused by bleeding disorders and blood vessel fragility. Palpable purpura is caused by vascular inflammation (i.e., vasculitis). The differential diagnosis of purpura is broad and is summarized in Table 31.1. A detailed history and physical examination as well as blood counts and coagulation studies can help in differentiating these causes of purpura.

When should a skin biopsy be obtained?

A skin biopsy is warranted for all suspected neoplastic lesions and, all bullous disorders, and to clarify a diagnosis when there is a limited differential. For an inflammatory rash, lesions that show characteristic inflammatory changes should be biopsied first while avoiding very early and late lesions. Skin biopsy specimens should always be sent for both hematoxylin and eosin (H&E) staining and direct immunofluorescence to help determine the pattern of vasculitis.

The results of laboratory testing are shown in Table 31.2. A skin biopsy is performed and shows leukocytoclastic vasculitis with evidence of fibrinoid necrosis of the small venules, intense neutrophilic infiltrate, and variable mononuclear inflammation (Figs. 31.2 and 31.3).

BASIC SCIENCE/CLINICAL PEARL **STEP 1/2/3**

Both erythrocyte sedimentation rate (ESR) and C-reactive protein (CRP) are nonspecific measures of inflammation in the body and can be elevated in a wide variety of inflammatory diseases, including autoimmune conditions, infection, and malignancy. CRP is a more accurate reflection of the acute phase of inflammation than is the ESR (Fig. 31.3). The high-sensitivity CRP (hs-CRP) measures low levels of CRP and can be predictive of coronary artery disease.

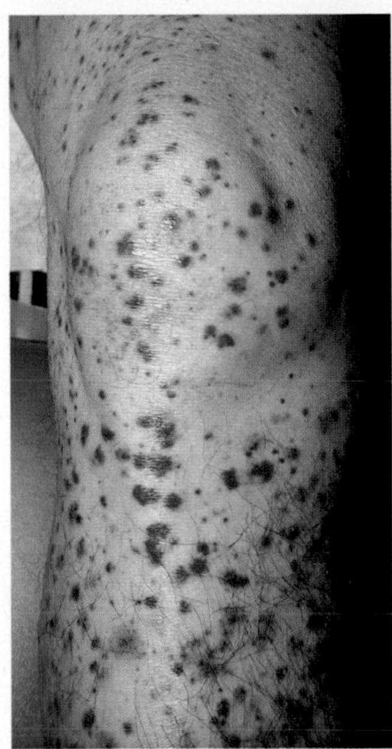

Fig. 31.1 Palpable purpura. (From James, W., & Berger, T. (2006). *Andrews' diseases of the skin: Clinical dermatology* (10th ed.). Elsevier.)

TABLE 31.1 ■ **Differential Diagnosis of Purpura**

Infectious	Malignant	Autoimmune	Other
Bacterial endocarditis Meningococcemia Rocky Mountain spotted fever Influenza Infectious mononucleosis HIV Other infections	Leukemia Lymphoma Myeloma Solid tumors Myelodysplastic syndromes	Polyarteritis nodosa Granulomatosis with polyangiitis Microscopic polyangiitis Eosinophilic granulomatosis with polyangiitis Systemic lupus erythematous IgA vasculitis Anti-GBM disease Juvenile rheumatoid arthritis Kawasaki disease Familial Mediterranean fever Inflammatory bowel disease Cryoglobulinemic vasculitis	Coagulopathies Acute hemorrhagic edema Leukocytoclastic vasculitis Thrombocytopenic purpura Hemolytic uremic syndrome Drug reactions

GBM, Glioblastoma multiforme; *HIV*, human immunodeficiency virus; *IgA*, immunoglobulin A

BASIC SCIENCE/CLINICAL PEARL **STEP 1/2/3**

Some autoimmune diseases can cause acquired hypocomplementemia via complement activation with accelerated consumption by immune complexes. Cryoglobulinemia is associated with low C4 but normal to mildly decreased C3 levels. Systemic lupus erythematosus is associated with low C3 and C4. Membranoproliferative glomerulonephritis usually has a low C3.

TABLE 31.2 ■ **Laboratory Tests**

Leukocyte count	17,100/μL (17 × 10^9/L)
Hematocrit	35%
Platelet count	540,000/μL (540 × 10^9/L)
Serum creatinine	0.9 mg/dL
Urinalysis	Normal
Erythrocyte sedimentation rate	90 mm/h
C-reactive protein	10 mg/L
RF	Positive
Cryoglobulin	Positive
C4	8
C3	120
c-ANCA	Negative
p-ANCA	Negative
Antiproteinase-3 antibodies	Negative
Antimyeloperoxidase antibodies	Negative
Hepatitis C Ab	Positive
Hepatitis C RNA	1,000,000 IU/mL

ANCA, Antineutrophil cytoplasmic antibody; *c-ANCA*, cytoplasmic pattern ANCA; *p-ANCA*, perinuclear pattern ANCA; *RF*, rheumatoid factor.

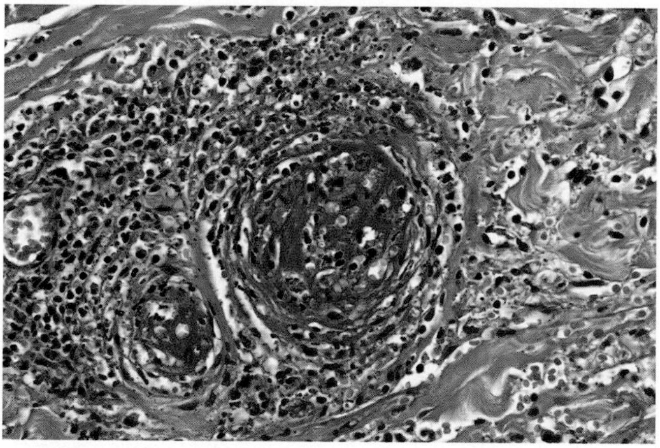

Fig. 31.2 Leukocytoclastic vasculitis. (From Calonje, J. E., Brenn, T., Lazar, A., & Billings, S. (2020). *McKee's pathology of the skin* (5th ed.). Elsevier).

What is leukocytoclastic vasculitis?

Leukocytoclastic vasculitis is a histopathologic term that describes the microscopic changes seen in small vessel vasculitis of the skin, mostly involving arterioles or postcapillary venules. This finding can develop from a variety of causes including systemic autoimmune disease, infection, drugs, and malignancy. Patients with small vessel vasculitis of the skin do not necessarily have a systemic vasculitis.

When should systemic vasculitis be suspected as a diagnosis?

Systemic vasculitis should be suspected as a diagnosis in patients presenting with constitutional symptoms (e.g., fever, fatigue) along with evidence of single or multiorgan disease involvement

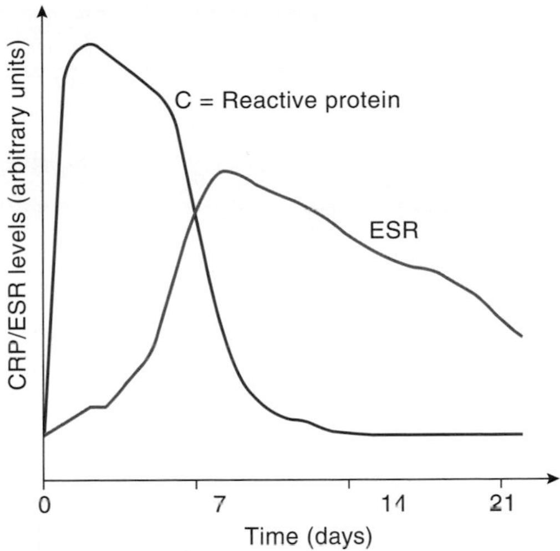

Fig. 31.3 Time course of inflammation markers. *CRP*, C-reactive protein; *ESR*, erythrocyte sedimentation rate. (From White, G., Vanbergen, O., Helbert, M., Singh, V., Datta, S., & Xiu, P. (2020). *Crash course: haematology and immunology* (5th ed.). Elsevier.)

(e.g., proteinuria with red blood cell (RBC) casts indicating renal involvement). However, in evaluating for a potential vasculitis, care must be taken to evaluate thoroughly for and rule out common mimickers of vasculitis, such as infection or malignancy.

Vasculitides can be classified based on the size of the vessels involved into small, medium, and large vessel vasculitis (Fig. 31.4). Small vessel vasculitis can be further differentiated between antineutrophil cytoplasmic antibody (ANCA)-associated vasculitis and immune complex small vessel vasculitis. This is summarized in Table 31.3. The many vasculitides can be differentiated based on knowledge of the clinical characteristics of each disease entity. Characteristic angiographic findings and pathology can be key in making a diagnosis of systemic vasculitis (see Fig. 31.5).

BASIC SCIENCE/CLINICAL PEARL **STEP 1/2/3**

In ANCA-associated vasculitis, there are two major immunofluorescence patterns. With the cytoplasmic pattern (c-ANCA), there is diffuse staining throughout the cytoplasm. In most cases, antibodies directed against proteinase 3 (PR3) cause this pattern. With the perinuclear ANCA (p-ANCA) pattern, there is staining around the nucleus. In most cases, antibodies against myeloperoxidase (MPO) cause this pattern. The typical staining pattern of c-ANCA is seen in Fig. 31.5A and the typical staining pattern of p-ANCA is seen in Fig. 31.5B.

What is your differential diagnosis for this case?

This is a 46-year-old female with a history of untreated hepatitis C who presents with fatigue, weakness, arthralgia, and purpura. Laboratory studies show positive cryoglobulin, elevated rheumatoid factor (RF), and low C4. Skin biopsy shows evidence of cutaneous small vessel vasculitis.

Although cutaneous small vessel vasculitis is not always associated with a systemic vasculitis and can also be caused by infections and medications, the presence of constitutional and articular symptoms would make a systemic vasculitis more likely. In the context of hepatitis C infection

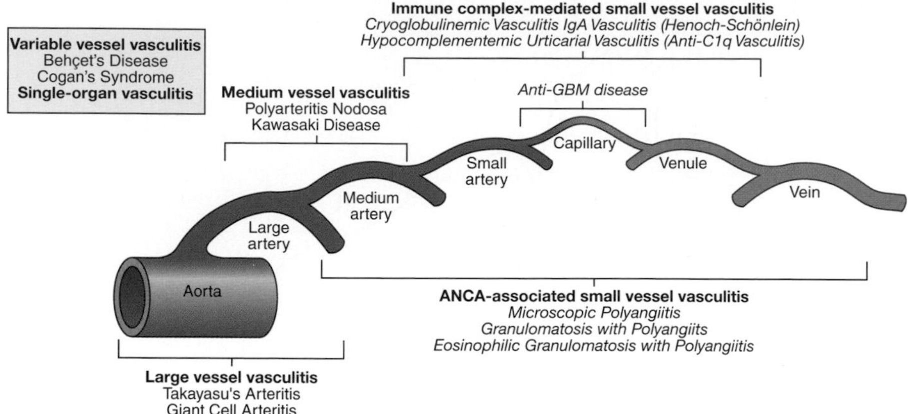

Fig. 31.4 Classification of vasculitides by blood vessel size. *ANCA*, Antineutrophil cytoplasmic antibody; *c-ANCA*, cytoplasmic pattern ANCA; *p-ANCA*, perinuclear pattern ANCA; *GBM*, glioblastoma multiforme. (From Firestein, G., Gabriel, S. E., McInnes, I. B., O'Dell, J., & Koretzky, G. (2021). *Firestein and Kelley's textbook of rheumatology* (11th ed.). Elsevier.)

TABLE 31.3 ■ **Classification and Clinical Features of Systemic Vasculitides**

Systemic Vasculitis	Common Presenting Features/Associations
Large Vessel Vasculitis	
Giant cell/temporal arteritis	Age >50 years, headache, jaw claudication, vision changes
Takayasu's arteritis	Age <40 years, claudication of the extremities, bruits
Medium Vessel Vasculitis	
Polyarteritis nodosa	Angiographic abnormalities of visceral arteries, neuropathy, hepatitis B
Kawasaki disease	Conjunctival injection, rash, strawberry tongue
ANCA-associated small vessel vasculitis	
Granulomatosis with polyangiitis	Nasal or sinus inflammation, pulmonary nodules or infiltrates, glomerulonephritis, c-ANCA/PR3
Eosinophilic granulomatosis with polyangiitis	Asthma, eosinophilia, neuropathy, pulmonary infiltrates, p-ANCA/MPO
Microscopic polyangiitis	Pulmonary hemorrhage, glomerulonephritis, p-ANCA/MPO
Immune complex small vessel vasculitis	
Cryoglobulinemic vasculitis	Constitutional symptoms, arthralgia, rash, hepatitis C
IgA vasculitis	Age <20 years, purpura, bowel angina, IgA deposits on histopathology

ANCA, Antineutrophil cytoplasmic antibody; *c-ANCA*, cytoplasmic pattern ANCA; *p-ANCA*, perinuclear pattern ANCA; *MPO*, myeloperoxidase; proteinase 3 (PR3), immunoglobulin A (IgA).

and positive cryoglobulin, the diagnosis of hepatitis C virus (HCV)-associated cryoglobulinemic vasculitis would be correct.

If a similar patient had presented with fatigue, weakness, arthralgia, and biopsy-proven cutaneous vasculitis without positive cryoglobulin, the differential diagnosis would be much broader. In such a patient, the majority of the systemic vasculitides and infection should be included on the

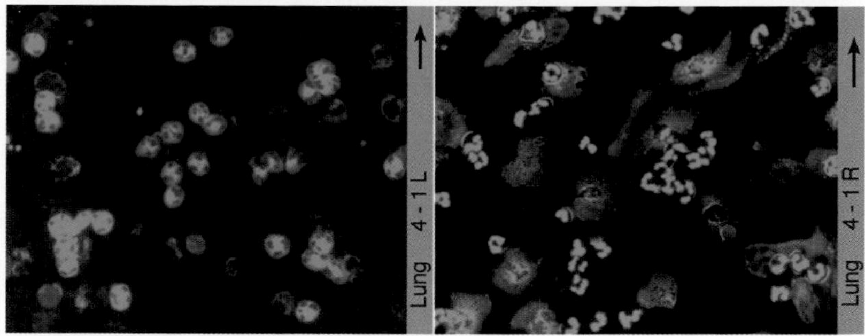

Fig. 31.5 p-ANCA and c-ANCA staining patterns. (From Leslie, K., & Wick, M. (2018). *Practical pulmonary pathology: a diagnostic approach* (3rd ed.). Elsevier.)

differential diagnosis list. The patient's age would make certain systemic vasculitides (i.e., giant cell arteritis, Takayasu's arteritis, IgA vasculitis) less likely. A careful history and physical examination would be crucial in helping to differentiate these diagnoses (e.g., sinusitis could be a feature of granulomatosis with polyangiitis). Although ANCA studies would be helpful in diagnosing one of the ANCA-associated vasculitides, it is imperative to note that a negative ANCA does not necessarily rule out these diagnoses and an ANCA-associated vasculitis can still be diagnosed in the correct clinical scenario with negative antibody studies.

Diagnosis: HCV-associated cryoglobulinemic vasculitis.

BASIC SCIENCE/CLINICAL PEARL **STEP 1/2/3**

Cryoglobulins are immunoglobulins or immunoglobulin complexes that precipitate at temperatures less than 37°C. They cause pathologic findings by hyperviscosity and immune complex deposition leading to complement fixation and vascular inflammation. Underlying etiologies including infections, inflammatory diseases, and malignancies.

How do you classify cryoglobulins?

Cryoglobulins can be classified into three types as noted in Table 31.4.

What are the clinical and laboratory features of cryoglobulinemic vasculitis?

Cryoglobulinemic vasculitis is seen most commonly in middle-aged women. About 50% of hepatitis C (HCV) patients will have positive cryoglobulin, but of these only 5%–10% develop vasculitis. Patients with hepatitis B, human immunodeficiency virus (HIV), or other autoimmune diseases can also have positive cryoglobulin without the development of vasculitis.

Cryoglobulins must be present for the diagnosis of cryoglobulinemic vasculitis. Other laboratory features include low C4 with normal to mildly decreased C3. Approximately two-thirds of patients will have elevated RF levels. Other nonspecific laboratory features indicative of chronic inflammation may also be seen, such as elevated inflammatory markers (i.e., ESR and CRP), leukocytosis, thrombocytosis, and normocytic anemia.

The clinical features associated with cryoglobulinemic vasculitis are caused by vasculitic involvement of organs. The most common presenting features are palpable purpura, arthralgia or arthritis, and weakness. Additional clinical features of cryoglobulinemic vasculitis are summarized in Table 31.5.

TABLE 31.4 ■ **Cryoglobulin Classification Groups**

Classification	Immunoglobulin Type	Association
Type 1	Single monoclonal immunoglobulin (most commonly IgM)	B cell proliferative disorders (e.g., multiple myeloma, Waldenström's macroglobulinemia)
Type II	Monoclonal IgM or IgG or IgA) and polyclonal Ig	Hepatitis C (80%–98% of cases) Less commonly associated with hepatitis B and human immunodeficiency virus (HIV)
Type III	Polyclonal IgG and polyclonal IgM	Autoimmune diseases (e.g., lupus, Sjögren's syndrome Hepatitis C Lymphoproliferative diseases

TABLE 31.5 ■ **Clinical Features of Cryoglobulinemic Vasculitis**

Organ/System	Frequency	Manifestations
Dermatologic	Common	Pruritic macules and papules Acrocyanosis Skin necrosis Skin ulcers Livedo reticularis
Musculoskeletal	Common	Arthralgia Raynaud's phenomenon
Renal	20%–40%	Hematuria Proteinuria
Neurologic	50%–80%	Peripheral neuropathy
Pulmonary	Rare	Interstitial lung disease Alveolar hemorrhage
Hyperviscosity	Rare	Headaches Transient ischemic attack Chest pain Heart failure
Other	Common	Fatigue Malaise

CLINICAL PEARL **STEP 2/3**

Raynaud phenomenon (RP) is characterized by fingers or toes that change color in the cold or with stress (most commonly, white, blue, and then red). It is caused by vasoconstriction of the digital arteries, causing impaired blood flow to the affected extremity. RP can be considered primary if the symptoms occur alone without an underlying disorder or secondary if there is an underlying disorder. Many autoimmune rheumatic disorders (e.g., scleroderma, systemic lupus erythematosus, vasculitis) can cause secondary RP.

The patient receives prednisone 1 mg/kg daily as the initial therapy. She is also given IV rituximab for remission induction of cryoglobulinemic vasculitis. After the first 2 months of steroid therapy, hepatitis C treatment is initiated and completed with 12 weeks of sofosbuvir-velpatasvir. The patient has sustained virologic response with viral load reported as undetectable.

How do you approach the treatment for cryoglobulinemic vasculitis?

Treatment for cryoglobulinemic vasculitis has two primary objectives: treatment of the underlying disease and immunosuppressive therapy. In patients with an underlying infection, antiviral therapy should be initiated with the ongoing immunosuppressive therapy. In patients with more severe disease, rituximab along with tapering doses of steroids is indicated. Patients presenting with organ-threatening manifestations of their disease (e.g., severe glomerulonephritis, alveolar hemorrhage) may require very high doses of steroids (e.g., "pulse" dose methylprednisolone 1000 mg for 3 days) and plasmapheresis followed by rituximab therapy. Plasmapheresis can be effective in removing the viral particles and cryoprecipitating proteins. Cyclophosphamide is an option for refractory patients but tends to have more adverse effects.

BASIC SCIENCE/CLINICAL PEARL **STEP 1/2/3**

Rituximab is a monoclonal antibody directed against the protein CD20, which is found on the surface of B cells. It is used in the treatment of certain autoimmune diseases and malignancies. Notable side effects include infusion reaction, reactivation of hepatitis B in previously infected patients, progressive multifocal leukoencephalopathy, and toxic epidermal necrosis.

CLINICAL PEARL **STEP 2/3**

Cyclophosphamide is used to treat certain autoimmune diseases and malignancies. It is a teratogenic. Other adverse drug reactions include nausea and vomiting, bone marrow suppression, cytopenia, infection, hemorrhagic cystitis, and cancer. The risk of bladder bleeding can be decreased with adequate fluid intake, intravenous administration of cyclophosphamide instead of oral use, and the use of mesna (2-mercaptoethanesulfonic acid).

After 6 months of being on tapering doses, prednisone was discontinued. The patient's symptoms resolved and there was no further recurrence of the petechial rash.

Case Summary

- **Complaint/History:** A 46-year-old female presents with a 4-month history of fatigue, weakness, and arthralgia and a 2-week history of bilateral lower extremity palpable purpura.
- **Findings:** Examination reveals purpuric macules and papules on the bilateral lower extremities and symmetric polyarthralgia.
- **Lab Results/Tests:** Lab tests reveal leukocytosis, thrombocytosis, elevated erythrocyte sedimentation rate of 90 mm/h, positive hepatitis C viral load, low C4, positive RF, and positive cryoglobulin. Notably, c-ANCA/PR3 and p-ANCA/MPO antibodies are negative. Urinalysis is normal, indicating no renal involvement. Skin biopsy shows leukocytoclastic vasculitis.

Diagnosis: HCV-associated cryoglobulinemic vasculitis.

- **Treatments:** The patient received prednisone 1 mg/kg daily as the initial therapy. She was also given IV rituximab for remission induction of cryoglobulinemic vasculitis. After the first 2 months of steroid therapy, hepatitis C treatment was initiated and completed with 12 weeks of sofosbuvir-velpatasvir. The patient had sustained virologic response with viral load reported as undetectable. After 6 months of being on tapering doses, prednisone was discontinued. The patient's symptoms resolved and there was no further recurrence of the petechial rash.

BEYOND THE PEARLS

- In patients with type 1 (monoclonal) cryoglobulin, treatment is directed toward the underlying malignancy and aimed at reducing the risk of hyperviscosity syndrome. The latter can be achieved with prompt plasmapheresis to remove the circulating IgM.
- Many medications can cause a drug-induced ANCA-associated vasculitis. The most common medications implicated are propylthiouracil, minocycline, allopurinol, D-penicillamine, hydralazine, sulfasalazine, penicillins, and cephalosporins. Treatment includes withdrawal of the offending agent.
- In the absence of vasculitis, ANCA can be positive in many other rheumatic disorders (e.g., lupus, scleroderma, reactive arthritis), autoimmune gastrointestinal disorders (e.g., ulcerative colitis and Crohn's disease), cystic fibrosis, and subacute bacterial endocarditis. In most of these cases, the immunofluorescence pattern is often p-ANCA or atypical ANCA.
- Patients with vasculitis and other autoimmune diseases often have prolonged exposure to glucocorticoids. These patients should be routinely monitored for common adverse effects of glucocorticoid use including osteoporosis, infection, hyperglycemia, and cataracts/glaucoma.
- In cryoglobulinemic vasculitis, mean survival is 70% at 10 years after the onset of symptoms. The most common causes of death are infection and cardiovascular disease. Poor prognostic markers include renal failure and the development of a lymphoproliferative disorder.

Bibliography

Damoiseaux, J. (2014). The diagnosis and classification of the cryoglobulinemic syndrome. *Autoimmunity reviews*, *13*(4-5), 359–362.

Ghetie, D., Mehraban, N., & Sibley, C. H. (2015). Cold hard facts of cryoglobulinemia: updates on clinical features and treatment advances. *Rheumatic Diseases Clinics of North America*, *41*(1), 93-108, viii-ix.

Jennette, J. C., Falk, R. J., Bacon, P. A., Basu, N., Cid, M. C., Ferrario, F., … Watts, R. A. (2013). 2012 revised International Chapel Hill Consensus Conference Nomenclature of Vasculitides. *Arthritis and Rheumatism*, *65*(1), 1–11.

Radice, A., Bianchi, L., & Sinico, R. A. (2013). Anti-neutrophil cytoplasmic autoantibodies: Methodological aspects and clinical significance in systemic vasculitis. *Autoimmunity reviews*, *12*(4), 487–495.

Reamy, B. V., Williams, P. M., & Lindsay, T. J. (2009). Henoch-Schönlein purpura. *American Family Physician*, *80*(7), 697–704.

Roane, D. W., & Griger, D. R. (1999). An approach to diagnosis and initial management of systemic vasculitis. *American Family Physician*, *60*(5), 1421–1430.

Stevens, G. L., Adelman, H. M., & Wallach, P. M. (1995). Palpable purpura: an algorithmic approach. *American Family Physician*, *52*(5), 1355–1362.

Walport, M. J. (2001). Complement. First of two parts. *The New England Journal of Medicine*, *344*(14), 1058–1066.

CASE 32

A 65-Year-Old Male With Acute Monoarticular Arthritis

Noopur Goel ■ Sophia Li

A 65-year-old male presents to your clinic with severe right wrist pain and swelling for the previous 5 days. His past medical history is significant for diabetes mellitus managed with metformin and hypertension managed with diet and exercise alone. He works as a plumber and the wrist pain is limiting his work. He tried over-the-counter acetaminophen for pain but the medication helps minimally. He denies any known triggers or recent trauma to his wrist. The patient reports occasional pain in his hands, knees, and feet after work but states the wrist pain is different from his previous pain. His wife reports a similar episode of pain and swelling 7 months ago affecting the left wrist that resolved spontaneously after a few days.

On physical examination, swelling and tenderness is noted over the dorsal aspect of the right wrist. There is mild erythema and warmth. Range of motion is restricted secondary to pain. The rest of his joint examination is normal.

How does the history help narrow down your differential diagnosis?

The differential diagnosis for joint pain can be narrowed down based on onset of symptoms, pattern of joint involvement, duration of symptoms, and absence or presence of morning stiffness. A thorough history will help differentiate inflammatory from noninflammatory arthritis or other causes. Sudden onset of symptoms is typically seen in crystal arthritis, infectious arthritis, and trauma-related arthritis whereas gradual onset of symptoms is typically seen in osteoarthritis, rheumatoid arthritis, psoriatic arthritis, and ankylosing spondylitis. In a patient with acute, monoarticular arthritis, septic arthritis must be ruled out.

Which physical examination findings help narrow down the differential diagnosis in this patient?

Physical examination findings such as swelling, warmth, and erythema of the overlying skin point toward the presence of an inflammatory arthritis. In noninflammatory arthritis, pain and restricted range of motion are the most common features. Nodules can be seen in patients with rheumatoid arthritis commonly on the extensor surfaces. Tophi are pathognomic for gout.

CLINICAL PEARL **STEP 2/3**

Fever is not specific to septic arthritis and can also be seen in crystal arthritis.

When should a synovial fluid analysis be performed?

Aspiration and microscopic examination of the synovial fluid is the gold standard in diagnosis of crystal arthritis. Synovial fluid should always be sent for Gram stain, culture, cell count, and crystal analysis prior to initiation of treatment. In a patient with new onset joint swelling or worsening of previously controlled inflammatory arthritis, it is important to perform an arthrocentesis to rule out an underlying infection.

> Blood-tinged synovial fluid (5 ml) is aspirated from the patient's wrist joint. Laboratory analysis reveals synovial fluid leukocyte count is 20,000 (85% polymorphonuclear cells) with 13 red blood cells (RBCs) and 2 lymphocytes. Gram stain is negative for bacteria. Synovial fluid culture results are pending. Polarized light microscopy reveals several rod-shaped weakly positive birefringent intracellular and extracellular crystals.
>
> Diagnosis: Acute calcium pyrophosphate dihydrate crystal deposition disease (CPPD) arthritis or "pseudogout."

Why is it called "pseudogout"?

The condition is termed "pseudogout" because the clinical presentation is similar to that of an acute gout attack. Patients can present with sudden onset pain, swelling, and erythema of the affected joint. CPPD commonly affects the knees, wrists, shoulders, hips, and elbows. Overlying erythema is less marked compared with gout. Patients will often complain of severe pain to the extent of impaired mobility of the affected joints. Symptoms can last up to 2 or 3 weeks before spontaneous resolution. Patients are asymptomatic between attacks. Chronic CPPD arthritis can mimic rheumatoid arthritis and present as a symmetrical arthritis affecting the small joints of the hands (see Fig. 32.1).

What differentiates gout from pseudogout?

Calcium pyrophosphate deposition (CPPD) crystals are composed of calcium and are rod/rhomboid shaped, negatively or weakly birefringent under polarized light microscopy. Gout crystals are composed of uric acid and are needle shaped, negatively birefringent under polarized light microscopy.

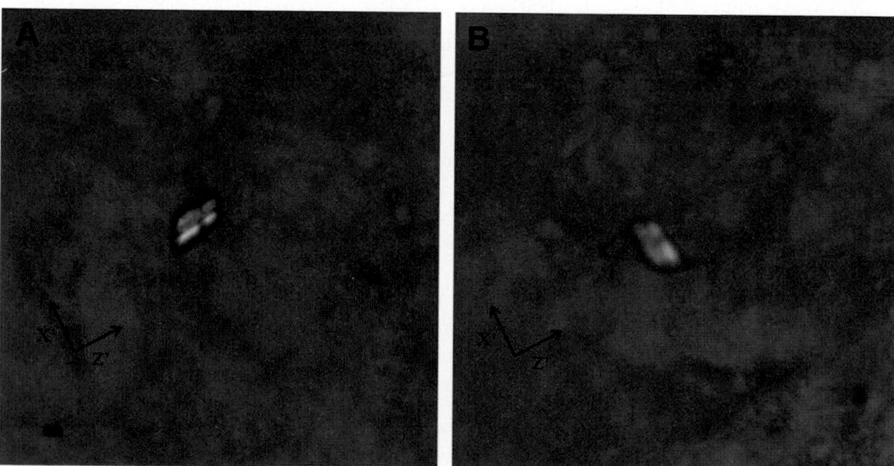

Fig. 32.1 Compensated polarizing light microscopic finding of CPPD crystal. (From Ryu, K., Iriuchishima, T., Oshia, M., Kato, Y., Saito, A., Imada, M., Aizawa, S., Tokuhashi, Y., & Ryu, J. (2014). *Osteoarthritis and Cartilage*, 22, (7), 975–979.)

TABLE 32.1 ■ **Synovial Fluid Analysis**

Synovial Fluid	Gout	Gout/Pseudogout	Septic Arthritis
WBC count	2000–20,000/mm^3	2000–20,000/mm^3	>20,000/mm^3
Crystals	Uric acid: needle shaped, negatively birefringent	Calcium pyrophosphate dihydrate, rod/rhomboid shaped, positive birefringence	Negative
Gram stain/ culture	Negative	Negative	Positive

WBC, White Blood Cells

What is inflammatory versus noninflammatory synovial fluid?

Synovial fluid is normally clear yellow and moderately viscous. Drops of synovial fluid at the tip of a syringe will form a string a few inches long before breaking off. Gross appearance of synovial fluid in crystal arthritis tends to be turbid and occasionally blood tinged. Turbidity increases as the synovial fluid white count increases.

Table 32.1 shows the difference between synovial fluid findings in inflammatory and noninflammatory arthritis.

CLINICAL PEARL **STEP 2/3**

Crystal arthritis and septic arthritis may coexist; therefore, it is important to send synovial fluid for cell count, crystal analysis, Gram stain, and culture, especially in cases of monoarticular arthritis.

Which conditions are commonly associated with CPPD?

CPPD is more common with advancing age; it is rarely seen in patients younger than 60 years of age. There is no gender predominance. There is strong evidence of association with metabolic diseases such as hyperparathyroidism, hemochromatosis, hypomagnesemia, and hypophosphatasia. Therefore, workup for secondary causes of CPPD includes testing for serum magnesium, calcium, phosphorus, iron levels, and parathyroid hormone. Situations that may trigger CPPD arthritis include direct trauma to the joint, medical illness, surgery (parathyroidectomy), blood transfusion, and joint lavage.

CLINICAL PEARL **STEP 2/3**

Metabolic or familial predisposition should particularly be considered in younger patients (<55 years) and if there is florid polyarticular chondrocalcinosis.

CLINICAL PEARL **STEP 2/3**

Hereditary hemochromatosis arthropathy can continue to develop even after initiation of phlebotomy.

Which radiologic findings can be seen in a patient with crystal arthritis?

Calcium crystals build up in the fibrocartilage and hyaline cartilage in CPPD, known as chondrocalcinosis. It is seen as thick linear deposits parallel to and separate from the bone surface on

X-ray imaging. This is especially seen in the knee menisci, wrist triangular fibrocartilage, symphysis pubis, and hip labrum. Computed tomography is useful in evaluating CPPD of the spine. Ultrasound can demonstrate CPPD in hyaline and fibrocartilage and around tendons. CPPD appears as linear hyperechoic deposits within the hyaline articular cartilage and as rounded/amorphous deposits in fibrocartilage.

In contrast, uric acid crystals deposited in gout appear as linear hyperechoic deposits on the surface of hyaline articular cartilage. X-ray imaging in gout will show characteristic articular surface erosions with overhanging edges. Tophi may be seen as cloudy hyperlucent deposits in and around the synovial tissue (see Fig. 32.2).

CLINICAL PEARL **STEP 2/3**

The joints most frequently affected by chondrocalcinosis are knees, wrists, hips, symphysis pubis, and metacarpophalangeal joints in descending order.

CLINICAL PEARL **STEP 2/3**

Currently, there is no treatment that modifies calcium pyrophosphate dihydrate crystal formation or dissolution and no treatment is required for asymptomatic chondrocalcinosis (CC).

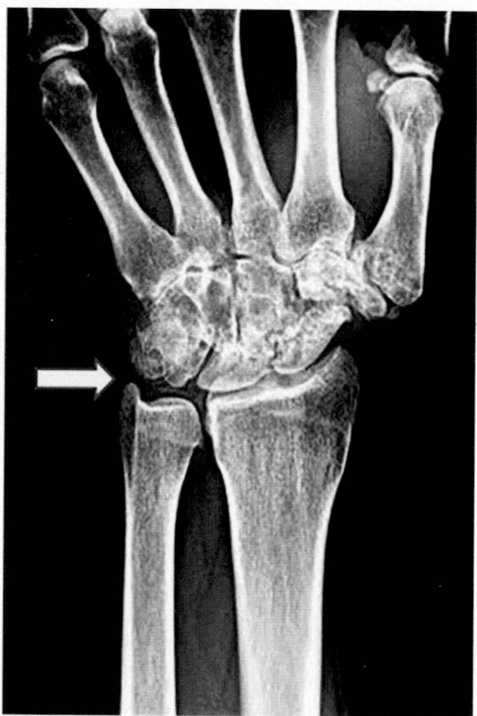

Fig. 32.2 Wrist radiograph of an affected patient showing chondrocalcinosis *(arrow)*. From Ryu, K., Iriuchishima, T., Oshia, M., Kato, Y., Saito, A., Imada, M., Aizawa, S., Tokuhashi, Y., & Ryu, J. (2014). The prevalence of and factors related to calcium pyrophosphate dihydrate crystal deposition in the knee joint. *Osteoarthritis and Cartilage, 22*(7), 975–979.;Williams, C. J., Qazi, U., Bernstein, M., Charmiak, A., Gohr C., Mittlon-Fitzgerald, E., Ortiz, A., Cardinal, L., Kaell, A.T., & Rosenthal, A. K. (2018). Mutations in osteoprotegerin account for the CCAL1 locus in calcium pyrophosphate deposition disease. *Osteoarthritis and Cartilage, 26*(6), 797–806.

How do you approach management of CPPD?

Management of CPPD arthritis depends on the acuity and number of joints involved. In an acute flare with only one or two joints involved, joint aspiration and intraarticular glucocorticoid administration is the treatment of choice, unless contraindicated. Systemic treatment is preferred with involvement of more than two joints. Options include nonsteroidal antiinflammatory drugs (NSAIDs), colchicine, or systemic oral glucocorticoids. Rest, application of ice, and non-weight-bearing of affected joints are also advised until symptoms disappear. IL-1 inhibitors can also be effective, although they have not yet been approved by the FDA.

CLINICAL PEARL **STEP 2/3**

The most common side effect of colchicine is diarrhea. Given similar efficacy and a lower risk of adverse effects, low-dose colchicine is preferable to high-dose colchicine.

The patient receives an intraarticular glucocorticoid injection. His symptoms resolve the next day and he is able to restart work. Eight weeks later he revisits your office, complaining of repeat episodes of pain and swelling in bilateral wrists. He has experienced two similar episodes since his last clinic visit. You clinically suspect CPPD flare and prescribe oral NSAIDs.

How can recurrence of CPPD flares be prevented?

In patients with recurrent symptoms, oral NSAIDs and/or low-dose colchicine can be used in prevention of future attacks. Low-dose corticosteroids are another option to consider in patients who continue to suffer flares. Hydroxychloroquine (HCQ) is a common antirheumatic agent used with some success in patients resistant to NSAIDs, colchicine, or steroids. Typically, treatment requires administration of HCQ for 6 months or longer to demonstrate efficacy.

Case Summary

- **Complaint/History:** A 65-year-old male presents with a 5-day history of sudden onset right wrist pain and swelling.
- **Findings:** Examination reveals swelling and tenderness of the right wrist with decreased range of motion.
- **Lab Results/Tests:** Synovial fluid analysis shows leukocytosis, with elevated neutrophils and weakly positive birefringent crystals on polarizing microscopy.

Diagnosis: Calcium pyrophosphate crystal deposition disease.

- **Treatments:** The patient received an intraarticular glucocorticoid injection. After 24 hours, his symptoms disappeared and he was completely pain free after 48 hours. Given recurrent episodes, he was treated with daily colchicine. The patient continued to be asymptomatic at the next follow-up visit 6 months later.

BEYOND THE PEARLS

- Periodontoid deposition of CPPD crystals can lead to crowned dens syndrome. It presents with severe neck pain, stiffness, and atlantoaxial synovial calcification. It can be misdiagnosed as meningitis unless there is a high degree of clinical suspicion. CT scan is the gold standard for visualizing ligamentous calcifications in crowned dens syndrome.
- Enhanced production or decreased removal of inorganic pyrophosphate (PPi) in the cartilage leads to binding with calcium and precipitation of excess PPi in the joint tissue, which is a key determinant for CPP crystal formation.

- CPP crystals elicit formation of the NOD-like receptor pyrin domain containing 3 (NLRP3) inflammasome. This triggers caspase-1 activation and the initiation of an inflammatory cascade, including release of IL-1 and IL-18.
- Mutations in the ankylosis human (*ANKH*) gene are a cause of some cases of familial CPPD.
- Use of cytochrome P450 (CYP450) 3A4 inhibitors such as clarithromycin concurrently with colchicine can lead to life-threatening bone marrow toxicity.

Bibliography

Abhishek, A., & Doherty, M. (2016). Update on calcium pyrophosphate deposition. *Clinical and Experimental Rheumatology*, *34*(4 Suppl 98), S32–S38.

Hochberg, M., Silman, A., Smolen, J., Weinblatt, M., & Weisman, M. (2016). Calcium pyrophosphate crystal associated arthropathy. *Rheumatology*, *6*(2), 1584–1593.

Iqbal, S. M., Qadir, S., Aslam, H. M., & Qadir, M. A. (2019). Updated treatment for calcium pyrophosphate deposition disease: an insight. *Cureus*, *11*(1), e3840.

Zamora, E. A., & Naik, R. (2019 Jann). *Calcium pyrophosphate deposition disease* (CPDD): *StatPearls [Internet]*. Treasure Island (FL): StatPearls Publishing.

CASE 33

A 22-Year-Old Female With Easy Bruising, Joint Hypermobility, and Arthralgia

Patil Injean ■ Christina Downey

A 22-year-old female presents to the clinic with pain in multiple joints including hands, knees, and elbows bilaterally. She has been experiencing the pain on and off since her teenage years. However, the pain has been more bothersome and has occurred every day for the last few months. She states she has always been "double jointed" since she was a child. Her past medical history is significant for shoulder dislocation while holding a strap hanger on a subway. She states she has anxiety surrounding shoulder movement because of constant fear of instability and dislocation. Family history includes a mother with similar symptoms. There is no family history of autoimmune disease or sudden death.

On physical examination, vital signs are normal. Skin has multiple bruises in extremities, scarring of skin particularly over joint surfaces, and a few scattered open wounds. In addition, the patient's skin is hyperextensive. Joint exam does not reveal erythema, warmth, or swelling. There is mild tenderness in the knees bilaterally. She exhibits hypermobility in the first and fifth digits of her hands, elbows, and knees bilaterally where she primarily feels joint pain without any swelling. She has preserved range of motion in all joints. Active range of motion of shoulders is inhibited secondary to fear of dislocation. Passive range of motion is met with voluntary resistance.

What are some causes of polyarticular pain?

Pain in multiple joints is a commonly encountered complaint in the outpatient setting. Important elements of the history when evaluating joint pain include symmetry, whether the pain is better or worse with movement, swelling of joints, and age when symptoms began. There are many potential causes for polyarticular pain including rheumatoid arthritis, connective tissue diseases, osteoarthritis, infections, and psoriatic arthritis. A summary of these conditions is highlighted in Table 33.1.

Many causes of polyarticular pain can be associated with joint swelling, joint stiffness, and limited range of motion resulting from pain. Additionally, patients often report unintended weight loss, fevers, and fatigue. Polyarticular pain can also be associated with hypermobility of joints because of repetitive microtrauma of dislocations and ligament and tendon injuries without systemic features.

CLINICAL PEARL **STEP 2/3**

Inflammatory arthritis will cause pain that is worse upon waking and after rest and better with activity. Joints involved may be swollen or, tender on examination, or show periarticular osteopenia or erosions on radiographs. There is associated morning stiffness, which is often associated with fatigue, unintended weight loss, and fevers, and blood inflammatory markers are elevated. If any of these are present, an inflammatory arthritis workup should be initiated.

TABLE 33.1 ■ **Differential Diagnosis for Joint or Extremity Pain**

Rheumatologic	JIA; SLE; juvenile dermatomyositis; polyarteritis; scleroderma; Sjögren syndrome; Behçet disease; granulomatosis with polyangiitis; sarcoidosis; HSP; chronic recurrent multifocal osteomyelitis; juvenile ankylosing spondylitis; psoriatic arthritis
Infectious	Bacterial: *Staphylococcus aureus, Streptococcus pneumoniae, Neisseria gonorrhoeae, Haemophilus influenzae* Viral: parvovirus, rubella, mumps, EBV, hepatitis B fungal Other: spirochetes, mycobacterial, endocarditis, Lyme
Immunodeficiencies	Hypogammaglobulinemia; IgA deficiency; HIV
Congenital and metabolic	Gout and pseudogout; mucopolysaccharidoses; hypothyroidism or hyperthyroidism; vitamin C or D deficiency; connective tissue disease; lysosomal storage diseases: Fabry and Farber diseases; familial Mediterranean fever
Bone and cartilage	Trauma; patellofemoral syndrome; osteochondritis dissecans and avascular necrosis; SCFE; hypertrophic osteoarthropathy
Inflammatory and reactive	Kawasaki syndrome; IBD; acute rheumatic fever; reactive arthritis; toxic synovitis; serum sickness
Neurologic and pain syndromes	Peripheral neuropathy; carpal tunnel syndrome; Charcot joints; fibromyalgia; depression with somatization; reflex sympathetic dystrophy
Neoplastic	Leukemia and lymphoma; neuroblastoma; histiocytosis; synovial tumors Bone tumors: osteosarcoma, Ewing sarcoma, osteoid osteoma

EBV, Epstein-Barr virus; *HIV*, human immunodeficiency virus; *HSP*, Henoch-Schönlein purpura; *IBD*, inflammatory bowel disease; *IgA*, immunoglobulin A; *JIA*, juvenile idiopathic arthritis; *SCFE*, slipped capital femoral epiphysis; *SLE*, systemic lupus erythematosus.

Modified from Kliegman, R. M., Stanton, B. F., St. Geme, J. W., Schor, N., & Behrman, R. (2011). *Nelson textbook of pediatrics* (19th ed.). Philadelphia: Elsevier.

In this particular patient, no joint swelling was exhibited. Her active and passive range of motion were preserved. She did not complain of joint swelling or morning stiffness. Her joints did exhibit hypermobility. A C-reactive protein level was <0.03 and an erythrocyte sedimentation rate was 8, making inflammatory arthritis very unlikely. Radiographs of the affected joints were normal.

What is the best way to evaluate this patient's hypermobility?

The Beighton score is an easily reproducible and reliable way to determine joint hypermobility (see Table 33.2 and Figs. 33.1 and 33.2). The test evaluates the range of motion of the first and fifth digits, elbows, knees, and spine. A point is added for every joint that exceeds the normal range of motion. A score greater than 4 is a sign that there is generalized joint hypermobility. A positive Beighton score is defined as >6 in prepubertal children, >5 in postpubertal individuals, and >4 in patients older than 50. The International Classification of the Ehlers-Danlos Syndromes recognizes the Beighton score to determine hypermobility in the diagnosis of EDS.

This patient had hypermobility in her thumb and fifth digit, elbows, and knees bilaterally where she primarily felt joint pain without any swelling, giving her a Beighton score of 8.

What is the best way to elicit the cause of this patient's joint hypermobility?

A carefully obtained history of previous injuries, fractures, dislocations, and level of activity will help narrow down the differential diagnosis. A detailed family history can help identify any

TABLE 33.2 ■ **The Nine-Point Beighton Hypermobility Score**

The Ability to:	Right	Left
1. Passively dorsiflex the fifth metacarpophalangeal joint to ≥90 degrees	1	1
2. Oppose the thenar aspect of the thumb to the volar aspect of the ipsilateral forearm	1	1
3. Hyperextend the elbow to ≥10 degrees	1	1
4. Hyperextend the knee to ≥10 degrees	1	1
5. Place hands flat on the floor without bending the knees	1	

One point may be gained for each side for maneuvers 1–4, so the hypermobility score will have a maximum of 9 points if all are positive.
Hakim, A., & Grahame, R. (2003). Joint hypermobility. *Best Practice and Research in Clinical Rheumatology, 17*, 989–1004 (Table 1).

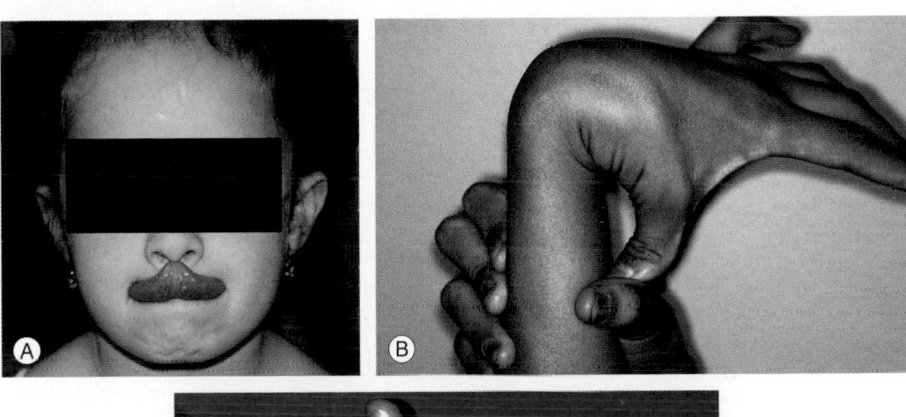

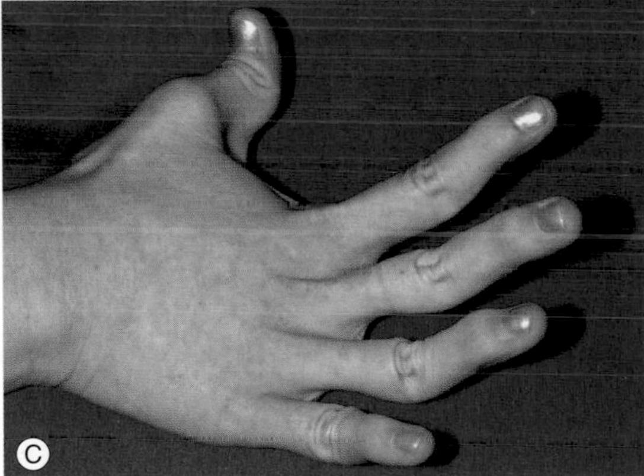

Fig. 33.1 (A) Ehlers–Danlos syndrome (EDS). Gorlin sign is five times more common in EDS than in normal individuals. Note the scars on the forehead. (B) Despite joint hyperextensibility, this patient does not meet Beighton score criteria for the extreme hypermobility seen with hypermobile EDS. (C) EDS. Hyperextensible joints may result in double-jointed fingers, as seen in this girl. (From A and C Paller, A. S., & Mancini, A. J. (2022). *Hurwitz clinical pediatric dermatology: a textbook of skin disorders of childhood and adolescence* (6th ed.). Elsevier; (B) Wilson, K. M., et al. (2020). In R. M. Kliegman, & J. W. St. Geme (Eds.), *Nelson textbook of pediatrics* (21st ed.). Elsevier.)

1. Passive dorsiflexion of the fifth metacarpophalangeal joint. Score is positive if ≥ 90°

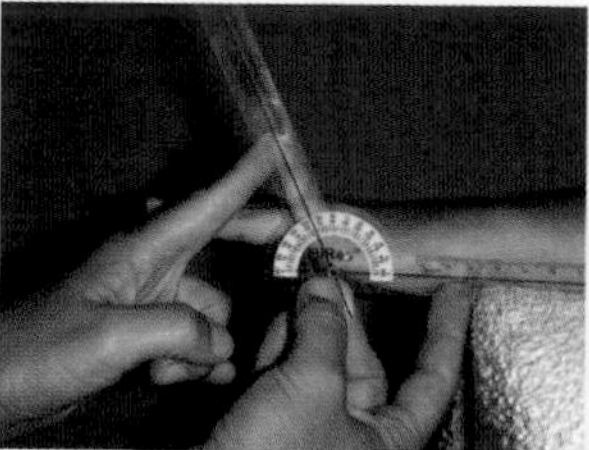

4. Passive apposition of the thumb to the flexor side of the forearm, while shoulder is 90° flexed, elbow extended and hand pronated. Score is positive if the whole thumb touches the flexor side of the forearm.

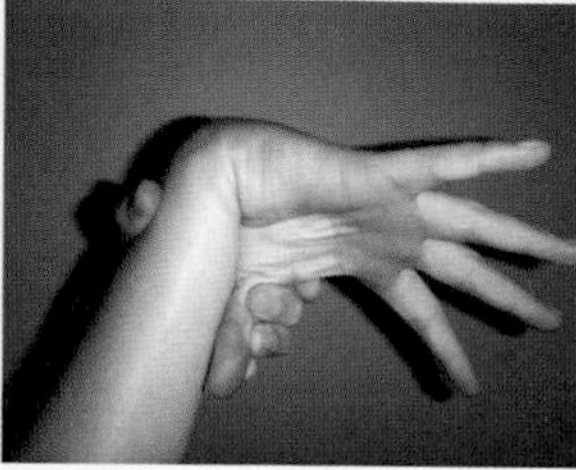

Score: Positive

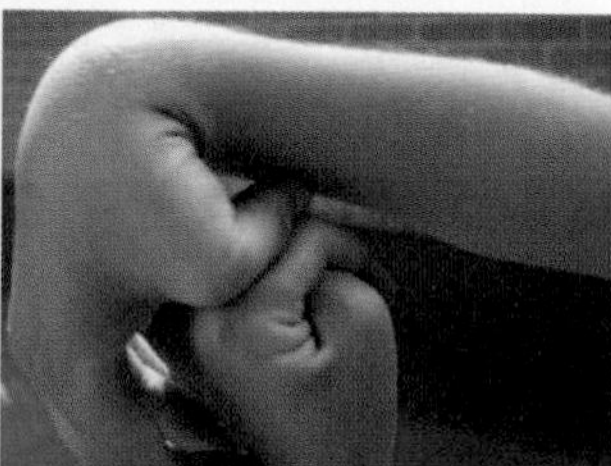

Score: Negative

2. Passive hyperextension of the elbow. Score is positive if ≥ 10°

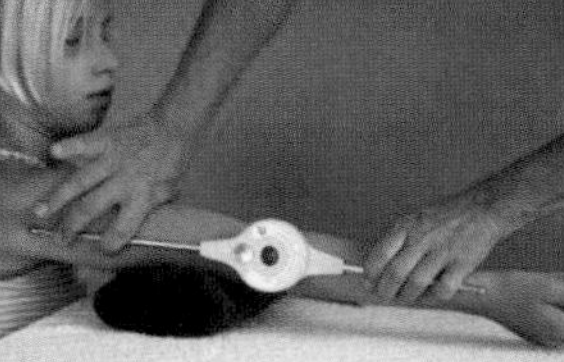

5. Forward flexion of the trunk, with the knees straight. Score is positive if the hand palms rest easily on the floor.

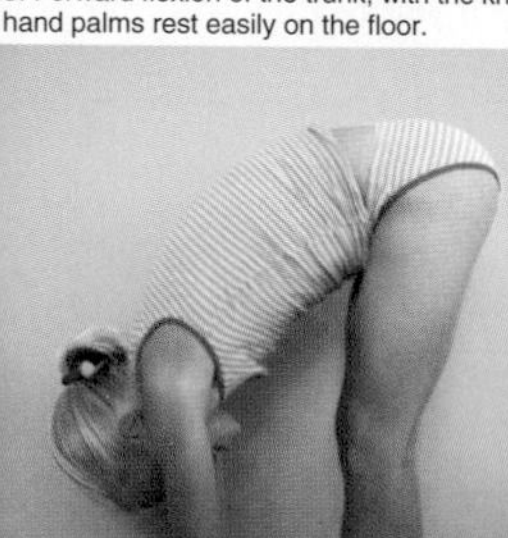

3. Passive hyperextension of the knee. Score is positive if ≥ 10°

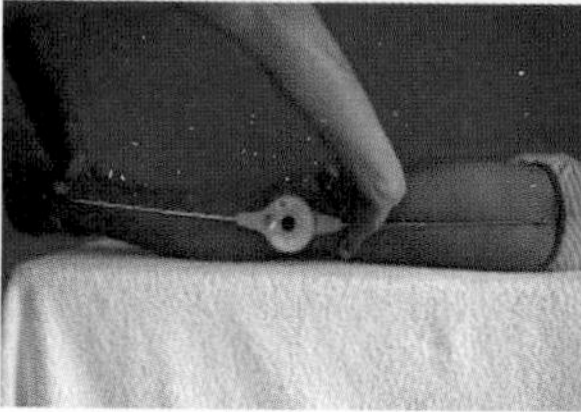

*Males positive if > 180° for measure 2. and 3.

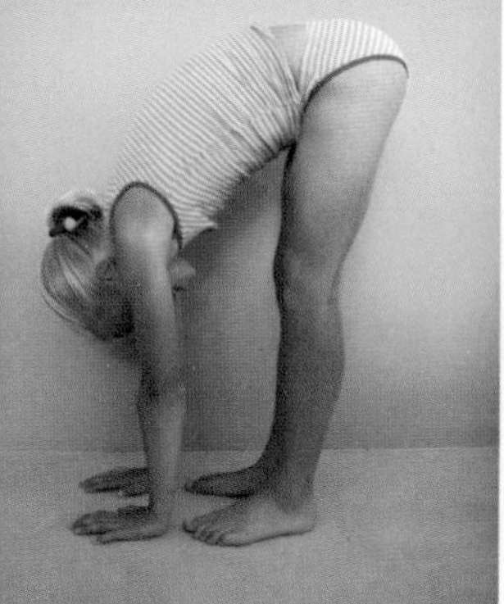

Score: Positive

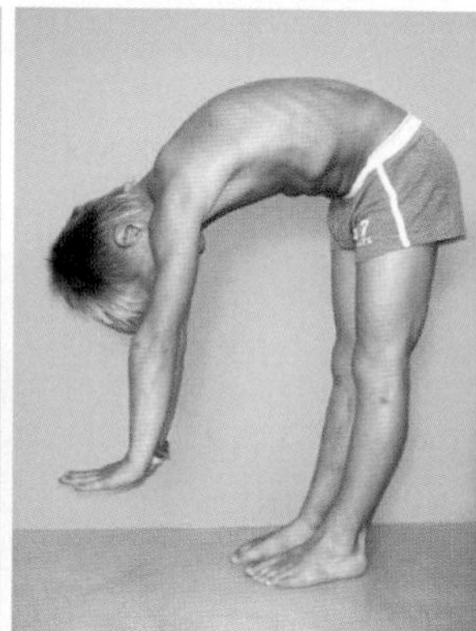

Score: Negative

Fig. 33.2 Beighton score. The range of motion of several key small and large joints is measured to provide an overview of joint hypermobility. Instability is not assessed. Scoring: 2 points for each bilateral measure in nos. 1 to 4 and 1 point for no. 5, equaling a total possible score of 9. Hypermobility is considered significant with a score of ≥6 between the ages of 6 and 35 years. (From Wilson, K. M., et al. (2020). In R. M. Kliegman, & J. W. St. Geme (Eds.), *Nelson textbook of pediatrics* (21st ed.). Elsevier.)

inheritance patterns of hypermobility, fractures, or skin scarring. A detailed physical examination is needed to evaluate the patient's skin, joints, and other organ systems that can be affected by collagen malformation.

Radiographs of joints and bones assess for fractures, bone mineralization defects, or signs of arthritis. Generally, radiographs are normal in patients with Ehlers-Danlos syndrome (EDS); however, this is a cost-effective method of eliminating other diagnoses as a source of the pain.

The history of low trauma shoulder dislocation and family history of hypermobility point toward an inherited cause of joint hypermobility. Hyperextensible skin points toward a collagen disorder.

What is your differential diagnosis?

Osteogenesis imperfecta is a heterogenous heritable connective tissue disorder of type I collagen. It can present with different phenotypes. Patients usually present with a history of multiple fractures secondary to minimal trauma. Clinical manifestations include brittle bones, blue sclerae, basilar skull deformities, hearing loss, intrasutural bones, and easy bruisability. Patients usually present with hypercalciuria and elevated alkaline phosphatase caused by irregular bone mineralization. There is no definitive test to diagnose osteogenesis imperfecta.

Marfan's syndrome is an autosomal dominant connective tissue disease resulting from a mutation in the fibrillin-1 gene that may present with variable severity. Patients may present with arachnodactyly, dolichostenomelia (unusually long limbs), increased skin stretching, pectus deformity, and/or aortic root dilation. The Ghent nosology can be used to diagnose Marfan's syndrome. The classification system assigns points based on specific clinical features with the most emphasis placed on aortic root dilation and ectopia lentis. Many of the other features included in the systemic score, including joint hypermobility, scoliosis, mitral valve prolapse, and skin striae, are similar to those of EDS.

Loeys-Dietz syndrome is a autosomal dominant mutation of the transforming growth factor-beta receptor (TGFBR) gene. Patients typically present with widely spaced eyes, bifid uvula, cleft palate, vascular aneurysms, dissections, and torturous arteries. In approximately 10% of cases, this mutation can present with features of Marfan's syndrome. Vascular Ehlers-Danlos is also caused by a mutation in the *TGFBR* gene. A specific distinguishing characteristic between the two is patients with Loeys-Dietz syndrome generally have better outcomes with surgical repair of aortic vasculature.

EDSs are rare heritable connective tissue diseases. The syndrome is characterized by joint hypermobility, skin hyperextensibility, and tissue fragility. Most of the mutations are identified in genes encoding collagen, or collagen modifying enzymes.

BASIC SCIENCE/CLINICAL PEARL **STEP 1/2/3**

Marfan's syndrome is an autosomal dominant connective tissue disease caused by a mutation in the fibrillin-1 gene.

Loeys-Dietz syndrome is an autosomal dominant connective tissue disease associated with mutations of the transforming growth factor-beta receptor gene.

Vascular type EDS is a defect in the *COL3A1* gene leading to an abhorrent collagen type III.

How do you establish a diagnosis of EDS?

EDS is primarily a clinical diagnosis because there are no reliable serological tests, imaging, or genetic testing that can confirm the diagnosis. The 2017 International Classification of Ehlers-Danlos Syndromes describes clinical diagnostic criteria. All three diagnostic criteria must be present in order to diagnose hypermobility EDS.

Criteria 1: Joint hypermobility as characterized by the Beighton score

Criteria 2: Two or more features from the following:

Feature A:

1. Unusually soft skin; velvety skin
2. Skin hyperextensibility
3. Striae of back, groins, thighs, breast, abdomen without explanation and without a history of significant weight loss
4. Piezogenic papules (soft, skin-colored papules found on the feet and wrists) of the heel bilaterally
5. Recurrent abdominal hernias
6. Atrophic scarring
7. Uterine, rectal, pelvic floor prolapse in children or nulliparous women without obesity
8. Dental crowding and high or narrow palate
9. Arachnodactyly as defined in one or more of the following: (i) positive wrist sign (Steinberg sign) on both sides; (ii) positive thumb sign (Walker sign) on both sides
10. Arm span-to-height >1.05

11. Mitral valve prolapse based on echocardiograph
12. Aortic root dilation with Z-score >+2

Feature B: A family history of first-degree relatives meeting diagnostic criteria for EDS

Feature C: Musculoskeletal complications that includes at least one of the following:

1. Daily musculoskeletal pain for at least 3 months in two or more limbs
2. Chronic pain for ≥3 months
3. Atraumatic recurrent joint dislocations or joint instability

Criteria 3: All must be present.

1. Absence of unusual skin fragility
2. Exclusion of other connective tissue diseases
3. Exclusion of other causes of joint hypermobility

This patient meets all three criteria.

CLINICAL PEARL **STEP 2/3**

EDS is a clinical diagnosis, meaning there are no tests to confirm the diagnosis. There is genetic heterogeneity in this syndrome and genetic testing is not required to make a diagnosis, though a careful family history may aid in diagnosis.

What are the different subtypes of EDS?

The Villefranche nosology currently identifies six different types of EDS based on inheritance pattern and phenotype.

- Type I or II, classic type, is characterized by skin hyperextensibility, joint hypermobility, and widened atrophic scarring.
- Hypermobility type II is described as generalized joint hypermobility with only mild skin involvement.
- Vascular type IV is characterized as excessive bruising; thin skin; and arterial, intestinal, or uterine fragility or rupture.
- Kyphoscoliotic type VI has muscular hypotonia, joint laxity, kyphoscoliosis at birth, scleral fragility, and rupture of the ocular globe.
- Athrochalasia type VIIa or VIIb has severe generalized joint hypermobility with subluxations and congenital bilateral hip dislocations.
- Dermatosparaxis type VIIc presents with severe skin fragility; sagging, redundant skin; and excessive bruising.

The 2017 International Classification of Ehlers-Danlos Syndromes identifies 13 subtypes. The different subtypes are summarized in Table 33.3. Identification of the particular subtype in each patient is important because some subtypes have implications for the cardiovascular system and pregnancy outcomes.

This patient experienced easy bruising in addition to hyperextensible skin, a family history of hypermobility, and a positive Beighton score. She should therefore be screened for vascular complications with aortic ultrasound and echocardiogram and she probably has type IV vascular type.

CLINICAL PEARL **STEP 2/3**

EDS is a clinical diagnosis, meaning there are no tests to confirm the diagnosis. There is genetic heterogeneity in this syndrome and genetic testing is not required to make a diagnosis, although a careful family history may aid in reaching a diagnosis.

What are the causes of musculoskeletal pain in patients with EDS?

Chronic joint pain is common in patients with EDS. A majority of pain is secondary to microtrauma caused by dislocations, subluxations, and subsequent soft tissue injury such as ligament, tendon, and muscle damage. Accumulated microtrauma developed from recurring connective tissue damage and impaired healing can be a significant source of chronic pain.

Chronic pain can begin as early as childhood, following acute joint trauma.

Patients also complain of growing pains and are described as clumsy. Additionally, they are noted to have decreased proprioception, which leads to secondary musculoskeletal pain. Joint hypermobility may lead to damage of proprioceptive receptors as a result of microscopic injuries from repetitive joint trauma or pain itself leads to a diminished proprioception. Patients with EDS have also been noted to have central sensitization, in which small insults to joints can be experienced as an exorbitant amount of pain similar to patients with fibromyalgia.

Chronic fatigue is another common finding in patients with EDS, which can lead to further debilitation and poor quality of life. Sleep disturbances are commonly present and can lead to worsening chronic pain. Psychological disturbances such as anxiety and depression are also prevalent in this population, probably stemming from psychological trauma of frequent joint dislocations and pain.

This patient experiences chronic joint pain and anxiety related to her condition.

How do you approach treatment?

There are no current guidelines for targeted treatment of joint pain. However, treatment should encompass a multidisciplinary approach. This can be divided into medications, physical therapy, surgery, and psychotherapy.

Pain management can be difficult because there are no medications approved for pain control specifically in patients with EDS, given the limited amount of evidence on this subject. The recommendation is to use nonsteroidal antiinflammatory drugs if pain is suspected to be secondary to inflammation. However, there must always be caution for gastrointestinal and renal adverse effects, in addition to cardiovascular and cerebrovascular health in older patients. Long-term opioid therapy is generally not recommended, although short periods of opioids for acute injuries can be considered with caution.

For neuropathic pain, low-dose tricyclic antidepressant medication, anticonvulsant medication, and selective norepinephrine reuptake inhibitors can be considered. Steroid injections into joints have not shown benefit in EDS-related joint pain. In addition, EDS patients have shown increased resistance to local anesthetic injections. Muscle relaxants have also not shown benefit during routine use and carry the risk of increasing joint instability, and these medications are therefore not recommended.

There is poor quality evidence to support the utility of physical therapy in EDS. The goal of physical therapy is to reduce disability and improve quality of life. Stretching should generally be avoided because of the increased risk of dislocations. EDS patients routinely use splints, braces, and massage therapy for pain management, although there are no data to suggest its efficacy. In 2010, a randomized control trial done in children showed strengthening symptomatic joints improves pain control. Bathen et al. reported that multiple uncontrolled clinical studies have shown core stability exercises can improve pain management. In 2008, a randomized control trial in adults showed improved pain control in the knee with exercises directed at proprioception compared with a control group with no exercise. There is also no evidence that recommends a specific type of exercise.

Well-recognized comorbidities of EDS are psychiatric disorders, insomnia, and fatigue disorders. The international consortium international consortium on the Ehlers–Danlos syndromes

TABLE 33.3 ■ **Ehlers-Danlos Syndrome Subtypes**

Type	Mode of Inheritance	OMIM Condition	Estimated Incidence	Genetic Basis (Common Pathologic Variants)	Protein Affected	Characteristic Primary Clinical Features
Classical	AD	130000, 130010	1 per 20,000 to 40,000	*COL5A1*, *COL5A2*	Type V collagen (rarely type I collagen)	Skin hyperextensibility; atrophic scarring; generalized joint hypermobility; easy bruising; doughy, soft, velvety skin
Classical-like	AR	606408	Very rare	*TNXB*	Tenascin XB	Skin hyperextensibility with velvety texture and absence of atrophic scarring; generalized joint hypermobility; easy bruising
Cardiac-valvular	AR	225320	Very rare	*COL1A2*	Type I collagen	Severe progressive cardiac-valvular problems (aortic and mitral valve); skin hyperextensibility; atrophic scarring; thin skin; easy bruising; generalized or small joint hypermobility
Vascular	AD	130050	1 per 50,000 to 100,000	*COL3A1*	Type III collagen (rarely type I collagen)	Small joint hypermobility; easy bruising; translucent, thin skin; arterial rupture at young age; spontaneous sigmoid colon rupture; uterine rupture during third trimester and severe peripartum perineal tears; atraumatic carotid-cavernous sinus fistula formation; positive family history

(Continued)

TABLE 33.3 ■ **Ehlers-Danlos Syndrome Subtypes—(Cont'd)**

Type	Mode of Inheritance	OMIM Condition	Estimated Incidence	Genetic Basis (Common Pathologic Variants)	Protein Affected	Characteristic Primary Clinical Features
Hypermobile	AD	130020	1 per 5000 to 20,000	Unknown	Unknown	Generalized joint hypermobility with musculoskeletal complications; no significant or severe skin fragility; easy bruising; mild skin hyperextensibility; frequent (2 or more) associated conditions/systemic manifestations (e.g., sleep disturbance, fatigue, chronic pain, dysautonomia, anxiety, depression, functional gastrointestinal disorders); positive family history; lack of other connective tissue disorders
Arthrochalasia	AD	130060	Very rare	*COL1A1, COL1A2*	Type I collagen	Congenital bilateral hip dislocation; severe generalized joint hypermobility with dislocation/subluxation; skin hyperextensibility
Dermatosparaxis	AR	225410	Very rare	*ADAMTS2*	*ADAMTS-2*	Extreme cutaneous manifestations present at birth (e.g., skin fragility, bruisability, redundant skin); dysmorphic features; umbilical hernia
Kyphoscoliotic	AR	225400, 614557	Rare	*PLOD1, FKBP14*	*LH1, FKBP22*	Congenital muscular hypotonia; congenital or early onset kyphoscoliosis; generalized joint hypermobility with dislocation/subluxation; easy bruising and tissue fragility; fragility of globe

(Continued)

TABLE 33.3 ■ **Ehlers-Danlos Syndrome Subtypes—(Cont'd)**

Type	Mode of Inheritance	OMIM Condition	Estimated Incidence	Genetic Basis (Common Pathologic Variants)	Protein Affected	Characteristic Primary Clinical Features
Brittle cornea syndrome	AR	229200, 614170	Very rare	*ZNF469, PRDM5*	*ZNF469, PRDM5*	Thin cornea with or without rupture; blue sclera; early onset progressive keratoconus and/or keratoglobus
Spondylodysplastic	AR	130070, 615349, 612350	Very rare	*B4GALT7, B4GALT6, SLC39A13*	β4GalT7, β3GalT6, *ZIP13*	Progressive short stature; muscular hypotonia; bowing of limbs
Musculocontractural	AR	601776, 615539	Very rare	*CHST14, DSE*	*D4ST1, DSE*	Multiple congenital contractures; dysmorphic craniofacial features; cutaneous manifestations (e.g., skin hyperextensibility, easy bruising, fragility with atrophic scarring)
Myopathic	AD or AR	616471	Very rare	*COL12A1*	Type XII collagen	Congenital muscular hypotonia and/or atrophy (improves with age); proximal joint contractures; hypermobility of distal joints
Periodontal	AD	130080	Very rare	*C1R*	C1r	Early onset, severe, intractable periodontitis; lack of attached gingiva; pretibial plaques; positive family history

AR, autosomal recessive; *AD*, autosomal dominant; *OMIM*, Online Mendelian Inheritance in Man

recommends cognitive behavioral therapy (CBT) for EDS patients. There is evidence that suggests CBT is beneficial for EDS-related anxiety, depression, and fibromyalgia. CBT has also been shown to help patients cope with living with a chronic disease. Lifestyle modifications are considered to be the most successful strategy for pain management of EDS patients. Education about joint injury prevention, ergonomics, decreasing overuse, weight control, and sleep hygiene are helpful tools to decrease the chronic pain. Although surgical options are available such as joint replacement, reconstruction, and cuff tightening, none of these procedures have shown to decrease joint pain.

This patient was treated with physical therapy, duloxetine, and cognitive behavioral therapy. On follow-up she reported a decrease in her pain level and in her anxiety levels.

CLINICAL PEARL **STEP 2/3**

There are no FDA-approved medications for treatment of EDS. This is a chronic condition with lifelong pain, and nonpharmacologic management should therefore be the focus of treatment plans.

Case Summary

- **Complaint/History:** A 22-year-old woman complains of pain in multiple joints that is not consistent with inflammatory arthritis by history or examination. She also has hyperextensible skin and joints with a family history of the same in her mother.
- **Findings:** No joint swelling, minimal joint tenderness, and a positive Beighton score. Her skin is hyperextensible with multiple scars and bruises.
- **Lab Results/Tests:** Inflammatory markers are normal and radiographs are normal.

Diagnosis: Presentation mostly consistent with EDS, type I/II or IV.

- **Treatment:** There is no specific treatment for EDS. Duloxetine and physical and cognitive behavioral therapy were offered and led to improvement in symptoms.

BEYOND THE PEARLS

- Polyarticular pain can be associated with joint swelling, joint stiffness, and limited range of motion because of pain but can also be associated with hypermobility of joints resulting from repetitive microtrauma of dislocations and ligament and tendon injuries without systemic features.
- The Beighton score is an easily reproducible and reliable way to determine joint hypermobility. Positive Beighton scores are >6 in prepubertal children, >5 in postpubertal individuals, and >4 in patients older than 50 years.
- A carefully obtained history of previous injuries, fractures, dislocations, and level of activity will help narrow the differential diagnosis.
- The diagnosis of EDS can be made utilizing the 2017 International Classification of Ehlers-Danlos Syndromes. This classification system identifies 13 subtypes of EDS, which are summarized in Table 33.3.
- The treatment of EDS is multidisciplinary and targeted toward decreasing pain, strengthening joints, managing anxiety and depression, and lifestyle modifications.

Bibliography

Balmuri, N. (2018). *Harriet Lane Handbook, 26*, 688–706.

Bathen, T., Hångmann, A. B., Hoff, M., Andersen, L. Ø., & Rand-Hendriksen, S. (2013). Multidisciplinary treatment of disability in Ehlers-Danlos syndrome hypermobility type/hypermobility syndrome: A pilot study using a combination of physical and cognitive-behavioral therapy on 12 women. *American Journal of Medical Genetics Part A, 161A*, 3005–3011.

Chopra, P., Tinkle, B., Hamonet, C., et al. (2017). Pain management in the Ehlers–Danlos syndromes. *American Journal of Medical Genetics, 175*, 212–219.

Colombi, M., et al. (2015). Differential diagnosis and diagnostic flow chart of joint hypermobility syndrome/ Ehlers-Danlos syndrome hypermobility type compared to other heritable connective tissue disorders. *American journal of medical genetics. Part C, Seminars in medical genetics, 169C*(1), 6–22.

Engelbert, R. H., Juul-Kristensen, B., Pacey, V., et al. (2017). The evidence-based rationale for physical therapy treatment of children, adolescents, and adults diagnosed with joint hypermobility syndrome/hypermobile Ehlers–Danlos syndrome. *American journal of medical genetics. Part C, Seminars in medical genetics, 175*, 158–167.

Hakim, A., & Grahame, R. (2003). Joint hypermobility. *Best Practice and Research. Clinical Rheumatology, 17*, 989–1004.

Kliegman, R. M., Stanton, B. F., St. Geme, J. W., Schor, N., & Behrman, R. (2011). *Nelson textbook of pediatrics* (ed 19). Philadelphia: Saunders.

Loeys, B. L., et al. (2006). Aneurysm syndromes caused by mutations in the TGF-beta receptor. *The New England Journal of Medicine, 355*, 788–798.

Malfait, F., et al. (2017). The 2017 International Classification of the Ehlers–Danlos Syndromes. *American journal of medical genetics. Part C, Seminars in medical genetics, 175C*, 8–26.

Paller, A. S., & Mancini, A. J. (2016). *Hunwitz clinical pediatric dermatology: A textbook of skin disorders of childhood and adolescence* (ed 5). Philadelphia: Elsevier.

Reginato, A. M. (2020). Ehlers-Danlos Syndrome. *Ferri's Clinical Advisor* 482.e2-482.e12.

Smits-Engelsman, B., Klerks, M., & Kirby, A. (2011). Beighton Score: A valid measure for generalized hypermobility in children. *The Journal of Pediatrics, 158*(1). 119-123.e4.

Tinkle, B. T., Bird, H. A., Grahame, R., Lavallee, M., Levy, H. P., & Sillence, D. (2009). The lack of clinical distinction between the hypermobility type of Ehlers–Danlos syndrome and the joint hypermobility syndrome (a.k.a. hypermobility syndrome). *American Journal of Medical Genetics Part A, 149A*, 2368–2370.

Zhou, Z., Rewari, A., & Shanthanna, H. (2018). Management of chronic pain in Ehlers-Danlos syndrome. *Medicine, 97*(45), e13115.

CASE 34

A 70-Year-Old Female With Bilateral Shoulder Pain

Kelli Kam ■ Kevin Kaplowitz ■ Sophia Li

A 70-year-old female presents to her primary care physician with bilateral shoulder pain and stiffness. She has been experiencing pain and stiffness in her shoulders for the past 3 months. She has also been having difficulty getting off her couch after sitting for a while. The stiffness is typically worse in the morning and lasts for 1 hour or longer. She also notes that she has felt more fatigued over the past few months. On presentation, the patient is afebrile with a temperature of 98.6°F (37°C), pulse rate and respirations are within normal range, and blood pressure is 130/78 mmHg.

What is the significance of the location and distribution of this patient's joint pain?

The location and distribution can help to differentiate between the many causes of joint pain and can implicate certain diagnoses over others. Shoulder pain has many etiologies and requires a thorough history and physical examination to help narrow the differential diagnoses. Table 34.1 outlines some of the more common causes of bilateral shoulder pain to keep in mind during the initial encounter with a patient with shoulder pain.

Upon further discussion with the patient, she mentions that she has noticed stiffness in her neck and lower back, particularly after long periods of inactivity. She denies any other joint pain in her wrists, ankles, and feet. The patient's physical examination reveals decreased range of motion in her bilateral shoulders and hips as well as her cervical spine. She is also unable to perform active abduction of her shoulders beyond 90 degrees without experiencing pain. The decision is made to order some laboratory tests and refer her to a rheumatologist.

CLINICAL PEARL **STEP 2/3**

When checking range or motion (ROM) of the shoulders, it is important to complete both passive and active ROM. Sometimes patients will have decreased restricted ROM because of pain; therefore, it is important to establish whether or not they have true decreased ROM. If a patient has decreased active ROM, it is important to complete a thorough shoulder exam to pinpoint areas that may have a possible tear or tendonitis.

Although this patient only endorses shoulder pain on initial presentation, it is important to take a thorough history to determine whether other joints are involved to make an accurate diagnosis. Different disease processes have a predilection for affecting different joints. Examples of these are given in Table 34.2.

TABLE 34.1 ■ **Differential Diagnoses of Bilateral Shoulder Pain**

Inflammatory Conditions	Musculoskeletal	Other
Rheumatoid arthritis	Degenerative joint disease	Statin-associated myopathy
Gout/pseudogout	Subacromial bursitis	Thyroid or parathyroid disorders
Polymyalgia rheumatica	Rotator cuff tendinopathy	Malignancy (e.g., multiple myeloma)
Vasculitis	Adhesive capsulitis	Metabolic bone disease
Inflammatory myositis	Fibromyalgia	Depression
Spondyloarthropathy (e.g., ankylosing spondylitis, psoriatic arthritis, inflammatory bowel disease (IBD) associated arthritis)	Chronic pain syndromes	

TABLE 34.2 ■ **Distribution of Joint Pain**

	Rheumatoid Arthritis	Osteoarthritis	Psoriatic Arthritis	Gout/ Pseudogout	Polymyalgia Rheumatica
Large joints	Knees and shoulders; hips in well-established disease	Hips, knees	Knees and shoulders, can be asymmetric	Knees	Shoulders and hips
Small/ Intermediate joints	MCP and PIP joints in the hands, wrists, elbows, MTP joints in the feet MTP joints in the feet	DIP, PIP, and first CMC joints in the hands; first MTP joint in the feet	Frequently DIP joints along with nail involvement	Hands, wrists, elbows, first MTP joint	Sometimes involves wrists and MCP joints.
Spine	Cervical spine	Cervical spine and LS spine	LS spine and SI joints	Rarely	Cervical and/ or lumbar tenderness

CMC, Carpometacarpal; *DIP*, distal interphalangeal; *LS*, lumbosacral; *MCP*, metacarpophalangeal; *MTP*, metatarsophalangeal; *PIP*, proximal interphalangeal; *SI*, sacroiliac.

What is the importance of the duration of her morning stiffness?

Duration of morning stiffness can help to differentiate inflammatory arthritis, noninflammatory arthritis, or other causes of joint pain. Inflammatory arthritis is typically associated with 30 minutes to over an hour of morning stiffness. The stiffness also tends to occur after periods of inactivity. In contrast, patients with osteoarthritis will usually have resolution of morning stiffness in less than 20 minutes.

Which laboratory tests would be important at this time to help narrow your differential diagnosis?

When ordering laboratory tests, it is important to keep in mind that the studies being ordered should help narrow the differential diagnosis and establish a baseline for monitoring therapy depending on the underlying disease process.

Initial laboratory testing should include a complete blood count (CBC), erythrocyte sedimentation rate (ESR), and C-reactive protein (CRP). Rheumatoid factor (RF) and anti-cyclic citrullinated peptide (anti-CCP) antibodies should be ordered if there is concern for inflammatory arthritis. Additional studies that can be considered in the workup depending on the presentation include blood glucose, serum creatinine, liver functions tests, a bone profile with calcium, vitamin D and alkaline phosphatase, as well as urinalysis. Creatinine kinase should also be ordered if the patient is presenting with muscle weakness, possibly indicating myopathy.

BASIC SCIENCE/CLINICAL PEARL **STEP 1/2/3**

A positive RF is a biomarker for rheumatoid arthritis (RA) and is present in 26% to 90% of RA patients. However, a positive RF can also be found in many other conditions. Common causes of a positive RF include advanced age, systemic lupus erythematosus, systemic lupus erythematosus, Sjögren's syndrome), polymyositis, mixed cryoglobulinemia types II and III, chronic hepatis C infection, tuberculosis, smoking, and syphilis.

How would you summarize the findings and the most likely differential diagnosis?

In summary, this is an elderly female who presents with chronic, symmetric joint pain affecting primarily her shoulders, hips, and cervical spine.

Polymyalgia rheumatica (PMR) is the most likely diagnosis, given the involvement of bilateral shoulders and hips, morning stiffness that lasts for more than 1 hour, and lack of muscle weakness or other joint involvement. Ankylosing spondylitis (AS) can also present with neck pain, hip pain, and elevated inflammatory markers. However, AS typically presents initially with lower back pain and onset before the age of 45. AS can be associated with other extraarticular manifestations such as uveitis. Rheumatoid arthritis can also present with symmetric large joint pain and morning stiffness lasting longer than 1 hour. However, there is typically involvement of small joints, such as the metacarpophalangeal and proximal interphalangeal joints of the hands, in addition to large joints.

What are typical laboratory findings in PMR?

Marked elevation in ESR and/or CRP, thrombocytosis, and mild anemia are characteristic findings in PMR. However, both ESR and CRP are nonspecific inflammatory markers and can be found in many other inflammatory conditions. There are no specific biomarkers thus far that have been identified for PMR. The absence of RF and anti-CCP are helpful in ruling out inflammatory arthritis.

A mild normocytic anemia may be present, although typically white blood cell count is usually normal. A thrombocytosis may also be present as a result of a generalized acute inflammatory response.

If ESR and/or CRP are only minimally elevated, what further testing can be done to help distinguish PMR from other inflammatory and noninflammatory shoulder and hip conditions?

Ultrasound or magnetic resonance imaging (MRI) can help to identify conditions such as subdeltoid bursitis (Fig. 34.1A,B), biceps tenosynovitis, rotator cuff tendonitis, or trochanteric bursitis (Fig. 34.1C,D). Diagnostic criteria formulated by the American College of Rheumatology (ACR) and European League Against Rheumatism (EULAR) were previously only based on physical examination and laboratory findings. The addition of ultrasonography in 2012 to the EULAR/ACR classification scoring algorithm improved the specificity to 81% for differentiating PMR from non-PMR patients and to 89% in discriminating PMR from other shoulder disorders.

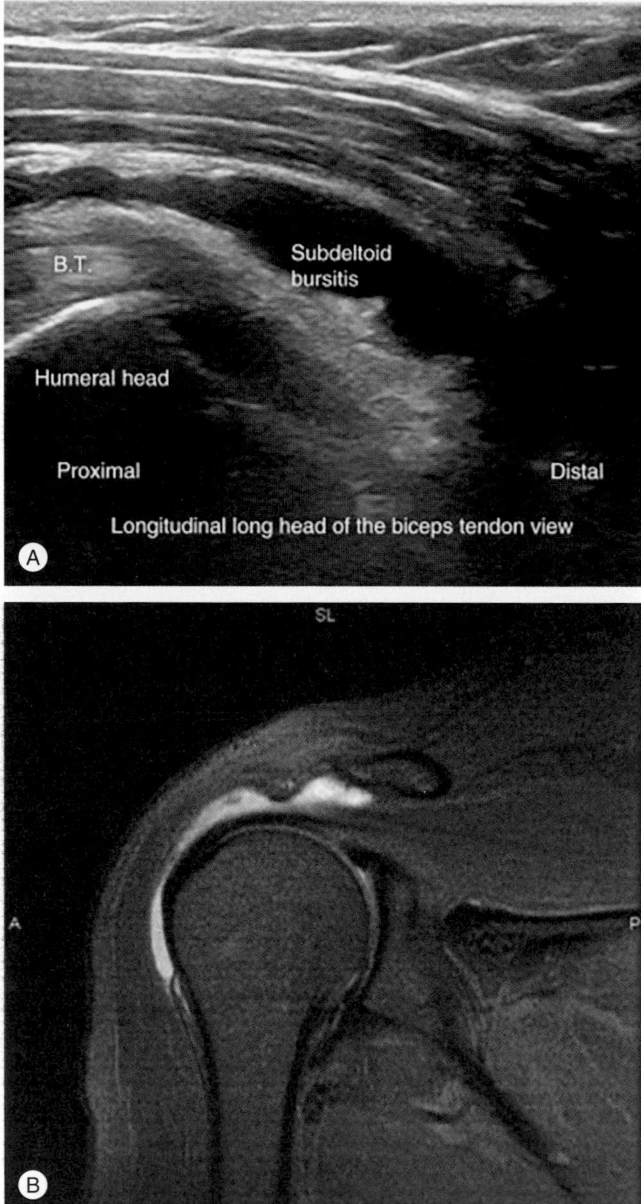

Fig. 34.1 Subdeltoid and trochanteric bursitis on ultrasound and magnetic resonance imaging (MRI). (A) Longitudinal ultrasound image demonstrating subdeltoid bursitis. (B) Subacromial (subdeltoid) bursitis by MRI. (continued)

What are the classification criteria for PMR?

See Table 34.3.

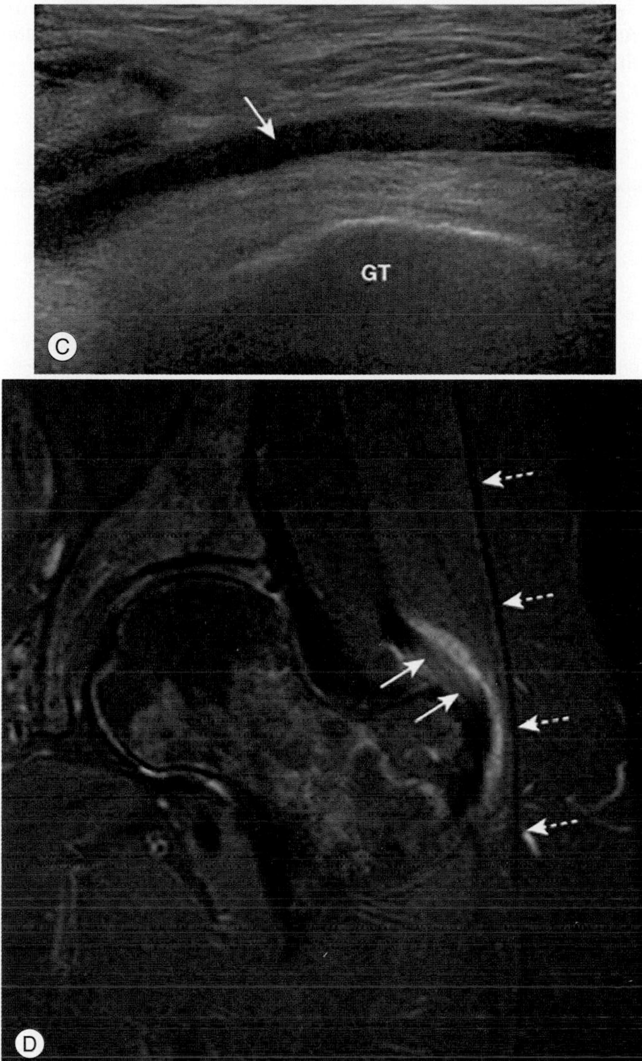

Fig. 34.1 (Cont'd) (C) Axial ultrasound image shows anechoic distention of the trochanteric bursa *(arrow)* adjacent to the greater trochanter. (D) MRI image of a patient with lateral hip pain and trochanteric bursitis with high-SI fluid lying between the iliotibial tract *(broken white arrows)* and the gluteus minimus tendon *(white arrows)*. *B.T.*, Biceps tendon; *GT*, greater trochanter.

The patient brings her labs to her rheumatology appointment. The results are significant for an elevated erythrocyte sedimentation rate (ESR) of 75 mm/h, elevated C-reactive protein (CRP) of 30 mg/L, negative RF, and negative anti-CCP. The complete blood count shows a mild normocytic anemia with hemoglobin of 10.5 and mean corpuscular value (MCV) of 85 fL. What is your differential diagnosis at this point?

If any patient begins to develop symptoms of new-onset headache, unilateral visual impairment, or jaw claudication, there should be a high suspicion for concomitant giant cell arteritis (GCA). About 15% of patients with PMR develop GCA and approximately 50% of patients with GCA present with PMR either before, during, or after a diagnosis of the vasculitis. All patients with a diagnosis of PMR should be educated about and clinically monitored for signs and symptoms of GCA.

TABLE 34.3 ■ **American College of Rheumatology and European League Against Rheumatism Provisional Classification Criteria for Polymyalgia Rheumatica**

Required Criteria
- Age ≥50 years
- Bilateral shoulder pain
- Abnormal erythrocyte sedimentation rate and/or C-reactive protein

Clinical Criteria	Points
Morning stiffness lasting >45 minutes	2
Hip pain or restricted range of motion	1
Negative rheumatoid factor and anti-citrullinated protein antibody	2
Absence of other joint involvement	1

Ultrasound criteria	Points
≥1 shoulder with subdeltoid bursitis, biceps tenosynovitis, or glenohumeral synovitis	1
AND	
≥1 hip with synovitis or trochanteric bursitis	
Both shoulder with subdeltoid bursitis, biceps tenosynovitis, or glenohumeral synovitis	1

According to the provisional ACR-EULAR classification criteria for polymyalgia rheumatica, a diagnosis requires that in addition to the mandatory criteria, there must be a score of 4 or more points for additional criteria without ultrasonographic findings (diagnostic sensitivity and specificity, 68% and 78%, respectively) and a score of more than 5 points with ultrasonographic findings (diagnostic sensitivity and specificity, 66% and 81%, respectively.

TABLE 34.4 ■ **ACR Classification Criteria for Giant Cell Arteritis**

At least three criteria must be met:
Age at disease onset ≥50 years
New headache, either new onset or new type of localized pain in the head
Abnormal temporal artery, with tenderness to palpation or decreased pulsation
Elevated ESR, >50 mm/h during first hour of testing (Westergren method)
Biopsy evidence of vasculitis with predominance of mononuclear-cell infiltration of granulomatous inflammation, usually with multinucleated giant cells.

Diagnosis: GCA in addition to PMR

What is GCA and how is it diagnosed?

GCA is an inflammatory vasculitis that typically affects medium- or large-sized arteries. The arteries most commonly involved include external carotid branches; ophthalmic and vertebral, distal subclavian, axillary arteries; and the thoracic aorta. GCA is diagnosed based on a combination of medical history, clinical evaluation, and laboratory and imaging tests. Confirmation of GCA requires histologic findings on biopsy. ACR classification criteria for GCA are outlined in Table 34.4.

BASIC SCIENCE PEARL **STEP 1**

GCA has been found to have an association with HLA-DRB*04. The mechanism of GCA has also been found to be centered around activation of IL-6.

Biopsy is most often taken from the temporal artery. It is recommended that a long-segment biopsy specimen of >1cm is obtained. Characteristic histological findings include a transmural inflammatory infiltrate comprised of lymphocytes, macrophages, and giant cells inflammation of the arterial wall with fragmentation and disruption of the internal elastic lamina. Inflammation of the arterial wall with fragmentation and disruption of the internal elastic lamina is seen (Fig. 34.2). However, given that the temporal artery is not always involved, a negative biopsy does not always rule out GCA.

In patients who have biopsy-confirmed GCA, noninvasive vascular imaging can be obtained to assess the extent of large vessel involvement (Fig. 34.3). In patients with suspected GCA but a negative temporal artery biopsy, magnetic resonance angiography (MRA) or CTA of the neck/chest/abdomen/pelvis can be completed to provide additional evidence of disease. F-fluorodeoxyglucose (FDG) positron emission tomography (PET) is a nuclear medicine technique that is also being utilized, typically in conjunction with CTA, to assess the extent of vascular involvement. In active large-vessel vasculitis there will be a demonstration of increased FDG uptake in areas of inflammation within the vessel wall. It is usually seen as a smooth linear pattern, as demonstrated in Fig. 34.4.

What are other signs and symptoms of GCA?

Cranial GCA:

- New-onset headache
- Constitutional symptoms
- Jaw claudication
- Scalp tenderness
- Tongue claudication
- Temporal artery tenderness or decreased pulse
- Stroke
- Acute visual deficits

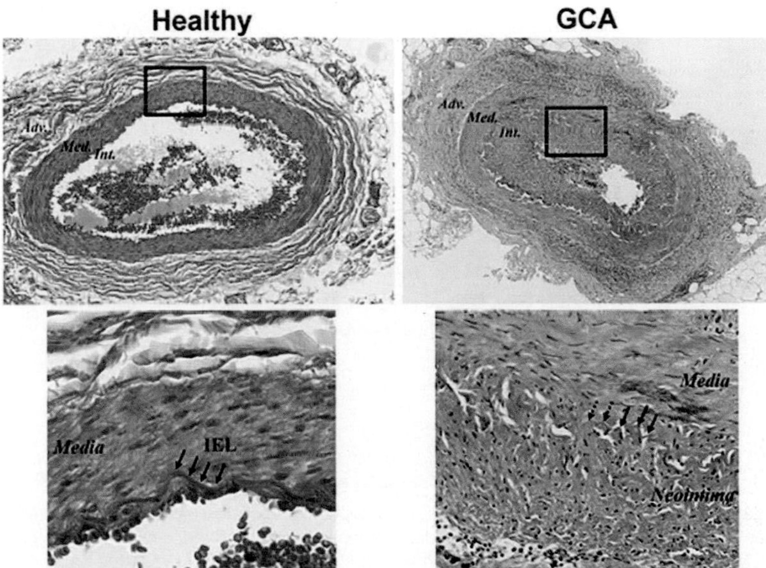

Fig. 34.2 Hematoxylin eosin safran staining of a healthy artery and of an artery affected by giant cell arteritis (GCA). The healthy artery is characterized by a well-structured media and a thin intima separated by a preserved internal elastic lamina (IEL). In the healthy artery, the artery wall is free of inflammatory cells and its lumen is large. By contrast, many mononuclear inflammatory cells infiltrate the three layers of the artery affected by GCA (panarteritis). The media and the IEL are destroyed, thus allowing the migration and proliferation of vascular smooth muscle cells in the intima, leading to intimal hyperplasia and vascular occlusion. Magnification ×40. *Adv*, Adventitia; *IEL*, internal elastic lumina; *int*, intima; *med*, media.

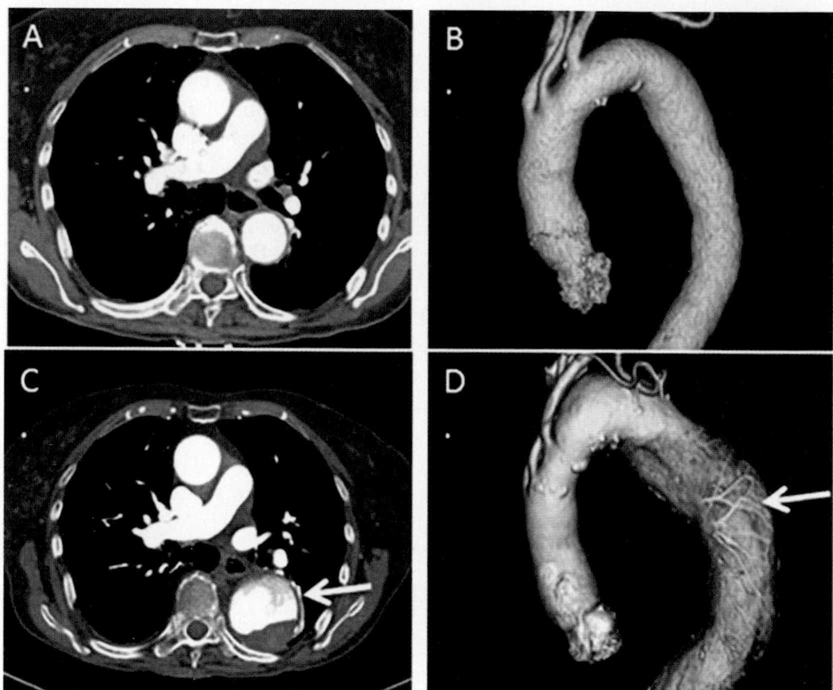

Fig. 34.3 Development of aneurysm in giant cell arteritis (GCA). Computed tomography angiography (CTA) demonstrating a normal caliber aorta in an 84-year-old female with GCA, temporal arteritis, and hypertension on (A) axial and (B) CT reconstruction imaging. Six years later repeat CTA noted fusiform aneurysmal involvement of the entire descending thoracic aorta *(arrows)* with thrombus present as noted in the (C) axial and (D) CT reconstruction images.

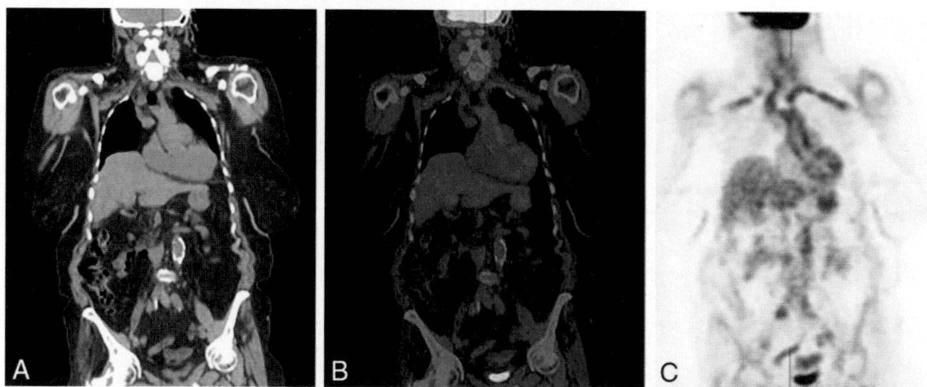

Fig. 34.4 Large vessel vasculitis in a patient with unexplained inflammatory syndrome. Persistently elevated acute phase reactants were found in a 79-year-old woman who had ended for three months corticosteroid treatment for "isolated" polymyalgia rheumatica. A temporal artery biopsy, guided by the patient's history and a typical picture of large vessel vasculitis on PET study yielded giant cell arteritis. (A, B, C): frontal images (CT imaging, coregistered PET/CT imaging, PET imaging). (From Liozon, É., & Monteil, J. (2008). Place de la tomographie par émission de positons (TEP) au [18F]FDG dans l'exploration des vascularites. *Médecine Nucléaire*, 32(10), 511-522.)

Extracranial GCA:

- Constitutional symptoms
- Ischemic signs and symptoms of extremities:
  - Limb claudication
  - Pulse asymmetry
  - Arterial pressure asymmetry
  - Peripheral arterial bruits
  - Distal necrosis or gangrene

CLINICAL PEARL **STEP 2/3**

For any patient where there is a high suspicion of GCA, it is imperative to start high-dose prednisone immediately in order to prevent irreversible vision loss.

What are the ocular signs of GCA?

The eye exam can be completely normal. Some acute visual deficits associated with GCA include amaurosis, diplopia (double vision) or severe vision loss. Vision loss can be caused by an arteritic anterior ischemic optic neuropathy, which may appear as chalky white disc edema with or without disc hemorrhages. If the ischemia is instead localized to the retina, a central retinal artery occlusion can occur, where the retinal edema is identifiable as a cherry red spot.

What is the recommended initial treatment for PMR and GCA?

Initial therapy for both PMR and GCA is glucocorticoid monotherapy. The dose for PMR is between prednisone 15–25 mg per day, whereas the dose of prednisone for GCA is higher with 1 mg per kilogram of body weight per day. If there is onset of any clinical signs or symptoms of unstable blood flow affecting the eyes or central nervous system, intravenous glucocorticoid pulse therapy is warranted (e.g., 500–1000 mg of methylprednisolone per day for 3 days). Timely administration of intravenous glucocorticoids is important to prevent irreversible vision loss from tissue necrosis.

In any patient started on a prolonged duration of glucocorticoids, prophylactic treatments should also be considered. Dietary or supplemental intake of calcium and vitamin D is recommended in order to prevent glucocorticoid-induced osteoporosis. *Pneumocystis jirovecii* pneumonia prophylaxis should also be considered in patients on prednisone 20 mg or more daily and a second immunosuppresant.

Which alternative therapies are available if the patient does not respond or has intolerance to initial therapies?

Currently there are two glucocorticoid-sparing agents that have been approved or well studied for the treatment of PMR and GCA. The two main glucocorticoid-sparing therapies that have been studied are methotrexate and tocilizumab. Tocilizumab was approved by the FDA in May 2017 for use in treatment of GCA. Tocilizumab has been shown in several studies to lead to rapid and maintained improvement, as well as decreased cumulative dose of glucocorticoids required by patients. Other agents that are available but have not been widely studied include abatacept, azathioprine, ustekinumab, cyclophosphamide, dapsone, and leflunomide (see Table 34.5).

BASIC SCIENCE/CLINICAL PEARL **STEP 1/2/3**

Methotrexate (MTX) acts on the S-phase of the cell cycle, which is when DNA synthesis occurs. MTX irreversibly binds to dihydrofolate reductase, which in turn prevents reduction of dihydrofolate to tetrahydrofolate, which is an essential cofactor needed to synthesize DNA precursor dTMP. Tetrahydrofolate can be synthesized via a second pathway through conversion of dietary folate. As cells continue to be synthesized, dietary folate becomes more rapidly repleted. This can lead to side effects seen often in folate deficiency such as gastrointestinal symptoms, hepatic transaminitis, stomatitis, and sores in the mouth. To avoid this from happening, patients on MTX must be started on folate supplementation.

TABLE 34.5 ■ **Glucocorticoid-Sparing Treatments for GCA and PMR**

	Mechanism of Action	Side Effects
Tocilizumab	Anti-IL-6 receptor antibody	• Risk of opportunistic infections • Risk of infection-related complications e.g., stroke secondary to infective endocarditis
Methotrexate	Inhibits dihydrofolic acid reductase	• Bone marrow suppression • Hepatotoxicity • Pulmonary fibrosis and interstitial disease • Acute renal failure • Risk of opportunistic infections

GCA, Giant cell arteritis; *PMR*, polymyalgia rheumatica.

Case Summary

- **Complaint/History:** A 70-year-old female who presents with bilateral shoulder pain and stiffness, new onset of headache, diplopia, and fatigue.
- **Findings:** Decreased range of motion of bilateral shoulders and hips.
- **Lab Results/Tests:** Elevated ESR and CRP, negative RF, negative anti-CCP, and mild normocytic anemia.

Diagnosis: Polymyalgia rheumatica and GCA.

- **Treatments:** The patient received intravenous (IV) pulse glucocorticoids for 3 days and a subsequent oral glucocorticoid taper. Her symptoms improved but she reported visual changes again when her prednisone was tapered to 30mg daily. Tocilizumab was added in addition to her glucocorticoids and her disease remained in remission.

BEYOND THE PEARLS

- In any patient with GCA or suspected GCA who presents with visual changes, they should immediately receive intravenous glucocorticoid pulse therapy with 500–1000 mg of methylprednisolone per day for 3 days to prevent irreversible vision loss.
- While less than 10% of all ischemic optic neuropathies are caused by temporal arteritis, of those patients with temporal arteritis who do lose vision, the majority are due to arteritic ischemic optic neuropathy.
- When prednisone is tapered, the patient is at high risk of relapse. It is important to obtain baseline ESR and CRP prior to initiating therapy and to monitor both biomarkers continuously during the taper. Pneumocystis carinii (jiroveci) pneumonia (PCP) can be a potentially fatal complication of immunosuppressive therapy for systemic vasculitis, particularly for those who receive cyclophosphamide and/or high-dose glucocorticoids. PCP prophylaxis with either trimethoprim-sulfamethoxazole or atovaquone is administered in this setting.
- Peripheral manifestations commonly occur with PMR, which can include arthritis, distal extremity swelling with pitting edema, carpal tunnel syndrome, and distal tenosynovitis. The arthritis associated with PMR does not lead to erosions or bony deformities, which is a key difference compared with rheumatoid arthritis.

Bibliography

Cantini, F., Salvarani, C., Olivieri, I., et al. (2000). Erythrocyte sedimentation rate and C-reactive protein in the evaluation of disease activity and severity in polymyalgia rheumatica: A prospective follow-up study. *Seminars in Arthritis and Rheumatism*, *30*(1), 17–24.

Dasgupta, B., Cimmino, M. A., Kremers, H. M., et al. (2012). Provisional classification criteria for polymyalgia rheumatica: A European League Against Rheumatism/American College of Rheumatology collaborative initiative. *Arthritis and Rheumatism*, *64*(4), 943–954.

Dejaco, C., Singh, Y. P., Perel, P., et al. (2015). Recommendations for the management of polymyalgia rheumatica: A European League Against Rheumatism/American College of Rheumatology collaborative initiative. *Annals of the Rheumatic Diseases*, *74*(10), 1799–1807.

González-Gay, M. A., Pina, T., Prieto-Peña, D., Calderon-Goercke, M., Gualillo, O., & Castañeda, S. (2019). Treatment of giant cell arteritis. *Biochemical Pharmacology*, *165*, 230–239.

Maz, M., Chung, S.A., Abril, A., et al. (2021). American College of Rheumatology/Vasculitis Foundation Guideline for the Management of Giant Cell Arteritis and Takayasu Arteritis. *Arthritis Rheumatol*, *73*(8),1349–1365.

Muratore, F., Pipitone, N., Salvarani, C., & Schmidt, W. A. (2016). Imaging of vasculitis: State of the art. *Best Practice & Research: Clinical Rheumatology*, *30*, 688–706.

Salvarani, C., Pipitone, N., Versari, A., & Hunder, G. (2012). Clinical features of polymyalgia rheumatica and giant cell arteritis. *Nature Reviews Rheumatology*, *8*(9), 509–521.

Weyand, C. M., & Goronzy, J. J. (2014). Clinical practice: Giant-cell arteritis and polymyalgia rheumatica. *The New England Journal of Medicine*, *371*(1), 50–57.

Bibliography

SECTION 8

Gastroenterology

CASE 35

A 44-Year-Old Female With Acute Onset Epigastric Pain

Evan Mosier ■ Daniel Chao

A 44-year-old female presents to the emergency department with acute onset epigastric pain for the past 2 days, constant, with radiation to the back. Her eyes and skin "turned yellow" 1 day ago. She denies any fevers. The patient drinks one or two beers per week, does not smoke, denies nonsteroidal antiinflammatory drug (NSAID), use and is not on glucocorticoids. She denies any heartburn or acid reflux symptoms. She had right upper quadrant (RUQ) abdominal pain that was colicky and worsened with food intake 1 week before, which resolved spontaneously after 1 day and she therefore did not seek medical attention. Her blood pressure is 118/55 mmHg, pulse rate is 105/min, respiration rate is 20/min, oxygen saturation is 97% on room air, and body mass index is 38. Her skin is noted to be jaundiced and scleral icterus is present. Murphy's sign is negative.

What is your differential diagnosis for the patient's abdominal pain?

Epigastric pain can be caused by conditions such as peptic ulcer disease (PUD), acute or chronic pancreatitis, and gastroesophageal reflux disease (GERD). Less typical but important etiologies to consider include acute myocardial infarction, aortic dissection, mesenteric ischemia, and choledocholithiasis. Causes of abdominal pain based on location are given in Table 35.1. Always consider causes of right upper quadrant (RUQ) and left upper quadrant (LUQ) abdominal pain in your differential diagnosis for epigastric pain given that the location of the pain is not always an accurate reflection of the anatomic location of the pathology.

In this patient, the history of jaundice and scleral icterus raises concern for hepatobiliary pathology, including cholecystitis and choledocholithiasis with obstruction. The negative Murphy's sign is encouraging but does not rule out acute cholecystitis, and imaging of the gallbladder should therefore be obtained. Liver biochemical tests should be checked to determine the severity of hyperbilirubinemia, and imaging of the common bile duct to check for stones and bile duct dilation is needed. The quality and location of the pain are consistent with acute pancreatitis, which needs to be investigated further because acute pancreatitis can lead to biliary obstruction. The negative history for NSAID and glucocorticoid use is helpful because both can lead to PUD. It is also rare for PUD to cause jaundice. The patient has no known cardiovascular disease but an initial workup with an electrocardiogram may be reasonable. She is relatively young for mesenteric ischemia and aortic dissection and has no known risk factors for premature atherosclerosis (e.g., smoking) and thromboembolic events (e.g., hypercoagulable disorders); therefore, these are less likely to be the cause.

The results of laboratory testing are shown in Table 35.2. An abdominal ultrasound reveals common bile duct dilation to 15 mm, but without a visible stone. Small gallstones were noted in the gallbladder without evidence of cholecystitis as seen in Fig. 35.1 (i.e., pericholecystic fluid or gallbladder wall thickening).

TABLE 35.1 ■ **Differential Diagnosis for Acute Abdominal Pain**

Right Upper Quadrant	Left Upper Quadrant	Epigastric	Right Lower Quadrant	Left Lower Quadrant
Gallstones	Splenomegaly	Ulcers	Appendicitis	Constipation
Cholecystitis	Pyelonephritis	Pancreatitis	Colitis	Colitis
Cholangitis	Ulcers	GERD	Diverticulitis	Diverticulitis
Hepatitis	GERD	Gastropathy	Inguinal hernia	Inguinal hernia
Pyelonephritis	Gastropathy	Cholangitis	Kidney stones	Kidney stones
Ulcers	Pancreatitis	Choledocholithiasis	Pyelonephritis	Pyelonephritis
Myocardial infarction	Myocardial infarction	Myocardial infarction	Ovarian torsion	Ovarian torsion
Aortic dissection	Aortic dissection	Aortic dissection	Pelvic inflammatory disease	Pelvic inflammatory disease
Mesenteric ischemia	Mesenteric ischemia	Mesenteric ischemia	Ectopic pregnancy	Ectopic pregnancy

GERD, Gastroesophageal reflux disease.

TABLE 35.2 ■ **Laboratory Results**

Leukocyte count	18,000
Hemoglobin	16.2 (baseline 14)
Hematocrit	48.6
Platelet count	355
Blood urea nitrogen (BUN)	30
Creatinine	1.1
Lipase	1354 (ULN 55)
Amylase	1844 (ULN 45)
Lactate	2.0
Troponin	<0.01
Alkaline phosphatase	155
Aspartate transaminase	677
Alanine transaminase	1022
Total bilirubin	3.1
Direct bilirubin	2.7
Triglycerides	325
Urinalysis	No white or red blood cells

ULN, upper limit of normal.

CLINICAL PEARL **STEP 2/3**

Because gallstones are high density and calcified, they do not absorb ultrasound waves. Therefore, the waves bounce off the gallstones and are reflected back at the probe, resulting in a shadow over the areas deep to the stone. This shadowing effect helps differentiate gallstones from gallbladder polyps, which do not cause shadowing because the soft tissue that comprises polyps absorbs ultrasound waves.

CLINICAL PEARL **STEP 1/2/3**

Cholelithiasis can occur at any age and usually consists of cholesterol. Risk factors include female gender, age 40 years or older, being overweight, and high estrogen states (premenopausal or oral contraceptive use). Remember the 4 Fs: Forty, Female, Fat, and Fertile.

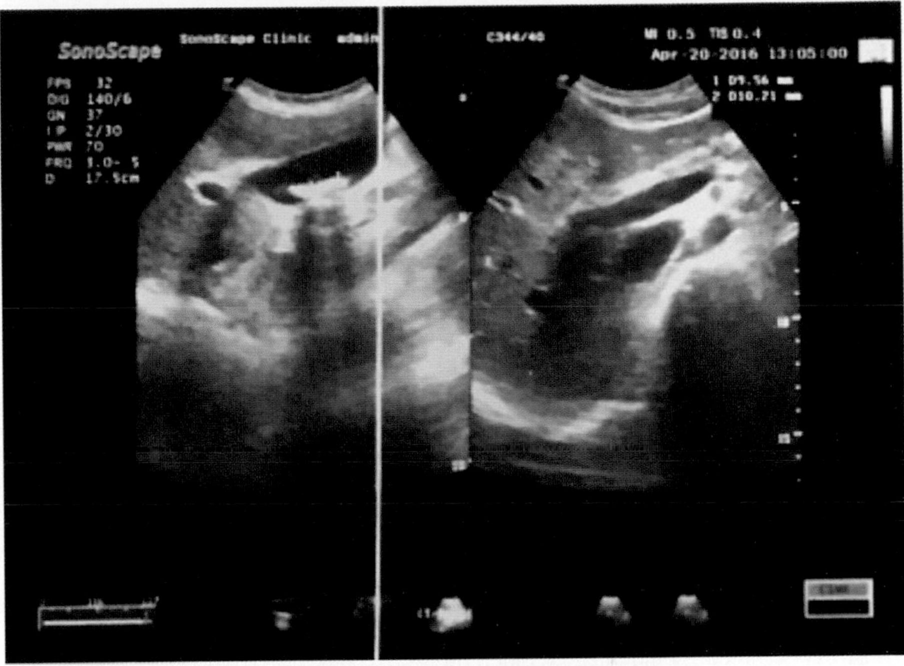

Fig. 35.1 Cholelithiasis on ultrasound without evidence of cholecystitis. (Adapted from Avdaj, A., Fanaj, N., Osmani, M., Bytyqi, A., & Cake, A. (2015). Case report of cholelithiasis in a patient with type 1 Gaucher disease. *International Journal of Surgery Case Reports*, *29*, 227–229.)

How do you diagnose acute pancreatitis?

Acute pancreatitis requires TWO of the following three criteria to be met:

1. Epigastric or LUQ abdominal pain, constant with radiation to the back
2. Lipase and/or amylase >3× upper limit of normal
3. Cross-sectional abdominal imaging consistent with acute pancreatitis

BASIC SCIENCE PEARL **STEP 1/2/3**

Lipase and amylase are both markers of acute pancreatitis but differ greatly in their response. Lipase rises within a few hours of symptom onset and can stay elevated for 3–5 days. Serum amylase levels also rise quickly from symptom onset. However, it normalizes much more quickly, which can lead to missed diagnoses if relied upon. Lipase is more specific to the pancreas. Amylase levels can be elevated in many other conditions such as salivary gland disorders, chronic kidney disease, peptic ulcer disease, appendicitis, and cholecystitis.

This patient meets the first and second criteria listed, and she therefore meets clinical criteria for acute pancreatitis. Cholelithiasis is the most common cause of acute pancreatitis and is probably the etiology given the gallstones seen on abdominal ultrasound and the lack of other obvious causes.

Diagnosis: Acute gallstone pancreatitis.

What are some other causes of acute pancreatitis?

Alcohol is the other common cause of acute pancreatitis and a thorough history of consumption is important. For women, low-risk drinking is considered no more than three standard drinks on any single day and no more than seven drinks per week. For men, it is defined as no more than four standard drinks on any single day and no more than 14 drinks per week. The accepted definition for one standard drink is 14 g of alcohol, which is the equivalent to 12 oz of beer, 5 oz of wine, and 1.5 oz of hard liquor. Rarer causes of pancreatitis are found in Table 35.3.

Given the patient's mild alcohol use, it is unlikely to be the main contributing factor to her pancreatitis. However, alcohol cessation during her recovery is a reasonable recommendation.

How do we assess the severity of this patient's acute pancreatitis?

Most cases of acute pancreatitis are mild with no complications. Moderate pancreatitis is characterized by local pancreatic complications (pseudocysts, pancreatic necrosis) or transient organ failure. Severe pancreatitis is defined as persistent end organ failure for 3 days that can have a mortality as high as 40%. Clinical scoring systems such as the APACHE II score and Ranson's criteria can help identify patients at greater risk of complications. Limitations of the APACHE II score and Ranson's criteria are the use of 17 and 11 variables, respectively, including those that require more invasive testing to obtain; these factors limit their practical utility. The Bedside Index of Severity in Acute Pancreatitis (BISAP) score uses fewer and more routinely available variables and is validated for risk stratifying low and high mortality in acute pancreatitis. Acute pancreatitis with BISAP scores of 0–2 indicate lower mortality (<2%) and BISAP scores 3–5 indicate higher mortality (>15%). BISAP should be calculated at the time of diagnosis (see Table 35.4).

You explain to the patient that her BISAP score is 2 (pulse rate >90 and white blood cell count >12,000) on presentation, placing her in a lower mortality risk category of acute pancreatitis, and she feels relieved. The patient then asks what the treatment plan is.

TABLE 35.3 ■ **Causes of Acute Pancreatitis**

Gallstones	40%
Chronic alcohol abuse	35%
Endoscopic retrograde cholangiopancreatography	4%
Medications (e.g., azathioprine, furosemide)	2%
Other	Rare
Annular pancreas	
Pancreas divisum	
Sphincter of Oddi dysfunction	
Autoimmune disorders	
Hereditary pancreatitis	
Hypercalcemia	
Hypertriglyceridemia (TG >1000)	
Infections	
Toxins (scorpion or snake bites)	
Tumors	
Vascular abnormalities (ischemia, vasculitis)	

TABLE 35.4 ■ **Variables to Calculate the Bedside Index of Severity in Acute Pancreatitis (BISAP)**

BUN >25 mg/dL	1 point
Abnormal mental status with Glasgow coma score <15	1 point
Evidence of SIRS[a]	1 point
Age >60 years	1 point
Imaging with pleural effusion	1 point

BUN, blood urea nitrogen; *SIRS*, Systemic inflammatory response syndrome.
[a]SIRS criteria: two or more of the following: (1) temperature <36°C or >38°C, (2) respiration rate >20/min, (3) heart rate >90/min, (4) WBC <4000 or WBC>12,000 or more than 10% bands on blood smear.

CLINICAL PEARL **STEP 2/3**

Hematocrit and blood urea nitrogen (BUN) are both quick markers for assessing severity of pancreatitis, because both tend to be elevated in severe pancreatitis. During acute pancreatitis, third-spacing of fluid occurs, leading to intravascular volume depletion and hemoconcentration represented by increased hematocrit and BUN levels. Goal hematocrit levels should be between 25% and 35% with down-trending BUN levels 12 hours after presentation.

How do we manage the patient's acute pancreatitis?

Early aggressive intravenous (IV) fluid resuscitation (250–500 cc/h) with isotonic crystalloid should be started upon presentation, with the most benefit occurring within the first 12 to 24 hours for preventing end organ failure and reducing mortality. Fluids should be titrated to maintain a normal heart rate, urine output, and, if being monitored, mean arterial pressure and central venous pressure. Hemoconcentration is a sign of worsening intravascular depletion and is a poor prognostic factor; therefore, hemoglobin and hematocrit can be monitored at regular intervals to ensure that adequate IV hydration is being provided. In patients with mild pancreatitis and controlled symptoms, early enteral nutrition (nutrition through the gastrointestinal tract including oral or tube feeds) is recommended rather than nil per os (NPO). For patients unable to tolerate oral nutrition because of the severity of their disease, placement of a nasogastric tube for administration of enteral feeds is preferred over total parenteral nutrition (TPN).

Given that the patient has evidence of hemoconcentration on her admission lab tests, 2 L of lactated Ringer's at bolus rate is administered followed by maintenance fluid at 250 cc/h. Hemoglobin 4 hours after the bolus is 14 and an additional 1 L bolus is given, after which hemoglobin decreases to 13 with no evidence of bleeding. The maintenance fluid is continued at the same rate. The patient is able to tolerate a clear liquid diet but is still requiring IV morphine to reduce her pain. Repeat lab results 24 hours after admission are shown in Table 35.5.

The patient's lab results show that she received adequate fluid resuscitation. Her heart rate is now normal and she has remained afebrile. Her abdominal pain has greatly improved. However, the patient remains jaundiced and her serum bilirubin is unchanged. She is concerned about her yellow eyes and wonders why this is happening.

What further investigation should be performed for the hyperbilirubinemia?

In a patient with persistently elevated bilirubin levels and dilated common bile duct on imaging with known cholelithiasis, there is concern for obstruction of the common bile duct by a gallstone (choledocholithiasis). Endoscopic ultrasound (EUS) or magnetic resonance

TABLE 35.5 ■ **Laboratory Results After 24 Hours**

Leukocyte count	8000
Hemoglobin	13.2
Hematocrit	39.6
Platelet count	280
Blood urea nitrogen	15
Creatinine	0.9
Lactate	0.7
Alkaline phosphatase	290
Aspartate transaminase	711
Alanine transaminase	800
Total bilirubin	3.8
Direct bilirubin	3.4

cholangiopancreatography (MRCP) are the tests of choice to confirm choledocholithiasis. If a stone is identified in the common bile duct, endoscopic retrograde cholangiopancreatography (ERCP) can be considered for stone removal to relieve the obstruction. Surgical management of choledocholithiasis is the only alternative and carries a higher rate of complication than ERCP.

When would you consider going straight to ERCP without performing EUS or MRCP to confirm choledocholithiasis?

When cholangitis is clearly present, urgent biliary decompression is necessary to prevent septic shock and death. Other indications to proceed straight to ERCP are confirmed choledocholithiasis on prior imaging or total bilirubin levels greater than 4.0 with symptoms consistent with choledocholithiasis.

CLINICAL PEARL **STEP 2/3**

Cholangitis is inflammation of the bile ducts often from bacteria, which can be precipitated by biliary obstruction such as gallstones. Charcot's triad (right upper quadrant pain, jaundice, and fever) and Raynaud's pentad (right upper quadrant pain, jaundice, fevers, hypotension, and altered mental status) are useful constellations of symptoms that suggest cholangitis, which would warrant urgent ERCP for biliary decompression.

The patient's lack of fever, hypotension, and confusion; improving abdominal pain; and normalization of leukocytosis all suggest against cholangitis. Therefore, antibiotics are not indicated. Total bilirubin is not high enough to proceed straight to ERCP and imaging is not conclusively showing choledocholithiasis. Therefore, she undergoes MRCP, which shows a stone in the distal common bile duct, as seen in Fig. 35.2.

ERCP is performed nonurgently after her epigastric pain resolves, with successful removal of the gallstones from her common bile duct. Fig. 35.3 shows the ERCP findings. Given the significant risk of recurrence of gallstone pancreatitis, cholecystectomy is performed prior to her discharge from the hospital.

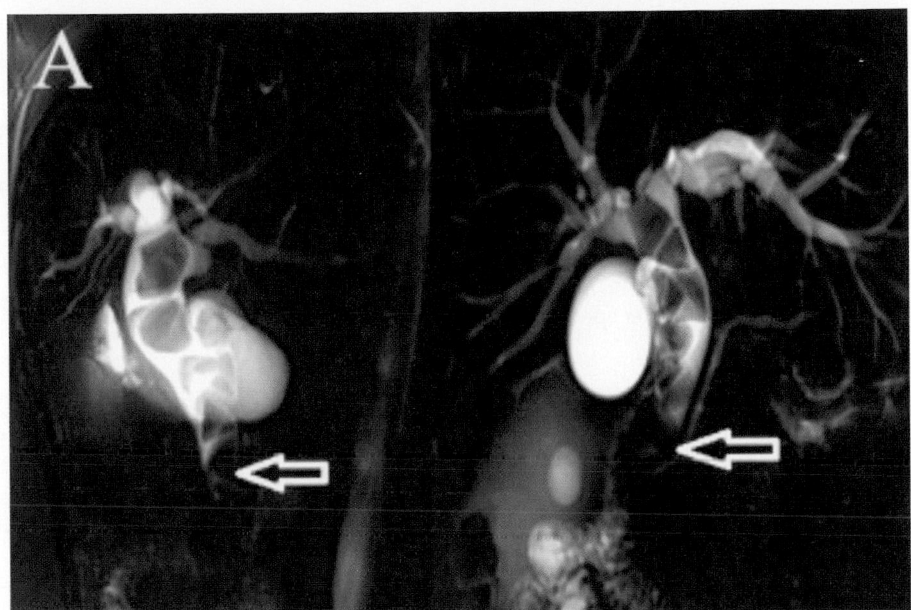

Fig. 35.2 Magnetic resonance cholangiopancreatography showing choledocholithiasis *(arrows)*. (Adapted from Yang, C., & Wang, H. (2019). Treatment of incarcerated choledocholithiasis. *Asian Journal of Surgery, 42*(10), 932–934.)

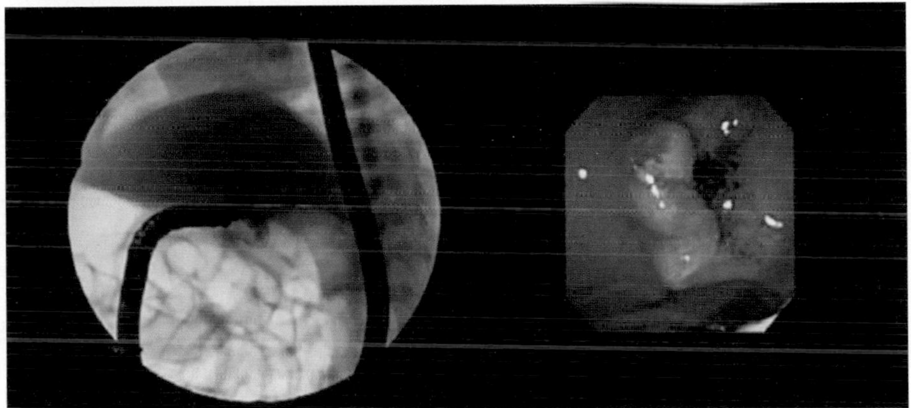

Fig. 35.3 Choledocholithiasis with biliary obstruction on fluoroscopy *(left)* and choledocholithiasis visualized at the ampulla of Vater on endoscopic retrograde cholangiopancreatography *(right)*. (Adapted from Yu, P. T., Fenton, S. J., Delaplain, P. T., Vrecenak, J., Adzick, N. S., Nance, M. L., & Guner, Y. S. (2018). Management of choledocholithiasis in an infant. *Journal of Pediatric Surgery Case Reports, 29*, 52–58.)

What are some complications of acute pancreatitis to consider, especially if the patient had not improved clinically?

Early complications of acute pancreatitis include pseudocyst formation and pancreatic necrosis, but neither cause clinical worsening. If the necrosis becomes infected, antibiotics, drainage of abscesses, or even removal of infected tissue may be necessary. Patients can develop ascites from a disrupted pancreatic duct. Intraabdominal inflammation can lead to portal vein and splenic vein thrombosis. Pancreatic and splenic artery pseudoaneurysms can also develop.

CLINICAL PEARL **STEP 3**

Computed tomography (CT) scan of the abdomen should be considered if the diagnosis of acute pancreatitis is uncertain, such as when only one of the two other diagnostic criteria are met. If the patient's clinical status is not improving, especially in the first 48–72 hours, CT should be considered or repeated to evaluate for abdominal complications. Be aware that pancreatic inflammation may be missed on early CT scans because of intravascular depletion and findings only appear after adequate volume resuscitation.

CLINICAL PEARL **STEP 2/3**

Prophylactic antibiotics are not indicated for severe pancreatitis or necrotizing pancreatitis. There is no evidence that antibiotics improve the rate of organ failure, length of hospital stay, or mortality. Antibiotics should be used when there is concern for infected necrosis or cholangitis.

Case Summary

- **Complaint/History:** A 44-year-old female presenting with epigastric pain radiating to the back, with preceding recurrent episodes of RUQ pain complicated by jaundice.
- **Findings:** Examination reveals epigastric tenderness on palpation without rigidity or rebound tenderness. Jaundice and scleral icterus are present. No fever, hypotension, or confusion.
- **Lab Results/Tests:** Labs show leukocytosis along with elevated lipase more than three times the upper limit of normal. Hematocrit and BUN are both elevated, suggesting volume depletion. Abdominal ultrasound shows evidence of cholelithiasis with common bile duct dilation and peripancreatic inflammation. MRCP shows choledocholithiasis.

Diagnosis: Acute gallstone pancreatitis with choledocholithiasis.

- **Treatments:** The patient received aggressive intravenous fluid resuscitation and early enteral nutrition. Later during the hospitalization, ERCP was performed to remove the gallstone from her common bile duct. To prevent recurrent pancreatitis, the patient underwent cholecystectomy prior to discharge.

BEYOND THE PEARLS

- The incidence of acute pancreatitis ranges from 5 to 30 cases per 100,000 and has an overall mortality of 5%.
- The most common causes of recurrent acute pancreatitis is still gallstones and alcohol, but for those with early onset disease and a family history of pancreatitis, hereditary pancreatitis conditions should be considered. These can be diagnosed through genetic testing.
- Recurrent acute pancreatitis, especially when alcohol induced, may lead to chronic pancreatitis, which is a consequence of permanent damage to the pancreas and can manifest with exocrine pancreatic insufficiency (malabsorption due to poor fat digestion), endocrine pancreatic insufficiency (diabetes mellitus), and evidence of structural abnormalities on imaging.

Bibliography

Aggarwal. A. (2014). Fluid resuscitation in acute pancreatitis. *World Journal of Gastroenterology*, *20*(48), 18092–18103.

Ammann. R. W. (2001). The natural history of alcoholic chronic pancreatitis. *Internal Medicine*, *40*, 368–375.

Cartwright. S. L. (2008 Apr 1). Evaluation of acute abdominal pain in adults. *American Family Physician*, *77*(7), 971–978.

Clavien, P. A., Robert, J., Meyer, P., et al. (1989). Acute pancreatitis and normoamylasemia. Not an uncommon combination. *Annals of Surgery*, *210*, 614–620.

Crockett. S. D. (2018). American college of gastroenterology guideline: Management of acute pancreatitis. *Gastroenterology*, *154*, 1096–1101.

Kumar. A. H. (2018). A comparison of APACHE II, BISAP, ranson score, and modified CTSI in predicting severity of acute pancreatitis. *Gastroenterology Report*, *6*(2), 127–131.

Millen, B. (2015). U.S. Department of health and human services dietary guidelines for americans, 2015-2020. Available from: https://health.gov/dietaryguidelines/2015/guidelines/appendix-9/

Quinlan. J. D. (2014). Acute pancreatitis. *American Family Physician*, *90*(9), 632–639.

Winslet, M., Hall, C., & London, N. J. M. (1992). Relation of diagnostic serum amylase levels to aetiology and severity of acute pancreatitis. *Gut*, *33*, 982–986.

Wu, B. U., Johannes, R. S., Sun, X., et al. (2008). The early prediction of mortality in acute pancreatitis: a large population-based study. *Gut*, *57*(12), 1698–1703.

Wu. B. U. (2011). Blood urea nitrogen in the early assessment of acute pancreatitis. *Archives of Internal Medicine*, *171*(7), 669–676.

CASE 36

A 26-Year-Old Female With Chronic Hepatitis B

Chuong Tran ■ Daniel Chao

A 26-year-old female with no significant medical history presents with hepatitis B diagnosed 6 months ago from routine laboratory testing. She is asymptomatic. Review of systems is negative for abdominal pain, nausea/vomiting, abdominal distension, jaundice, melena, or hematochezia. She has never had a blood transfusion, tattoos, or any history of incarceration. Social history reveals no history of alcohol use, tobacco use, or illicit drug use. She is not married and has never been sexually active. The patient emigrated from Vietnam with her family when she was a child. Her mother and one of her siblings have chronic hepatitis B (CHB). There is no family history of liver cancer. Her vital signs and physical examination are normal.

Who should be screened for hepatitis B?

Hepatitis B virus (HBV) accounts for about 15% of chronic viral hepatitis in the United States. The prevalence is highest among immigrants from countries where chronic HBV infection is endemic (where prevalence is as high as 25%) and those with high-risk behaviors. Transmission of HBV is via perinatal, percutaneous, and sexual exposure, and by close prolonged contact (presumably by open cuts and sores) with infected individuals. In countries with high prevalence of CHB, perinatal transmission (also referred to as vertical transmission) is the most common. Screening tests for HBV infection include hepatitis B surface Ag (HBsAg), hepatitis B surface antibody (anti-HBs), and hepatitis B core antibody (anti-HBc) (see Tables 36.1–36.3).

CLINICAL PEARL **STEP 2/3**

When screening for HBV infection, HBsAb should be included in the test panel to determine the immunization status of the patient and to provide vaccination if needed.

CLINICAL PEARL **STEP 1/2/3**

HBsAg establishes the presence of active HBV infection. Chronic hepatitis B is defined as the presence of serum HBsAg for at least 6 months.

Additional tests are obtained and the results are shown in Table 36.4. An abdominal ultrasound shows normal appearance of liver contour and echotexture without hepatomegaly or splenomegaly and no ascites. The portal vein is patent with blood flow toward the liver.

TABLE 36.1 ■ **Countries With High or Intermediate Prevalence of HBV**

- All African countries
- All North, Southeast, and East Asia
- South Pacific (except Australia and New Zealand)
- Middle East (except Cyprus and Israel)
- Eastern Europe (except Hungary)
- Western Europe: Malta, Spain, Greenland indigenous populations
- North America: indigenous populations of Alaska and Northern Canada
- Central America: Guatemala and Honduras
- South America: Venezuela, Ecuador, Guyana, Suriname
- Caribbean (Antigua-Barbuda, Dominica, Grenada, Haiti, Jamaica, Saint Kitts and Nevis, Saint Lucia, and Turks and Caicos Islands)

HBV, Hepatitis B Virus.

Does the patient need to be started on antiviral therapy?

For an individual to have chronic hepatitis B (CHB), HBsAg must remain positive for at least 6 months. There are three main phases of CHB and knowing which phase a patient is in is critical for determining whether anti-HBV medications are indicated. This is because there is no cure for CHB, and the goal of antiviral therapy is viral suppression to prevent complications such as fulminant hepatic failure, cirrhosis of the liver, and hepatocellular carcinoma (HCC). Viral activity and, consequently, the risk of complications of infection, is evaluated using the alanine aspartate (ALT), a measure of liver inflammation, the hepatitis B viral load (HBV DNA), and the hepatitis B envelope antigen and antibody (HBeAg and HBeAb, respectively). These are all blood tests. Immune-tolerant CHB patients often have very high viral load (typically >1 million IU/mL) and positive HBeAg, but minimal to no inflammation and fibrosis of the liver; their ALT usually remains normal. If the patient develops biochemical or histological evidence of active hepatitis, the patient may have transitioned to the immune-active phase, which has two subtypes based on whether HBeAg is positive or negative. Immune-active CHB criteria are met when ALT is greater than twice the upper limit of normal (ULN) and HBV DNA is greater than 20,000 IU/mL in HBeAg-positive individuals, and greater than 2000 IU/mL in HBeAg-negative individuals. Patients are said to have inactive chronic hepatitis B when they are HBeAg negative and anti-HBe positive; HBV DNA is less than 2000 IU/mL, with ALT less than twice the ULN; and there is no evidence of inflammation on liver biopsy. The ULN for ALT is 30 for males and 19 for females, which can differ significantly from laboratory reference ranges.

BASIC SCIENCE PEARL **STEP 1**

Although HBV is a DNA virus, replication occurs through a pregenomic RNA and requires reverse transcriptase, which is the main target of antiviral therapy.

Current guidelines from the American Association for the Study of Liver Diseases (AASLD) recommend anti-HBV therapy for any individual with immune-active CHB. It is important to remember that other causes of ALT elevation should be ruled out before attributing the elevation to CHB. Serial monitoring of ALT, HBV DNA, and HBeAg is recommended for individuals who do not meet the criteria for starting therapy (see Table 36.5).

CLINICAL PEARL **STEP 2/3**

When a patient with chronic hepatitis B develops an elevated ALT, the next step is to assess for causes other than HBV infection; this should be done before initiating anti-HBV therapy.

TABLE 36.2 ■ **Who Should Be Screened for HBV in the United States**

- Individuals born in regions of high or intermediate prevalence[a]
- US-born unvaccinated individuals whose parents were born in high/intermediate prevalence regions
- Intravenous drug users
- Men who have sex with men
- Individuals needing immunosuppressive therapy
- Individuals with elevated liver enzymes of unknown etiology
- Donors of blood, organs, and semen
- Persons with end-stage renal disease who will require any method of dialysis
- Pregnant women
- Infants born to HBsAg-positive mothers
- Individuals with chronic liver disease
- Individuals with HIV infection
- Household, needle-sharing, and sexual contacts of HBV-positive individuals
- Individuals with more than one sexual partner in the last 6 months
- Individuals seeking evaluation for sexually transmitted infections
- Health care and public safety workers with potential occupational exposure
- Residents of health facilities
- Inmates of correctional facilities
- Travelers to countries with high/intermediate prevalence of HBV
- Unvaccinated individuals with diabetes between the ages of 19 and 59 years

HBsAg, Hepatitis B surface antigen; *HIV*, human immunodeficiency virus.
[a]A high-prevalence or endemic geographic region is defined as prevalence of HBsAg positivity in ≥8% of the population, and intermediate-prevalence is defined as prevalence of HBsAg positivity in 2% to 7% of the population.

TABLE 36.3 ■ **HBV Screening Tests Interpretation**

HBsAg	Anti-HBs	Anti-HBc	Interpretation
+	–	+	Chronic hepatitis B
–	+	+	Prior HBV infection with development of immunity from de novo infection (but NOT reactivation)
–	–	+	Prior HBV infection without active infection or development of immunity
–	+	–	Immunity with no prior exposure (vaccinated)
–	–	–	Unaffected, not immune

HBsAg, Hepatitis B virus surface antigen; *anti-HBs*, antibody to Hepatitis B surface antigen; *anti-HBc*, antibody to Hepatitis B core antigen.

TABLE 36.4 ■ **Laboratory Test Results**

Hepatitis B surface antigen (HBsAg)	Positive
Hepatitis B core antibody (anti-HBc)	Positive
Hepatitis B surface antibody (anti-HBs)	Negative
Hepatitis B viral load (HBV DNA)	1.57 million IU/mL
Hepatitis B e antigen (HBeAg)	Positive
Hepatitis B e antibody (anti-HBe)	Negative
Alanine aminotransferase (ALT)	20 U/L
Aspartate aminotransferase (AST)	18 U/L
Alkaline phosphatase	57 IU/L
Total bilirubin	0.9 mg/dL
Albumin	3.8 g/dL
Prothrombin time (PT)	12 seconds
International normalized ratio (INR)	1.0

TABLE 36.5 ■ **Chronic Hepatitis B Definitions**

Status	Definition	When to Treat	Duration of Treatment
Immune-tolerant	– HBsAg positive for at least 6 months – HBeAg positive – HBV DNA levels high, typically >1 million IU/mL – ALT level <1.5 times the ULN[a] – Liver biopsy or noninvasive tests show no inflammation and no fibrosis	Treat when there is evidence of necroinflammation or fibrosis	Indefinitely for advanced fibrosis
Immune-active	– HBsAg positive for at least 6 months – HBV DNA >20,000 IU/mL in HBeAg-positive individuals, and >2000 IU/mL in HBeAg-negative individuals – ALT level intermittently or persistently elevated – Liver biopsy or noninvasive tests show chronic hepatitis with necroinflammation – [a]Fibrosis may or may not be present	HBeAg negative: when HBV DNA >20,000 IU/mL and ALT >2 times ULN HBeAg positive: when HBV DNA >2000 IU/mL and ALT >2 times ULN	Indefinitely for HBeAg-negative individuals For HBeAg-positive individuals, treat through HBeAg seroconversion[b] and may discontinue after 12 months of consolidation therapy[c]
Inactive	– HBsAg positive for at least 6 months – HBeAg negative, anti-HBe positive – HBV DNA levels low (<2000 IU/mL) – Persistently normal ALT level – Liver biopsy or noninvasive tests show no necroinflammation – Fibrosis may or may not be present	May consider treatment in those with high-risk virus or increased risk of HCC	Indefinitely

ULN, Upper limit of normal; *ALT*, alanine transaminase; *HCC*, hepatocellular carcinoma.
[a]ULN for ALT is defined as 29–33 U/L for adult males and 19–25 U/L for adult females.
[b]HBeAg seroconversion: loss of HBeAg and detection of anti-HBe in an individual who was previously HBeAg positive and anti-HBe negative.
[c]Consolidation therapy period: normal ALT and undetectable HBV DNA for 12 months under therapy after seroconversion.

CLINICAL PEARL **STEP 1/2/3**

The upper limit of normal for ALT is defined by the AASLD as 29–33 U/L for adult males and 19–25 U/L for adult females. Beware that the normal range of ALT varies widely between clinical laboratories and may be different from these definitions.

Based on the laboratory tests, you determine that the patient has immune-tolerant CHB and is not cirrhotic; therefore, anti-HBV therapy is not recommended at this time. You explain this to the patient and instruct her to return in 6 months with repeat liver function tests, HBV DNA, and HBeAg. Before the end of the visit, the patient asks you which treatment options are available for her should she need it in the future.

Which treatment options are available for CHB?

There are two broad categories of anti-HBV medications: interferon and nucleoside/nucleotide analogs. Nucleoside/nucleotide analogs are generally preferred because they are administered orally, are well tolerated, and have potent inhibition of viral replication, and newer generations carry low risk of drug resistance. Entecavir and tenofovir disoproxil fumarate (TDF) are the preferred first-line agents; lamivudine and adefovir have fallen out of favor because of high rates of resistance and adefovir has limited potency. The primary concern with entecavir is a 3% rate of viral resistance with long-term use. Nephrotoxicity is the primary concern for TDF, although the rate is less than 2%.

BASIC SCIENCE PEARL **STEP 1**

Nucleoside/nucleotide analogs are reverse transcriptase inhibitors. They work by interfering with the HBV DNA polymerase activity, resulting in inhibition of viral replication. These drugs were initially developed for HIV treatment.

The main advantages of interferon are a finite duration of therapy (typically less than 1 year) and lower rates of biochemical and virological relapse. However, it has a high rate of adverse effects, must be administered via subcutaneous injection, and can lead to hepatic decompensation in patients with cirrhosis. These are the reasons patients older than 60 years and the presence of significant medical comorbidities, including advanced liver fibrosis, are relative contraindications for its use. As a result, interferon is primarily reserved for young, healthy individuals who do not wish to be on long-term treatment.

CLINICAL PEARL **STEP 2/3**

Entecavir and tenofovir disoproxil fumarate (TDF) are the recommended first-line monotherapy agents in hepatitis B treatment because of their efficacy and low rates of viral resistance.

The patient returns for follow-up after 6 months. She is doing well and remains asymptomatic. Laboratory testing shows that she is still immune tolerant. The patient happily announces that she is pregnant. She has many questions about how CHB can affect the pregnancy and how to prevent perinatal transmission.

How does CHB affect pregnancy?

CHB does not affect fertility and does not appear to have any effect on fetal development. Most studies have shown that HBV DNA levels do not change significantly over the course of pregnancy. However, there appears to be an increased incidence of HBV-related hepatitis (defined as elevation in ALT to three to five times the ULN) in the postpartum period. Postpartum flares usually resolve spontaneously and are thought to be related to reconstitution of the immune system after delivery.

CLINICAL PEARL **STEP 2/3**

During pregnancy, certain examination findings (e.g., palmar erythema, edema) and laboratory changes (e.g., decrease in albumin and hematocrit) may mimic progression of liver disease. These are normal physiologic changes related to pregnancy; there is no evidence to suggest that pregnancy is associated with progression of liver disease.

What can be done to prevent perinatal transmission?

All pregnant women should be routinely screened for hepatitis B at their initial visit. Without intervention, perinatal transmission of HBV is as high as 90%. Hepatitis B immune globulin (HBIG) and HBV vaccine given to the newborn within 12 hours of delivery has been shown to reduce the perinatal transmission rate to 3%–7%.

Mothers with CHB and HBV DNA >200,000 IU/mL during the second trimester should also be given anti-HBV therapy during the third trimester to reduce the risk of perinatal transmission. TDF is the agent of choice because of its safety profile in pregnancy, potency, and lack of drug resistance.

Antiviral therapy started during the third trimester to prevent perinatal transmission is usually stopped at the time of delivery or within 4 weeks postpartum. Breastfeeding is not prohibited while taking antiviral therapy, despite drug labels not recommending it. Although there are small amounts of the drugs excreted into breast milk, clinical studies have not revealed any safety concerns.

HBV vaccination is safe and effective during pregnancy and is recommended in pregnant women who are not immune and not infected with HBV.

You recommend that the patient obtain an HBV DNA level at the end of the second trimester, with the plan to start TDF in the third trimester if the viral load is >200,000 IU/mL. You also recommend that the newborn be given HBIG and HBV vaccine within 12 hours of delivery. The patient agrees with your recommendations. Before the conclusion of the visit, the patient asks you about her risk of liver cancer and whether screening is necessary.

When is hepatocellular carcinoma (HCC) screening indicated in CHB?

HCC screening is recommended for all patients with cirrhosis. In patients with CHB who are not cirrhotic, HCC screening is recommended for subgroups in which the annual incidence of HCC exceeds 0.2%, which is the threshold above which screening is cost effective. These subgroups are identified in Table 36.6. The recommended tools for screening are abdominal ultrasound with or without serum alpha-fetoprotein (AFP) every 6 months. The use of AFP alone is not recommended.

TABLE 36.6 ■ **Chronic HBV Subgroups Without Cirrhosis Recommended to Undergo HCC Surveillance**

- Active hepatitis (e.g., elevated ALT) and HBV DNA >20,000 IU/mL
- Family history of HCC
- Asian males over 40 years of age
- Asian females over 50 years of age
- Africans and African Americans

HCC, Hepatocellular carcinoma.

CLINICAL PEARL **STEP 2/3**

In clinical practice, liver protocol computed tomography (CT) can be used for HCC surveillance and when there is increased clinical suspicion of HCC (i.e., normal ultrasound but elevated AFP level), but it is not recommended for routine screening because of the risks of radiation exposure.

The patient reports no family history of liver cancer. Therefore, if she continues to be in the immune-tolerant phase and does not progress to cirrhosis, she will not need HCC surveillance until she is 50 years old.

Case Summary

- **Complaint/History:** A 26-year-old woman from Vietnam with no significant past medical history presents to your clinic with a new diagnosis of CHB that is in the immune-tolerant phase, and she later becomes pregnant.
- **Lab Results/Tests:** Laboratory testing reveals high HBV DNA, normal liver function tests, and positive HBeAg.

Diagnosis: Immune-tolerant CHB infection with no cirrhosis of the liver. She probably acquired HBV via perinatal transmission, by far the most common mode of transmission in countries with high prevalence of HBV such as Vietnam.

- **Management:** Since the patient was in the immune-tolerant phase, antiviral therapy was not indicated. At her return visit, she announced she was pregnant. You recommended that her newborn receive HBIG and HBV vaccine within 12 hours of delivery and, for her high viral load, she might need antiviral therapy during the third trimester to prevent perinatal transmission. She will need to begin HCC screening starting at the age of 50 years unless her disease state changes.

BEYOND THE PEARLS

- The following ultrasonographic features suggest advanced fibrosis of the liver: nodular liver contour and shrunken liver. The following features suggest portal hypertension: splenomegaly, ascites, reversal of flow of the portal vein, and cavernous transformation of the portal vein. These features are useful in clinical practice to evaluate for cirrhosis and the resulting portal hypertension. However, these findings lack sensitivity, and if a study does not demonstrate these findings, it does not rule out cirrhosis.
- HBV infection is the most common cause of HCC worldwide, accountable for up to 54% of all liver cancers. In endemic countries, it is estimated to account for up to 80% of HCC. In the United States, only about 10%–16% of HCC cases are attributed to HBV.
- There are 10 genotypes of hepatitis B. In the United States, genotypes A, B, and C are most prevalent. Genotyping can be useful in specific clinical scenarios (for example, genotype A is known to have higher rates of HBeAg and HBsAg loss with interferon therapy) but is not routinely indicated.
- Patients who are HBsAg positive or anti-HBc IgG positive are at risk of HBV reactivation when sufficiently immunosuppressed or immunocompromised, even if HBV DNA is initially undetectable.
- Isolated anti-HBc IgG positivity suggests prior de novo infection with clearance of the virus from the blood. However, there is an undetectable reservoir of viral covalently closed circular DNA (cccDNA) within hepatocytes that can reactivate, leading to acute HBV infection and in some cases fulminant liver failure in the setting of immunosuppression.

- In mothers with CHB, the risks of transmission from invasive procedures such as amniocentesis is unclear; studies suggest that high viremia (>1 million IU/mL) may correlate with higher rates of transmission.
- Extending third trimester antiviral therapy up to 12 weeks postpartum does not offer protection against postpartum flare.

Bibliography

Bruix, J., & Sherman, M. (2005). Management of hepatocellular carcinoma. *Hepatology, 42*, 1208–1236.

Bzowej. N. H. (2012). Optimal management of the hepatitis B patient who desires pregnancy or is pregnant. *Current Hepatology Reports, 11*, 82–89.

Center for Disease Control and Prevention. (2011). Use of hepatitis B vaccination for adults with diabetes mellitus: Recommendations of the Advisory Committee on Immunization Practices (ACIP). *MMWR. Morbidity and Mortality Weekly Report, 60*, 1709–1711.

Chang, C. Y., Aziz, N., Poongkunran, M., et al. (2016). Serum alanine aminotransferase and hepatitis B DNA flares in pregnant and postpartum women with chronic hepatitis B. *The American Journal of Gastroenterology, 111*, 1410–1415.

Chayanupatkul, M., Omino, R., Mittal, S., et al. (2017). Hepatocellular carcinoma in the absence of cirrhosis in patients with chronic hepatitis B virus infection. *Journal of Hepatology, 66*, 355–362.

Giles, M., Visvanathan, K., Lewin, S., et al. (2015). Clinical and virological predictors of hepatic flares in pregnant women with chronic hepatitis B. *Gut, 64*, 1810–1815.

Lok, A. S., McMahon, B. J., Brown, R. S., et al. (2016). Antiviral therapy for chronic hepatitis B viral infection in adults: a systemic review and meta-analysis. *Hepatology, 63, 284–306.*

Society for Maternal-Fetal Medicine (SMFM), Dionne-Odom, J., Tita, A. T., & Silverman, N. S. (2016). #38: Hepatitis B in pregnant screening, treatment, and prevention of vertical transmission. *American Journal of Obstetrics and Gynecology, 214, 6–14.*

Terrault, N. A., Bzowej, N. H., Chang, K. M., et al. (2016). AASLD guidelines for treatment of chronic hepatitis B. *Hepatology, 63, 261–283.*

Terrault, N. A., Lok, A. S., McMahon, B. J., et al. (2018). Update on prevention, diagnosis, and treatment of chronic hepatitis B: AASLD 2018 hepatitis B guidance. *Hepatology, 67*(4), 1560–1599.

Weinbaum, C. M., Williams, I., Mast, E. E., et al. (2008). Recommendations for identification and public health management of persons with chronic hepatitis B virus infection. *MMWR: Recommendations and Reports, 57*, 1–20.

CASE 37

A 24-Year-Old Male With Elevated Liver Function Tests

Daniel Chao

A 24-year-old male presents to the emergency department with 3 days of "yellow eyes" and generalized fatigue. The patient has no known medical history, no history of surgery, and no family history of hepatobiliary disease. He reports no medication use, does not smoke or drink alcohol, and reports no use of illicit substances. Review of systems is otherwise negative. On physical examination, blood pressure is 115/68 mmHg, pulse rate is 81/min, respiration rate is 8/min, and oxygen saturation is 99% on room air. He is afebrile. Scleral icterus is present. The remainder of the examination is normal. Blood work is significant for total bilirubin (Tbili) 8, aspartate aminotransferase (AST) 694, alanine aminotransferase (ALT) 585, and alkaline phosphatase (ALP) 217.

What is the initial approach to evaluation of elevated liver function tests (LFTs)?

LFTs can be organized into liver biochemical tests (Tbili, AST, ALT, and ALP) and tests of hepatic synthetic function (albumin and prothrombin time). It is important to analyze results both individually and collectively. Elevated AST and ALT indicate hepatocellular injury. Hyperbilirubinemia can be caused by increased breakdown of hemoglobin from red blood cells, which causes an oversupply of bilirubin that has not yet been processed by the liver (unconjugated bilirubin). Elevated total bilirubin can also be caused by impaired hepatic metabolism and release from damaged hepatocytes or bile ducts, which results in increased levels of conjugated bilirubin. Therefore, the first step whenever Tbili is elevated is to fractionate it by obtaining a direct (conjugated) bilirubin level. An elevated direct bilirubin indicates that hepatobiliary disease is present.

When hyperbilirubinemia and elevated AST and ALT are present, causes can be categorized as either bile duct obstruction or hepatitis with cholestasis and initial workup should include both types of diseases. A condensed initial differential diagnosis for elevated LFTs is shown in Table 37.1.

The patient is found to have an elevated direct bilirubin. Over the next 3 hospital days, AST and ALT trend upward, with both peaking around 1000. Tbili increases to 10.7. Available results of the initial workup can be seen in Table 37.2. Ultrasound of the abdomen shows a normal caliber common bile duct of 4 mm, a smooth liver contour, and spleen size within normal limits. He reports no abdominal pain, nausea, or vomiting, and his white blood cell count, prothrombin time, and international normalized ratio (INR) are normal. HIV test is negative. He is questioned again regarding medication, alcohol, and illicit substance intake, and he does not recall taking anything of significance and reiterates that he takes no medication daily. A decision is made to perform a liver biopsy.

TABLE 37.1 ■ **Causes of Elevated Total Bilirubin, Alanine Aminotransferase, and Aspartate Aminotransferase**

Biliary Obstruction	Hepatocellular Injury With Cholestasis
Choledocholithiasis	Acute alcoholic hepatitis
Cholangiocarcinoma	Acute viral hepatitis (including HSV, CMV, EBV)
HIV cholangiopathy	Autoimmune hepatitis
Pancreatic head cancer	Congestive hepatopathy (i.e., from heart failure)
Parasitic infections	Cirrhosis with active liver injury
Primary sclerosing cholangitis	Drug-induced liver injury
	Hypoperfusion (shock liver)
	Infiltrative liver disease (e.g., lymphoma, tuberculosis)
	Wilson disease

CMV, Cytomegalovirus; *EBV*, Epstein-Barr virus; *HSV*, herpes simplex virus.

TABLE 37.2 ■ **The Patient's Initial Serological Workup**

Disease	Test(s)	Result
Acute hepatitis A	HAV IgM	Negative
Acute hepatitis B	HBsAg (surface antigen)	Negative
	HBsAb (surface antibody)	Negative
	HBc IgM (core antibody)	Negative
Acute hepatitis C	Anti-HCV Ab	Negative
	HCV RNA (viral load)	Negative
Autoimmune hepatitis	Antismooth muscle antibody	Pending
	Antimitochondrial antibody	Pending
Wilson disease	Ceruloplasmin	34 (within normal limits)

HAV, Hepatitis A Virus; *HCV*, Hepatitis C Virus

What should be part of this patient's daily clinical monitoring?

The lack of right upper quadrant pain, fevers, leukocytosis, and bile duct dilation on imaging indicate that bile duct obstruction and cholangitis are unlikely. Therefore, this is probably a case of severe hepatocellular injury with cholestasis that is acutely progressing.

This patient is at risk of developing fulminant hepatic failure, which is defined as the presence of encephalopathy and an elevated INR in the setting of acute liver injury. The daily physical examination should include assessment of alertness, orientation, communication, and basic cognitive skills as well as evaluation for asterixis. INR should be monitored daily. For a patient who is relatively young with no obvious contraindications, a liver transplant evaluation should be initiated if he were to develop fulminant liver failure.

CLINICAL PEARL **STEP 2/3**

Hepatitis C virus (HCV) antibody seroconverts from negative to positive between day 15 and month 3 of infection; therefore, if very recent, acute infection should be suspected and a viral load (HCV RNA) should be checked. Anyone with a detectable viral load has active HCV infection. The virus genotype is obtained in those with active HCV infection to help determine the appropriate treatment regimen, although the most recently developed antiviral medications work across all genotypes.

CLINICAL PEARL **STEP 2/3**

It is important to recognize cholangitis early because patients can decompensate if they do not receive prompt treatment. Early treatment includes resuscitation and antibiotics and relief of biliary obstruction should be achieved within 24 hours of presentation.

Charcot's triad describes the clinical manifestations that should raise concern for ascending cholangitis.

1. Fever
2. Jaundice
3. Right upper quadrant pain

CLINICAL PEARL **STEP 2/3**

Examination for asterixis is performed by asking the patient to hold their arms out straight in front of them with the wrists extended so that the fingers are perpendicular to the ground. They should then hold this position for several seconds. Asterixis is described as a "flapping tremor," where the hands fall toward the ground as the wrists lose their extension suddenly. This was first described in hepatic encephalopathy but can occur in any form of toxic-metabolic encephalopathy (Figs. 37.1 and 37.2).

Why is a liver biopsy indicated?

The diagnostic plan is always dependent on the differential diagnosis. Focusing on the causes of hepatocellular injury with cholestasis (Table 37.1), the lab results in Table 37.2 allow us to eliminate acute hepatitis A, hepatitis B, and hepatitis C. Because the patient has no significant alcohol history, acute alcoholic hepatitis is not suspected at this point. There are no findings to suggest heart failure, no history of hypotension or shock, and no evidence of cirrhosis; therefore, these are also less likely etiologies. A normal ceruloplasmin and elevated ALP do not indicate Wilson disease. This leaves autoimmune hepatitis (AIH), drug-induced liver injury (DILI), and infiltrative liver disease. The best way to differentiate among these entities is through liver histology.

The liver biopsy shows a combination of lobular hepatitis with necrosis (Fig. 37.3), interface hepatitis (Fig. 37.4), and cholestasis (Fig. 37.5). This is suggestive of DILI, with features of AIH.

One week after admission, the patient remembers that he was taking medication that he obtained from a friend because he had hurt his back at work about 6 weeks prior to the onset of his

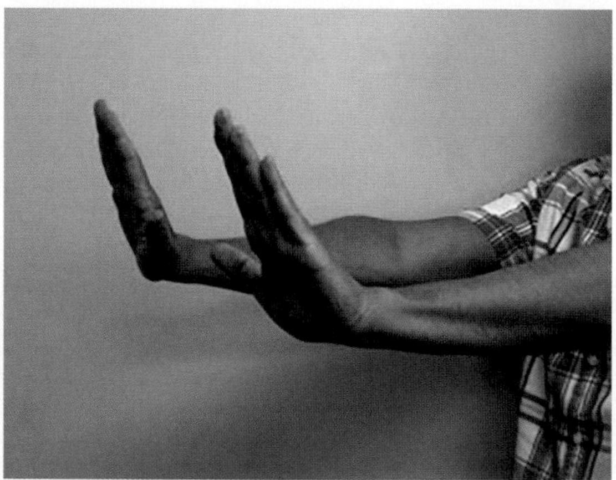

Fig. 37.1 Physical examination for asterixis: The patient is asked to hold their arms out straight in front of them with the wrists extended so that the fingers are perpendicular to the ground.

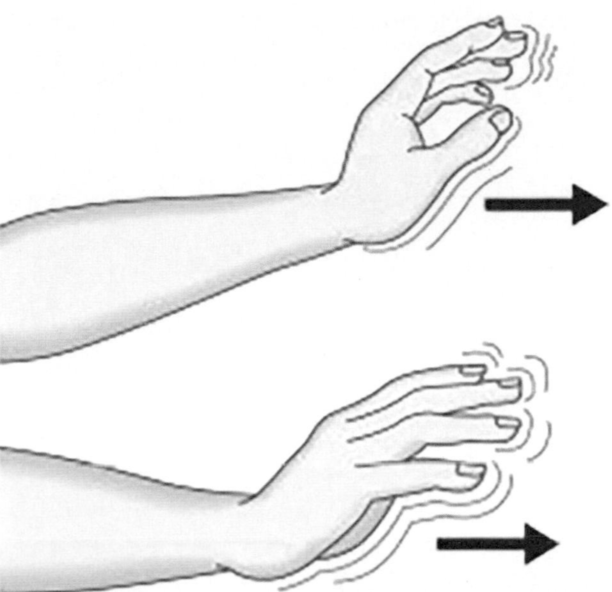

Fig. 37.2 Asterixis is described as a "flapping tremor". The examiner will observe the patient being unable to maintain the wrists in flexed position, exhibiting a repetitive wrist drop that is followed by return to the original position.

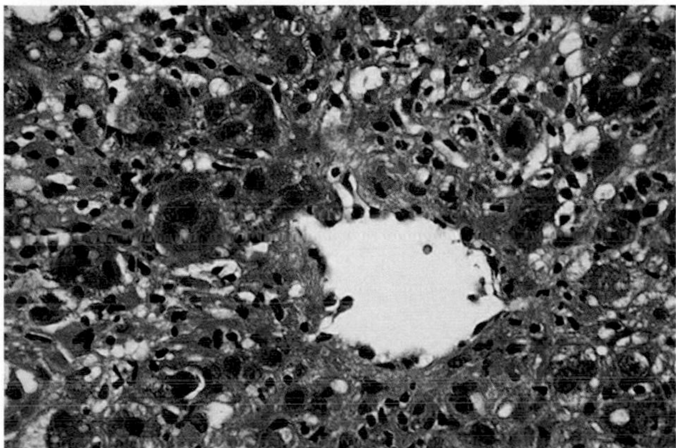

Fig. 37.3 Liver biopsy: Lobular hepatitis with necrosis.

symptoms. His family was able to bring in the bottle and the medication was identified as diclofenac. He cannot remember how many pills he was taking each day, but consumption was daily for at least 1 week. DILI caused by diclofenac was thus determined to be the most likely diagnosis.

The patient did not receive any nonsteroidal antiinflammatory drug (NSAID) for the duration of his hospitalization, but despite this his Tbili plateaus at 10, and does not decrease for the next 3 days. AST and ALT have improved to 217 and 254, respectively, but also plateau. Antismooth muscle antibody (SMA) has now resulted and is positive. Antimitochondrial antibody is negative.

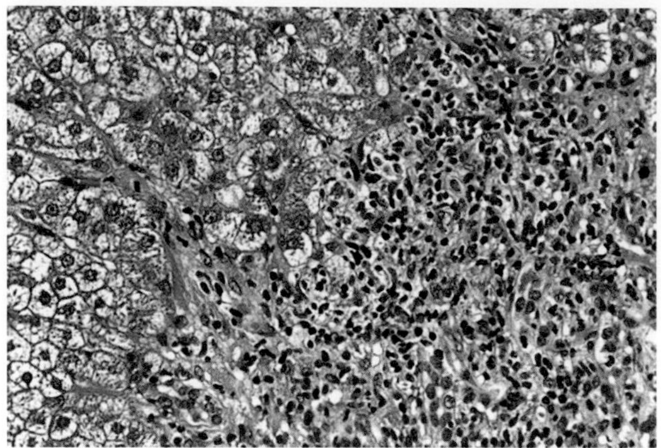

Fig. 37.4 Liver biopsy: Interface hepatitis.

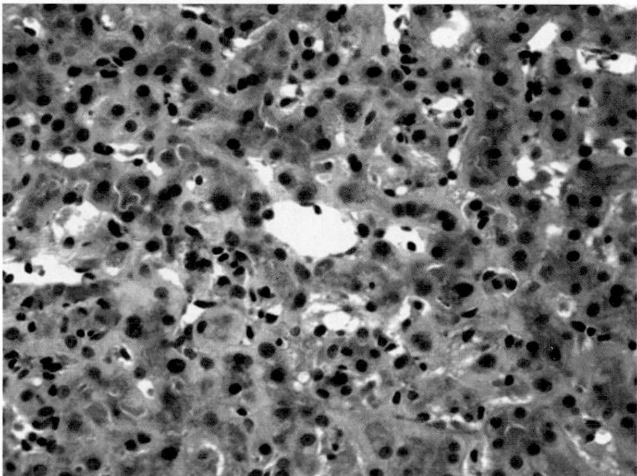

Fig. 37.5 Liver biopsy: Cholestatic liver injury.

What is the most appropriate next step in management?

Given that NSAIDs are some of the most widely used medications in the world, the overall incidence of acute hepatotoxicity is relatively rare. However, the reaction is idiosyncratic rather than dose dependent and the consumption history can therefore sometimes seem underwhelming. Patients also often forget to mention their use, because it may be temporary and weeks or months prior to the adverse event. Therefore, repeated questioning is important in the setting of liver injury of unclear etiology.

As the biopsy in this case demonstrates, DILI can cause different types of liver injury. Interface hepatitis and a positive SMA is suggestive of an AIH-like presentation. Although most cases of diclofenac-associated DILI resolve relatively quickly upon withdrawal of the medication, this patient stopped improving and therefore immunosuppression with glucocorticoids should be considered.

The patient's AST, ALT, and Tbili began to improve within 24 hours of initiating IV methylprednisolone, and he is transitioned to oral prednisone at discharge with a gradual taper. At the clinic follow-up 4 weeks later, all liver biochemical tests were normal.

Case Summary

- **Complaint/History:** A 24-year-old male presents with jaundice and elevated liver biochemical tests.
- **Findings:** Examination reveals scleral icterus but is otherwise unremarkable.
- **Lab Results/Tests:** The patient had severe acute hepatitis with cholestasis and antismooth muscle antibody was positive. All other serological tests for acute and chronic liver disease were negative. Imaging showed no evidence of bile duct obstruction. Liver biopsy showed features consistent with drug-induced liver injury with autoimmune hepatitis-like features.

Diagnosis: Diclofenac-associated hepatotoxicity with autoimmune hepatitis-like features.

- **Treatment:** Supportive care, clinical monitoring for fulminant hepatic failure, and withdrawal of the offending agent. The autoimmune hepatitis component eventually required immunosuppression with glucocorticoids to enable full recovery.

BEYOND THE PEARLS

- Other than diclofenac, other medications known for causing DILI with AIH-like features include statins, hydralazine, methyldopa, minocycline, nitrofurantoin, and procainamide.
- Histological features for DILI with AIH-like features are similar to AIH, including interface hepatitis and plasma cell infiltrates. Serological tests for both diseases can also be similar, with positive antinuclear antibodies (ANA) and/or SMA and elevated total IgG.
- DILI with AIH-like features may respond faster to glucocorticoid therapy than AIH and there is no recurrence if the drug is not reintroduced.
- Table 37.3 provides a list of some important causes of DILI and key considerations for each cause.

TABLE 37.3 ■ **Important Causes of Drug-Induced Liver Injury**

Drug Name or Family	Important Points to Consider
Acetaminophen	Can lead to acute liver failure; low levels can be toxic if time of ingestion was many hours earlier.
Antibiotics	Onset of hepatotoxicity may be 1–3 weeks after administration; risks and benefits of stopping the medication depend on the severity and acuity of the liver injury and the alternative treatments available for the infection.
Dietary supplements and herbals	Data may be limited and lack of evidence does not rule these out as causes; these should be stopped whenever DILI is suspected.
Immune checkpoint inhibitors	Can lead to severe hepatitis with cholestasis and liver failure; high dose corticosteroid therapy is usually needed to help resolve the liver injury.
Lipid lowering agents	Combination therapy with niacin, statins, and/or fibrates can lead to severe hepatitis with cholestasis.
Neuropsychiatry treatments	Many antidepressants, antiepileptics, antipsychotics, and addiction therapy medications can cause hepatotoxicity; stopping these can cause patients to destabilize, so make sure Psychiatry is involved in management.
NSAIDs	Patients may forget or be unaware they have been taking these over the counter; ask about specific drugs.

DILI, Drug-induced liver injury; *NSAIDs*, nonsteroidal antiinflammatory drugs.

Bibliography

Banks, A. T., Zimmerman, H. J., Ishak, K. G., & Harter, J. G. (1995). Diclofenac-associated hepatotoxicity: Analysis of 180 cases reported to the Food and Drug Administration as adverse reactions. *Hepatology, 22*(3), 820–827.

deLemos, A. S., Foureau, D. M., Jacobs, C., Ahrens, W., Russo, M. W., & Bonkovsky, H. L. (2014). Drug-induced liver injury with autoimmune features. *Seminars in Liver Disease, 34*, 194–204.

Febres-Aldana, C. A., Alghamdi, S., Krishnamurthy, K., & Poppiti, R. J. (2019). Liver fibrosis helps to distinguish autoimmune hepatitis from DILI with autoimmune features: A review of twenty cases. *Journal of Clinical and Translational Hepatology*, 7(1), 21–26.

Lefkowitch, J. H. (2016). Drugs and toxins. *Scheuer's liver biopsy interpretation* (9th ed.). Elsevier. Ch 8:127-144.

Manns, M. P., Czaja, A. J., Gorham, J. D., Krawitt E. L., Mieli-Vergani G., Vergani D., and Vierling J. M. (2010). AASLD Practice Guidelines: Diagnosis and management of autoimmune hepatitis. *Hepatology, 51*(6), 2193–2213.

Meunier, L., & Larrey, D. (2018). Recent advances in hepatotoxicity of non-steroidal anti-inflammatory drugs. *Annals of hepatology: official journal of the Mexican Association of Hepatology, 17*(2), 187–191.

O'Connor, N., Dargan, P. I., & Jones, A. L. (2003). Hepatocellular damage from non-steroidal anti-inflammatory drugs. *QJM: Monthly Journal of the Association of Physicians, 96*, 787–791.

Pratt, D.S., Feldman, M., Friedman, L. S., & Brandt, L. J. (2010). Liver chemistry and function tests. In *Sleisenger and Fordtran's gastrointestinal and liver disease: Pathophysiology, diagnosis, management* (9th ed.). Saunders/Elsevier. Ch 73:1227-1234.

Scully, L. J., Clarke, D., & Bar, J. (1993). Diclofenac induced hepatitis: 3 cases with features of autoimmune chronic active hepatitis. *Digestive Diseases and Sciences, 38*, 744–751.

Weber, S., Benesic, A., Rotter, I., & Gerbes, A. L. (2019). Early ALT response to corticosteroid treatment distinguishes idiosyncratic drug-induced liver injury from autoimmune hepatitis. *Liver International: Official Journal of the International Association for the Study of the Liver, 39*(10), 1906–1917.

CASE 38

A 54-Year-Old Female With Dysphagia

Lillian Dawit ■ Christina S. Gainey ■ Ara Sahakian

A 54-year-old female presents with difficulty swallowing over the past 4 years that occurs with both solid foods and liquids. Her symptoms have progressed to the point that she frequently regurgitates food contents and experiences chest discomfort associated with swallowing. Previously, she was diagnosed with gastroesophageal reflux disease, for which she takes a proton pump inhibitor without relief. Currently, she maintains a liquid diet. She also reports unintentional weight loss of 15 lb over the past year. On physical examination, her temperature is 98.5 °F, pulse is 82 beats/min, respiratory rate is 18 breaths/min, blood pressure is 126/78, and oxygen saturation is 99% on room air. The physical examination is otherwise unremarkable. A chest radiograph (Fig. 38.1) shows a retrocardiac air-fluid level in the mediastinum at the level of the aortic arch.

What are some causes of dysphagia?

Dysphagia is defined as difficulty with swallowing. When considering the differential diagnosis for dysphagia, it is important to determine the site of origin (Fig. 38.2).

Oropharyngeal dysphagia is characterized by difficulty transferring digested food from the mouth to the esophagus. Most commonly, this is seen in neuromuscular disorders such as stroke, multiple sclerosis, and dementia. However, structural abnormalities of the oropharynx, including Zenker's diverticulum and malignancies, can also lead to this type of dysphagia.

Esophageal dysphagia occurs when there is difficulty with passing food and/or liquid from the esophagus to the stomach. Mechanical obstruction by a stricture in the esophagus is the most common cause. Esophageal strictures can be either malignant or benign stenoses. Nevertheless, motility disorders such as achalasia, diffuse esophageal spasm, jackhammer esophagus, and gastroesophageal reflux must be considered when evaluating esophageal dysphagia (Table 38.1).

What are key aspects of the history that can help differentiate between the types of dysphagia?

Symptomatology is important for distinguishing features between the many types and causes of dysphagia (Table 38.2). Oropharyngeal dysphagia is described as difficulty with swallow initiation. Patients often report coughing or choking upon eating and may have associated nasopharyngeal regurgitation. In addition, they may experience changes in voice, including nasal tone or hoarseness, known as dysphonia.

Esophageal dysphagia is described as the sensation of food getting "stuck" in the throat or chest. It is important to elicit whether a patient is having difficulty swallowing solids, liquids, or both to help narrow the differential diagnosis. In the setting of mechanical obstruction, patients often report difficulty swallowing solid foods alone. Progression of dysphagia from solid, and foods to liquids over time may suggest the presence of an enlarging tumor. In motility disorders, the patient will generally present with difficulty swallowing both solids and liquids. Associated symptoms must also be considered. Although gradual weight loss is seen in many patients with dysphagia as a result of chronically reduced oral intake, rapid weight loss raises concern for malignancy, as would a history of heavy alcohol use or smoking.

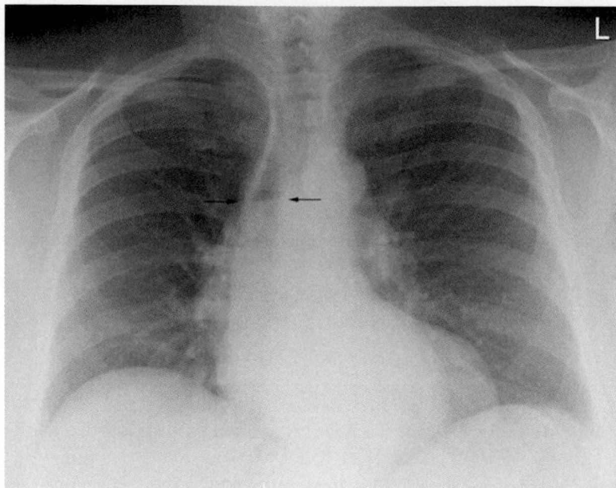

Fig. 38.1 Chest radiograph showing a retrocardiac air-fluid level in the mediastinum at the level of the aortic arch. (From Maher MM, Dixon AK, Grainger & Allison's diagnostic radiology, ed 6. London, Elsevier, 2016.)

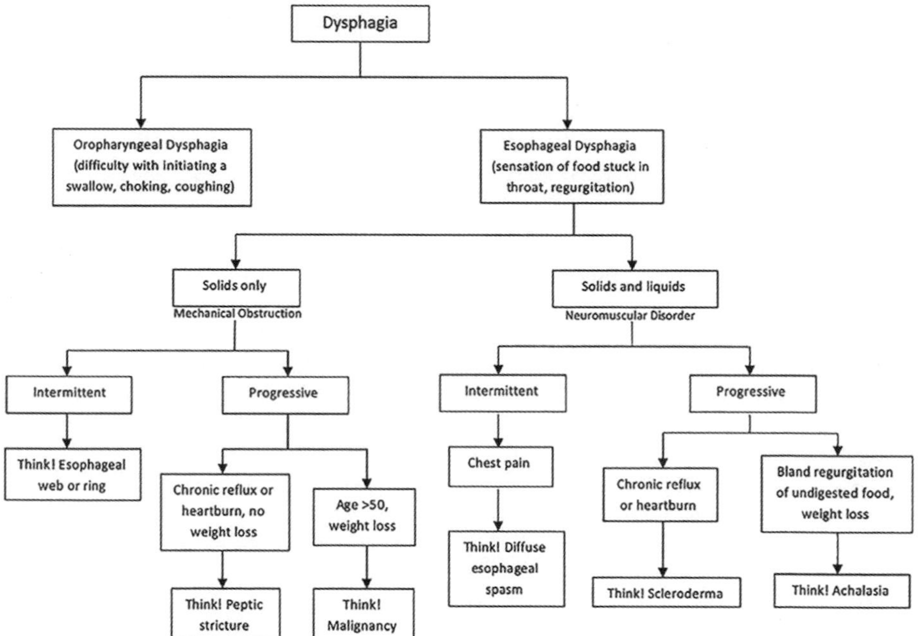

Fig. 38.2 Dysphagia differential flowchart.

Eosinophilic esophagitis is an autoimmune inflammatory disorder that can result in both motility disturbances and mechanical obstruction caused by rings or strictures. Although generally uncommon, eosinophilic esophagitis should be placed higher on the differential diagnosis for dysphagia in a younger patient with a history of food or seasonal allergies, asthma, or atopic dermatitis.

TABLE 38.1 ■ **Causes of Esophageal Dysphagia**

Motility	Mechanical
Diffuse esophageal spasm	Esophagitis
Achalasia	Malignancy
Diabetes mellitus	Peptic stricture
Scleroderma/mixed connective tissue disease	Schatzki's ring
Diffuse esophageal spasm	Extrinsic compression from surrounding structures

TABLE 38.2 ■ **Symptoms of Dysphagia**

Symptoms	Possible Etiology
Coughing, choking while eating, dysphonia, nasopharyngeal regurgitation	Oropharyngeal dysfunction
Trouble swallowing solids only	More likely mechanical obstruction: ring, web, stricture, or, rarely, malignancy
Trouble swallowing both solids and liquids	Motility disorder, especially achalasia
Acid reflux, heartburn	GERD
Recent onset, rapidly progressive, weight loss	Malignancy
History of food or seasonal allergies, asthma, atopic dermatitis	Eosinophilic esophagitis
Alcohol, smoking history	Esophageal cancer

GERD, Gastroesophageal reflux disease.

What are the main diagnostic studies used to evaluate dysphagia?

Imaging and endoscopic techniques are commonly used to evaluate dysphagia and distinguish between structural and motility disorders. The primary imaging studies utilized include esophagogastroduodenoscopy (EGD), barium esophagram swallowing study, and high-resolution esophageal manometry.

For most patients, the best initial test is an EGD (Fig. 38.3) because it allows direct visualization of strictures, masses, mucosal features of eosinophilic esophagitis, or sequelae of gastroesophageal reflux disease (GERD) such as Barrett's esophagus or erosive esophagitis. If no significant endoscopic findings are encountered, biopsies should be obtained from the proximal and distal esophagus to evaluate for eosinophilic esophagitis. Histologic examination of biopsy samples can distinguish eosinophilic esophagitis from GERD, whereby eosinophilia occurs in the distal esophagus in GERD but occurs both proximally and distally in eosinophilic esophagitis. Any mass lesion must be biopsied. Additionally, retroflexion should be performed in the stomach to evaluate for pseudoachalasia, a condition caused by a mass at the gastric cardia or gastroesophageal junction that can masquerade who was as achalasia.

The barium esophagram swallowing study and found is a less invasive diagnostic modality for evaluating dysphagia (Fig. 38.4). First, the patient is instructed to swallow barium sulfate contrast to coat the esophagus. Next, the radiologist takes a series of X-ray images as the barium moves from mouth to stomach to assess for structural abnormalities in the esophagus. The dynamic nature of this study can also help identify motility disorders. An esophagram may be obtained first in a patient at high risk of complications with procedures or if EGD might be considered difficult to perform (e.g., presence of proximal obstruction, tight strictures, inability to exclude oropharyngeal causes, etc.).

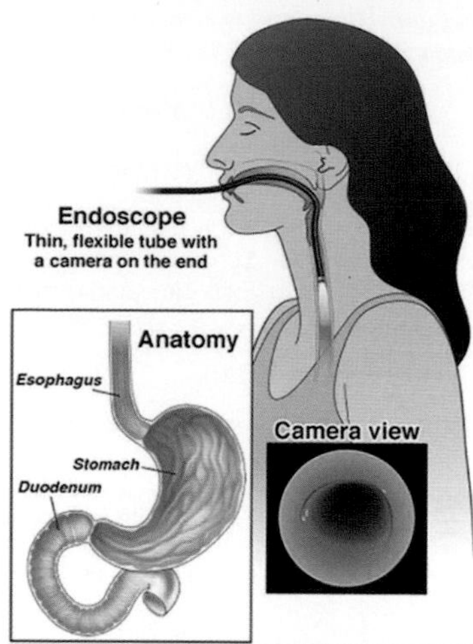

Fig. 38.3 Esophagogastroduodenoscopy.

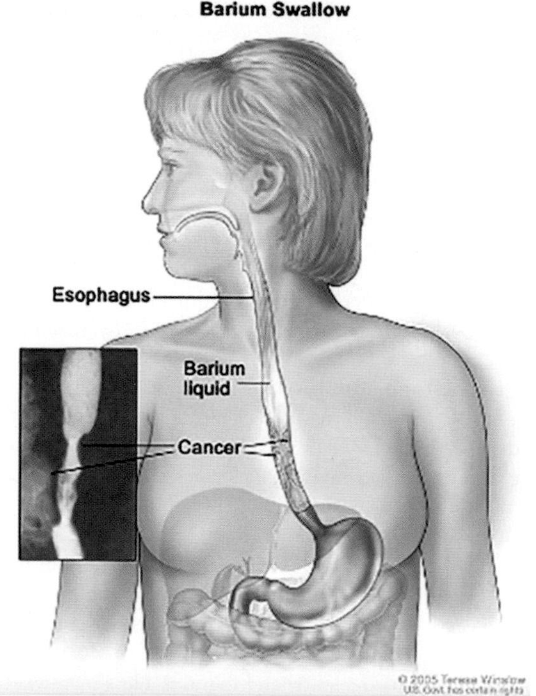

Fig. 38.4 Patients Barium swallow.

The gold standard for diagnosing motility disorders is high-resolution manometry (Fig. 38.5). A flexible catheter with pressure sensors arranged at 1-cm intervals is placed through the patient's nose to rest in the esophagus with the distal tip in the stomach. The patient then performs multiple swallows as the catheter records and measures esophageal pressures along the catheter. This

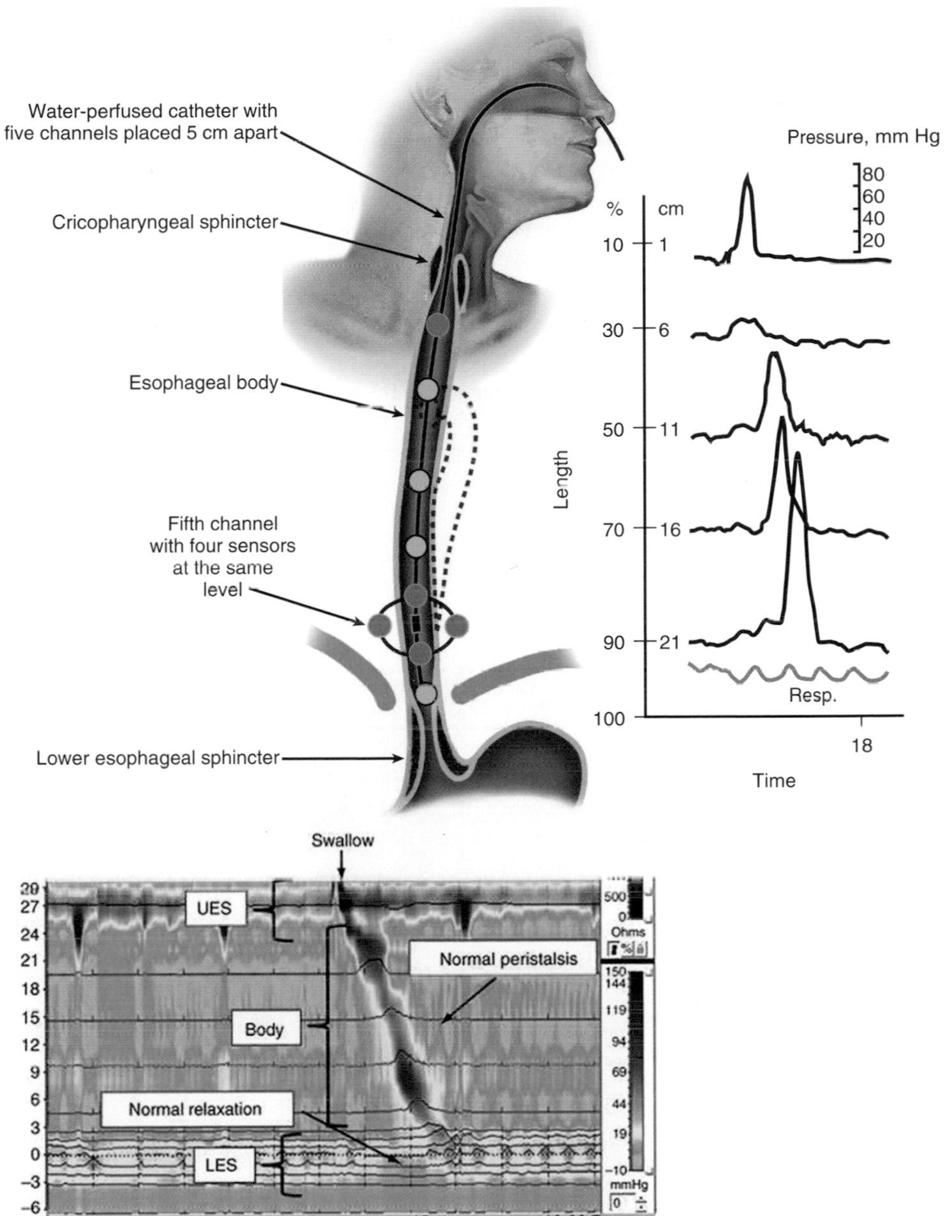

Fig. 38.5 (A) Esophageal manometry. (B) High-resolution esophageal manometry. *LES*, Lower esophageal sphincter; *UES*, upper esophageal sphincter. (From (A) Cameron, J.L. (2017). *Current surgical therapy*, (12th ed.). Elsevier; (B) Yates, R. B., Oelschlager, B. K., & Pellegrini, C. A. (2017). Gastroesophageal reflux disease and hiatal hernia. In C. M. Townsend, R. D. Beauchamp, B. M. Evers, & K. L. Mattox, (Eds.), *Sabiston textbook of surgery* (20th ed.). Elsevier.)

allows pressure patterns to be visualized as a color-coded pressure map of the esophagus and interpreted for diagnosis.

A barium esophagram is performed. The resulting image is shown in Fig. 38.6.

What diagnosis does this suggest and why?

This image is a classic esophagram of a patient with achalasia. Given the absence of peristalsis and lack of relaxation at the lower esophageal sphincter, food and liquid contents will build up and cause dilation proximal to the gastroesophageal junction. The result is a dilated esophagus that narrows at the distal esophagus, creating a typical "bird's beak" appearance. In late-stage achalasia, the esophagus can develop sigmoid tortuosity as seen in Fig. 38.7.

An EGD is performed and there is no sign of obstruction or inflammation in the esophagus. The endoscopist notes difficulty passing the endoscope from the esophagus into the stomach. However, the stomach was also normal in appearance tendineae. The barium esophagram demonstrated a dilated esophagus with stasis of contrast.

What is the next best step to establish a diagnosis?

An esophageal manometry study to evaluate for a motility disorder would be the next best diagnostic step (Table 38.3). Manometry is considered the gold standard imaging for achalasia and

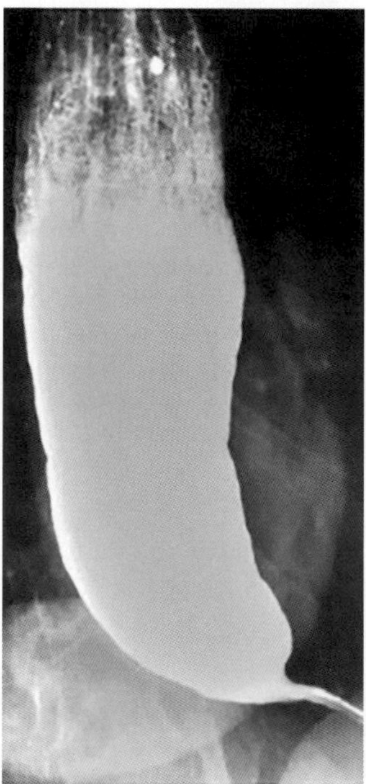

Fig. 38.6 Barium esophagram showing a lower esophageal narrowing with proximal dilation, creating a "bird's beak" image on radiograph, which is pathognomonic for achalasia.

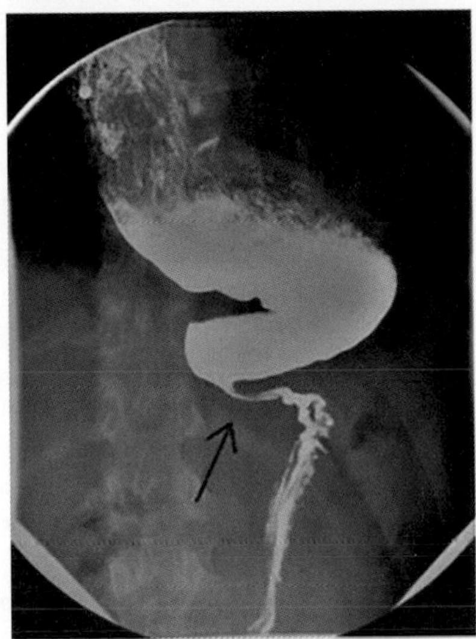

Fig. 38.7 Barium esophagram showing "sigmoid esophagus" (massive dilation of the esophagus with a tortuous configuration and distal tapering), which can result from long-standing achalasia. Interventional therapies may be limited once sigmoidization occurs.

TABLE 38.3 ■ **Esophageal Manometric Findings in Normal Patients and in Patients With Motility Disorders**

Finding	Normal	Achalasia	Diffuse Esophageal Spasm	Nutcracker Esophagus	Ineffective Esophageal Motility
Basal lower esophageal sphincter (LES) pressure	10–45 mmHg	Normal or high	Normal	Normal	Low or normal
LES relaxation, with swallow	Complete	Incomplete	Normal	Normal	Normal
Wave progression	Peristalsis	Aperistalsis	Peristalsis with at least 20% simultaneous contractions	Normal	30% or more failed nontransmitted contractions
Distal wave amplitude	30–180 mmHg	Usually low (may be normal or high)	Normal	High	30% or more <30 mmHg

https://www.clinicalkey.com/-!/content/book/3-s2.0-B9780323611794000685?scrollTo=%23t0010

is required for diagnosis. There are two types of manometry: conventional manometry and high-resolution manometry (Fig. 38.5). High-resolution manometry is preferred because it enables categorization of achalasia subtypes, which can guide management.

Manometry showed multiple areas in the esophagus with simultaneously increased pressure readings upon swallowing, which is described as a spastic pattern.

Integrating the history and workup thus far, what is the most likely diagnosis?

Achalasia, a primary esophageal motility disorder characterized by the patient of esophageal peristalsis and inability of the lower esophageal sphincter to relax.

What is the pathophysiology of achalasia?

Primary achalasia is an autoimmune, neurodegenerative motility disorder of the esophagus. The pathologic, consequence of the disease is **degeneration of ganglion cells in the myenteric plexus** of the esophageal body and the lower esophageal sphincter (LES). Although the etiology of the degenerative processes remains unclear, the consequence of the inflammatory process is loss of inhibitory neurotransmitters such as nitrous oxide and vasoactive intestinal peptide. Imbalance between the excitatory and inhibitory neurons results in **unopposed cholinergic activity that leads to incomplete relaxation of the LES and aperistalsis**.

BASIC SCIENCE/CLINICAL PEARL **STEP 1/2/3**

The LES is under tonic contraction by acetylcholine. After swallowing and as the food bolus descends, the LES relaxes through the release of nitric oxide (NO) and VIP, allowing for the food bolus to pass into the stomach.

Secondary achalasia can be caused by Chagas disease from *Trypanosoma cruzi* or from pseudoachalasia.

What are the classic presenting symptoms of achalasia? Achalasia should be suspected in patients with:

- Dysphagia to solids and liquids
- Heartburn symptoms unresponsive to a trial of proton pump inhibitors for 4 weeks

The classic triad of presenting symptoms of achalasia consists of **dysphagia, regurgitation, and weight loss**. Lack of LES relaxation causes patients to have dysphagia with both solids and liquids. Eating becomes a difficult process, whereby patients must eat slowly and drink large volumes of liquid to help wash tendineae into the stomach (due to absent peristalsis). Mounting pressure from water buildup can cause severe retrosternal chest pain to occur and persist until the LES opens, which leads to prompt relief. Patients with spastic achalasia frequently report chest pain. Regurgitation of undigested, foul-smelling food is common, and with progressive disease, aspiration can become life threatening.

What are some diseases associated with achalasia?

Most cases of achalasia are sporadic. However, achalasia can be seen in several genetic disorders such as familial dysautonomia, familial glucocorticoid insufficiency, triple A syndrome, and Pierre-Robin sequence. Additionally, patients with achalasia are at increased risk of developing esophageal malignancy. Currently, there are no guideline recommendations regarding cancer screening in patients with achalasia.

How do we score a patient's clinical symptoms in achalasia?

The Eckhardt score (Table 38.4) is based on the summation of four symptoms (dysphagia, regurgitation, chest pain, weight loss) that are graded according to severity, and treatment success is a score ≤ 3.

TABLE 38.4 ■ **Eckhardt Score: Clinical Scoring System for Achalasia**

Score	Weight Loss (kg)	Dysphagia	Retrosternal Pain	Regurgitation
0	None	None	None	None
1	<5	Occasional	Occasional	Occasional
2	5–10	Daily	Daily	Daily
3	>10	Each meal	Each meal	Each meal

BASIC SCIENCE/CLINICAL PEARL **STEP 1/2/3**

The upper one-third of the esophagus consists of striated muscle whereas the lower two-thirds is made up of smooth muscle.

BASIC SCIENCE/CLINICAL PEARL **STEP 1/2/3**

Upper endoscopy should be the first test performed to evaluate new-onset dysphagia because it combines the ability to detect most structural causes of dysphagia with the ability to obtain biopsies.

How do we classify the different types of achalasia?

Achalasia is classified into three subtypes based on manometry findings. The Chicago Classification of Motility Disorders was created to differentiate these subtypes (Fig. 38.8). All three subtypes exhibit abnormal peristalsis and failure of LES relaxation. They differ by locations and mechanisms underlying abnormal peristalsis of the esophagus.

In type I achalasia, the LES displays increased pressurization, but minimal or complete lack of contractility or peristalsis of the esophageal body. Type II achalasia is characterized by pan-esophageal pressurization on manometry. This means that there is equally increased nonpropulsive pressure throughout the entire length of the esophagus. Type III achalasia, also known as spastic achalasia, occurs when there are multiple simultaneous spastic contractions of different areas of the distal esophagus. Treatment options are often guided by the achalasia subtype present.

After reviewing these studies, a diagnosis of type III achalasia was made. The patient was started on oral nifedipine 10 mg daily prior to meals and continued on a liquid diet for symptomatic management. She was scheduled for definitive treatment with peroral endoscopic myotomy (POEM) and sent home.

BASIC SCIENCE/CLINICAL PEARL **STEP 1/2/3**

In achalasia, there is degeneration of the myenteric plexus, also known as Auerbach's plexus. This is a group of ganglion cells that provide motor innervation to both the longitudinal and circular muscle layers of the gastrointestinal tract.

BASIC SCIENCE/CLINICAL PEARL **STEP 1/2/3**

Secondary achalasia can mimic primary achalasia but is commonly caused by a mechanical obstruction, such as malignancy, Chagas disease, strictures, neurofibromatosis type 1, and sarcoidosis.

What are the treatment options for achalasia?

Pharmacologic treatments for achalasia

Medical management of achalasia is often used for short-term symptom relief in patients who cannot tolerate or are waiting for definitive, procedural management. Calcium channel blockers, nitrates, and phosphodiesterase inhibitors are commonly used therapies that facilitate esophageal emptying by transiently reducing lower esophageal sphincter pressure via smooth muscle relaxation. However, medical therapy is limited by poor efficacy and side effects.

Botulinum toxin injections are also utilized, whereby inhibition of acetylcholine release from cholinergic nerve endings blocks unopposed cholinergic stimulation of the LES without any impact on myogenic tone. These injections provide symptomatic relief in over two-thirds of patients receiving them, but many patients require repeat injections within 6 months to 1 year with reports of diminished efficacy with each subsequent injection. Botulinum toxin injections are generally reserved for elderly patients or patients who are poor candidates for invasive interventions.

BASIC SCIENCE/CLINICAL PEARL **STEP 1/2/3**

Eosinophilic esophagitis (EoE) is a chronic, allergic inflammatory disease of the esophagus that can present similarly to achalasia. EoE is a result of eosinophilic accumulation throughout the esophagus resulting in symptoms such as dysphagia, pain, and reflux. Mechanical obstruction from strictures can also occur in EoE.

Nonpharmacologic treatments for achalasia

Surgical and endoscopic approaches are preferred for definitive management of achalasia. These include pneumatic balloon dilation, laparoscopic or open Heller myotomy, and POEM. Choice of treatment modality is multifactorial, including achalasia subtype, patient comorbidities, and patient preference. Pneumatic dilation and POEM have faster recovery compared with surgical myotomy in patients and may be preferred in older patients or patients with comorbidities. Pneumatic dilation involves uncontrolled disruption of the LES with a large balloon and the perforation rate may approach 4% when larger diameter balloons are used. Repeat dilations are often required. POEM may be preferred in patients with type III achalasia because of longer myotomy proximally into the esophagus. The complication rate of POEM is also lower than surgical myotomy. However, development of GERD is common after POEM, occurring in up to 50% of patients. Most patients will require acid suppressive medication after POEM. The surgical approach allows fundoplication concurrently, which decreases the incidence of GERD compared with POEM. These approaches are summarized in Table 38.5.

The patient returns for follow-up several weeks after her procedure and reports significant improvement in dysphagia. She is now able to tolerate liquids and solids easily and expresses relief and gratitude.

Case Summary

- **Complaint/History:** A 54-year-old female presents with difficulty swallowing solids and liquids over the past four years.
- **Findings:** Temperature is 98.5; Physical exam was unrevealing.
- **Lab Results/Tests:** Labs reveal _. Chest x-ray shows a retrocardiac air-fluid level in the mediastinum at the level of the aortic arch. Upper endoscopy showed no signs of obstruction or inflamation in the esophagus, although it was difficutl for the ednoscopist to pass the endscope from the esophagus to the stomach which was normal in appearance. Manometry

showed multiple areas of the esophagus with increased pressure readings simultaneously as the patient swallowed.

Diagnosis: Type III Achalasia.

- **Treatment:** The patient was started on Nifedipine 10mg before meals and a liquid diet for symptomatic management. She was scheduled for definitive treatment wiht peroral endoscopic myotomy (POEM).

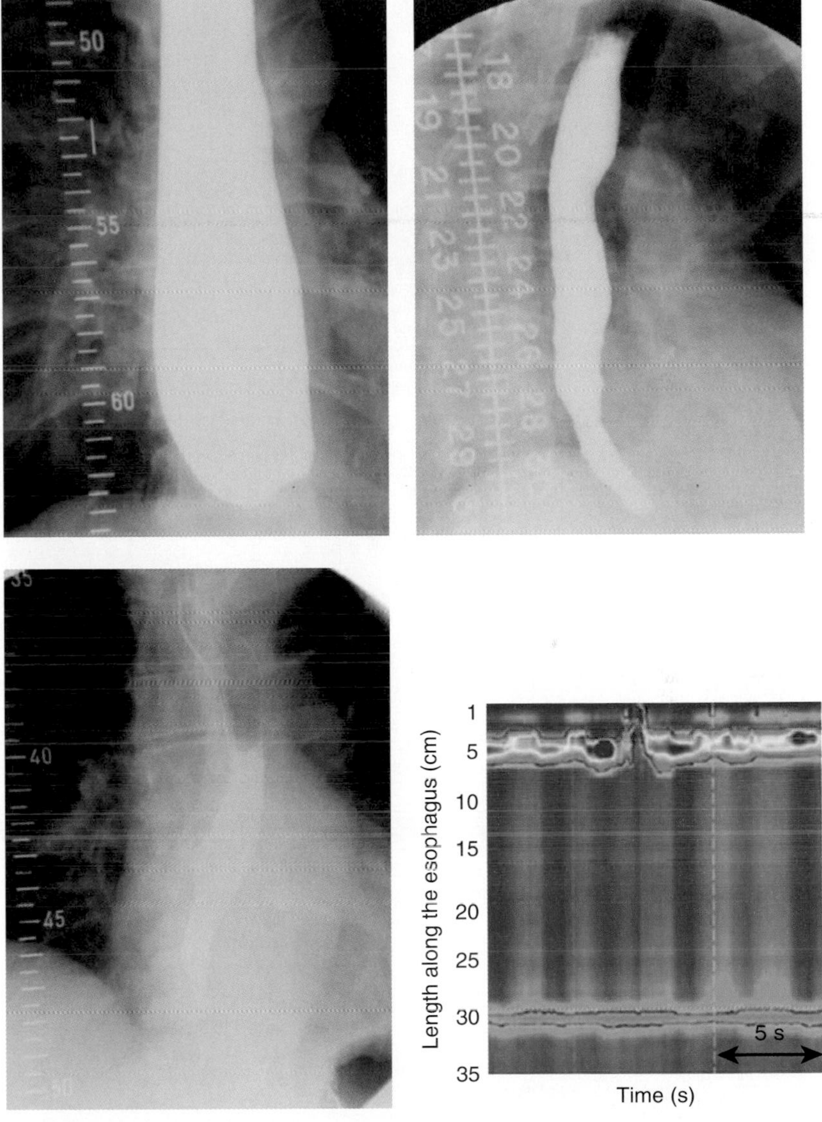

Fig. 38.8 Summary of Chicago Classification of Motility Disorders v3.0: Characteristics and treatment options for achalasia. (From Etchill, E. W., & Yang, S. C. (2020). Achalasia of the esophagus. In J. L. Cameron, & A. M. Cameron (Eds.), *Current surgical therapy* (13th ed.). Elsevier. https://www.clinicalkey.com/#!/content/book/3-s2.0-B9780323640596000086?scrollTo=%23t0015.)

TABLE 38.5 ■ **Nonpharmacologic Treatments for Achalasia**

Pneumatic Dilation (PD)	Laparoscopic Heller's Myotomy (LHM) + Partial Fundoplication	Peroral Endoscopic Myotomy (POEM)
Pneumatic dilation of the gastroesophageal junction. (A) Placement of the balloon across the gastroesophageal junction. (B) Inflation of the balloon, leading to the disruption of the fibers of the LES. (C) Relieved obstruction of the LES.	Line of incision into constricted section of muscle A and B, Esophagomyotomy (Heller's procedure) is the surgical procedure of choice when a segment of esophagus narrows and causes functional obstruction. From (A) Black, J. M., Hokanson, J. H., Malarvizhi, S., Renuka, K.: *Black's medical-surgical nursing: clinical management for positive outcomes* (1st South Asia ed.); (B and C) Yates, R. B., Oelschlager, B. K., & Pellegrini, C. A. (2017). Gastroesophageal reflux disease and hiatal hernia. In C. M. Townsend, R. D. Beauchamp, B. M. Evers, & K. L. Mattox, (Eds.) *Sabiston textbook of surgery* (20th ed.). Philadelphia; Elsevier.	The four steps of PerOral Endoscopic Myotomy (POEM): mucosal incision and tunnel entry (A), submucosal tunneling (B), myotomy (C), and closure of mucosal entry (D). From Rosch T., Sethi A., Khashab M.A., Alessandro Repici (2019). How to perform a high-quality peroral endoscopic myotemy? *Gastroenterology*, *157*(5), 1184–1189.

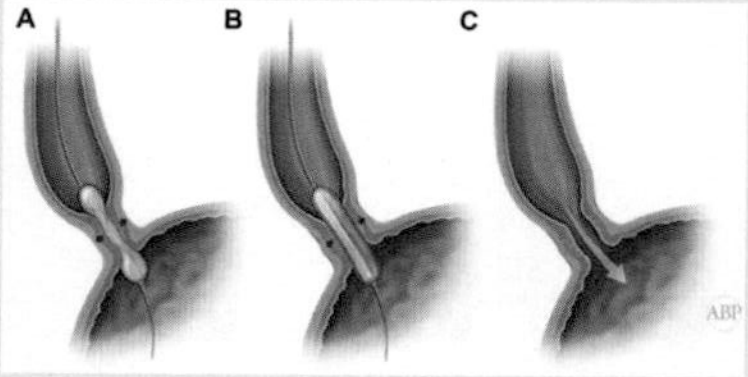

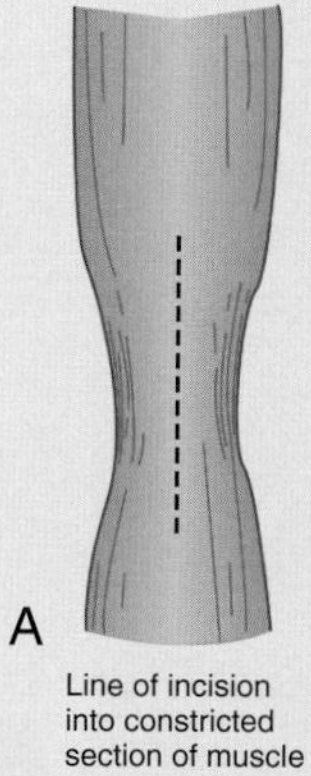

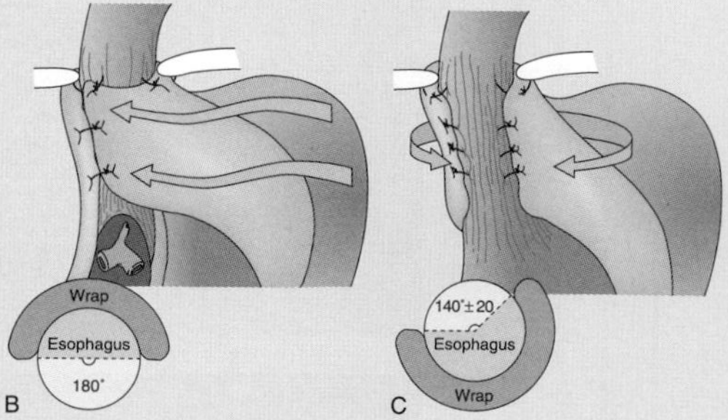

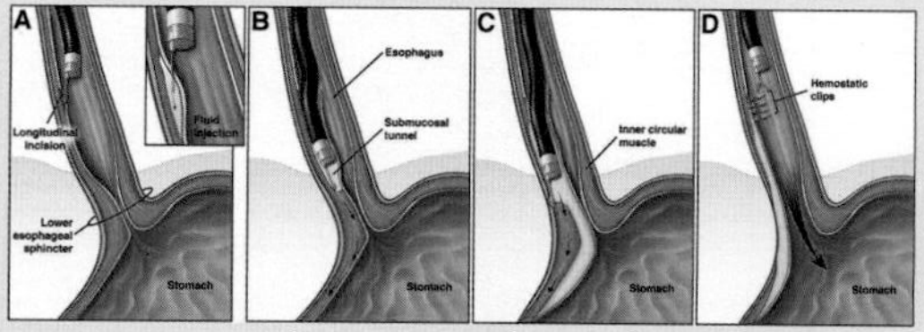

TABLE 38.5 ■ **Nonpharmacologic Treatments for Achalasia—con'd**

	Pneumatic Dilation (PD)	Laparoscopic Heller's Myotomy (LHM) – Partial Fundoplication	Peroral Endoscopic Myotomy (POEM)
Procedure	Endoscopic balloon is used to dilate the lower esophageal sphincter	Laparoscopic surgical operation which consists of dividing muscles of the LES, followed by a partial fundoplication to prevent acid reflux.	Combination of endoscopic and surgical technique. A myotomy of the LES is performed using an endoscopic approach.
Pros	– Cost-effective – Minimally invasive	– Definitive surgical treatment with good long-term results – Fundoplication helps prevent GERD	– Primary therapy for type III achalasia – Endoscopic approach allows for access to the full length of the esophagus – Safe and well-tolerated – Low complication rate and rapid recovery
Cons	– Requires serial dilations – About one-third of patients will have recurrent symptoms and will need repeat within 5 years – Risk of esophageal rupture or perforation (2%–4%) – Complications include GERD, hematoma, esophagitis	– Morbidity/complications associated with surgery – Laparoscopic approach gives access to a limited length of the esophagus	– Approximately ½ one-half patients may subsequently develop reflux disease as this approach does not include fundoplication

GERD, Gastroesophageal reflux disease; *LES*, lower esophageal sphincter.

BEYOND THE PEARLS

- Primary achalasia is an uncommon disease of unknown etiology in which there is loss of normal peristalsis in the esophagus and failure of the LES to relax with swallowing.
- Progressively worsening dysphagia for solids and liquids along with regurgitation of food are the most common symptoms in patients with achalasia. Other signs/symptoms include weight loss, chest pain, heartburn, and difficulty belching.
- Upper endoscopy is performed to exclude pseudoachalasia. Those without obstruction for the GE junction should undergo a contrast esophagram and esophageal manometry to confirm the diagnosis of achalasia.
- The three different types of achalasia can be differentiated based on manometry findings. Diagnosing the correct subtype can guide treatment more appropriately.
- Pharmacologic management of achalasia includes the use of botulinum toxin injections, calcium channel blockers, and nitrates. Medical treatments are limited in efficacy and botulinum toxin injection provides only temporary symptomatic relief.
- Interventional management of achalasia provides more definitive treatment. Endoscopic, laparoscopic, and open approaches are all available for patients. Achalasia subtype, comorbidities, and patient preference may help guide treatment choice.

Bibliography

Eckardt, V. F., Aignherr, C., & Bernhard, G. (1992). Predictors of outcome in patients with achalasia treated by pneumatic dilation. *Gastroenterology*, *103*(6), 1732–1738.

Kavitt, Robert, T., Vaezi, , & Michael, F. (2021). Diseases of the esophagus. Cummings otolaryngology. *Head and Neck Surgery*, *68*, 964–991.e3.

Kim, J. P., & Kahrilas, P. J. (2019). How I approach dysphagia. *Current Gastroenterology Reports*, *21*(10), 49. Published 2019 Aug 20.

Nassri, A., & Ramzan, Z. (2015). Pharmacotherapy for the management of achalasia: Current status, challenges and future directions. *World Journal of Gastrointestinal Pharmacology and Therapeutics*, *6*(4), 145–155.

Spieker. M. R. (2000 Jun 15). Evaluating Dysphagia. *American Family Physician*, *61*(12), 3639–3648.

Torresan, F., Ioannou, A., Azzaroli, F., & Bazzoli, F. (2015 Jul-Sep). Treatment of achalasia in the era of high resolution manometry. *Annals of Gastroenterology*, *28*(3), 301–308.

Werner, Y. B., Hakanson, B., Martinek, J., Repici, A., von Rahden, B., Bredenoord, A. J., Bisschops, R., Messmann, H., Vollberg, M. C., Noder, T., Kersten, J. F., Mann, O., Izbicki, J., Pazdro, A., Fumagalli, U., Rosati, R., Germer, C. T., Schijven, M. P., Emmermann, A., von Renteln, D., & Rösch, T. (2019]). Endoscopic or Surgical Myotomy in Patients with Idiopathic Achalasia. *The New England Journal of Medicine*, *381*(23), 2219–2229. https://doi.org/10.1056/NEJMoa1905380.

Wolf. D. C. (1990). Dysphagia. In H. K. Walker, W. D. Hall, & J. W. Hurst (Eds.), *Clinical methods: The history, physical, and laboratory examinations* (3rd ed.). Boston: Butterworths. Chapter 82.

CASE 39

A 25-Year-Old Male With Chronic Diarrhea

Patrick Lee ■ Liam Hilson ■ Sarah Sheibani

A 25-year-old male presents with diarrhea for the previous 6 weeks. He describes having non-bloody stools with significant mucous output approximately four times per day. Associated symptoms include left-sided, crampy abdominal pain with no radiation that is worse prior to bowel movements, urgency, and tenesmus. Also, he reports fatigue and unintentional weight loss of 5 lb. He denies rashes and joint pain. He has never been diagnosed with any medical conditions, has not traveled recently, and takes no medications.

Currently, he is a graduate student in Florida. On physical examination, blood pressure is 123/72 mmHg, pulse rate is 91/min, respiration rate is 16/min, and oxygen saturation is 98% on room air. He has mild tenderness to palpation of the left lower quadrant with no rebound or guarding. The remainder of the examination is unremarkable.

What are some causes of chronic diarrhea?

Chronic diarrhea is defined as increased stool frequency for >4 weeks. There are numerous causes of chronic diarrhea as described in Table 39.1. It is important to obtain a thorough history, including medication and travel history. Antibiotic use may also help narrow the etiology of chronic diarrhea to medication side effects or *Clostridium difficile*. Greasy, malodorous stools that float may indicate fat malabsorption.

What is the best way to evaluate the cause of this patient's chronic diarrhea?

Stool tests, including a culture and *C. difficile* polymerase chain reaction, should be checked to evaluate for enteric infections. Serum electrolytes may help determine the severity of the diarrhea. Nonspecific inflammatory markers such as erythrocyte sedimentation rate, C-reactive protein (CRP), and fecal calprotectin can be ordered, but those lab tests can be elevated in both infectious and inflammatory colitis.

CLINICAL PEARL **STEP 1, 2, 3**

Fecal calprotectin is a protein that is elevated in the setting of increased neutrophils in the intestinal mucosa. It can be used to help differentiate inflammatory bowel disease from irritable bowel syndrome.

BASIC SCIENCE PEARL

Serologic markers, including positive perinuclear antineutrophil cytoplasmic antibodies (pANCAs) and negative anti-*Saccharomyces cerevisiae* antibody, can help establish a diagnosis of ulcerative colitis (UC).

TABLE 39.1 ■ **Differential Diagnosis for Chronic Diarrhea**

- Irritable bowel syndrome
- Inflammatory bowel disease (Crohn's disease and ulcerative colitis)
- Microscopic colitis
- Malabsorption (lactose intolerance, chronic pancreatitis, celiac disease, small intestinal bacterial overgrowth)
- Chronic infections (*Clostridium difficile*, *Giardia*, *Campylobacter*, Whipple's disease)
- Medications

TABLE 39.2 ■ **Laboratory Tests**

Leukocyte count	10,000/μL (10×10^9/L)
Hemoglobin	12 g/dL
Platelet count	350,000/μL (350×10^9/L)
Serum creatinine	1.0 mg/dL
C-reactive protein (CRP)	7 mg/L
Stool culture	No growth to date
Stool *Clostridium difficile* toxin	Negative
Stool ova and parasite	No growth to date
Fecal calprotectin	170 μg/g

The results of the lab tests are shown in Table 39.2.

What is your differential diagnosis?

This is a 25-year-old male with no past medical history who presents with a 6-week history of several episodes of nonbloody diarrhea daily with urgency, mucus, and an unintentional 5-lb weight loss with lab results revealing an elevated CRP.

Inflammatory bowel disease (IBD), particularly ulcerative colitis, is highest on the differential diagnosis at this point given his constellation of clinical symptoms and the workup that revealed an elevated CRP and fecal calprotectin. UC can be diagnosed in all age groups, but it is predominately diagnosed between the ages of 15 and 30 years.

His stool tests were negative for an infection. Noninflammatory conditions, such as irritable bowel syndrome, are less likely given the elevated CRP and fecal calprotectin.

How do you establish a diagnosis of IBD, particularly in this case?

The diagnosis of ulcerative colitis requires a lower gastrointestinal examination (complete colonoscopy with evaluation of the terminal ileum) with histologic confirmation. A routine upper endoscopic evaluation is not required unless the patient has upper intestinal symptoms.

It can be challenging to distinguish ulcerative colitis from Crohn's disease (CD). Some of the clinical, endoscopic, and histologic differences are described in Table 39.3.

A colonoscopy showed continuous inflammation in the rectum and sigmoid colon, characterized by loss of normal vascular markings, mild granularity, and erosions (Fig. 39.1). The mucosa proximal to the sigmoid colon appeared normal. The terminal ileum was normal.

Biopsies showed evidence of neutrophils infiltrating crypt epithelium (cryptitis) with collections of neutrophils within crypt lumens (crypt abscesses). There were also signs of chronicity defined by crypt architectural distortion and Paneth cell metaplasia in the left colon.

Diagnosis: Ulcerative colitis.

TABLE 39.3 ■ **Clinical Presentations of Crohn's Disease and Ulcerative Colitis**

	Crohn's Disease	Ulcerative Colitis
Location	Noncontiguous involvement of the gastrointestinal tract (mouth to anus), more commonly in the terminal ileum	Colonic inflammation involving the rectum that can extend proximally to the cecum
Endoscopic findings	Creeping fat, deep ulcers, fissures, and cobble-stoning	Continuous inflammation involving the rectum and extending proximally, with features of friable mucosa, deep ulcerations, and erosions
Radiologic findings	Barium swallow: "String sign"	"Lead pipe" appearance because of loss of haustra
Histologic findings	• Transmural inflammation • Noncaseating granulomas	• Mucosal and submucosal inflammation • Crypt abscesses • Ulcers • No granulomas
Complications	• Fistulas • Abscess • Strictures	• Toxic megacolon (Fig. 39.2) • Fulminant colitis • Increased risk of colon cancer

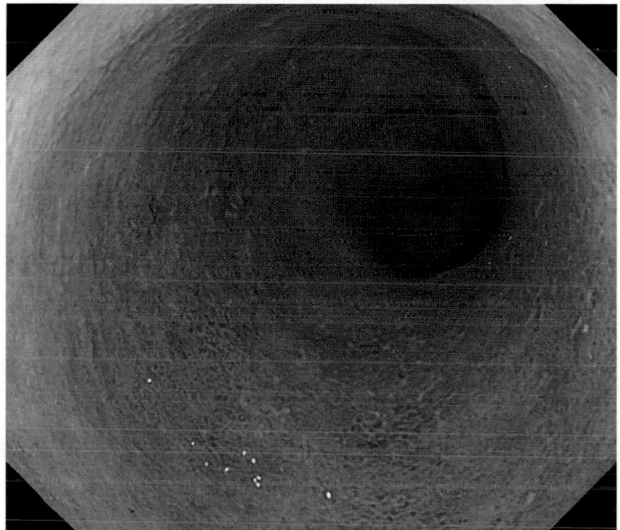

Fig. 39.1 An endoscopic picture showing mild colitis. (From Matsumoto, T., Kudo, T., Jo, Y., Esaki, M., Yao, T., & Iida, M. (2007). *Gastrointestinal Endoscopy*, *66*(5), 957–965.)

CLINICAL PEARL **STEP 1**

Cigarette smoking is protective against developing ulcerative colitis.

Upon discussion of the biopsy results and diagnosis, the patient asks whether there are other symptoms associated with UC.

What are some extraintestinal manifestations of IBD?

Extraintestinal involvement (EIM) is seen in up to 47% of patients and may occur before or after IBD. The common EIMs seen in patients with IBD are listed in Table 39.4.

CLINICAL PEARL **STEP 1, 2, 3**

Approximately 75% of patients with primary sclerosing cholangitis (PSC) have IBD, mainly UC. The presence of PSC is a risk factor for the development of colorectal dysplasia and/or cancer in patients with IBD.

The patient asks about his treatment options and treatment duration.

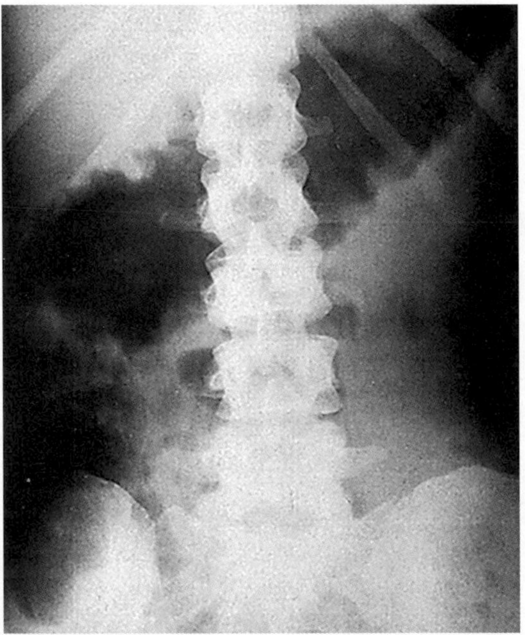

Fig. 39.2 An abdominal radiograph showing toxic megacolon. (From Rougas, S. (2020). Toxic megacolon. In F. F. Ferri (Ed.), *Ferri's clinical advisor* (pp. 1381–1382.e1). Elsevier.)

TABLE 39.4 ■ **Extraintestinal Manifestations of Inflammatory Bowel Disease**

Skin	• Pyoderma gangrenosum (Fig. 39.3) • Psoriasis
Eyes	• Uveitis • Episcleritis
Mouth	• Aphthous ulcers
Liver	• Primary sclerosing cholangitis (more commonly seen in ulcerative colitis)
Kidney	• Calcium oxalate nephrolithiasis (more commonly seen in Crohn's disease)
Musculoskeletal	• Spondylarthritis • Peripheral arthritis

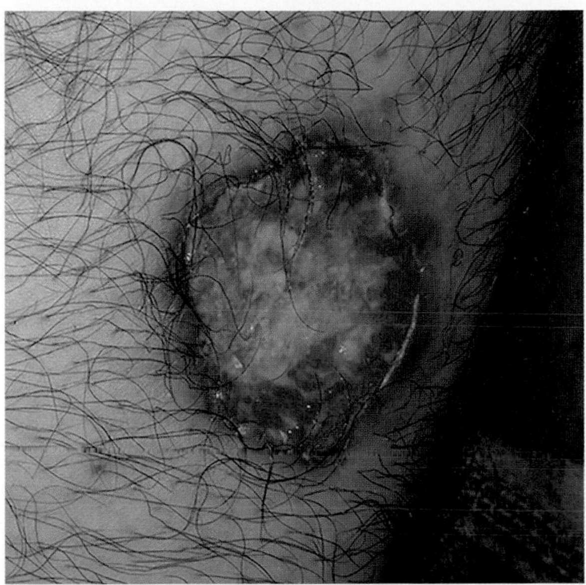

Fig. 39.3 An example of pyoderma gangrenosum on the leg of a patient. (From Najem, C.E. (2020). Pyoderma gangrenosum. In F. F. Ferri (Ed.), *Ferri's clinical advisor* (pp. 1184.e2–1184.e3). Elsevier.)

TABLE 39.5 ■ **Overview of the Treatment for Inflammatory Bowel Disease**

Crohn's Disease	Ulcerative Colitis

• Glucocorticoids
• Immunomodulators (azathioprine)
• Biologics
  • Anti-TNFα
    • Infliximab
    • Adalimumab
    • Certolizumab
  • Anti-integrin
    • Vedolizumab
  • Anti-IL12/IL23
    • Ustekinumab
	• Glucocorticoids
	• 5-aminosalicylate (5-ASA)
	• Immunomodulators (azathioprine)
	• Biologics
	  • Anti-TNFα
	    • Infliximab
	    • Adalimumab
	    • Golimumab
	  • Anti-integrin
	    • Vedolizumab
	  • Anti-IL12/IL23
	    • Ustekinumab
	• Janus kinase inhibitor (tofacitinib)
	• Colectomy

IL, Interleukin; *TNF*, tumor necrosis factor.

How do you approach treatment for IBD?

Treatment options for patients with UC are guided by the severity of the disease. In patients with mildly active UC, oral 5-aminosalicylates (5-ASA) should be used. Rectal 5-ASA can be used in left-sided colonic disease.

In more moderate to severe disease, immunosuppressant medications can be initiated. Since UC is confined to the colon, colectomy can be considered in disease refractory to medical therapy.

The commonly used therapies for CD and UC are listed in Table 39.5.

The patient was diagnosed with mild left-sided ulcerative colitis. He was started on therapy with 5-aminosalicylates: oral (2 g/day) and rectal (1 g/day). After about 2 weeks, he noted an improvement in the diarrhea and urgency. A repeat fecal calprotectin checked about 3 months after initiating therapy showed improvement. He was maintained on therapy with oral 5-aminosalicylates.

Case Summary

- **History:** A 25-year-old male presents with 6 weeks of approximately four episodes of non-bloody diarrhea per day associated with mucus, urgency, and tenesmus.
- **Findings:** Weight loss of 5 lb; mild tenderness to palpation in the left lower quadrant.
- **Lab Results/Tests:** Lab tests revealed mild anemia, elevated CRP, and fecal calprotectin. A colonoscopy showed continuous inflammation in the rectum and sigmoid colon, characterized by loss of normal vascular markings, mild granularity, and erosions; biopsies showed neutrophils infiltrating crypt epithelium (cryptitis) with crypt abscesses and Paneth cell metaplasia.

Diagnosis: Ulcerative colitis.

- **Treatment:** Patient was started and maintained on oral (2 g/day) and rectal (1 g/day) 5-aminosalicylates.

BEYOND THE PEARLS

- Tofacitinib, an orally administered small molecule that is a nonselective inhibitor of the Janus kinase enzyme, has been recently approved for the treatment of moderate to severe UC. As opposed to biologic agents, this is an oral agent with no risk of developing immunogenicity.
- Patients with inflammatory bowel disease are at increased risk of venous thromboembolism, which is more common in patients with more severe inflammation. DVT prophylaxis should be used in hospitalized patients.
- Surveillance colonoscopy to evaluate for dysplasia in patients with UC should begin 8 years after diagnosis.
- Restorative proctocolectomy with ileal pouch-anal anastomosis is the surgical procedure recommended for medically refractory UC.
- Because of concerns for reactivation, screening for hepatitis B and latent tuberculosis should be performed before initiation of anti-TNF therapy.

Bibliography

Grainge, M. J., West, J., & Card, T. R. (2010). Venous thromboembolism during active disease and remission in inflammatory bowel disease: A cohort study. *Lancet*, *375*, 657–663.

Lutgens, M.W.M.D., Vleggar, F.P., Schipper, M.E.I., Stokkers, P.C.F., van der Woude, C.J., Hommes, D.W., de Jong, D.J., Dijkstra, G., van Bodegraven, A.A., Oldenburg, B., & Samsom, M. (2008). High frequency of early colorectal cancer in inflammatory bowel disease. *Gut*, *57*, 1246–1251.

Mahid, S. S., Minor, K. S., Soto, R. E., Hornung, C. A., & Galandiuk, S. (2006). Smoking and inflammatory bowel disease: a meta-analysis. *Mayo Clinic Proceedings*, *81*, 1462–1471.

Mosli, M.H., Zou, G.Y., Garg, S.K., Feagan, S.G., MacDonald, J.K., Chande, N., Sandborn, W.J., & Feagan, B.G. (2015). C-reactive protein, fecal calprotectin, and stool lactoferrin for detection of endoscopic activity in symptomatic inflammatory bowel disease patients: A systematic review and meta-analysis. *The American Journal of Gastroenterology*, *110*, 802–819.

Plevy, S., Silverberg, M.S., Lockton, S., Stockfisch, T., Croner, L., Stachelski, J., Brown, M., Triggs, C., Chuang, E., Princen, F., & Singh, S. (2013). Combined serological, genetic, and inflammatory markers differentiate non-IBD, Crohn's disease, and ulcerative colitis patients. *Inflammatory Bowel Diseases*, *19*, 1139–1148.

Rubin, D.T., Ananthakrishnan, A.N., Siegel, C.A., Sauer, B.G., & Long, M.D. (2019). ACG clinical guidelines: ulcerative colitis in adults. *The American Journal of Gastroenterology*, *114*, 384–413.

Vavricka, S.R., Schoepfer, A., Scharl, M., Lakatos, P.L., Navarini, A., & Rogler, G. (2015). Extraintestinal manifestations of inflammatory bowel disease. *Inflammatory Bowel Diseases, 21,* 1982–1992.

SECTION 9

Infectious Diseases

CASE 40

A 29-Year-Old Male With a Headache

Fernando Dominguez ■ Emily Blodget

A 29-year-old male presents to the emergency department with 3 weeks of progressive headache. He also complains of bilateral ear fullness, blurry vision, posterior neck pain, headache, nausea, vomiting, and fever. He lives in Los Angeles and has sex with men. A review of his medical records shows a positive fourth generation human immunodeficiency virus (HIV) screening test done 4 weeks earlier when he initially established care with his primary care doctor. On physical examination, his temperature is 38°C (100.4°F), blood pressure is 128/92 mmHg, heart rate is 92 beats/min, respiratory rate is 16 breaths/min, and oxygen saturation is 98% on room air. He is thin and in moderate distress. Cardiac auscultation reveals normal heart sounds and lungs are clear to auscultation. Abdominal exam is benign. Funduscopic exam shows bilateral papilledema, but otherwise he has no evidence of focal neurologic deficits.

What are some causes of increased intracranial pressure (ICP) in patients with acquired immunodeficiency syndrome (AIDS)?

The presence of papilledema is indicative of elevated intracranial pressure. In an immunocompromised patient, particularly one with HIV, this represents an emergency condition that requires further evaluation. The differential for elevated ICP in this subpopulation is broad; however, in this patient *Cryptococcus* disease should be strongly suspected (see Table 40.1).

BASIC SCIENCE PEARL **USMLE STEP 2**

Cryptococcus gattii tends to cause cryptococcomas more commonly than *Cryptococcus neoformans*, and it is also more likely to cause disease in immunocompetent patients rather than immunocompromised patients where *C. neoformans* is more common.

What would be the recommended next step when evaluating this patient?

An immunocompromised patient with symptoms of increased ICP should have neuroimaging with computerized tomography (CT) scan prior to lumbar puncture to assess the risk of cerebral herniation. Additional diagnostics would include peripheral blood cultures and serum cryptococcal antigen. The microorganism can be isolated from standard blood cultures in approximately two-thirds of patients with AIDS-related meningoencephalitis. A serum cryptococcal antigen has an excellent sensitivity of approximately 99% in patients with AIDS and would be a valuable rapid diagnostic test while awaiting further studies.

Based on his clinical presentation, suspicion is raised of a central nervous system (CNS) pathologic process, which could be infectious or noninfectious (see Table 40.2). The patient's CD4 count, not yet available at this point, would also help stratify the patient's likelihood for an HIV/AIDS-related opportunistic intracranial process.

No intracranial lesion is identified via imaging and a lumbar puncture (LP) is performed with the following values: opening pressure of 32 cm, glucose of 40 mg/dL, protein 78 mg/dL, and cell count of 40 cells/μL (60% monocytes).

TABLE 40.1 ■ **Etiologies of Headache in Patients With HIV**

Infectious	Noninfectious
Primary HIV-related • Aseptic HIV meningitis • Chronic HIV meningitis Secondary HIV-related • Cryptococcal meningoencephalitis • Cerebral toxoplasmosis • Tuberculous meningitis • Meningovascular syphilis • Viral encephalitis (CMV, HSV) Nonopportunistic • Bacterial meningitis • Viral meningitis • Acute sinusitis	Primary CNS lymphoma Lymphomatous meningitis Medication-induced headache Tension headache Migraine headache

AIDS, Acquired immunodeficiency syndrome; *CMV*, cytomegalovirus; *CNS*, central nervous system; *HIV*, human immunodeficiency virus; *HSV*, herpes simplex virus.

TABLE 40.2 ■ **CSF Findings of Meningitis Etiologies**

	Cell Count (cells/μL)	Cell Count Differential	Glucose (mg/dL)	Protein (mg/dL)
Bacterial	100–1000	Neutrophils	<10–40	100–500
Viral	5–1000	Lymphocytes	10–40	50–300
Tuberculosis	5–1000	Lymphocytes	<10	50–300
Cryptococcosis	<50	Monocytes	10–75	50–150

Which infectious etiologies are suggested by the cerebrospinal fluid analysis?

Cerebrospinal fluid with a low cell count with monocyte predominance, low glucose, and mildly elevated protein is suggestive of cryptococcal meningoencephalitis. However, a normal profile can be seen in approximately 25%–30% of patients with a positive cerebrospinal fluid (CSF) cryptococcal culture. Increased opening pressure (greater than or equal to 25 cm) can also commonly be seen and may suggest a higher fungal disease burden.

Based on the patient's clinical history, risk factors, and preliminary diagnostics, cryptococcal meningoencephalitis is the most likely diagnosis (see Table 40.2).

What is cryptococcosis and why are patients with AIDS at increased risk?

Cryptococcus spp. is an encapsulated yeast commonly found in soil, especially in areas where there is an abundance of birds. Most of the cases are seen in patients with AIDS with CD4 of less than 100 cells/μL. Impaired cellular immunity such as seen in patients with AIDS is the greatest risk factor for development of disease. Cryptococcus disease is also well described to occur in patients with cellular immunodeficiency including cirrhotic patients and transplant recipients.

CLINICAL PEARL **USMLE STEP 2**

Most patients with cryptococcosis have underlying immunodeficiency. Besides AIDS, other predisposing factors include liver disease, sarcoidosis, steroid use, biologic agents, malignancy, and solid organ recipients.

What testing is available for diagnosis of cryptococcal meningoencephalitis?
Diagnostic testing includes direct microscopy, antigen detection, and culture. Staining of CSF with India ink was historically the only available method for rapid detection of yeast; however, it has mostly been replaced by cryptococcal antigen. Visualization on India ink staining offers the benefit of more rapidly establishing a diagnosis when compared with other confirmatory testing modalities; however, sensitivity is around 85% and is dependent on CSF fungal burden.

BASIC SCIENCE PEARL **USMLE STEP 1**

India ink preparation from CSF showing halo around cell indicating presence of polysaccharide capsule.

From McPherson, R. A., & Pincus, M. R. (2022). *Henry's clinical diagnosis and management by laboratory methods* (24th ed.). Elsevier.

The detection of cryptococcal antigen (CrAg) is recommended to be performed on all patients with suspected cryptococcal meningitis. Three techniques are currently available: latex agglutination, ELISA, and lateral flow assay (LFA).

Latex agglutination and ELISA have been the most common methods but LFA is increasingly used in resource-limited settings. Sensitivity of spinal fluid CrAg ranges from 93% to 100% and specificity from 93% to 98% with latex agglutination; similar performance values have been achieved with LFA in Africa. In patients with AIDS, the sensitivity of serum CrAg is more than 99% when CSF CrAg is detectable.

In high resource settings, the use of molecular testing with multiplex polymerase chain reaction (PCR) is more commonly performed. The reported sensitivity of PCR for cryptococcus is in excess of 95%.

The diagnostic gold standard is that CSF should be sent for fungal culture; however, it requires laboratory and microbiologic support, which can be challenging in developing countries. It can also be falsely negative with low fungal burden (see Table 40.3).

CLINICAL PEARL **USMLE STEP 3**

The prevalence of asymptomatic cryptococcal antigenemia from several cohort studies in South Asia and sub-Saharan Africa ranges from 4% to 12%. Studies have shown that the presence of asymptomatic antigenemia is associated with increased mortality and increased incidence of progression to cryptococcal meningitis. The World Health Organization (WHO) recommends screening all patients with HIV and a CD4 count <100 cells/μL with serum cryptococcal antigen testing. All asymptomatic patients with antigenemia require CSF evaluation and, if negative, initiation of preemptive antifungal therapy with fluconazole.

TABLE 40.3 ■ **Sensitivity and Specificity of Diagnostic Techniques in Spinal Fluid of Patients With HIV**

Test	Sensitivity	Specificity
India ink	85%	95%
Latex agglutination	95%	95%
PCR	95%	>90%
Culture	90%	>95%

HIV, Human immunodeficiency virus.

In this patient, CSF CrAg was positive, which established the diagnosis of cryptococcal meningitis.

How should this patient's elevated ICP be managed?

Aggressive management of elevated ICP is required. Increased ICP is defined as a CSF opening pressure greater than or equal to 25 cm. This patient had symptoms consistent with elevated ICP and an opening pressure obtained duration lumbar puncture of 32 cm of CSF.

Current recommendations suggest reduction by either 50% of CSF pressure or to a pressure of 20 cm in order to reduce the risk for complications caused by rapid decreases in intracranial pressure. Persistently elevated CSF pressures may require serial lumbar puncture for therapeutic reduction in ICP until pressure and symptoms have been stable for more than 2 days. Advanced options in refractory cases include placement of lumbar drain, ventriculostomy, or ventriculoperitoneal shunt.

The patient's ICP was elevated for one additional day but subsequently decreased to 15 cm of CSF after a repeat LP. His symptoms also improved.

How should you treat cryptococcal meningoencephalitis?

The preferred regimen for individuals with HIV is divided into induction, consolidation, and maintenance phases:

Induction: Guidelines recommend amphotericin (either deoxycholate or liposomal) plus flucytosine for a minimum of 2 weeks. Alternatives, especially in resource-limited countries or related to toxicity, include amphotericin plus fluconazole, fluconazole plus flucytosine, and high-dose fluconazole alone. Combination therapy has been shown to increase survival and to decrease relapse rates.

Consolidation: High-dose fluconazole of 6–12 mg/kg for 8 weeks.

Maintenance: Fluconazole for a minimum of 12 months; in the HIV population antifungals can be discontinued if the CD4 >100 cells/μL and HIV viral load is undetectable for at least 3 months.

Note: There are alternative regimens in resource-limited settings that can be found in the Infectious Disease Society of America (IDSA) website. Other specific recommendations for transplant recipients and non-HIV/nontransplant patients are also available.

THERAPEUTIC PEARL **USMLE STEP 3**

Amphotericin has been well recognized as a medication with significant nephrotoxicity risk, especially with older formulations (deoxycholate). The risk of renal injury is lower with lipid and liposomal formulations.

Renal function and electrolytes should be monitored carefully because abnormal kidney function with impaired clearance can lead to increased levels of flucytosine, which can cause bone marrow suppression with liver and gastrointestinal adverse effects, which can be life threatening.

The patient was started on induction therapy with liposomal amphotericin B plus oral flucytosine and was closely monitored for appropriate tolerance of therapy. His vision and headache symptoms improved.

Fungal culture from CSF shows growth of* C. neoformans*—should you repeat LP?

In patients with growth of *Cryptococcus* on CSF culture, it would be appropriate to repeat lumbar puncture after 2 weeks of induction therapy to assess for CSF sterilization via fungal culture. Persistence of a positive fungal culture would support a potential benefit for an extended duration induction regimen. Remember that the presence of India ink does not reflect disease activity other than identifying the polysaccharide capsules of dead yeast.

In this patient, a repeat lumbar puncture was performed and subsequent CSF fungal culture was negative. Therefore, the patient was transitioned to consolidation therapy with fluconazole.

CLINICAL PEARL **USMLE STEP 3**

Serum cryptococcal antigen should not be used for monitoring disease response and therefore serial posttreatment checks are not necessary.

When should you start antiretroviral therapy (ART)?

Guidelines recommend initiation of ART between 2 and 10 weeks after initiation of antifungal therapy (induction phase), but it is unclear exactly when. The risk of initiation of ART should be weighed against the risk of immune reconstitution inflammatory syndrome (IRIS) and should be tailored to the individual patient and other factors including access to healthcare and subsequent follow-up. There is evidence from a randomized clinical trial in Africa that early initiation of ART (within 1 to 2 weeks after diagnosis) resulted in increased 6-month mortality (45% versus 30%) compared with deferred ART (until 5 weeks). It was hypothesized that increased mortality could be attributed to IRIS, which is why it is generally recommended to delay ART initiation as long as possible in patients with increased ICP such as this patient.

Case Summary

- **Complaint/History:** A 29-year-old male with recent positive HIV screening presents with 3 weeks of progressive headache.
- **Findings:** Temperature is 38°C (100.4°F); funduscopic exam shows bilateral papilledema without evidence of focal neurologic deficits.
- **Lab Results/Tests:** Neuroimaging does not reveal intracranial mass. Lumbar puncture shows opening pressure of 32 cm, pleocytosis with monocyte predominance, low glucose, and mild elevated protein with positive cerebrospinal fluid cryptococcal antigen consistent with cryptococcal meningitis.

Diagnosis: AIDS-related cryptococcal meningoencephalitis.

- **Treatment:** Repeat lumbar puncture to decrease ICP below 25 cm of CSF with induction therapy with liposomal amphotericin B plus flucytosine for 2 weeks followed by fluconazole.

Bibliography

Abassi, M., Boulware, D. R., & Rhein, J. (2015). Cryptococcal meningitis: Diagnosis and management update. *Curr Trop Med Rep*, *2*(2), 90–99.

Panel on Guidelines for the Prevention and Treatment of Opportunistic Infections in Adults and Adolescents with HIV. Guidelines for the prevention and treatment of opportunistic infections in HIV-infected adults and adolescents: recommendations from the Centers for Disease Control and Prevention, the National Institutes of Health, and the HIV Medicine Association of the Infectious Diseases Society of America. Available at http://aidsinfo.nih.gov/contentfiles/lvguidelines/adult_oi.pdf.

Perfect, J. R., Dismukes, W. E., Dromer, F., Goldman, D. L., Graybill, J. R., Hamill, R. J., Harrison, T. S., Larsen, R. A., Lortholary, O., Nguyen, M., Pappas, P. G., Powderly, W. G., Singh, N., Sobel, J. D., & Sorrell, T. T. C. (2010). Clinical practice guidelines for the management of cryptococcal disease: 2010 Update by the Infectious Diseases Society of America. *Clinical Infectious Diseases*, *50*, 291–322.

WHO. (2011). *Rapid advice: diagnosis, prevention and management of cryptococcal disease in HIV-infected adults, adolescents and children*. World Health Organization. PMID: 26110194.

CASE 41

A 45-Year-Old Male With Knee Pain

Chitra Punjabi ■ Priya Nori

A 45-year-old male with diabetes and hypertension on hydrochlorothiazide and metformin presents for evaluation of right knee pain. He reports that 2 weeks ago he underwent arthroscopic repair for a meniscal tear and recovered well from the surgery. He was asymptomatic until 2 days ago when he woke up with knee pain. There was no preceding trauma or change in his medications and no history of intravenous (IV) drug use. He took ibuprofen but the pain has progressed, making walking very difficult. He is afebrile on presentation. His right knee is larger than the left, warm to touch, with pain on passive and active flexion and extension.

How do we approach monoarticular arthritis? What are the differential diagnoses?

Monoarticular arthritis can have many causes. Historical information and acuity of illness can give clues to the etiology.

For instance, use of diuretics, alcohol binging, and history of hyperparathyroidism can indicate crystal arthritis. Trauma in a hemophiliac or in a patient on anticoagulants can indicate hemarthrosis.

Infections can present variably, but an acutely affected joint, IV drug use, immunosuppression, or a contiguous site of infection raises concern for bacterial (pyogenic) arthritis. Young, sexually active patients should be evaluated for gonococcal arthritis and residence in or travel to an area endemic for Lyme disease can indicate this as the cause. Fungal and tubercular arthritis are typically more indolent and often considered in those who have been in areas endemic for these diseases. Soil contact is also a historical clue for fungal arthritis.

CLINICAL PEARL **USMLE STEP 2/3**

Septic arthritis is a rheumatologic and orthopedic emergency and should be high on the differential diagnosis in a patient presenting with acute knee pain, swelling, and difficulty with range of motion. Nongonococcal bacterial arthritis causes rapid destruction of cartilage within days of onset and can result in high morbidity.

Are there any clinical features or physical findings to help establish or exclude the diagnosis of septic arthritis?

Classic findings of fever, chills, and an acutely inflamed joint are not specific and do not distinguish etiologies of inflammatory arthritis. Likewise, the absence of fever does not preclude the diagnosis of septic arthritis, being present in only 50% of cases.

CLINICAL PEARL **USMLE STEP 1/3**

The absence of fever does not rule out septic arthritis.

CLINICAL PEARL **USMLE STEP 2/3**

The diagnostic yield of synovial fluid cultures is increased by inoculation into aerobic blood culture bottles.

In a patient suspected of having septic arthritis, which diagnostic tests can be pursued?

Blood cultures are positive in approximately 50% of cases and up to 80% when there is polyarticular septic arthritis. Elevated peripheral white blood count, erythrocyte sedimentation rate, and C-reactive protein are often seen but are nonspecific for the diagnosis. Radiographs are frequently normal in acute disease (<2 weeks). Computerized tomography (CT) or magnetic resonance imaging (MRI) can show synovial thickening or joint effusion; however, they are often not necessary, unless a contiguous abscess is suspected. Synovial fluid analysis remains the cornerstone for the diagnosis.

Which tests are done on synovial fluid? What are the typical findings seen for the different causes of arthritis in synovial fluid analysis?

Synovial fluid should be sent for a white blood cell (WBC) count and differential, microscopic exam for crystals, Gram stain, and culture. Synovial fluid protein and glucose are not helpful in establishing the etiology. Table 41.1 gives the usual findings for different etiologies.

Arthrocentesis is performed yielding 10 cc of cloudy fluid. Synovial fluid analysis shows WBC count of 85,000 cells/µL with 92% PMN. Negatively birefringent crystals are noted. Gram stain is pending.

TABLE 41.1 ■ **Typical Findings for Different Arthritis Etiologies**

Diagnosis	WBC Count Cells/µL	% Polymorphonuclear Neutrophils (PMNs)	Other Findings
Normal	<200	<25	
Noninflammatory (e.g., osteoarthritis)	200–2000	<25	
Inflammatory, noncrystalline	2000–100,000	>50	
Inflammatory, crystalline	2000–100,000	>50	Crystals seen
Infectious: bacterial	>50,000	>75	Gram stain (+) in 60%–80%; cultures (+)
Infectious: gonococcal	30,000–70,000	>75	Gram stain and culture variably positive Urine/mucosal NAAT test of choice
Infectious: Lyme	3000–100,000	>50	Serum serology (+); synovial PCR (+) in 85% cultures are not routinely available

From Horowitz, D. L., Katzap, E., Horowitz, S., & Barilla-labarca, M. L. (2011). Approach to septic arthritis. *American Family Physician*, 84(6), 653–660.

How do we interpret the synovial fluid result of this patient?

The crystals seen in synovial fluid indicate the possibility of a crystalline arthritis. At the same time, however, the WBC count and differential should still raise concern for septic arthritis. Synovial fluid WBC counts >50,000 and >100,000 were found to have positive likelihood ratios of 7.7 and 28, respectively, for the diagnosis of septic arthritis, and a PMN differential of >90% had a positive LR of 3.4 for septic arthritis.

CLINICAL PEARL **USMLE STEP 2/3**

Crystal arthropathies can coexist with septic arthritis, therefore the presence of crystals on synovial fluid exam does not rule out coexisting infection.

CLINICAL PEARL **USMLE STEP 2/3**

In a patient with a synovial fluid WBC count of >50,000 or PMN of >75%, antibiotics should be started empirically while awaiting culture results.

What are the causes of infectious arthritis?

The most common etiological agent of all septic arthritis cases (excluding gonococcal arthritis in the United States) is *Staphylococcus aureus*, causing almost half of all cases (44%) and up to 71% of cases in IVDU. *Streptococcus spp*. are the next most common cause, with *Streptococcus pneumoniae* and *Streptococcus pyogenes* the most often reported. Gram-negative bacilli account for approximately 10% to 20% of cases especially in elderly patients, particularly those with a history of intravenous drug abuse, an immunocompromising condition, or trauma. *Pseudomonas* is most common in the immunocompromised or in IVDU (caused by use of contaminated water sources).

CLINICAL PEARL **USMLE STEP 2/3**

Empiric therapy when the Gram stain is negative is directed toward most common organisms and guided by patient risk factors.

- Vancomycin can be used as monotherapy in the absence of any additional risk factors listed. It provides reliable coverage against MRSA, other staphylococcal species, and streptococci.
- Vancomycin and a third-generation cephalosporin (e.g., ceftriaxone) should be used for the elderly, in the setting of trauma, or in patients with risks for Gram-negative infections (i.e., recurrent UTIs, recent abdominal surgery).
- Vancomycin and an antipseudomonal agent (e.g., cefepime or ceftazidime) should be used for those with IVDU or those who are immunocompromised (e.g., on chronic steroids or chemotherapy for malignancy, organ transplan recipients, etc.)

Gram stain of the fluid is as shown in Fig. 41.1.

Based on this Gram stain, what is the likely organism involved? Which antibiotic should be prescribed?

Gram-positive cocci (GPCs) are seen on the Gram stain; thus, staphylococci or streptococci are the likely etiologic agent. In this smear, clusters of GPCs are seen; thus, this is probably *Staphylococcus aureus*, given our patient has a native knee joint. If this patient had a prosthetic joint infection, coagulase-negative staphylococci may also be the culprit. Streptococci would usually be seen as pairs or chains on the Gram stain. Vancomycin should be started, pending identification and susceptibility results.

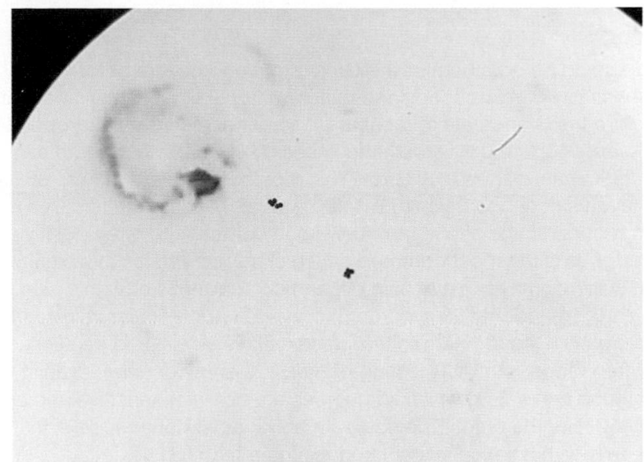

Fig. 41.1 Gram stain showing Gram-positive cocci.

How should septic arthritis be managed?

Septic arthritis should be managed aggressively; both appropriate antibiotics and adequate joint drainage are essential. Joint drainage relieves joint pressure and removes cartilage destructive enzymes produced by the bacteria. Drainage can be achieved with arthrocentesis (often repeated until cultures are negative), arthroscopy, or open drainage. Antibiotics are tailored toward the causative organism and continued for approximately 3–4 weeks in septic arthritis of a native joint, although a recent trial (Gjika. E., et al., 2019) suggests 14 days may be sufficient in an immunocompetent host with native joint disease.

CLINICAL PEARL **USMLE STEP 1,2,3**

Classically, open surgical drainage is recommended when adequate drainage is not achievable by either arthroscopic or needle aspiration because of penetrating trauma with a foreign body or joint effusion persists despite serial needle aspiration.

The patient is scheduled for urgent surgical incision and drainage. Operative cultures confirm growth of methicillin-resistant *Staphylococcus aureus*. The patient is continued on intravenous vancomycin for 4 weeks and has a satisfactory recovery course.

Case Summary

- **Complaint/History:** A 45-year-old male with acute onset monoarticular right knee pain 2 weeks after arthroscopic repair.
- **Findings:** Right knee effusion with warmth and discomfort on both active and passive range of motion.
- **Lab Results/Tests:** Synovial fluid analysis with a white-blood count of 85,000 and 92% mononuclear cells. Negatively birefringent crystals are noted; however, the Gram stain indicates concurrent Gram-positive cocci indicative of *Staphylococcus* species. Methicillin resistant *Staphylococcus aureus* grows in cultures.

Diagnosis: Postsurgical native right knee septic arthritis.

- **Treatments:** Operative joint irrigation and debridement followed by intravenous vancomycin for 4 weeks.

BEYOND THE PEARLS

- Synovial fluid should be obtained for the Gram stain and culture before the initiation of antibiotics. Sensitivity of microscopy and cultures drops significantly if patients receive antibiotics before the Gram stain and culture. Microscopy sensitivity dropped from 58% to 12% (native knees: 46% to 0%; prosthetic knees: 72% to 27%). Culture sensitivity dropped from 79% to 28% (native knees: 69% to 21%; prosthetic knees: 91% to 36%).
- Polyarticular involvement occurs in 15% to 20% of all septic arthritis cases and has higher mortality than monoarticular septic arthritis. Blood cultures are often positive.
- Gonococcal arthritis is the most common cause of septic arthritis in sexually active young adults. Patients may present with oligoarticular arthritis or with a skin rash and tenosynovitis (arthritis–dermatitis syndrome) or have monoarticular involvement. High index of suspicion is needed and a thorough sexual history should be elicited. The diagnosis is often made with PCR testing of mucosal areas or urine, even in the absence of symptoms in these areas. Synovial fluid cultures are not very sensitive and are positive only approximately 50% of the time. Empiric treatment against gonococcal arthritis should be started in patients with a sexual history suggesting a high STI risk.
- In the United States, Lyme disease is usually seen in highly endemic areas: the Northeast, the Midwest, Northern California, and Oregon. Patients presenting from these areas with septic arthritis and in whom cultures have been negative should have serologic testing for Lyme and synovial fluid PCR for *Borrelia burgdorferi*. Empiric treatment against Lyme arthritis can be started in patients at high risk while awaiting results of serologic testing.

Bibliography

Gjika, E., Beaulieu, J.-Y., Vakalopoulos, K., Gauthier, M., Bouvet, C., Gonzalez, A., Morello, V., Steiger, C., Hirsiger, S., Lipsky, B. A., & Uçkay, I. (2019). Two weeks versus four weeks of antibiotic therapy after surgical drainage for native joint bacterial arthritis: A prospective, randomised, non-inferiority trial. *Annals of the Rheumatic Diseases*, *78*, 1114.

Hindle, P., Davidson, E., & Biant, L. C. (2012). Septic arthritis of the knee: the use and effect of antibiotics prior to diagnostic aspiration. *Annals of the Royal College of Surgeons of England*, *94*(5), 351–355.

Horowitz, D. L., Katzap, E., Horowitz, S., & Barilla-labarca, M. L. (2011). Approach to septic arthritis. *American Family Physician*, *84*(6), 653–660.

Hu, L. (2005). Lyme arthritis. *Infectious Disease Clinics of North America*, *19*(4), 947–961.

Margaretten, M. E., Kohlwes, J., Moore, D., & Bent, S. (2007). Does this adult patient have septic arthritis? *The Journal of the American Medical Association*, *297*(13), 1478–1488.

Rice, P. A. (2005). Gonococcal arthritis (disseminated gonococcal infection). *Infectious Disease Clinics of North America*, *19*(4), 853–861.

Ross, J. J. (2005). Septic arthritis. *Infectious Disease Clinics of North America*, *19*(4), 799–817.

CASE 42

A 70-Year-Old Male With Fever and Diarrhea

Rachel Bartash ■ Priya Nori

A 70-year-old man with a medical history of diabetes, hypertension, and coronary artery disease and who underwent a coronary artery bypass grafting 6 months previously is admitted to the hospital with complaints of watery diarrhea and abdominal discomfort for 3 days. He denies any fevers, chills, nausea, vomiting, or urinary symptoms. He reports no recent travel, sick contacts, or change in oral intake. He reports receiving a 7-day course of amoxicillin 2 weeks before for a suspected dental infection. Other medications include metoprolol, metformin, aspirin, atorvastatin, and omeprazole. On examination he is afebrile and is noted to have mild tenderness to palpation in the left lower quadrant. Blood work shows a leukocytosis of 15,000 cells/uL.

What is the differential diagnosis for infectious causes of acute onset diarrhea?

Acute diarrhea, which is defined as >3 watery or loose bowel movements per day, is caused by both infectious and noninfectious etiologies. The first step in evaluating patients with acute diarrhea is taking a detailed history to determine those at highest risk of complications of acute diarrhea (hospitalization, organ failure, etc.). This includes patients with immunocompromising conditions, history of recent travel, exposure to young children or daycare settings, and recent antibiotic use or healthcare exposure. In terms of infectious causes, the differential diagnosis is broad and includes bacterial, viral, and parasitic infections depending on a patient's exposure history (see Table 42.1).

What is* Clostridioides difficile*?

Clostridioides difficile is a spore and toxin producing anaerobic Gram-positive bacillus. The organism is ubiquitous and found in water, soil, healthcare surfaces, and human and animal feces. *C. difficile* infection occurs when there is proliferation and toxin production in the colon resulting in an acute diarrheal illness, which is also known as pseudomembranous colitis. *C. difficile* infection is estimated to cause about 200,000 infections in hospitalized patients and 12,000 deaths per year according to the Centers for Disease Control and Prevention's (CDC's) 2019 Antibiotic Resistant Threats report.

CLINICAL PEARL — **USMLE STEP 2/3**

Clostridioides difficile colonization is common especially in infants, patients with prior hospital exposures, and patients with prior episodes of *C. difficile* infection. The presence of the organism in the colon in the absence of symptoms does not indicate an active infection and does not warrant treatment.

TABLE 42.1 ■ **Possible Infectious Causes of Acute Onset Diarrhea**

Bacterial	Viral	Parasitic
Enterotoxigenic *Escherichia coli*	Norovirus	*Giardia lamblia*
Enteropathogenic *Escherichia coli*	Rotavirus	*Strongyloides stercoralis*
Enterotoxigenic *Escherichia coli*	Cytomegalovirus	*Cryptosporidium parvum*
Enteroinvasive *Escherichia coli*		*Cyclospora cayetanensis*
Escherichia coli O157		*Entamoeba histolytica*
Shigella		
Salmonella		
Shigella dysenteriae		
Vibrio cholerae		
Noncholera *Vibrio cholerae*		
Campylobacter		
Clostridioides difficile		

CLINICAL PEARL **USMLE STEP 2/3**

Although *Clostridioides difficile* infection remains a common hospital acquired infection, increasing numbers of community onset cases are being seen, according to the CDC (2).

CLINICAL PEARL **USMLE STEP 2/3**

The primary contributing risk factor of *C. difficile* infections is prior antibiotic exposure. Although antibiotics are needed to treat other bacterial infections such as urinary tract infections, cellulitis, and pneumonia, studies show that these antibiotic courses are often too long or have a too broad spectrum, which can increase the risk of developing *C. difficile* infection. Effective hand hygiene and environmental cleaning of hospital environments are also crucial for preventing the spread of infection from one patient to another.

How is* C. difficile *transmitted and what is the pathogenesis of infection?

C. difficile can be acquired via fecal-oral route through contact with the environment, through contact with contaminated hospital surfaces, or from direct contact with infected or colonized patients. Transmission from healthcare workers because of poor hand hygiene remains common. Not all individuals who have direct contact with *C. difficile* will develop an active infection. Many patients will become colonized, but active disease typically occurs in those with some degree of immunosuppression or disruption to the normal colonic microbiota from antibiotic exposure.

The two main virulence factors for infection are toxin A and toxin B. Both toxins are responsible for activating an inflammatory response composed predominantly of neutrophils, which results in direct damage to colonic epithelial cells. The histopathologic changes associated with this inflammatory reaction are called pseudomembranes. Notably, not all strains of *C. difficile* produce toxins; these are called nontoxigenic strains of *C. difficile* and rarely cause symptomatic infection.

CLINICAL PEARL **USMLE STEP 2/3**

A hypervirulent strain of *C. difficile* called NAP1/B1/027 was recognized in the last decade and is associated with higher mortality and rate of recurrence.

Which infection control measures should be taken to prevent the spread of* C. difficile*?

All patients with suspected or documented *C. difficile* infection should be placed in a private isolation room with a private bathroom to prevent transmission to others (contact isolation). All healthcare personnel entering the room should wear protective gowns and gloves and dedicated equipment should be used to examine the patient. Hand hygiene is required before and after all patient encounters as transmission can occur via healthcare workers to other patients. For routine use, hand hygiene with either soap and water or an alcohol-based hand sanitizer is acceptable; however, alcohol-based hand sanitizers are not sporicidal, and therefore are not recommended as effective hand hygiene after contact with patients with known *C. difficile* infection.

CLINICAL PEARL **USMLE STEP 2/3**

Washing with soap and water is preferred to alcohol-based hand sanitizers when there is direct contact with fecal material or an area possibly contaminated with fecal material because using soap and water improves the removal of spores. In the hospital setting, this method of hand hygiene is preferred because fecal contamination of the environment is assumed even if not visibly apparent.

CLINICAL PEARL **USMLE STEP 2/3**

Sporicidal agents (e.g., bleach) are needed to clean hospital rooms previously occupied by patients with *C. difficile*. Treatment of the room with ultraviolet light as part of a "terminal cleaning" procedure is also highly effective at removing *C. difficile* spores.

What are the symptoms of* C. difficile *infections?

The most common symptoms are watery diarrhea, abdominal pain, and fever. Diarrhea can be profuse, occurring >10–15 times per day. Nausea, vomiting, anorexia, and lack of appetite can also be seen. Leukocytosis >15,000 cells/mL and serum creatinine >1.5 mg/dL are indicative of severe *C. difficile* infection. Elderly patients over the age of 65 years are at increased risk of severe infection. In fulminant *C. difficile*, the symptoms mentioned occur along with hypotension, shock, or ileus. Toxic megacolon, which is a marked dilation of the colon, can also be seen in fulminant *C. difficile* and can lead to colonic perforation and death if not treated appropriately.

What are key risk factors for* C. difficile *infection?

Antibiotic exposure is the main risk factor for the development of *C. difficile* infection. Although almost all antibiotics can cause this infection, the most commonly implicated antibiotics include clindamycin, amoxicillin, cephalosporins, and fluoroquinolones. Other risk factors for symptomatic infection include advanced age, underlying immunocompromising conditions, and prolonged hospitalization. Patients with inflammatory bowel disease, particularly ulcerative colitis, are also at increased risk. Proton pump inhibitors have been shown to be associated with *C. difficile* infection, possibly as a result of disruption of healthy microbiota in the presence of increased intestinal pH.

CLINICAL PEARL **USMLE STEP 2/3**

Antimicrobial stewardship programs are important for ensuring appropriate use of antibiotics (e.g., "the right drug for the right bug" and for the "right" duration) and decreasing rates of *C. difficile* infections.

Which diagnostic tests should be performed for the workup of* C. difficile *infection?
Stool samples should be sent for *C. difficile* testing for patients with acute onset of three or more watery bowel movements daily, especially in the setting of the risk factors mentioned. Because of high rates of colonization, testing should not be performed in asymptomatic patients because this may lead to unnecessary treatment. Microbiology lab tests should only be performed if liquid stool specimens are received (specimens should conform to the shape of the container and not be solid).

The gold standard for diagnosis is either toxigenic culture or cell cytotoxicity, but these are mainly used by research laboratories and rarely used in clinical practice. Enzyme immunoassays (EIAs), nucleic acid amplification tests (NAATs), or polymerase chain reaction (PCR) tests, or a combination of these in either two- or three-step testing, are licensed for *C. difficile* testing by clinical laboratories. EIAs are used to identify glutamate dehydrogenase (GDH) or toxin A or B. GDH is an enzyme that is present in all strains of *C. difficile*, but it is not specific to this pathogen and does not differentiate between toxigenic and nontoxigenic strains. Based on these limitations, it is often coupled with EIA testing for toxin A and/or B in what is known as two-step testing. Two-step testing has an improved sensitivity and specificity over antigen testing alone for diagnosis of *C. difficile*. If there is a discrepancy between the GDH and toxin EIA, this is often followed by a confirmatory NAAT or PCR. When testing algorithms include all three tests (GDH EIA, toxin EIA, and NAAT/PCR), it is known as three-step testing. Two-step and three-step testing are outlined in Fig. 42.1.

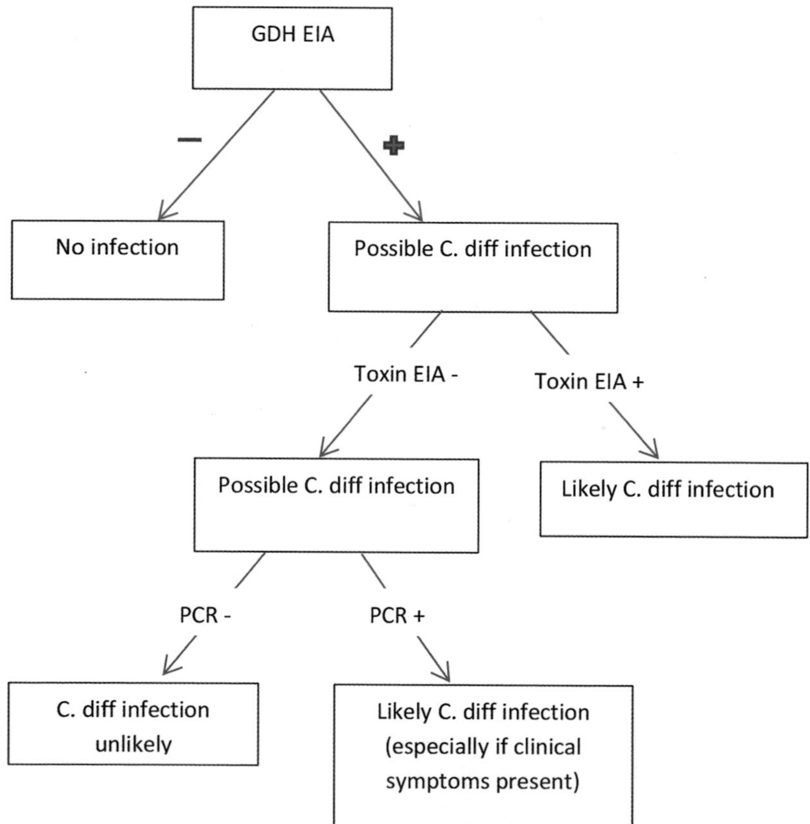

Fig. 42.1 Two- and three-step testing for *Clostridioides difficile. C. difficile, Clostridioides difficile*; *GDH*, glutamate dehydrogenase; *EIA*, enzyme immunoassays; *PCR*, polymerase chain reaction.

Nucleic acid amplification tests can also be performed in isolation as a diagnostic modality. However, NAATs are highly sensitive and may result in higher rates of false positive results in the setting of colonization (especially in patients without true diarrhea).

CLINICAL PEARL **USMLE STEP 2/3**

Tests of cure should not be performed once a patient has completed treatment for *C. difficile* because prolonged carriage of the bacteria can occur following clinical infection.

What are the treatment options for initial* C. difficile *infection?

The first step in treatment of *C. difficile* infection is discontinuing the causative antibiotic agent and mitigating any other modifiable risk factors (e.g., stopping proton pump inhibitors if not absolutely indicated, limiting immunosuppression if possible). Recommended treatment for initial episodes of non-fulminant *C. difficile* infection is oral fidaxomicin 200 mg twice daily. As this treatment may not be available due to cost and other resources, oral vancomycin 125 mg every 6 hours is an acceptable alternative. Treatment with either agent should be continued for 10 days.

Oral vancomycin is the treatment of choice in fulminant *C. difficile*, although higher doses (500 mg every 6 hours) are generally recommended, especially if ileus is present and there is concern for inadequate amount of medication reaching the colon. In these cases, rectal instillation of vancomycin and/or intravenous metronidazole should also be given concurrently. Early surgical consultation is recommended for fulminant cases because urgent colectomy can be needed for perforation, toxic megacolon, or failure to improve despite medical management.

What are the treatment options for recurrent* C. difficile *infection?

Fidaxomicin is also recommended for first recurrence of *C. difficile*. Alternatively, vancomycin can be used in this setting but is often given as in a prolonged taper over 6–8 weeks. For second or multiple recurrences, fidaxomicin or vancomycin tapers are recommended.

A monoclonal antibody directed at toxin B, bezlotuxumab, can also be considered for patients with recurrent *C. difficile* as an adjunct to standard of care. This agent is not used for treatment of infection but has been shown to decrease the risk of recurrence in high risk patients.

Fecal microbiota transplantation should also be considered in those with multiple recurrences as studies have shown good outcomes and higher rates of cure with this procedure compared with medications alone.

CLINICAL PEARL **USMLE STEP 2/3**

Bezlotuxumab should not be used in patients with a history of congestive heart failure.

What is the prognosis of this infection?

Recurrent infection is common, especially in the first month after treatment, because colonization with *C. difficile* can remain even after effective treatment and progression from colonized state to symptomatic illness is easily triggered. Systemic antibiotics should be avoided unless indicated to prevent recurrent infection.

Case Summary

- **Complaint/History:** Watery diarrhea and abdominal discomfort x 3 days in the setting of antibiotic use.
- **Findings:** Mild tenderness to palpation in the left lower quadrant

- **Labs Results/Tests:** Two-step *C. dificile* algorithm positive (GDH positive, toxin EIA positive)

Diagnosis: Antibiotic-associated diarrhea secondary to *Clostrioides difficile* infection

- **Treatment:** Fidaxomicin 200mg twice daily × 10 days

BEYOND THE PEARLS

- *Clostridioides difficile* is a common cause of antibiotic associated diarrhea and a significant cause of morbidity and mortality in hospitalized patients.
- Infection control measures with contact isolation, compliance with hand hygiene, and use of sporicidal cleaning agents are important in preventing the spread of infection in hospitalized patients.
- Appropriate and judicious use of antimicrobials can be improved by antimicrobial stewardship programs, which help prevent cases of *C. difficile* because of excess antibiotic use.
- Diagnosis typically involves enzyme immunoassays +/- nucleic acid amplification tests in two- or three-step testing.
- Isolated nucleic acid amplification may be overly sensitive and may identify cases of colonization rather than true infection.
- Treatment guidelines recommend using fidaxomin, if available, as initial therapy for non-fulminant disease with oral vancomycin as an alternative.
- For fulminant *C. difficile* infection, oral vancomycin is the treatment of choice and can be combined with rectal instillation of vancomycin and/or intravenous metronidazole.
- Fecal microbiota transplantation should be considered for patients with multiple recurrences of *C. difficile* infection because it is the only current option to cure this infection.
- Bezlotuxumb can be considered as an adjunct to standard of care therapy to help decrease the risk of recurrent infection.

Bibliography

Centers for Disease Control. (2019). Antibiotic resistance threats in the United States. https://www.cdc.gov/drugresistance/pdf/threats-report/2019-ar-threats-report-508.pdf

Gerding, D.,N., Young, V. B., & Donskey, C. J. (2000). *Clostridioides difficile (formerly Clostridium difficile)* infection. In J. E. Bennett, R. Donlin, M. J. Blaser (Ed.). (2020). *Mandell, Douglas, and Bennett's principles and practice of infectious diseases* (pp 2933–2947). Philadelphia, PA. Elsevier.

Hvas, C. L., Jorgensen, D., Jorgensen, S. P., Storgaard, M., Lemming, L., Hansen, M. M., Erikstrup, C., & Dahlerup, J. F. (2019). Fecal microbiota transplantation is superior to fidaxomicin for treatment of recurrent *Clostridium difficile* infection. *Gastroenterology*, *156*, 1324–1332.

Johnson, S., Lavergne, V., Skinner, A. M., Gonzales-Luna, A. J., Garey, K. W., Kelly, C. P., & Wilcox, M. H. Clinical practice guideline by the Infectious Diseases Society of America (IDSA) and Society for Healthcare Epidemiology of America (SHEA): 2021 focused update guidelines on management of *Clostridioides difficile* infection in adults. *Clinical Infectious Diseases*, 73(5), e1029-e1044.

McDonald, L. C., Gerding, D. N., Johnson, S., Bakken, J. S., Carroll, K. C., Coffin, S. E., Dubberke, E. R., Garey, K. W., Gould, C. V., Kerry, C., Loo, V., Shaklee Sammons, J., Sandora, T. J., Wilcox, M. H. (2018). Clinical practice guidelines for *Clostridium difficile* infection in adults and children: 2017 update by the Infectious Diseases Society of America (IDSA) and Society for Healthcare Epidemiology of America (SHEA). *Clinical Infectious Diseases*, *66*(7), e1–e48.

Wilcox, M. H., Gerding, D. N., Poxton, I. R., Kelly C., Nathan R., Birch, T., Cornely, O. A., Rahav, G., Bouza, E., Lee, C., Jenkin, G., Jensen, W., Kim, Y. S., Yoshida, J., Gabryelski, L., Pedley, A., Eves, K., Ripping, R., Guris, D., Kartsonis, N., & Dorr, M. B. (2017). Bezlotoxumab for prevention of recurrent *Clostridium difficile* infection. *NEJM*, *376*, 305–317.

World Health Organization (WHO). Diarrhoea. https://www.who.int/topics/diarrhoea/en//

CASE 43

A 30-Year-Old Female With Neutropenia and Fever

Patrick Wu ■ Darren Wong

A 30-year-old female with recently diagnosed refractory T-cell acute lymphoblastic leukemia who recently completed initial induction chemotherapy with cyclophosphamide, vincristine, doxorubicin, and dexamethasone (HyperCVAD) presents for diffuse pain. She had been discharged 2 weeks earlier after completing her most recent cycle of induction chemotherapy during which time she received granulocyte colony-stimulating factor (G-CSF) for neutropenia. She complains of diffuse hip and lower extremity bone pain, which is refractory to her home pain medications, in addition to subjective fevers and chills. On physical examination, vital signs reveal her temperature (oral) 38.3°C (101°F), blood pressure 122/65 mmHg, heart rate 98/min, respiratory rate 20/min, and oxygen saturation 99% on room air. There are scattered ecchymoses of the upper extremities bilaterally but no other rashes. The patient has no indwelling intravenous catheters. The remainder of the examination is unremarkable.

Which aspects of the history and physical examination will be most important to include on your initial assessment?

The likely clinical diagnosis in this case is neutropenic fever because of the history of hematologic malignancy with recent induction chemotherapy and history of neutropenia requiring G-CSF support.

On initial assessment, patients with neutropenic fever should be questioned regarding any organ-specific symptoms, such as dermatologic (catheter site inflammation, swelling, pain or erythema, other rashes or skin lesions, e.g., necrotic or nonnecrotic ulcers, vesicles, or nodules), genitourinary (vaginal discharge, urinary frequency, hematuria, dysuria), pulmonary (cough, shortness of breath, sputum production), or gastrointestinal (diarrhea, constipation, rectal pain or bleeding). Other important elements of the history to gather in the febrile neutropenia patient include medical comorbidities, time since last chemotherapy administration, medications, recent antibiotic use including prophylaxis therapies or treatment courses, history of documented infections, especially with antibiotic-resistant organisms, and relevant epidemiologic exposure history (travel, pets, sick contacts, sexual history, history of testing for HIV or other sexually transmitted infections).

A careful physical examination of mucosal barriers should also be investigated, particularly indwelling catheter sites, oropharynx (including gingiva), lungs, abdomen, and perineal area. A detailed list of potential infection-related signs and symptoms in neutropenic fever are listed in Table 43.1.

CLINICAL PEARL **STEP 2/3**

The definition of neutropenia may vary across centers but, most commonly, severe neutropenia is defined as an absolute neutrophil count (ANC) of <500/μL. Fever in neutropenic patients is defined as a single oral temperature of ≥38.3°C (101°F) or a temperature of ≥38.0°C (100.4°F) sustained over a 1-hour period.

TABLE 43.1 ■ **Signs and Symptoms of Infection From Febrile Neutropenia**[2]

Fever
Chills and sweats
Change in cough or new cough
Sore throat or new mouth sore
Shortness of breath
Nasal congestion
Stiff neck
Burning or pain with urination
Unusual vaginal discharge or irritation
Increased urination
Redness, soreness, or swelling in any area, including surgical wounds and ports
Diarrhea
Vomiting
Pain in abdomen or rectum
New onset of pain
Changes in skin, urination, or mental status

BASIC SCIENCE PEARL **STEP 1**

In addition to the paucity of granulocytes, disruption of the mucosal and mucociliary barriers of the gastrointestinal, genitourinary, and sinopulmonary tracts, a component of the innate immune system, is another predisposing factor to infection in neutropenic patients.

Which tests should be ordered on initial presentation?

At a minimum, the following lab tests should be ordered:

- **Complete blood cell count with differential:** Determination of the presence and severity of any cytopenia is vital to determine whether the patient requires transfusion support or any immediate intervention, including empiric antibiotics.
- **Complete metabolic panel:** Significant metabolic derangement, including metabolic acidosis, hepatic insufficiency, or acute kidney injury, may increase the diagnostic likelihood of sepsis caused by infection with end-organ dysfunction and will necessitate aggressive volume resuscitation. Liver function test abnormalities may also indicate infectious or noninfectious etiologies of fever, such as cholecystitis, cholangitis, or drug-induced liver injury.
- **Blood culture:** At least two sets of blood cultures should be ordered to assess for bacteremia. If the patient has an indwelling central venous catheter such as a port catheter or peripherally inserted central venous catheter, sets of blood cultures should be drawn from each lumen of the indwelling catheter in addition to a peripheral vein.

Depending on the clinical presentation, additional tests and imaging should be ordered based on the relevant focused history of illness and physical examination. For example, a chest radiography may be ordered if there are clinical signs or symptoms of an underlying pneumonia; stool studies including *Clostridium difficile* studies may be ordered for diarrhea.

CLINICAL PEARL **STEP 2/3**

The sensitivity of two sets of blood cultures in detecting a bloodstream pathogen in a critically ill patient is 80%–90%; the sensitivity rises to 96% if three sets of blood cultures are obtained. However, a negative blood culture result(s) should be interpreted in context, especially as only 23% of febrile neutropenic episodes are associated with bacteremia.

The patient's initial laboratory data on presentation are shown in Table 43.2.

What is the differential diagnosis for this patient's neutropenic fever?

The most common causes of neutropenic fever include bacterial infections, namely catheter-associated infections and neutropenic enterocolitis (typhlitis) with Gram-positive (coagulase-negative staphylococci, *Staphylococcus aureus*, enterococci) and Gram-negative (enteric organisms including *Escherichia coli*, *Klebsiella*, and *Enterobacter* as well as *Pseudomonas aeruginosa*) bacteremia, as well as noninfectious etiologies including superficial thrombophlebitis, deep venous thrombosis and/or pulmonary embolism, drug-related fever, and underlying malignancy. Since neutropenia blunts host immune response, infections can often be subclinical in presentation, only presenting with fever.

Viral infections including seasonal infections such as influenza and parainfluenza, respiratory syncytial virus (RSV), and West Nile virus, reactivation herpes viruses (e.g., HSV-1 and -2, CMV, EBV, VZV, and HHV-6), and other viruses (adenovirus) should also be considered. Rarer causes of neutropenic fever include disseminated candidiasis, aspergillosis, and infections with other molds (e.g., Zygomycetes, *Fusarium*), tuberculosis, nontuberculous mycobacterial infections, cryptococcosis or endemic fungal infections (e.g., coccidioidomycosis, blastomycosis, histoplasmosis).

CLINICAL PEARL **STEP 3**

Neutropenic fever develops in roughly 10%–50% of patients with solid organ tumors and over 80% of patients with hematologic malignancies undergoing chemotherapy. However, most patients, approximately 70%–80% of febrile neutropenia cases, will not have a documented infectious etiology.

Does this patient need to be admitted to the hospital?

The decision of whether to admit a patient with neutropenic fever to the inpatient setting should be guided by evidence-based risk stratification. High-risk patients are characterized by prolonged neutropenia (≥7 days), "profound" neutropenia (ANC ≤100 cells/mm^3), clinical instability (e.g., hemodynamic compromise, inability to tolerate oral intake, encephalopathy, hypoxemia) or significant high-risk medical comorbidities (e.g., poor functional status or advanced age) (see Table 43.3). The Multinational Association for Supportive Care in Cancer (MASCC) scoring system (see Table 43.4) may be used to further distinguish high-risk from low-risk patients. A MASCC score of ≥21 (out of a maximum of 26) is indicative of a low-risk patient who may be managed as an outpatient with oral empiric antibiotics, whereas a patient with a score of <21 should be admitted and managed in the inpatient setting.

TABLE 43.2 ■ **Initial Laboratory Tests**

Leukocyte count	500/μL (60% neutrophils, 35% lymphocytes, 5% monocytes)
Absolute neutrophil count	300/μL
Hemoglobin	7.9g/dL
Platelet count	32,000/μL
Peripheral smear	76% blasts indicative of uncontrolled T-cell acute lymphoblastic leukemia
Complete metabolic panel	All values within normal limits

TABLE 43.3 ■ **Risk Stratification in Neutropenic Fever**

High Risk	Low Risk
MASCC Risk Index ≤21[a] Profound neutropenia • Duration of neutropenia >7 days • ANC ≤100 cells per microliter Clinically unstable Medical comorbidities[b] Hepatic insufficiency Renal insufficiency Poor functional status Advanced age Disease type Intensity of chemotherapy	MASCC Risk Index >21[a] Duration of neutropenia ≤7 days Clinically stable No active medical comorbidity

[a]Scored by burden of febrile neutropenia based on presence of no, mild, or moderate symptoms; no hypotension, chronic obstructive pulmonary disease, solid tumor or hematologic malignancy with fungal infection presence, or dehydration requiring parenteral fluids; outpatient status; and age <60 years.
[b]Comorbidities include but are not limited to hemodynamic instability, gastrointestinal symptoms, new onset of neurological changes, intravascular catheter infection, and underlying chronic lung disease.
ANC, Absolute neutrophil count; *MASCC*, Multinational Association for Supportive Care in Cancer.

TABLE 43.4 ■ **The Multinational Association for Supportive Care in Cancer (MASCC) Scoring System**

Characteristic	Score
Burden of illness: no or mild symptoms	5
No hypotension	5
No chronic obstructive pulmonary disease	4
Solid tumor or no previous fungal infection	4
No dehydration	3
Burden of illness: moderate symptoms	3
Outpatient status	3
Age <60 years	2

Burden of febrile neutropenia refers to the general clinical status of the patient as influenced by the febrile neutropenic episode. It should be evaluated on the following scale: no or mild symptoms (score of 5); moderate symptoms (score of 3); and severe symptoms or moribund (score of 0). Scores of 3 and 5 are not cumulative.

This patient is high risk by MASCC criteria: her MASCC score is 17 based on age, hematologic malignancy, tachycardia signifying hypovolemia/dehydration, presence of moderate symptoms without hypotension, no history of chronic obstructive pulmonary disease, and outpatient status. Therefore, she should be admitted as an inpatient for further monitoring and diagnostic workup, as well as intravenous antibiotics.

CLINICAL PEARL **STEP 3**

Patients with neutropenic fever in the setting of prolonged neutropenia as a result of preconditioning for hematopoietic stem-cell transplantation (HSCT) or induction chemotherapy for acute myeloid leukemia (AML) should always be admitted to the inpatient setting.

Which empiric antimicrobials should be initiated in this patient?

The preferred initial empiric antibiotic of choice would be a broad-spectrum, antipseudomonal beta-lactam with wide Gram-positive and Gram-negative activity. Depending on local hospital-based protocols and epidemiology, this may consist of cefepime, piperacillin-tazobactam, or an antipseudomonal carbapenem, such as meropenem or imipenem-cilastatin. Further modification to the empiric antibiotic choice should subsequently be guided by any culture or imaging results, as well as clinical response to empiric therapy.

Vancomycin can be considered as expanded Gram-positive antibacterial therapy in patients with specific clinical indications: indwelling intravenous catheters, suspected pneumonia, hemodynamic instability, mucositis, and/or skin/soft tissue infections (see Table 43.5). If, however, blood cultures have demonstrated no growth of Gram-positive organisms after 48 hours of incubation, it is recommended to discontinue vancomycin. Continued administration of vancomycin in a patient with persistent fever who is otherwise asymptomatic and hemodynamically stable is not recommended.

If the patient has a history of resistant bacterial infections, such as vancomycin-resistant enterococci (VRE) or extended-spectrum beta-lactamase (ESBL) positive or carbapenemase-producing Enterobacteriaceae, empiric antibiotics would need to be tailored based on the prior isolated organism's in vitro susceptibility pattern.

CLINICAL PEARL **STEP 3**

Febrile neutropenia should be managed with the urgent initiation of empiric antibiotics, ideally within 2 hours of presentation. If managing neutropenic fever in a low-risk patient as an outpatient, the preferred empiric antibiotic regimen is ciprofloxacin plus amoxicillin-clavulanate. Ciprofloxacin should not be used as monotherapy for neutropenic fever because of its unreliable activity for viridans group streptococci. Utilizing a combination regimen inclusive of amoxicillin-clavulanate provides more effective Streptococcus spectrum.

Is this patient a candidate for antifungal prophylaxis?

Yes, the patient has recently received induction chemotherapy for acute myeloid leukemia, making her a candidate for the use of antifungal prophylaxis.

CLINICAL PEARL **STEP 2/3**

Select patient populations are at an elevated risk of invasive *Candida* infection. Patients who are status postallogeneic hematopoietic stem cell transplant (HSCT) and those undergoing induction chemotherapy for acute leukemia or myelodysplastic syndrome (MDS) are recommended for antifungal prophylaxis for the duration of their neutropenia. In these same high-risk groups, if a patient is herpes simplex (HSV) seropositive, acyclovir prophylaxis is also recommended.

TABLE 43.5 ■ **Indications for Addition of Expanded Gram-Positive Coverage in Neutropenic Fever**

- Hemodynamic instability or other evidence of severe sepsis
- Pneumonia documented radiographically
- Positive blood culture for Gram-positive bacteria pending identification and susceptibility results
- Clinically suspected serious catheter-related infection (e.g., chills or rigors with infusion through catheter and cellulitis around the catheter entry/exit site)
- Skin/soft tissue infection
- Colonization with MRSA, VRE, or penicillin-resistant *Streptococcus pneumoniae*
- Severe mucositis

MRSA, Methicillin-resistant *Staphylococcus aureus*; *VRE*, vancomycin-resistant enterococci

The patient is admitted and started on cefepime. She tolerates therapy without adverse effects with cessation of fever episodes. She also receives fluconazole for antifungal prophylaxis. However, on hospital day 5, she experiences another fever of 38.2°C (100.8°F). Blood cultures from admission remain negative and an additional two sets of blood cultures are ordered.

The same day, the patient also begins to complain of oral discomfort while taking her morning medications. On physical examination, she is discovered to have multiple new 1–2 cm ulcerative lesions on her tongue (see Fig. 43.1). Her clinical status is otherwise unchanged. An otolaryngology consultation is ordered for biopsy of the new tongue lesions.

When should empiric antimicrobials be adjusted to address potential fungal etiologies of neutropenic fever?

Persistent neutropenic fever despite 4–7 days of broad-spectrum antibacterial medication warrants consideration for fungal infection as the etiology of the patient's fever. In these patients, initiation of empiric broad spectrum antifungal therapy can be considered.

CLINICAL PEARL **STEP 2/3**

Early request of surgery consult for potential biopsy is of utmost importance in a patient with skin or mucosal lesions because of the risk of infection (especially necrotic lesions suggestive of fungal infections). Cutaneous ecthyma gangrenosum, a necrotic skin lesion, can be caused by Gram-negative organisms including *Pseudomonas aeruginosa* and molds including Zygomycetes. In the case of the latter, histopathology of biopsy specimens will show invasive fungal hyphae with invasion of the blood vessels and subcutaneous tissue. Early aggressive surgical excision and wide debridement of such lesions, along with systemic antifungal therapy, is the mainstay of therapy.

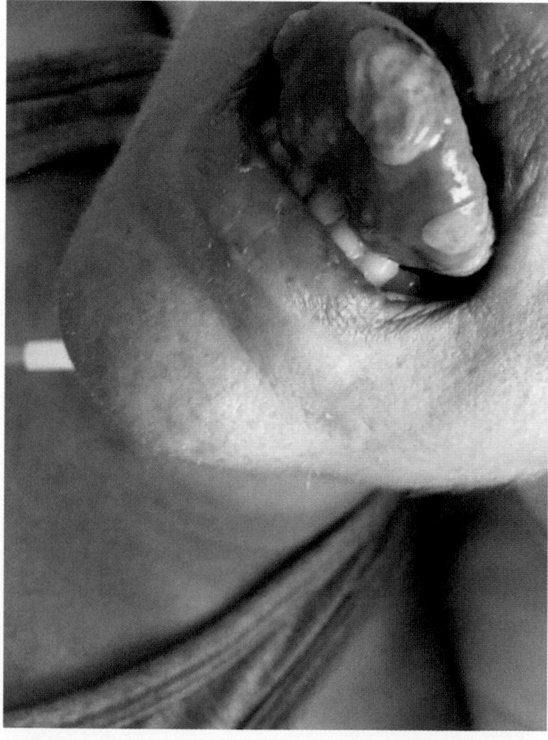

Fig. 43.1 Ulcerative tongue lesions.

What is the role of fungal biomarkers in this patient?

In some situations, serum galactomannan can be tested as a marker of invasive aspergillosis. Similarly, β-(1–3)-D-glucan can be tested as a serum marker of both invasive candidiasis and invasive aspergillosis. However, only patients who are at risk of invasive fungal infections including patients undergoing preparatory treatment for HSCT and those undergoing induction chemotherapy for acute leukemia should be routinely tested. These serologic tests are not recommended for low-risk patients.

CLINICAL PEARL **STEP 2/3**

The serum galactomannan assay as a marker of invasive aspergillosis may be falsely elevated in other infections (e.g., histoplasmosis and talaromycosis, the latter formerly known as penicilliosis) and administration of certain beta-lactam antibiotics. The β-(1–3)-D glucan detects infections caused by *Candida* species, *Aspergillus* species, *Pneumocystis jiroveci*, and *Fusarium* species. However, it will not detect infections caused by Zygomycetes (e.g., *Mucorales)* or *Cryptococcus* species, and false positive can occur in patients undergoing renal replacement therapy or receiving intravenous immunoglobulin (IVIg) therapy.

The patient's serum galactomannan is undetectable at <0.5 ng/mL; however, her serum beta-D-glucan returns were elevated at 270 pg/mL.

Which clinical entity is this patient at risk of given the clinical and laboratory findings?

Necrotizing ulcerations in the mouth and mucosal membranes in febrile neutropenia warrant evaluation for infectious etiologies, including viral, especially HSV; fungal infections; and noninfectious etiologies, namely malignant infiltration.

This patient's clinical presentation should raise concern for disseminated candidiasis, specifically with a fluconazole-resistant *Candida* species, such as *Candida krusei* or *Candida glabrata*, given that her symptoms began while she was receiving fluconazole. Her discomfort during oral intake and new tongue lesions are indicative of at least *Candida* mucosal colonization and probably tissue invasive disease. However, she is probably not a candidate for an invasive endoscopic procedure because of her thrombocytopenia and neutropenia, which place her at elevated risk of complications of bleeding and perforation. Therefore, if invasive fungal infection is suspected, chest and sinus imaging may be beneficial.

CLINICAL PEARL **STEP 2/3**

Disseminated candidiasis should be considered in patients with persistent or recurrent fever at the time of recovery from neutropenia. Investigation including routine blood cultures (fungal blood cultures are not needed because routine blood cultures are sufficient to isolate *Candida* species) liver function testing (elevated alkaline phosphatase), and imaging of the liver and spleen to assess for nodular lesions consistent with hepatosplenic candidiasis should be pursued in such patients.

The patient's tongue lesions are biopsied by otolaryngology. Histopathologic examination of the lesions demonstrates fungal elements and pseudohyphae indicative of *Candida* infection. *Candida krusei* develops from culture of the lesions. Her antifungal therapy is changed to micafungin. Eventually, the lesions resolve after completion of a course of micafungin. The patient's fever also resolves after several days of antiinfective therapy. She is monitored for recurrent fever but has none after 3 days.

What is your next step in treating this neutropenic patient who is now afebrile?
Discontinue cefepime and consider starting an antipseudomonal fluoroquinolone, such as levofloxacin or ciprofloxacin, for antibacterial prophylaxis if the patient's neutropenia is expected to persist for ≥7 days. Multiple studies have shown that empiric antibiotics can be safely de-escalated in patients with negative blood cultures who have demonstrated 48–72 hours of overall clinical stability and resolution of fever. Other criteria necessary for switch from intravenous to oral antibiotics in this patient include intact gastrointestinal absorption and tolerance of oral medications.

CLINICAL PEARL **STEP 2/3**

Among the fluoroquinolones active against *Pseudomonas aeruginosa*, levofloxacin has superior viridans group streptococcal activity and would be preferred instead of ciprofloxacin in patients with mucositis. However, ciprofloxacin is considered a preferred antipseudomonal quinolone in contrast to levofloxacin.

Case Summary

- **Complaint/History:** A 30-year-old female with neutropenic fever but a paucity of other symptoms.
- **Findings:** Initial physical examination is only significant for tachycardia and scattered ecchymoses but no other discrete rashes or skin lesions. Eventually, the patient is discovered to have multiple ulcerative lesions on her tongue.
- **Lab Results/Tests:** Complete blood count reveals severe neutropenia with an ANC of 300, as well as anemia and thrombocytopenia. Later, fungal serologic assays show an elevated β-(1–3)-D-glucan and a nondetectable serum galactomannan.

Diagnosis: Oropharyngeal candidiasis caused by *C. krusei.*

- **Treatment:** Micafungin.

BEYOND THE PEARLS

- Approximately 70%–80% of febrile neutropenia cases do not have any documented infectious etiology.
- The sensitivity of two sets of blood cultures in detecting a bloodstream pathogen in a critically ill patient is 80%–90%; the sensitivity rises to 96% if three sets of blood cultures are obtained.
- Vancomycin should not be routinely initiated as empiric therapy for neutropenic fever patients. Instead, it is recommended for suspected catheter-related infection or pneumonia, hemodynamic instability, mucositis, and/or skin/soft tissue infections. Once initiated, vancomycin can be safely discontinued if the patient remains clinically stable and no Gram-positive organism is identified on blood culture after 48 hours of inoculation.
- Patients with neutropenic fever should undergo daily assessment for any new signs or symptoms of infection, review of pertinent laboratory data and blood culture results, and evaluation of fever trend with determination of overall response to empiric antibiotic therapy.
- In cases of persistent neutropenic fever for 4–7 days without an identified pathogen diagnosis, there should be an investigation for invasive fungal infection and expanded antifungal therapy should be considered.
- Duration of antibiotic therapy depends on the site of infection, if one is identified, and the organism, if bacteremia is diagnosed. In general, a 10–14-day course of antibiotic therapy is considered sufficient to treat most cases of uncomplicated and/or catheter-associated bloodstream infections.

Bibliography

Aguilar-Guisado, M., Espigado, I., Martín-Peña, A., Gudiol, C., Royo-Cebrecos, C., Falantes, J., Vázquez-López, L., Montero, M. I., Rosso-Fernández, C., de la Luz Martino, M., Parody, R., González-Campos, J., Garzón-López, S., Calderón-Cabrera, C., Barba, P., Rodríguez, N., Rovira, M., Montero-Mateos, E., Carratalá, J., Pérez-Simón, J. A., & Cisneros, J. M. (2017). Optimisation of empirical antimicrobial therapy in patients with haematological malignancies and febrile neutropenia (How Long study): An open-label, randomised, controlled phase 4 trial. *The Lancet Haematology*, *4*, e573.

Freifeld, A. G., Bow, E. J., Sepkowitz, K. A., Boeckh, M. J., Ito, J. I., Mullen, C. A., Raad, I. I., Rolston, K. V., Young,, J. H., & Wingard, J. R. (2011). Clinical practice guideline for the use of antimicrobial agents in neutropenic patients with cancer: 2010 update by the Infectious Diseases Society of America. *Clinical Infectious Diseases*, *52*(4), e56–e93.

Klastersky. J. (2004). Management of fever in neutropenic patients with different risks of complications. *Clinical Infectious Diseases*, *39*(Suppl 1), S32–S37.

Klastersky, J., Ameye, L., Maertens, J., Georgala, A., Muanza, F., Aoun, M., Ferrant, A., Rapoport, B., Rolston, K., & Paesmans, M. (2007). Bacteraemia in febrile neutropenic cancer patients. *International Journal of Antimicrobial Agents*, *30*(Suppl 1), S51–S59.

Le Clech, L., Talarmin, J. P., Couturier, M. A., Ianotto, J. C., Nicol, C., Le Calloch, R., Dos Santos, S., Hutin, P., Tandé, D., Cogulet, V., Berthou, C., & Guillerm, G. (2018). Early discontinuation of empirical antibacterial therapy in febrile neutropenia: The ANTIBIOSTOP study. *Infectious Diseases (London, England)*, *50*, 539.

Marchetti, O., Lamoth, F., Mikulska, M., Viscoli, C., Verweij, P., & Bretagne, S. (2012). ECIL recommendations for the use of biological markers for the diagnosis of invasive fungal diseases in leukemic patients and hematopoietic SCT recipients. *Bone Marrow Transplantation*, *47*, 846–854.

NCCN Clinical Practice Guidelines in Oncology Prevention and Treatment of Cancer Related Infections version 1.2019. © 2018 National Comprehensive Cancer Network, Inc. Available at: NCCN.org.

Prattes, J., Schilcher, G., & Krause, R. (2015). Reliability of serum 1, 3-β-D-glucan assay in patients undergoing renal replacement therapy: A review of the literature. *Mycoses*, *58*, 4–9.

Taplitz, R. A., Kennedy, E. B., Bow, E. J., Crews, J., Gleason, C., Hawley, D. K., Langston, A. A., Nastoupil, L. J., Rajotte, M., Rolston, K., Strasfeld, L., & Flowers, C. R. (2018). Outpatient management of fever and neutropenia in adults treated for malignancy: American Society of Clinical Oncology and Infectious Diseases Society of America Clinical Practice Guideline Update. *Journal of Clinical Oncology*, *36*, 1443.

CASE 44

A 42-Year-Old Male With Fever and Malaise

Katharine Yang ■ Noah Wald-Dickler

A 42-year-old Ugandan male with no significant medical history who recently returned from a 1-month trip to Uganda presents to the emergency room with fever, shortness of breath, and fatigue for 5 days.

He was in his usual state of health until 5 days ago, when he started experiencing intermittent fevers. He returned from Uganda 9 days ago. He has no fever in the mornings, but fever starts around 3 p.m. every other afternoon and he breaks into sweats. He has been taking acetaminophen at dinner time, which offers some subjective improvement. However, he still reports going to bed feeling febrile, with improved condition upon awakening in the morning. During his febrile episodes, he reports headache, generalized weakness, shortness of breath, and poor appetite; he has only been eating one meal and one snack a day since his illness began.

Which questions should be asked of a returning traveler with fevers?

A good history is essential to building a complete and broad differential diagnosis for fever in a returning traveler. Make sure to ask about:

- Location of travel, season, day-by-day itinerary, living arrangement, travel activities
- Type of ingested foods (unpasteurized dairy foods are risk factors for infections with *Brucella*, *Mycobacterium bovis*, and diarrheal illnesses caused by *Campylobacter* and *Salmonella*), shellfish (*Vibrio*, enteric viruses), undercooked beef (*Toxoplasma*, *Campylobacter*, *Escherichia coli* O157:H7)
- Exposure to types of waters (fresh water is associated with schistosomiasis and leptospirosis and brackish water exposure is associated with *Vibrio* species infections)
- Mosquito/tick bites (malaria, dengue, Chikungunya, rickettsial infections, Zika virus)
- Sexual history (chlamydia, gonorrhea, HIV)
- Drug use (HIV, hepatitis)
- Animal contact (Q fever, anthrax)
- Pretravel prophylaxis (vaccines and malaria prophylaxis).

Understanding the timing and incubation periods of various infections also helps the clinician narrow the differential diagnosis (Table 44.1).

What are some noninfectious etiologies of recurrent fevers?

- Periodic fever syndromes: familial Mediterranean fever (FMF), tumor necrosis factor receptor-1 associated periodic syndrome (TRAPS), hyperimmunoglobulin D syndrome (HIDS) to name a few
- Malignancy
- Cyclic neutropenia
- Adult-onset Still's disease

TABLE 44.1 ■ **Infectious Differential Diagnosis for Fever in a Returning Traveler**

Short Incubation (<10 days)	Intermediate (10–21 days)	Long (>21 days)
Malaria (esp. falciparum)	Malaria	Malaria (esp. vivax)
Arboviruses (dengue)	Japanese encephalitis	Schistosomiasis
Typhoid	Acute HIV	Acute HIV
Bacterial pneumonia	Typhoid	Tuberculosis
Leptospirosis	Giardiasis	Viral hepatitis
Rickettsia (RMSF, typhus)	Amebiasis	*Coxiella* (Q fever)
Meningococcemia	Brucellosis	Secondary syphilis
Chikungunya	Measles	Mononucleosis (EBV, CMV)

CMV, Cytomegalovirus; *EBV*, Epstein-Barr virus; *RMSF*, Rocky Mountain spotted fever.

The patient denies any chest pain, nausea, vomiting, diarrhea, dysuria, or joint pains.

Two weeks earlier, the patient reports wading through a waist-deep swamp in Lake Kyoga to reach a small island in the middle of the lake. He reports some mosquito bites but states that he has always had mosquito bites when in this area and had no issues in the past. He denies exposure to farm animals. He also denies any history of infectious diseases, including HIV, tuberculosis, or malaria. He had not been taking malaria prophylaxis or received any pre trip vaccines. He reports being monogamous with his wife for the past 15 years.

On physical examination, his temperature is 38.8°C, blood pressure is 100/72 mmHg, pulse rate is 101 beats/min with respiratory rate of 20/min, and oxygen saturation is 88% on room air. He is alert and oriented, but tired, with scleral icterus, scattered petechiae on his limbs, conjunctival pallor, and palpable splenomegaly.

Which tests should be ordered next?

Routine blood work should be ordered including complete blood count, comprehensive metabolic panel including a liver panel, and an HIV screening test.

CLINICAL PEARL

An HIV test obtained early is crucial in a patient with a wide differential diagnosis, because a positive result will guide your thinking toward a different set of diagnostic considerations.

Routine lab results are notable for a normocytic anemia, mild thrombocytopenia, and an indirect bilirubinemia. A low haptoglobin level with an indirect bilirubinemia suggests a hemolytic process. As follows: white blood cells 6.9k (6,900)/mL, hemoglobin 13.1 g/dL, MCV 74.9 fL, platelets 104, 000/mL, sodium 135 mEq/L, potassium 4.3 mEq/L, chloride 99 mEq/L, bicarbonate 24 mEq/L, BUN 7 mg/dL, Cr 1.11 mg/dL, alkaline phosphatase 62 U/L, AST 48 U/L, ALT 56 U/L, total bilirubin 2.5 mg/dL, direct bilirubin 0.4 mg/dL, total protein 6.2 g/dL, albumin 3.3 g/dL, calcium 8.7 mg/dL, haptoglobin <10 mg/dL, LDH 339 U/L, and HIV antigen/antibody screen—negative.

What is the differential diagnosis for hemolytic anemia?

- Autoimmune
  - Cold agglutinin disease
  - Paroxysmal cold hemoglobinuria (PCH)
  - Warm autoimmune hemolytic anemia (AIHA)
- Congenital hemolytic anemias (i.e., thalassemia, hereditary spherocytosis)
- Disseminated intravascular coagulation (DIC)

- Drug-induced hemolytic anemias
- Transfusion-related hemolysis
- Other conditions
  - Clostridial sepsis
  - Mechanical hemolysis from abnormal heart valve
  - Osmotic lysis from hypotonic infusion
  - Paroxysmal nocturnal hemoglobinuria (PNH)
  - Intracellular parasite (e.g., malaria, babesia)
  - Snake bite
  - Thrombotic microangiopathy (TMA) such as thrombotic thrombocytopenic purpura (TTP) or hemolytic uremic syndrome (HUS)

What is included in the differential diagnosis for thrombocytopenia?

- Immune thrombocytopenia (ITP)/drug-induced ITP
  - Heparin, quinine, sulfa drugs, NSAIDs, H2 blockers, antibiotics
  - GP2b/3a inhibitors (abciximab, tirofiban, eptifibatide)
- Infections
  - HIV, Hep C, HBV, *Helicobacter pylori*, sepsis-induced DIC, intracellular parasites (malaria, babesia)
- DIC (sepsis, malignancy, trauma)
- Hypersplenism from chronic liver disease
- Alcohol
- Nutrient deficiencies (B^{12}, folate, copper)
- Rheumatologic/autoimmune disorders (SLE, RA)
- Pregnancy
  - Gestational thrombocytopenia
  - Pre-eclampsia
  - HELLP syndrome
- Other
  - Myelodysplasia
  - Cancer with bone marrow infiltration or suppression (lymphoma, leukemia, some solid tumors)
  - Paroxysmal nocturnal hemoglobinuria (PNH)
  - Thrombotic microangiopathy (TMA)
  - Antiphospholipid syndrome (APS)
  - Aplastic anemia
  - Hereditary thrombocytopenia
    - Von Willebrand disease
    - Wiskott-Aldrich syndrome
    - Alport syndrome
    - May-Hegglin anomaly
    - Fanconi syndrome
    - Bernard-Soulier syndrome
    - Thrombocytopenia absent radius syndrome

A unifying diagnosis that ties all symptoms and laboratory findings is something clinicians should strive to attain, although it does not always happen. A Venn diagram, such as the one in Fig. 44.1, tying in three important clinical features (hemolysis, thrombocytopenia, fever in a traveler) can help narrow your differential diagnosis.

At this point, which conditions are included in your differential diagnosis?

The differential diagnosis includes infectious, rheumatologic, and drug-induced etiologies.

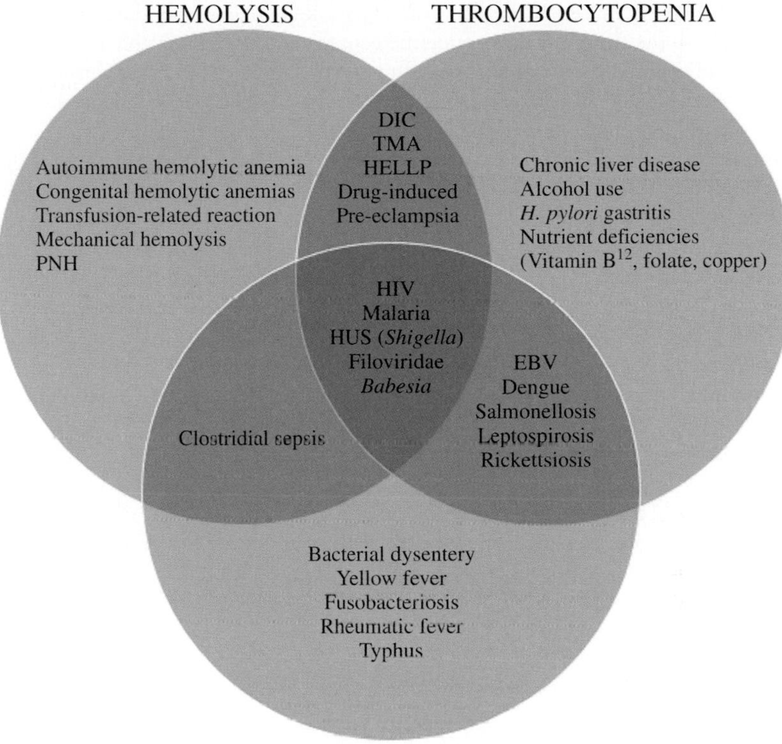

Fig. 44.1 Venn diagram of differential diagnoses.

Infectious. Given this patient's more diffuse constitutional symptoms rather than a focal organ system complaint, his disease process is probably systemic. However, specific organ systems to be considered include the central nervous system, heart, lungs, gastrointestinal tract, and abscesses in any specific organ such as liver, spleen, pancreas, prostate, etc.

In terms of organisms, we can consider bacterial, viral, fungal, and/or parasitic etiologies.

- Bacteria: Common bacterial infections include Gram-positive organisms such as staphylococci and streptococci, which are commonly implicated in skin structure and bloodstream infections, and Gram-negative rod infections such as *E. coli*, *Shigella*, and *Campylobacter*, which can be associated with traveler's diarrhea.
- In patients with significant travel history and exposures, it is important to consider typhus (*Rickettsia typhi*) particularly with centripetal rash with thrombocytopenia and liver derangements, leptospirosis with exposure to animal urine and fresh water, as well as typhoid fever, which is also associated with travel, organomegaly, and cytopenias.
- Viruses: An acute viral illness differential diagnosis should always include HIV. Given travel history and exposure to mosquitos, flaviviruses including dengue, West Nile virus, yellow fever, Zika, and Chikungunya should be included in the differential diagnosis. Also consider hepatitis viruses (A, B, C, D, and E) and hemorrhagic fever viruses (Ebola, Lassa, Marburg, or Junin).
- Fungi: Fungal infections such as histoplasmosis, coccidioidomycosis, and *Pneumocystis jirovecii* typically do not present in patients with new onset fevers. Symptomatology is usually more indolent and slowly progressive. Thus, fungal infection as the source of this patient's presentation is less likely.

- Parasites: Malaria, caused by the *Plasmodium* parasite, is high on our differential because the patient has come from a malaria-endemic country and the risk factors of being in murky waters and exposed to mosquito bites. Other bloodborne parasites to consider in returning travelers include less commonly *Onchocerca* and *Loa* filariasis, although these are often accompanied by significant peripheral eosinophilia.

Rheumatologic. At this point, the diagnosis is likely to be infectious because of its acute nature; however, if an infectious workup is negative and symptoms persist, we should consider diagnoses such as serum sickness, systemic lupus erythematosus, rheumatoid arthritis (if the patient has joint pain), inflammatory bowel disease (if he has gastrointestinal symptoms), and vasculitis (if he has any dermatologic findings).

Malignancy. Underlying malignancy—hematologic or oncologic—can also present in patients with fever and weight loss, like our patient. If this investigation does not yield any results, imaging such as a nuclear scan can shed more light on an undiagnosed malignancy.

Drug-related. Hypersensitivity is the most common cause of drug fever. Common medications that cause drug fever include anticonvulsants, minocycline, antimicrobial agents, allopurinol, and heparin. However, this patient has not been taking any of these agents.

What additional blood work should you order?

- Point-of-care blood glucose (patients with malaria are prone to hypoglycemia, which can contribute to fatigue/altered mental status)
- Coagulation tests including PT and INR, PTT
- Arterial blood gas if hypoxic
- Blood cultures
- Peripheral blood smear with Wright-Giemsa stain (to visualize bloodstream parasites)

CBC and CMP are performed. Blood sugar was 92.
Blood cultures collected at admission had no growth for 5 days.
Peripheral blood smear microscopy evaluation is made in the emergency department (Fig. 44.2).
The BinaxNOW test, an in vitro immunochromatographic assay for the qualitative detection of *Plasmodium* antigens, is positive for *Plasmodium falciparum*. A diagnosis of malaria is made.

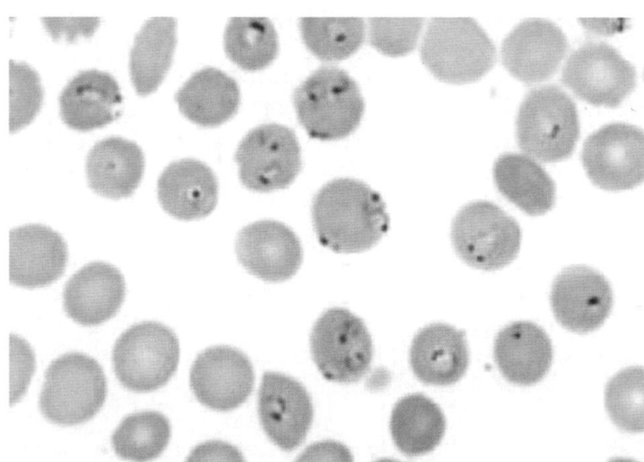

Fig. 44.2 Trophozoite rings of *Plasmodium falciparum* on thin smear. (From McPher, R.A., & Pinncus, M. (2022). *Henry's Clinical Diagnosis and Management by Laboratory Methods, 24th Edition, Chapter 65, pp. 1290–1351.e3. ClinicalKey, Elsevier.*)

CLINICAL PEARL

In 2018, malaria accounted for 405,000 deaths worldwide and over 228 million cases. Africa carries a disproportionately high burden of the global malaria burden with 93% of cases and 94% of deaths.

Diagnosis. To establish a diagnosis of malaria, the gold standard is detection of parasites on Giemsa-stained blood smear by light microscopy, which allows identification and quantification of parasitemia. It is, however, difficult to detect parasitemia that is less than 5–10 parasites/microliter. In low-resource settings without rapid access to microscopy, rapid diagnostic tests such as BinaxNOW Malaria are able to detect antibodies and establish diagnosis.

CLINICAL PEARL

Semi-immune individuals may have substantial parasitemia with few or no symptoms.

After living in nonmalaria endemic regions for a while, people from endemic regions who originally were asymptomatic but semi-immune can lose malaria immunity and develop symptoms after revisiting an endemic country and becoming reinfected.

What are some features of severe malaria that portend a worse prognosis and require expedited attention?

- **Decreased sensorium (Glasgow Coma Scale <11 in adults)**
- **Anemia (Hgb <5 g/dL),** which stems from hemolysis of parasitized RBCs, increased splenic sequestration of erythrocytes with diminished deformability, cytokine suppression of hematopoiesis, and shortened erythrocyte survival.
- **Acidosis (HCO_3 <15, venous plasma lactate >5),** which is one of the causes of death in severe malaria. Anaerobic glycolysis occurs in host tissues where sequestered parasites interfere with microcirculatory flow, induce increased lactate production, and decrease hepatic and renal lactate clearance.
- **Hypoglycemia (blood glucose <40 mg/dL)** also portends a poor prognosis, particularly in children and pregnant women.
- **Renal injury (Cr >3 mg/dL or BUN >20)** is found commonly in adults with severe falciparum malaria and may be related to erythrocyte sequestration interfering with renal microcirculation flow and metabolism. Patients can also have acute tubular necrosis.
- **Jaundice (serum total bilirubin >3 mg/dL)** from hemolysis, hepatocyte injury, and cholestasis
- **Noncardiogenic pulmonary edema (confirmed on radiograph or O_2 sat <92% on room air with RR >33)** is thought to be a result of sequestration of parasitized red cells in lungs and/or cytokine-induced leakage from pulmonary vasculature. ARDS may develop after several days of antimalarial therapy and can be aggravated by vigorous IVF administration. Greatest risk of severe ARDS is in nonimmune individuals, immunocompromised (asplenic) individuals, children, and pregnant women.
- **Hyperparasitemia >5% in *P. falciparum***

There are currently no clearly defined clinical diagnostic criteria for severe malaria; however, for most purposes, severe *P. falciparum* malaria is defined as at least one of the criteria mentioned, in the absence of an identified alternative cause, and in the presence of *P. falciparum* asexual parasitemia (the last not required if a different *Plasmodium* species is identified).

BASIC SCIENCE PEARL

It has been hypothesized that G6PD deficiency (possibly related to oxidant stress in G6PD-deficient erythrocytes that kills parasites). Severe hemoglobinopathies including sickle cell anemia may offer some protection against severe infection from *Plasmodium falciparum* through a variety of potential mechanisms.

If this patient had altered mental status, seizures, and/or focal neurological deficits, what diagnosis should you be concerned about and which test should you obtain?

Cerebral malaria. These patients may present with encephalopathy with impaired consciousness, delirium, seizures, unusual focal neurologic signs, and/or retinal hemorrhages. Other infections such as bacterial, viral, and fungal meningoencephalitis should also be considered.

A lumbar puncture (with head CT if there is concern for intraparenchymal mass) should be obtained with cerebrospinal fluid cell count with differential, protein, glucose, and culture. Mean opening pressure in patients with cerebral malaria is about 16 cm H_2O, with elevated protein and white cell count.

Risk factors for cerebral malaria include young or old age, pregnancy, poor nutritional status, HIV, host genetic susceptibility, and history of splenectomy.

How is malaria treated?

Several questions should be answered prior to deciding on antimalarial therapy:

1) What is the severity of the patient's malaria?
2) If the patient is female, what is her pregnancy status? If pregnant, what trimester?
3) If available, what type of *Plasmodium* species does the patient have (*Plasmodium falciparum, vivax, ovale, knowlesi,* or *malariae*)?
4) What is the availability of antimalarial medications at your institution?

The answers to these questions:

1) If the patient has severe malaria (regardless of pregnancy status or type of organism), first-line treatment is intravenous artesunate. After 24 hours and if the patient is able to take oral medications, artemisinin-based combination therapy (ACT) for 3 days.
2) If the patient is pregnant and malaria is uncomplicated, doxycycline is contraindicated. In uncomplicated malaria, artemisinin-based therapy is also not recommended in the first trimester but is recommended in the second and third trimesters.
3) When infections are uncomplicated, there are nuanced differences between the treatments of various malaria in different regions based on resistance patterns. Some regimens include:
   a. ACT 3-day regimen
   b. Atovaquone-proguanil for 3 days or
   c. Quinine with one of tetracycline/doxycycline/clindamycin for 7 days
   d. Uncomplicated *P. vivax/ovale/malariae*: chloroquine for 2 days
4) Alternate therapy for severe malaria includes intramuscular artemether injections or IV quinine infusions.

CLINICAL PEARL **USMLE STEP 1 AND 2**

Remember that *P. ovale and P. vivax* life cycles include hypnozoite forms, which can remain in the liver for months to years if untreated. Primaquine is required in the treatment of *P. ovale* and *P. vivax* because most other agents are only active for the erythrocytic stages of infection.

Hospital course

The Infectious Disease team wanted to treat this patient with artemisinin-based combination therapy (ACT), as per WHO recommendations. However, because of a lack of this medication at the institution, the patient was treated with an alternative combination of atovaquone-proguanil (Malarone). Three days later in the primary care clinic follow-up, the patient was functioning and mentating back to baseline.

What is the association with HIV and malaria?

HIV and malaria often coexist. Both induce cell-mediated immunodepression. Patients who have HIV with a CD4 count lower than 200 have a higher risk of contracting malaria. Patients with HIV and malaria will generally have lower CD4 counts than patients who have HIV without malaria, because malaria also plays a role in cell-mediated immunodepression. Acute infection with malaria is associated with a transient increase in HIV viral load, but it does not speed up progression to AIDS.

Case Summary

- **Complaint/History:** A 42-year-old male returning traveler from Uganda experiencing recurrent fevers, diaphoresis, poor appetite, and generalized weakness.
- **Findings:** Febrile with physical examination findings of scleral icterus, scattered petechiae of the extremities, conjunctival pallor, and palpable splenomegaly.
- **Lab Results/Tests:** Hemolytic anemia with thrombocytopenia. Peripheral Giemsa-stained blood smear with visualization of trophozoites consistent with malaria.

Diagnosis: *P. falciparum* malaria.

- **Treatments:** Atovaquone-proguanil therapy 1000 mg/400 mg for 3 days.

Bibliography

Arnold, D. M., & Cuker, A. (2020). Approach to the adult with unexplained thrombocytopenia. In T. Post (Ed.), *UpToDate*. Waltham, MA: UpToDate. www.uptodate.com.

Bomsztyk, M., & Arnold, R. W. (2013). Infections in travelers. *Medical Clinics of North America, 97*(4), 697–720.

Brodsky, R. A. (2020). Diagnosis of hemolytic anemia in the adult. In T. Post (Ed.), *UpToDate*. Waltham, MA: UpToDate. www.uptodate.com.

Franke, M. F., Spiegelman, D., Ezeamama, A., Aboud, S., Msamanga, G. I., Mehta, S., Fawzi, W. W. (2010). Malaria parasitemia and CD4 T cell count, viral load, and adverse HIV outcomes among HIV-infected pregnant women in Tanzania. *The American Journal of Tropical Medicine and Hygiene, 82*(4), 556–562.

Plewes, K., Leopold, S. J., Kingston, H. W., & Dondorp, A. M. (2019). Malaria. *Infectious Disease Clinics of North America, 33*(1), 39–60.

World Health Organization. (2014). Severe malaria. *TropMedInt Health, 19*(Suppl 1), 7–131.

A 19-Year-Old Female With Acute Abdominal Pain

Christopher Vo ■ Noah Wald-Dickler

A 19-year-old female with no medical history presents to the emergency department with acute abdominal pain. She reports that the pain began 1 day earlier in her right lower abdominal quadrant and describes the pain as persistent, severe, and sharp in nature. Shortly after the onset of pain, she developed a poor appetite, nausea, and vomiting. She denies any diarrhea, dysuria, or abnormal menses. She reports having her menstrual period about 10 days ago and reports being sexually active with one partner.

On physical examination, her temperature is 38.4°C, pulse rate is 115 beats/min, blood pressure is 110/60 mmHg, and oxygen saturation is 98% on room air. The patient appears to be in moderate acute distress. The cardiopulmonary examination is unremarkable. Her abdomen is firm with tenderness to palpation in the right lower quadrant (RLQ) and suprapubic region with guarding. Pelvic examination reveals no purulent discharge and no cervical wall motion tenderness or tenderness in her bilateral adnexa.

What is concerning about her physical examination?

This patient is displaying signs of an "acute abdomen," which refers to sudden and severe abdominal pain. It is often used synonymously with peritonitis, which manifests itself as rebound abdominal tenderness or abdominal rigidity. Patients who present in this fashion often require immediate surgical intervention.

What is your differential diagnosis?

The differential diagnosis for abdominal pain and intra-abdominal infections is broad and often guided by the anatomic location of pain. This includes appendicitis, acute mesenteric adenitis, cecal diverticulitis, viral gastroenteritis, inflammatory bowel disease flare, peptic ulcer disease, nephrolithiasis, cholecystitis, and urinary tract infection. In women, the following should be considered: pelvic inflammatory disease, ectopic pregnancy, ovarian torsion, tubo-ovarian abscesses, acute endometritis, and ruptured Graafian follicle (mittelschmerz). For men, the differential diagnoses should also include testicular torsion and epididymitis. All of these may present as a surgical emergency (Fig. 45.1).

CLINICAL PEARL **USMLE STEP 2**

The differential diagnosis for abdominal pain is extremely broad. Making the diagnosis can be difficult. In doing so, it is important to consider the location of the pain, the natural history, and to distinguish between anatomical differences between men and women.

How should you approach the workup of this patient?

All patients with abdominal pain should be triaged as either nonurgent or emergent, or in other words, nonsurgical or surgical. In this case, the patient's presentation is concerning for an acute

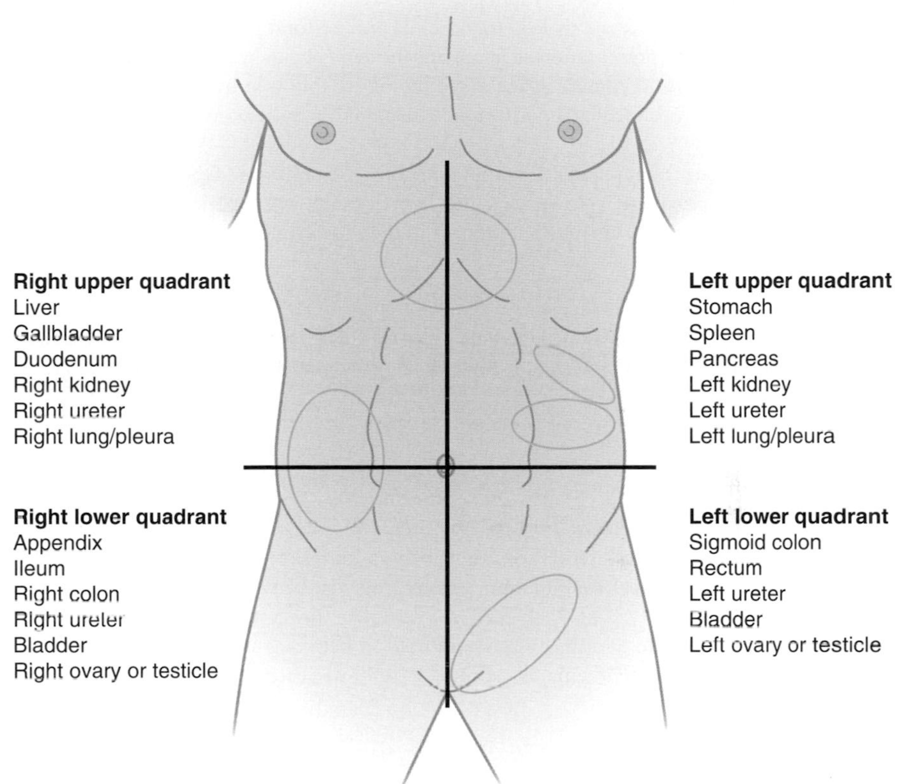

Fig. 45.1 Quadrants of abdomen. (From Townsend CM et al, Sabiston textbook of surgery, ed 21. Philadelphia, Elsevier, 2022.)

abdomen and requires an immediate surgical consult. Although the differential diagnosis for abdominal pain is expansive, the location of pain raises greater suspicion for acute appendicitis, right-sided nephrolithiasis, and any of the aforementioned syndromes that may be specific to female patients.

Basic routine laboratory tests should be started including a complete blood count (CBC) with a differential count, comprehensive metabolic panel (CMP), urinalysis, and a pregnancy test (where appropriate) to guide decision making. Imaging such as a CT abdomen can help differentiate between other abdominal pathologies, especially within an emergent setting or helping to triage a patient for surgery.

CLINICAL PEARL **USMLE STEP 2**

Patients with evidence of acute abdomen pain should be triaged appropriately and be considered for emergent surgery.

What is a typical presentation of appendicitis?

The development of appendicitis generally begins with luminal obstruction by a fecalith, lymphoid hyperplasia, or food matter. As a result of the obstruction, there is an increase in mucus secretion, venous and lymphatic congestion, and then eventual bacterial overgrowth and inflammation. If untreated, this process may lead to ischemia and perforation.

The classic history and presentation of acute appendicitis begins with vague pain in the periumbilical region, nausea, and vomiting. These symptoms are followed by localization of the pain in the RLQ associated with localized peritonitis. The patient may also present with fevers, chills, and anorexia.

Of note, the incidence of appendicitis is approximately 100 per 100,000 person-years in Europe and the Americas. Approximately 9% of men and 7% of women will experience an episode during their lifetime. Appendicitis occurs most commonly in the second and third decades of life.

CLINICAL PEARL **USMLE STEP 3**

Only approximately 50% of patients with acute appendicitis show the classic presentation of Murphy's triad with right lower abdominal pain (RLQ) with nausea, vomiting, and fever.

How do you diagnose appendicitis?

The diagnosis of acute appendicitis is frequently made on the basis of clinical history, physical findings, and laboratory data.

Patients with the classic presentation generally require only a thorough history and physical examination, a CBC with a differential count, urinalysis, and a pregnancy test (where appropriate) for diagnosis. On physical examination, patients may present with one of the findings in Table 45.1.

Historically, the Alvarado Scoring system was used to help diagnose appendicitis. A score of 7 or 8 indicates probable appendicitis. A score of 9 or 10 indicates a high probability for acute appendicitis (Table 45.2).

When patients present with an atypical history, physical examination, or laboratory findings, selective application of diagnostic imaging is indicated. In such a case, it is important to determine whether the atypical presentation is related to another disease process or to atypical positioning of the diseased appendix. The preferred imaging modality of choice for diagnosing appendicitis is CT imaging, which has a 95% accuracy in diagnosis, as well as ultrasonography, which may have greater sensitivity for gynecologic pathology, but is less sensitive for appendicitis. One may also consider clinical observation with serial physical exams and laboratory studies (Kasper et al., 1989; Baird et al., 2017) (Figs. 45.2 and 45.3).

TABLE 45.1 ■ **Different Physical Examination Findings Associated With Acute Appendicitis**

Physical Examination Maneuver	Physical Examination Finding
McBurney's sign	Point tenderness at the RLQ
Rovsing's sign	Pain in the RLQ with deep palpation of the LLQ
Psoas sign	RLQ pain with passive right hip extension that is associated with a retrocecal appendix
Obturator sign	RLQ pain elicited by the clinician flexing the patient's right hip and knee, followed by internal rotation of the hip, which is associated with a pelvic appendix

LLQ, Left lower quadrant; *RLQ*, right lower quadrant.

TABLE 45.2 ■ **Alvarado's Scoring System**

Signs	Points
Abdominal pain that migrates to the right lower quadrant	1
Anorexia	1
Nausea or vomiting	1
Tenderness to the right lower quadrant	1
Rebound tenderness	1
Fever of >37.3°C	1
Leukocytosis of >10,000/m^3	1
Neutrophilia (>75%)	1

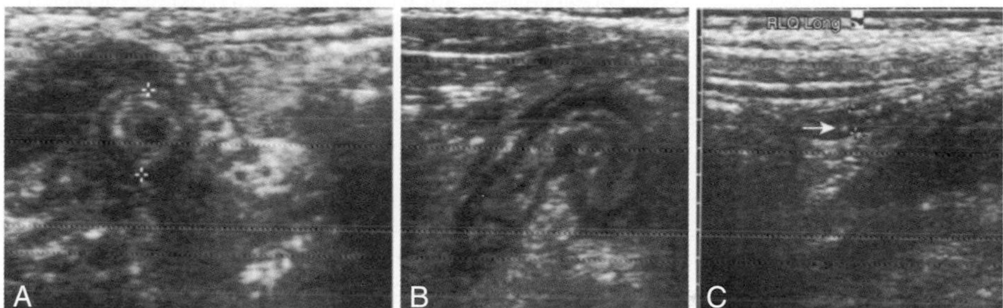

Fig. 45.2 Ultrasound examination of patients with appendicitis. (A) Transverse ultrasound scan of the appendix demonstrates the characteristic "target sign." In this case, the innermost portion is sonolucent, compatible with fluid or pus. (B) Longitudinal view of another patient demonstrates the alternating hyperechoic and hypoechoic layers with an outermost hypoechoic layer, suggesting periappendiceal fluid. (C) Longitudinal ultrasound scan of the right lower quadrant demonstrates a dilated, noncompressible appendix. The bright echo *(arrow)* within the appendix represents an appendicolith with acoustic shadowing. (From Kuhn, J. P., Slovis, T. L., & Haller, J.O. (2003). *Caffey's pediatric diagnostic imaging* (pp. 1684) (10th ed.). Philadelphia; Saunders/Elsevier.)

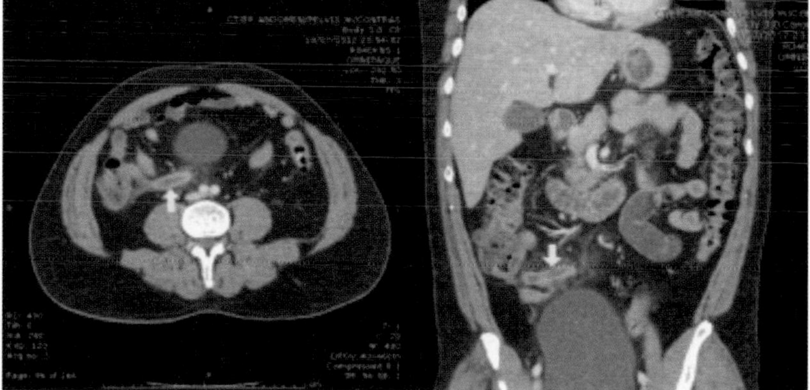

Fig. 45.3 Computed tomography scan images (axial and coronal sections) demonstrating a dilated appendix, with adjacent fat stranding, suggestive of acute appendicitis. *Arrows* on both images demonstrate a dilated appendix. (From Waldman, S. (2019). *Atlas of common pain syndromes* (pp. 306–310) (4th ed.). Elsevier.)

CLINICAL PEARL **USMLE STEP 2 AND 3**

The diagnosis of acute appendicitis can be made on the basis of clinical history, physical findings, and laboratory data. Imaging is helpful but not always necessary. Remember that pseudoappendicitis, an acute bacterial enteritis caused by *Yersinia enterocolitica*, mimics acute appendicitis clinically with surgical findings including ileal and periappendiceal inflammation but a generally normal-appearing appendix.

How do you treat appendicitis?

It should first be determined whether the patient's appendix is perforated. In patients with a perforated appendix, an appendectomy with possible percutaneous drainage should be performed without further delay. In stable patients without perforation, initial nonoperative management is indicated followed by eventual surgery within a reasonable time frame. Nonoperative management for all diagnoses of acute appendicitis includes intravenous antibiotics, electrolyte repletion, and fluids, such as lactated ringer solution. IV antibiotics are used as an adjunctive therapy to surgery.

The choice of antibiotics depends on the severity of the patient's presentation (Tables 45.3 and 45.4). Typically, antimicrobials are targeted at common causative agents such as the following enteric organisms: *Escherichia coli, Klebsiella, and Bacteroides*. Note that *Pseudomonas aeruginosa* is an exceedingly rare cause of community-acquired acute appendicitis. Inclusion of intravenous anti–pseudomonal active antibiotics where *Pseudomonas* is not a commonly implicated pathogen risks development of antibiotic resistance and adverse antibiotic events including *Clostridium difficile* colitis. Avoidance of agents active for methicillin-resistant *Staphylococcus aureus* and *Pseudomonas* is a cornerstone of effective antimicrobial stewardship (Solomon et al., 2010). Although enterococcal species are part of normal enteric flora, empiric enterococcal-directed therapy (e.g., vancomycin or linezolid) is not routinely required in otherwise clinically stable patients.

According to the Infectious Diseases Society of America practice guidelines, acute appendicitis without evidence of perforation, abscess, or local peritonitis requires only administration of narrow spectrum antibiotic regimens active against aerobic and facultative and obligate anaerobes.

TABLE 45.3 ■ **Infectious Diseases Society of America (IDSA) Practice Guidelines Recommended Antibiotics for Community-Acquired Infections in Pediatric Patients**

Regimen	Community-Acquired Infection in Pediatric Patients
Combination	Ceftriaxone or cefotaxime, each in combination with metronidazole

TABLE 45.4 ■ **Infectious Diseases Society of America (IDSA) Practice Guidelines Recommended Antibiotics for Community-Acquired Infections in Adult Patients**

	Community-Acquired Infection in Adults	
Regimen	Mild-to-moderate severity: perforated or abscessed appendicitis and other infections of mild-to-moderate severity	High risk or severity: severe physiologic disturbance, advanced age, or immunocompromised state
Single	Cefoxitin, moxifloxacin	N/A
Combination	Cefazolin, cefuroxime, ceftriaxone, cefotaxime, ciprofloxacin, or levofloxacin, each in combination with metronidazole	Ciprofloxacin or levofloxacin, each in combination with metronidazole

Most patients should ultimately undergo curative treatment for appendicitis with appendectomy as a source of definitive source control. The procedure can be performed either by an open approach or laparoscopic approach. Laparoscopic appendectomy is associated with less postoperative pain and improved recovery, but it is more costly than the open approach. Antibiotic therapy may generally be discontinued within 4 days of surgical source control. For noncomplicated cases, postoperative antibiotics are generally unnecessary and not recommended (see Tables 45.3 and 45.4).

CLINICAL PEARL **USMLE STEP 3**

Source control is essential in acute appendicitis. Regardless of severity, all patients should proceed to appendectomy.

What happens next?

Our 19-year-old female patient was revealed to have a WBC of >16,000/m^3. The patient's pregnancy test was negative. CT imaging of the abdomen indicated edema and inflammation of the appendix without perforation. The patient's clinical history, exam, laboratory, and imaging findings were sufficient to establish a diagnosis of acute appendicitis. She was started on intravenous cefoxitin and intravenous fluids, treated symptomatically for pain and nausea, and was scheduled for laparoscopic appendectomy within the next 24 hours. The patient's surgery was uncomplicated and she was discharged home within the next day.

Case Summary

- **Complaint/History:** A 19-year-old female with acute onset abdominal pain, nausea, and vomiting.
- **Findings:** Febrile with RLQ abdominal tenderness with guarding. Unremarkable pelvic examination.
- **Lab Results/Tests:** Leukocytosis with 16,000 cell/m^3 white blood count. Negative pregnancy test. Abdominal imaging indicating of an edematous appendix without perforation.

Diagnosis: Uncomplicated acute appendicitis.

- **Treatments:** Intravenous cefoxitin, antiemetics, analgesics, and surgical consult for laparoscopic appendectomy.

Bibliography

Alvarado, A. (1986). A practical score for the early diagnosis of acute appendicitis. *Annals of Emergency Medicine*, *15*(5), 557–564. https://doi.org/10.1016/s0196-0644(86)80993-3.

Baird, D. L. H., Simillis, C., Kontovounisios, C., Rasheed, S., & Tekkis, P. P. (2017). Acute appendicitis. *British Medical Journal*, *357*, j1703. doi: 10.1136/bmj.j1703. PMID: 28424152.

Jacobs, D. O. (2018). Acute appendicitis and peritonitis. In J. Jameson, A. S. Fauci, D. L. Kasper, S. L. Hauser, D. L. Longo, & J. Loscalzo (Eds.), *Harrison's principles of internal medicine*, 20th ed. McGraw Hill.

Kasper, D. L., Hauser, S. L., Jameson, J. L., Fauci, A. S., Longo, D. L., & Loscalzo, J. (2015). Acute appendicitis and peritonitis. In D. Jacobs (Ed.), *Harrison's principles of internal medicine* (19th ed., pp. 1985–1989). New York: McGraw Hill Education.

Solomkin, J. S., Mazuski, J. E., Bradley, J. S., Rodvold, K. A., Goldstein, E. J., Barron, E. J., O'Neill, P. J., Chow, A. W., Dellinger, E. P., Eachempati, S. R., Gorbach, S., Hilfiker, M., May, A. K., Nathens, A. B., Sawyer, R. G., & Bartlett, J. G. (2010). Diagnosis and management of complicated intra-abdominal infection in adults and children: Guidelines by the Surgical Infection Society and the Infectious Diseases Society of America. *Clinical Infectious Diseases*, *50*(2), 133–164. https://doi.org/10.1086/649554.

CASE 46

A 30-Year-Old Male With Shortness of Breath, Fatigue, and Weight Loss

Tyler Degener ■ Jean Gibb

A 30-year-old male presents to the emergency room with shortness of breath, fatigue, and weight loss. The patient states he first noticed his pants feeling loose about 2 months ago. This was associated with a decreased appetite and an unintentional 15-lb weight loss. His shortness of breath started 2 weeks prior to presentation; he characterizes it as constant, worsening over several weeks, and now present even at rest. He feels he has been more tired than normal during the day, but attributes this to sleeping less because of coughing episodes throughout the night. On further review of systems, he admits to intermittent subjective fevers and white phlegm with scant amounts of red blood.

How can the differential diagnosis be narrowed for a patient presenting with progressive weight loss and fever?

The primary categories of disease to consider with the constellation of fatigue, fever, and night sweats are infectious, rheumatologic, and oncologic, keeping in mind that more than one condition may be present. The collective symptoms of fever, unintentional weight loss, and night sweats are referred to as B symptoms, most traditionally used to describe disease stages of lymphoma. However, there are many infectious diseases, rheumatologic conditions, and malignancies that present this way (see Table 46.1).

Infectious diseases that lead to chronic fever and weight loss (generally considered to be greater than 2 weeks of symptoms) are the result of indolent pathogens. This clinical syndrome has historically been described as consumptive disease; the most classic example is infection with *Mycobacterium tuberculosis* (MTB). Other chronic infections that can lead to unintentional weight loss include infection with endemic fungal organisms such as coccidioidomycosis, histoplasmosis, and blastomycosis, as well as bacterial vector-borne and zoonotic pathogens.

Rheumatologic and autoimmune causes of unintentional weight loss and fever include inflammatory bowel disease and vasculitis that may affect the lungs, skin, kidneys, and gastrointestinal (GI) tract. A family history and thorough review of symptoms with a focus on sinopulmonary, gastrointestinal, and musculoskeletal symptoms can help decide on the likelihood of these etiologies.

Hematologic and oncologic malignancies may come to medical attention with nonspecific complaints of fatigue, night sweats, fever, and weight loss. Leukemia, lymphoma, aplastic anemia, multiple myeloma, and solid tumors are included in this differential. The likelihood of each can often be based on the age of the patient.

This list is not exhaustive. The differential diagnosis of fever and unintentional weight loss is broad; a thorough review of symptoms, family history, and epidemiologic risk factors will focus the approach.

TABLE 46.1 ■ **Differential Diagnosis of B Symptoms: Example Etiologies**

	Pathology	History	Social or Family History
Infectious	*Mycobacterium tuberculosis*	Prominent cough ± hemoptysis, night sweats	Birthplace in an endemic country, household MTB contact
	Endemic fungal infections	Cough, chronic headache, oligoarthritis, skin lesions	Birthplace and travel history to endemic regions
	Human immunodeficiency virus		History of intravenous drug use or high-risk sexual contacts
Rheumatologic/ autoimmune	Granulomatous polyangiitis	Frequent sinus infections, hematuria, hemoptysis, history of purpuric rash	
	Rheumatoid disease	Symmetric arthralgia	Family history of rheumatoid disease or arthritis symptoms
	Sarcoidosis		
	Inflammatory bowel disease	History of chronic abdominal pain, hematochezia, mouth or perianal lesions	Family history of inflammatory bowel disease
Hematologic	Leukemia	Easy bruising/bleeding	Family history of leukemia or lymphoma
	Lymphoma	Palpable lymphadenopathy	
	Multiple myeloma	Age >50 years	

CLINICAL PEARL **STEP 1**

Risk of disease with endemic fungi is largely based on the geography of long-term residence. *Coccidioides immitis* and *Coccidioides posadasii*, the agents of coccidioidomycosis or "valley fever," are endemic in the southwest of the United States and the western half of Texas. *Histoplasma* is present on every continent but within the United States it is concentrated in the Midwest and the Ohio River Valley. Blastomyces is endemic in the northeast of the United States and the eastern half of Canada. Multiple variants of *Histoplasma* are present in Central and South America and Africa. *Penicillium* is endemic in Thailand and its neighboring countries.

How can the review of systems be structured to help narrow the differential diagnosis?

When approaching a patient with chronic, nonspecific symptoms as described, the review of systems is important to identify localized complaints. Chronic infectious and rheumatologic syndromes often involve two or three primary symptoms or organ systems. Recognizing these patterns narrows the differential diagnosis from the initial broad categories of disease.

The patient reports that his cough has been relentless for the past few weeks. He has had loose, nonbloody stool three to five times daily for the past 2 months. He has no joint pain and has not noticed any easy bruising or bleeding. He reports no headaches, difficulty or pain with urination, rash, or skin lesions.

Vital signs include a temperature of 38.4°C (101.1 °F), heart rate 110 beats/min, blood pressure 122/85 mmHg, and respiratory rate 20 breaths/min. Oxygen saturation is 90% on room air and 97% on 2 L/min of supplemental O_2. Physical examination is significant for a thin, malnourished man at 114 lb (52 kg); BMI is 17. The patient has white mucocutaneous patches in the mouth and on the tongue, bilateral rales on auscultation of the lungs, and a napkin at bedside with white phlegm and a single streak of blood.

What important parts of this history and examination identify key differential diagnoses for his cough?

This patient has evidence of a lower respiratory tract infection (LRTI) with fever, cough, and hypoxia. The additional examination findings of oral thrush and cachexia raise suspicion of an underlying disease process that has precipitated a state of immune suppression; this broadens the differential of pneumonia pathogens to include opportunistic pathogens that take advantage of hosts with compromised immune systems.

Thrush is overgrowth of yeast (*Candida*) species on oropharyngeal mucous membranes. In the setting of severe immune suppression, *Candida* overgrowth can extend into the esophagus to cause esophageal candidiasis, which can present with nausea, vomiting, and odynophagia (Figs. 46.1 and 46.2).

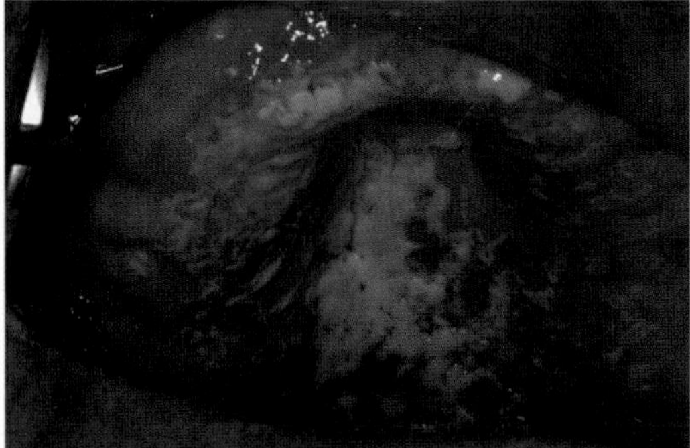

Fig 46.1 Thrush (overgrowth of yeast species on the hard palate; may also be seen on the tongue, uvula, and intra-oral mucous membranes). (From Huber, M.A., Tantiwongkosi, B. (2014). Oral and oropharyngeal cancer. *Medical Clinics of North America, 98*(6), 1299–1321, Figure 18).

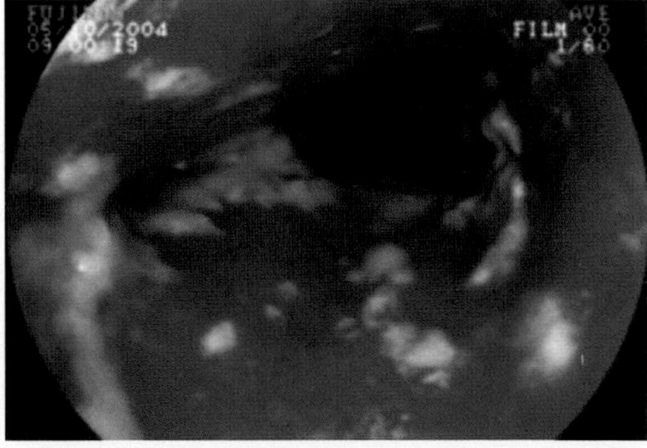

Fig 46.2 Esophageal candidiasis on endoscopy. (Courtesy Rembacken, B. (2022). In F. Ferri (Ed.), *Ferri's clinical advisor 2022*. Elsevier.) Candidiasis, Cutaneous. Philadelphia.

CLINICAL PEARL **STEP 2/3**

Thrush may occur in an immune competent host simply by way of altered normal oropharyngeal flora with systemic antibacterial agents, or by administering systemic glucocorticoids. In immune compromised hosts, thrush can occur more frequently, with greater severity, and progress to involve the esophagus.

A chest X-ray examination and basic lab tests are performed:

Leukocyte count 12,000/μL (75% neutrophils, 16% lymphocytes, 8% monocytes)
Hemoglobin 12.5 g/dL
Platelets 175/μL
Sodium 137 mEq/L
Potassium 3.8 mEq/L
Chloride 102 mmol/L
Bicarbonate 20 mmol/L
BUN 20 mg/dL
Creatinine 0.7 mg/dL
Liver function tests are within normal limits.

The chest X-ray image shows bilateral, diffuse interstitial infiltrates without any discrete consolidation, mass, cavitation, or pleural effusions. Laboratory studies indicate a mild leukocytosis with noted lymphopenia (Fig. 46.3).

The absence of discrete lobar consolidations makes a typical bacterial pneumonia less likely.

The emergency room triage staff is concerned because of the presence of blood in the sputum and asks about the appropriateness of isolation and evaluation for pulmonary tuberculosis.

Which features of a chest X-ray examination would raise suspicion of communicable MTB?

Active pulmonary tuberculosis can present with fever and hemoptysis. In cases of advanced disease, cavitary lesions may be visible on chest radiographs. However, up to 60% of patients

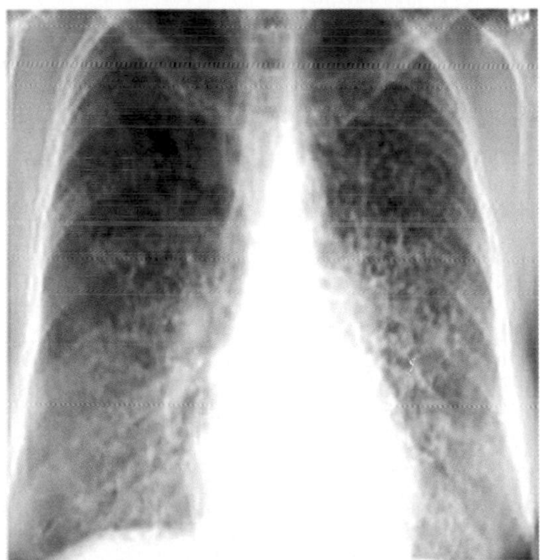

Fig 46.3 Chest radiography. (From Arze, S., Arze, L., & Abecia, C. (2016). Post-transplantation infections in Bolivia. *Transplantation Proceedings*, *48*,(2), 646–653.)

with communicable pulmonary tuberculosis may not have cavitary lesions. In immunocompromised hosts (and especially in the context of HIV coinfection) the chest radiograph pattern of infiltration can be diffuse or sometimes appear "miliary" in its pattern. The miliary pattern reflects hematogenous dissemination of MTB organisms throughout the lung parenchyma.

A detailed social history is required to evaluate for risk factors that heighten the suspicion of tuberculosis.

CLINICAL PEARL **STEP 2/3**

Classic epidemiologic risk factors for tuberculosis **exposure** include the following:

- Birthplace in an area with endemic tuberculosis
- A known household contact with someone with communicable tuberculosis (recent or in the past)
- Exposure to high-risk environments or populations such as healthcare facilities, jails, or homeless persons

Risk factors for tuberculosis **reactivation** include:

- Acquired immunosuppression: HIV infection, new onset diabetes mellitus, autoimmune disease, malnutrition
- Iatrogenic immunosuppression: long-term glucocorticoid use, solid organ transplant, bone marrow transplant, tumor necrosis factor alpha (TNF-alpha) inhibitors, other immunosuppressive therapies

The patient tells you he was born in New York City and has lived in the states of New York, New Jersey, and Georgia. He has never lived outside the United States. He is unsure if he has ever had an HIV test. His sexual partners are identified as men only; he engages in oral and anal receptive and penetrative intercourse. He estimates 10–12 partners in the past 6 months and more than 25 lifetime partners. He tells you he traded sex for money on one occasion. He estimates condom use about 50% of the time.

How will you evaluate the risk of HIV disease?

Everyone who is sexually active is at risk for HIV exposure. Taking a sexual history helps to assess individual risk. Aside from sexual transmission, the other main risk factor HIV acquisition is intravenous drug use. In terms of sexual exposure, not all sexual contacts carry equal risk. Anal intercourse is higher risk for HIV transmission in comparison to vaginal intercourse, with highest risk in receptive partners compared to penetrative partners. Oral sex is a relatively inefficient mode of HIV transmission, but higher risk when there are oral mucous membrane or cutaneous disruptions in the receptive partner. Other components in the sexual history that increase risk for HIV exposure is contact with multiple partners in a single encounter, condomless sexual contact with partners who work in the sex industry, and trading sex for money.

The patient is admitted to the hospital for closer monitoring, further diagnostic workup, and treatment. Because of the concern for pulmonary tuberculosis, he is placed in isolation and a workup for communicable tuberculosis is initiated. The HIV antibody test results positive.

CLINICAL PEARL **STEP 1**

There are three ways to detect evidence of HIV infection. The first detectable evidence of HIV following an exposure is HIV RNA in blood, detectable as soon as 7 days after exposure. The p24 antigen, a surface protein on the HIV virus, is detectable 10–14 days after exposure.

Antibodies are detectable about 3 weeks after exposure. The fourth generation HIV test combines the p24 and the antibody and is useful about 14 days after exposure. Testing for HIV that occurs <14 days from a potential exposure should be done with an HIV RNA polymerase chain reaction (PCR). This time course is highlighted in Fig. 46.4.

Now that you know the patient's HIV status, which pulmonary pathogens are added to your differential diagnosis?

Patients living with uncontrolled HIV are at risk of community-acquired pneumonia (CAP) (most often caused by *Streptococcus pneumoniae, Haemophilus influenzae, Moraxella* species, and atypical organisms such as *Mycoplasma* and *Chlamydia pneumophilia*) in addition to fungal and viral opportunistic pathogens. Fungal pneumonia with *Pneumocystis jiroveci* pneumonia (PJP) and *Cryptococcus* are of great concern in this patient who has lived primarily in urban settings; his environmental exposure to *Coccidioides, Histoplasma*, and *Blastomyces* is limited.

A note on seasonality: depending on the season, common viral respiratory infections are also to be considered. In general, testing for respiratory viruses is indicated when interventions can be made to treat it. This applies most to influenza and COVID-19, for which treatment with oseltamivir and dexamethasone, respectively, can be initiated. In the United States the flu season is December to March.

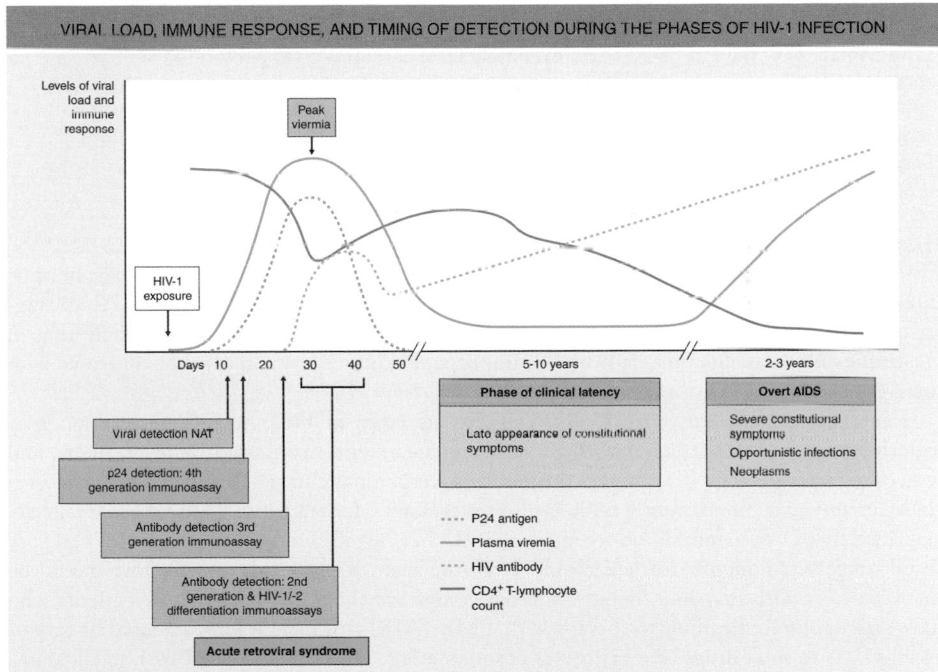

Fig 46.4 HIV diagnostics: detectable p24, viremia, and HIV antibodies over time. (From Chan, R.K.W., Chio, M.T.W., & Koh, H.Y. (2018). Dermatology. Elsevier. Philadelphia. Fourth edition. pp 1364–1382. Adapted from Bart PA, Pantaleo G. (2004). The immunopathogenesis of HIV-1 infection. In Cohen J, Powderly WG, *Infectious diseases*. Edinburgh: Mosby, 1236.)

While undergoing evaluation for pulmonary tuberculosis, antibiotics are started with a macrolide and third generation cephalosporin to treat community-acquired pneumonia. Several hours later the patient requires 4 L/min of supplemental oxygen. He continues to have tachypnea. The results of laboratory studies indicate a procalcitonin within normal limits, indicating that typical bacterial pneumonia is less likely.

How will you evaluate this patient for fungal pneumonia?

The risk of opportunistic infection in patients living with HIV is assessed based on the CD4 T-cell count and the HIV viral load. The risk of PJP escalates dramatically when the CD4 count is below 200 cells/mm^3. However, PJP can occur at any T-cell count in the setting of uncontrolled HIV viremia. The diagnosis of PJP is made with a combination of the patient's viral load, CD4 count, chest X-ray findings, and direct testing of the sputum. Sputum testing across all testing methods has higher sensitivity when obtained via bronchoscopy rather than expectorated sputum.

The two most commonly used laboratory tests for PJP are the PJP direct fluorescence antibody (DFA) and the PJP nucleic acid amplification test (NAAT). Both can be done on expectorated sputum and from bronchoalveolar lavage (BAL); sensitivity is higher on samples collected by BAL.

You order a T-cell count for your patient, the results of which will take several days. The pulmonary MTB evaluation results with three negative acid-fast sputum smears and two negative MTB PCRs from expectorated sputum. Your suspicion of PJP is increasing.

CLINICAL PEARL **STEP 2/3**

The sensitivity of the PJP DFA is approximately 60% and 80% on expectorated sputum and BAL specimens, respectively. The sensitivity of expectorated sputum varies widely with the quality of the sputum collected; specimens contaminated with saliva or oropharyngeal squamous cells are lower yield. The sensitivity of the PJP NAAT is 80%–90% and >90% on expectorated sputum and BAL specimens, respectively.

What are the treatment options for PJP?

First-line therapy for PJP is trimethoprim-sulfamethoxazole (TMP-SMX). Dosing must be optimized for effective therapy; the standard total daily dose is 15–20 mg/kg of TMP and 75–100 mg/kg of SMX in dividend dose every eight hours. Standard therapy is 21 days. Monitoring of creatinine and potassium on a daily basis is important; kidney injury can often be mitigated with intravenous fluids (IVFs).

First-line and alternative treatment regimens are given in Table 46.2. Some patients may experience a clinical worsening with initiation of treatment, manifested by fever, rigors, and worsening gas exchange. To mitigate this reaction, certain patients will benefit from corticosteroid therapy given concurrently with antibiotic therapy. Moderate and severe disease is characterized by pO_2 <70 mmHg on room air or PAO_2–PaO_2≥35mmHg. Patients in this category should receive adjunctive corticosteroids. It is important to note that every effort should be made to treat with first-line therapy; alternative options should be reserved for patients who have strict contraindications to therapy with TMP-SMX. This includes documented history of anaphylaxis to sulfa drugs or a history of desquamating skin rash associated with medications of the same class.

TABLE 46.2 ■ **Treatment Options for Pneumocystis jiroveci Pneumonia**

PCP Treatment Regimen	Dose	Potential Toxicity
Mild to Moderate Disease		
First line: TMP-SMX	15–20 mg/kg TMP and 75–100 mg/kg SMX divided q8hrs	Toxicity: leukopenia, hyperkalemia, rash, Stevens-Johnson syndrome
Alternative: dapsone + TMP	Dapsone 100 mg daily + TMP 15 mg/kg divided q8hrs	Toxicity: leukopenia, hyperkalemia, hemolysis (with G6PD deficiency)
Alternative: primaquine + clindamycin	Primaquine 30 mg PO daily + clindamycin 450 mg PO q6hrs or clindamycin 600 mg PO q8hrs	Toxicities: anemia (hemolytic anemia in G6PD deficiency), rash, diarrhea
Alternative: atovaquone	Atovaquone 750 mg PO BID	Hepatocellular liver function test abnormalities
Severe Disease		
First line: TMP-SMX	15–20 mg/kg TMP and 75–100 mg/kg SMX divided q8hrs	
Alternative: pentamidine	Pentamidine 4 mg/kg IV once daily	Toxicity: hemolysis, pancreatitis, leukopenia, cardiac arrhythmia
Alternative: primaquine + clindamycin	Primaquine 30 mg PO daily + clindamycin 600 mg PO q6hrs OR clindamycin 900 mg PO q8hrs	

BID, Twice a day; *PO*, by mouth; *TMP-SMX*, trimethoprim-sulfamethoxazole.

CLINICAL PEARL **STEP 1/2/3**

Corticosteroids improve survival in patients with HIV and PCP pneumonia with room air PO_2 <70 mmHg or PAO_2–PaO_2≥35 mmHg. Steroids should be initiated concurrently with antibiotic therapy. Typical dosing starts at 40 mg prednisone BID (about 0.5 mg/kg BID) and tapers over the 21-day course of therapy.

When can antiretroviral therapy (ART) be safely initiated in a patient with a new diagnosis of HIV?

With new HIV diagnoses it is generally preferred to start ART as soon as possible. For patients with CD4 200 and above, this uncommonly precipitates complications. Complications of ART initiation occur when the patient develops immune reconstitution inflammatory syndrome (IRIS), a clinical syndrome wherein recovery of immune function precipitates worsening symptoms related to a previously asymptomatic or paucisymptomatic infection. The severity of the IRIS syndrome is often inversely related to the rate of recovery in the CD4 count. In specific cases, delaying ART initiation is beneficial. The two best examples of this are in the setting of cryptococcal meningitis and MTB meningitis. In these conditions, intracranial inflammation precipitated by IRIS can be devastating and difficult to manage once it has started.

All patients with CD4<100 should be evaluated by an ophthalmologist for cytomegalovirus (CMV) retinitis before initiation with ART. CMV retinitis IRIS can lead to permanent vision loss and if CMV retinitis is present, it should be treated ideally before, but at minimum concurrently, with initiation of ART. Additionally, screening with a serum cryptococcal antigen is an excellent test screening for cryptococcal meningitis. Sensitivity is generally considered >95%. In PJP patients should start ART within 14 days of the diagnosis, provided there are no prohibitive coinfections.

The CD4 count is 85 and the viral load is 900,000 copies/mL. The cryptococcal serum antigen is negative. Over the next 3–4 days, the patient's oxygen requirements gradually decrease. He is evaluated by an ophthalmologist, who finds no evidence of CMV retinitis. After a discussion with the patient, he is interested in starting ART.

CLINICAL PEARL **STEP 1**

PJP prophylaxis is indicated for all patients with uncontrolled viremia and a CD4 count <200 or a CD4 percentage of <14%. Prophylaxis should be continued until the CD4 is >200 and CD4% > 14% for 3 months or when the CD4 is >100 and the viral load is suppressed for 3–6 months.

Case Summary

- **Complaint/History:** A 30-year-old male with shortness of breath, fatigue, and weight loss.
- **Findings:** Physical examination is notable for fever, tachycardia, and hypoxia. The patient is thin and has white patches in the mouth and on the tongue and diffuse pulmonary rales.
- **Lab Results/Tests:** Complete blood count reveals lymphopenia and chest x-ray produces evidence of diffuse, bilateral, interstitial infiltrate without discrete consolidation or pleural effusion. The HIV antibody test results positive.

Diagnosis: Acquired immunodeficiency syndrome secondary to human immunodeficiency virus with Pneumocystis jirovecii pneumonia.

- **Treatment:** TMP-SMX and anti-retroviral therapy.

Bibliography

Aberg, J.A., Gallant, J.E., Ghanem, K.G., Emmanuel, P., Zingman, B.S., & Horberg, M.A. (2014). Primary care guidelines for the management of persons infected with HIV: 2013 update by the HIV medicine association of the Infectious Diseases Society of America. *Clinical Infectious Diseases*, *58*, 1.

Huang, L., Cattamanchi, A., Davis, J.D., den Boon, S., Kovacs, J., Meshnick, S., Miller, Robert F., Walzer, P.D., Worodria, W., & Masur, H. (2011). International HIV-associated Opportunistic Pneumonias (IHOP) Study, Lung HIV Study. *Proceedings of the American Thoracic Society*, *8*, 3.

Lewinsohn, D.M., Leonard, M.K., LoBue, P.A., Cohn, D.L., Daley, C.L., Desmond, E., Keane, J., Lewinsohn, D.A., Loeffler, A.M., Mazurek, G.H., O'Brien, R.J., Pai, M., Richeldi, L., Salfinger, M., Shinnick, T.M., Sterling, T.R., Warshauer, D.M., & Woods, G.L. (2017). Official American Thoracic Society/Infectious Diseases Society of America/Centers for Disease Control and Prevention Clinical Practice Guidelines: Diagnosis of tuberculosis in adults and children. *Clinical Infectious Diseases*, *64,2*(15), e1–e33.

Mandell, L.A., Wunderink, R.G., Anzueto, A., Bartlett, J.G., Campbell, G.D., Dean, N.C., Dowell, S.F., File, T.M. Jr., Musher, D.M., Niederman, M.S., Torres, A., Whitney, C.G. (2007). Infectious Diseases Society of America/American Thoracic Society consensus guidelines on the management of community-acquired pneumonia in adults. *Clinical Infectious Diseases*, *1*, 44.

Panel on Antiretroviral Guidelines for Adults and Adolescents. *Guidelines for the Use of Antiretroviral Agents in Adults and Adolescents with HIV*. Department of Health and Human Services. Available at https://clinicalinfo.hiv.gov/en/guidelines/adult-and-adolescent-arv. Accessed January 28 2022.

Ramirez, J.A., Wiemken, T.L., Peyrani, P., Arnold, F.W., Kelley, R., Mattingly, W.A., Nakamatsu, R., Pena, S., Guinn, B.E., Furmanek, S.P., Persaud, A.K., Raghuram, A., Fernandez, F., Beavin, L., Bosson, R., Fernandez-Botron, R., Cavallazzi, R., Bordon, J., Valdivieso, & Carrico, R.M. (2017). Adults hospitalized with pneumonia in the United States: incidence, epidemiology, and mortality. *Clinical Infectious Diseases*, *13*(11), 65.

U.S. Department of Health and Human Services. HIV treatment: HIV and immunizations. AIDSinfo.nih.gov. 2019.

SECTION 10

Hepatology

CASE 47

A 60-Year-Old Female With Elevated Alkaline Phosphatase and Hypercalcemia

Ashwini Mulgaonkar ■ Liyun Yuan

A 60-year-old female with a history of type 2 diabetes mellitus, hypothyroidism, and hypercalcemia complicated by recurrent nephrolithiasis and recurrent urinary tract infections presents to the emergency department from her urology appointment with a blood pressure of 80/34 mmHg. Over the past few months, she has also experienced a 60 lb weight loss, shortness of breath, and generalized fatigue. She was admitted to the hospital where her lab tests were notable for hypercalcemia (16.6 mg/dL), elevated alkaline phosphatase (305 U/L), aspartate aminotransferase (52 U/L), alanine aminotransferase (24 U/L), and total bilirubin (0.8 mg/dL).

How should abnormal liver tests be evaluated?

There are three main patterns of liver enzymes that can help to refine the differential diagnosis: cholestatic, hepatocellular, and mixed picture.

In cholestatic liver disease, the primary lab test abnormalities are an elevated serum bilirubin (BR) and alkaline phosphatase (ALP), with proportionally lower elevations of the aminotransferase levels. ALP is a zinc metalloproteinase enzyme that is produced in five different organs: liver, kidney, bone, intestine (ileal mucosa), and placenta. Therefore, it is important to know that elevations in ALP can also occur in normal physiologic states, such as pregnancy. Within the liver, ALP is found in hepatocytes bound to the canalicular membrane. In cholestatic liver injury, the bile ducts are the main location of damage, which stimulate the hepatocytes to synthesize increased levels of ALP. Gamma glutamyl transpeptidase (GGT) is an enzyme in the tissue of liver, biliary tract, pancreas, brain, and heart. Therefore, a rise in in ALP with a concurrent rise in GGT is indicative of liver injury and primarily differentiates from a bone source. (Schreiner & Rockey, 2018; Woreta & Alqahtani, 2014).

In hepatocellular liver disease, the primary lab test abnormalities are an elevation in aminotransferase levels (aspartate aminotransferase, AS; alanine transaminase, ALT) greater than the elevation of ALP and BR. Levels of aminotransferases greater than 1000 IU/L are indicative of extensive hepatocellular injury extensive hepatocellular injury, commonly drug-induced injury, acute ischemic injury, or acute viral hepatitis. Aminotransferases are intracellular enzymes released following cell damage. ALT is produced primarily in the liver, making it a much more specific liver damage marker compared with AST, which is also produced in skeletal muscle and cardiomyocytes (Schreiner & Rockey, 2018; Woreta & Alqahtani, 2014).

Mixed-picture liver disease is a combination of cholestatic injury and hepatocellular injury usually with elevations of ALP, BR, AST, and ALT in similar proportions.

The liver injury pattern can be better characterized by the R-factor. It is a ratio of AST to ALP, which is normalized to the upper limit of normal (ULN) of each.

CLINICAL PEARL **STEP 1**

Identification of the pattern of liver injury (hepatocellular injury versus cholestatic injury) helps narrow the causes and differential diagnoses.

How should a differentiation be made between the main diagnoses in cholestatic injury via their clinical and biochemical profiles?

Cholestatic liver injury can be caused by several disease processes. Etiologies of cholestatic liver disease include primary biliary cholangitis (PBC), primary sclerosing cholangitis (PSC), drug-induced liver injury, biliary obstruction (biliary stones, strictures, cholangiocarcinoma and pancreatic cancers), hepatic infiltrative disease including hepatic sarcoidosis, tuberculosis (MTB), amyloidosis, and malignancy. Imaging is an important tool to help guide the differential. The presence of biliary ductal dilation on imaging suggests biliary obstruction and further imaging evaluation (Woreta & Alqahtani, 2014). A list of etiologies for cholestatic liver disease and associated clinical and diagnostic factors are shown in (Table 47.2).

How should a differentiation be made between the main diagnoses in hepatocellular injury via their clinical and biochemical profiles?

The approach to evaluate a patient with hepatocellular liver injury relies essentially on biochemical markers and history (Table 47.3).

TABLE 47.1 ■ **R-Factor Chart**

	R-Factor
Cholestatic injury	<2
Mixed injury	2–5
Hepatocellular injury	>5

TABLE 47.2 ■ **Differential Diagnosis of Cholestatic Liver Injury**

	Presentation	Diagnosis
PBC	• Women age 40 • Pruritis, jaundice, fatigue • Occasionally concomitant Sjögren's, vasculitis, and Raynaud's	• Biopsy is diagnostic: florid bile duct destruction • Serum: antimitochondrial antibody
PSC	• Fever, pruritis, jaundice • May have ulcerative coatis	• MRCP/ERCP: bead-string appearance (extrahepatic stricture) • Biopsy not indicated
Billary obstruction	• Cholangitis, pruritis, jaundice, abdominal pain	• MRCP: stricture, stones, mass • Biopsy not indicated
Infiltrative: TB, sarcold, amyloidosis, malignancy	• B symptoms: fever, night sweats, weight loss • Clinical history of TB, sarcoid, amyloid	• CT/MRCP: hepatomegaly, lymphadenopathy • Biopsy and staining are diagnostic

CT, Computed tomography; *ERCP*, endoscopic retrograde cholangiopancreatography; *MRCP*, magnetic resonance cholangiopancreatography; *TB*, tuberculosis.

TABLE 47.3 ■ **Differential Diagnoses of Hepatocellular Liver Injury**

Acute viral hepatitis: Hep A–E, HSV, CMV, VZV	• Recent exposure • ALT>1000 (ALT>AST) • Viral serologies
Drugs: Acetaminophen, Halothane, Minocycline, Isoniazid	• Temporal relation of ingestion or drug exposure (within weeks to 3 months) • For Tylenol toxicity, ALT could be >500 IU/L to 10,0001 U/L • Improvement after discontinuation of drugs
Ischemic injury	• Sepsis, hypotensive shock • AST>ALT, AST>500 IU/L • Rapid recovery within days with supportive care
Autoimmune hepatitis	• Women > men, presence of other autoimmune disorders • Positive serum autoimmune markers: antinuclear antibody (ANA), antismooth muscle antibody, IgG • Liver histology with characteristic portal/periportal predominance of necroinflammatory lesions with rosetting of hepatocytes in the area of interface hepatitis

ALT, Alanine transaminase; *AST*, aspartate aminotransferase.

Abdominal ultrasound was notable for a nodular liver. Computed tomography (CT) scan of the chest and abdomen revealed diffuse mediastinal lymphadenopathy and radiographic findings consistent with cirrhosis. A positron emission tomography (PET) scan showed hypermetabolism of the cardiophrenic and supraclavicular lymph nodes as well as within the spleen.

R value: 0.4, indicating cholestatic liver injury.

Further workup included negative infectious workup (viral serologies, MTB) and negative autoimmune workup (antineutrophil cytoplasmic antibody, antinuclear antibody, and antimitochondrial antibody AMA).

A percutaneous liver biopsy was performed, which confirmed the presence of nonnecrotizing granulomas in the portal tracts and septa as well as mild lymphoplasmacytic inflammatory infiltrate. There was also evidence of macrovesicular steatosis and advanced fibrosis. An excisional biopsy of a mediastinal lymph node was also performed, which showed nonnecrotizing granulomatous lymphadenitis.

What is a granuloma?

Granulomas are microscopic rounded collections of cells, primarily macrophages, CD4+ T lymphocytes, and fibroblasts. This formation of cell aggregates is thought to occur secondary to a chronic exposure to an antigen that results in cytokine secretion, thus activating the macrophages. Hepatic granulomas are thought to be a local response to a specific causative agent (bacterial or fungal infections) or reflect a more generalized systemic disease (sarcoidosis, tuberculosis). Sarcoid granulomas often present in clusters and have central fibrinoid necrosis. They are frequently found in the portal and periportal areas of the liver. Granulomas may eventually resolve without residua, although some undergo fibrosis leading to scarring (Culver et al., 2016; Lagana et al., 2010; Modaresi et al., 2015).

What are causes of granulomas in the liver and how can you distinguish them?

Although sarcoidosis is one of the more common causes of granulomatous liver disease, it is not the only cause (Modaresi et al., 2015). The main categories of conditions associated with hepatic granulomas include noninfectious immunologic insults, infection, foreign body reactions, drugs, and neoplasia. On biopsy, the morphology and location of the granulomas can help with the differential diagnoses. There are four main histological variants of hepatic granulomas: noncaseating,

caseating, fibrin-ring, and lipogranulomas. Other histological findings may help support the diagnoses—for example, Schaumann bodies, which are irregular, concentrically laminated, intracellular inclusion bodies consisting of calcified proteins. They are more commonly found in hepatic sarcoidosis but are not specific (Tables 47.4 and 47.5; Fig. 47.1) (Culver et al., 2016; You et al., 2012).

What is hepatic sarcoidosis?

Sarcoidosis is a multisystem disease that is characterized by noncaseating epithelioid granulomas in various organs. The liver is one of the most commonly involved extrapulmonary sites. Hepatic sarcoidosis has a broad range of presentations ranging from asymptomatic to nonspecific symptoms. They can have scattered, diffuse noncaseating granulomas with normal liver enzymes or a cholestatic pattern resulting in portal hypertension and cirrhosis. The most common clinical findings are usually hepatomegaly, splenomegaly, and jaundice. Occasionally patients can exhibit signs and symptoms of portal hypertension and cirrhosis. A classification system was established to divide patients with sarcoidosis and granulomatous liver disease into four broad categories (Ebert et al., 2008; Ibrahim et al., 2018; Tadros et al., 2013) (Table 47.6).

CLINICAL PEARL **STEP 2**

The diagnosis of systemic sarcoidosis can only be made if there are granulomas seen in two or more organs. It is important to note that histological confirmation of the second organ is not always required. For example, if a patient does not have a diagnosis of systemic sarcoidosis but is found to have hepatic granulomas and concomitant hilar lymphadenopathy, a biopsy of lymph nodes is not required.

How can hepatic sarcoidosis be diagnosed?

TABLE 47.4 ■ **Histological Variants of Granulomas**

Noncaseating	Nonnecrotic
Caseating	Area of central necrosis
Fibrin-ring	Epithelioid cells surround a vacuole within an encircling fibrin ring
Lipogranulomas	Contain a central lipid vacuole

TABLE 47.5 ■ **Differential Diagnoses of Hepatic Granulomas**

Disease	Histological Classification	Location of Granulomas
PBC	Noncaseating	Within portal tracts and with severe destruction of the bile ducts (segmental destructive cholangitis). Portal inflammation composed of lymphoid infiltrate, plasma cells, and often prominent eosinophils. Few periportal granulomas surrounding damaged bile ducts.
Sarcoldosis	Noncaseating	Granulomas found in any location in the liver—often cluster in periportal regions and produce dense hyaline fbrosis with the presence of epithelioid macrophages and multinudeated giant cells.
TB/MAC	Caseating	Immunocompromised—numerous organisms seen on AFB stain; immunocompetent—few organisms seen on AFB stain
Drugs: Amlodarone, Sulfonamides	Fibrin-ring	Located anywhere within the liver

TABLE 47.6 ■ **Maddrey Classification for Sarcoidosis of the Liver**

Group I	Incidental granulomas discovered on a random liver biopsy
Group II	Hepatomegaly and/or splenomegaty with mild derangement of hepatic function but no evidence of hepatic insufficiency or portal hypertension
Group III	Clinical and laboratory evidence of *hepatocellular* disease with or without portal hypertension
Group IV	Portal hypertension as the predominant clinical abnormality

TABLE 47.7 ■ **Imaging Findings for Hepatic Sarcoidosis**

Imaging Modality	Findings
Ultrasound	Hepatomegaly, retroperitoneal lymphadenopathy, parenchymal echogenicity, focal calcifications, nodularity of the liver
CT	Diffuse parenchymal heterogeneity, hepatomegaly, lymphadenopathy, focal low-attenuation liver lesions
MRI	Heterogeneous liver parenchyma, multiple diffuse densely packed nodular foci, irregular contour T2-weighted: decreased hepatic signal intensity MRCP: normal biliary ducts

MRCP, Magnetic resonance cholangiopancreatography.

The diagnosis of sarcoidosis requires granulomatous inflammation in at least two organs. Hepatic sarcoidosis is usually asymptomatic and is associated with elevated ALP, up to five times of the upper limit normal (ULN). Other laboratory tests that may be present include hypercalcemia, hypercalciuria, and elevation in angiotensin-converting enzyme (although it is not recommended to use this test in isolation to confirm a diagnosis of sarcoidosis) (Modaresi et al., 2015; Tadros et al., 2013).

Imaging is a useful tool to rule out other causes of the serum abnormalities but, unfortunately, sarcoid granulomas 100–200 μm (Table 47.7).

Biopsy is the diagnostic gold standard because serological markers and imaging techniques lack the necessary sensitivity or specificity to establish the diagnosis. Biopsy offers the benefits of confirmation of the diagnosis, but also allows other liver disease processes to be excluded, such as nonalcoholic fatty liver disease and drug-induced liver disease.

CLINICAL PEARL **STEP 2**

The diagnosis of hepatic granulomas cannot be made on imaging. A liver biopsy must be performed to identify the histology changes that are associated with sarcoidosis.

What is the management and treatment of hepatic sarcoidosis?

There is currently no standard of care in how to treat hepatic sarcoidosis. Treatment is usually reserved for patients with concomitant pulmonary sarcoidosis. Isolated, asymptomatic hepatic sarcoidosis is usually not treated but monitored via serum laboratory testing and imaging (Ebert et al., 2008; Modaresi et al., 2015).

CLINICAL PEARL **STEP 2**

Isolated, asymptomatic hepatic sarcoidosis is usually not treated but monitored via serum laboratory testing and imaging.

For patients who are symptomatic, have a substantial amount of granulomatous disease on biopsy, or have proven pulmonary sarcoidosis, the most studied treatment is glucocorticoids. Glucocorticoids have an antiinflammatory effect by inhibiting activation and proliferation of the T cells and macrophages. In the limited data published, steroids have been shown to improve clinical symptoms and improve liver enzymes but have not been proven to prevent the progression of hepatic sarcoidosis to cirrhosis (Cremers et al., 2012; Ebert et al., 2008; Modaresi et al., 2015).

CLINICAL PEARL **STEP 2**

Prior to initiating any glucocorticoid therapy, it is important to exclude infectious etiologies (particularly MTB or disseminated fungemia) and gastrointestinal bleed.

Alternative treatments have been trialed in various case studies for patients who cannot tolerate steroid treatment or for whom steroids were not effective. These treatments include budesonide and ursodeoxycholic acid (UDCA). These agents are of unknown benefit due to limited data but have been shown in various case studies to have few side effects. No treatment options thus far have shown histologically proven improvement of the disease course (Cremers et al., 2012; Modaresi et al., 2015).

The patient was diagnosed with pulmonary and hepatic sarcoidosis. She received prednisone 30 mg daily. Her symptoms stabilized and therefore treatment was discontinued after 1 month. Because the patient was asymptomatic for pulmonary sarcoidosis and had no evidence of decompensation from cirrhosis, the decision was made to follow a strategy of serial surveillance of liver enzymes and imaging instead of treating with further steroids.

Case Summary

- **Complaint/History:** A 60-year-old woman presents profound weight loss, shortness of breath and fatigue.
- **Lab Results/Tests:** Complete metabolic panel revealed hyperglycemia (16.6 mg/dL), elevated alkaline phosphatase (305 U/L). CT scan was notable for diffuse mediastinal lymphadenopathy, and a nodular liver. Further work up excluded atypical infection and AMA was negative. Both a liver biopsy and a biopsy of mediastinal lymph note revealed non-necrotizing granulomatous changes.

Diagnosis: Hepatic sarcoidosis.

- **Treatment:** Observe or Prednisone for concomitant pulmonary sarcoidosis.

Bibliography

Cremers, J. P., Drent, M., Baughman, R. P., Wijnen, P. A., & Koek, G. H. (2012). Therapeutic approach of hepatic sarcoidosis. *Curr Opin Pulm Med*, *18*(5), 472–482.

Culver, E. L., Watkins, J., & Westbrook, R. H. (2016). Granulomas of the liver. *Clin Liver Dis (Hoboken)*, *7*(4), 92–96.

Ebert, E. C., Kierson, M., & Hagspiel, K. D. (2008). Gastrointestinal and hepatic manifestations of sarcoidosis. *Am J Gastroenterol*, *103*(12), 3184–3192. quiz 3193.

Ibrahim, A. M., Bhandari, B., Soriano, P. K., et al. (2018). Hepatic involvement in systemic sarcoidosis. *Am J Case Rep*, *19*, 1212–1215.

Kaplowitz. N. (2004). Drug-induced liver injury. *Clin Infect Dis*, *38*(Suppl 2), S44–48.

Lagana, S. M., Moreira, R. K., & Lefkowitch, J. H. (2010). Hepatic granulomas: pathogenesis and differential diagnosis. *Clin Liver Dis.*, *14*(4), 605–617.

Manns, M. P., Lohse, A. W., & Vergani, D. (2015). Autoimmune hepatitis—Update 2015. *J Hepatol*, *62*(1 Suppl), S100–111.

Modaresi Esfeh, J., Culver, D., Plesec, T., & John, B. (2015). Clinical presentation and protocol for management of hepatic sarcoidosis. *Expert Rev Gastroenterol Hepatol*, *9*(3), 349–358.

Schreiner, A. D., & Rockey, D. C. (2018). Evaluation of abnormal liver tests in the adult asymptomatic patient. *Curr Opin Gastroenterol*, *34*(4), 272–279.

Tadros, M., Forouhar, F., & Wu, G. Y. (2013). Hepatic sarcoidosis. *J Clin Transl Hepatol*, *1*(2), 87–93.

Woreta, T. A., & Alqahtani, S. A. (2014). Evaluation of abnormal liver tests. *Med Clin North Am*, *98*(1), 1–16.

You, Z., Wang, Q., Bian, Z., et al. (2012). The immunopathology of liver granulomas in primary biliary cirrhosis. *J Autoimmun*, *39*(3), 216–221.

CASE 48

A 77-Year-Old Male With Progressive Jaundice and Pruritus

Ashwini Mulgaonkar ■ Liyun Yuan

A 77-year-old male with a history of sick sinus syndrome status post pacemaker placement, ulcerative colitis, hypertension, and type 2 diabetes mellitus was referred by his primary medical doctor for jaundice and pruritus.

His doctor noted newly elevated liver enzymes alkaline phosphatase (ALP) 672 U/L, total bilirubin (BR) 5.0 mg/dL, alanine aminotransferase (ALT) 77 U/L, and aspartate aminotransferase (AST) 63 U/L. When he presented to the liver clinic, his total bilirubin increased to 20 mg/dL.

On review of his records, a trend of abnormal liver enzymes was noted with no prior workup (Table 48.1).

How should these lab tests be evaluated?

An elevations in serum ALP and total BR is indicative of a cholestatic pattern of injury. This often results from an obstructive process which causes damage to the biliary ducts and eventual upstream damage to hepatocytes. ALP is a zinc metalloproteinase enzyme that is produced in numerous organs. Within the liver, ALP is found in hepatocytes bound to the canalicular membrane. Bilirubin, a breakdown product of heme, is processed within hepatocytes and, following conjugation is stored in the gallbladder. Conjugated bilirubin passes through the enterohepatic circulation with bile and may be excreted in urine or feces. Any biliary tree injury resulting in backflow within the bile duct may lead to an increased serum circulation of direct and indirect BR (Schreiner & Rockey, 2018; Woreta & Alqahtani, 2014).

Anatomy of the biliary system

When evaluating a patient with abnormal liver enzymes, pertinent organs that need to be assessed include the liver, gallbladder, and biliary tree (Fig. 48.1).

The biliary tree plays a small but important role in enterocolic circulation. Its main role is to connect the gallbladder, the organ responsible for the storage of bile, bile acids, and cholesterol, to the liver and the duodenum via the common bile duct (CBD). The CBD is divided into an extrahepatic and an intrahepatic portion. The intrahepatic portion includes both small and large ducts that collect bile from the liver parenchyma. The extrahepatic portion consists of three parts: the hepatic duct, the cystic duct, and the rest of the common bile duct. The hepatic duct connects from the liver hilum into the CBD. The cystic duct empties the gallbladder into the CBD. The CBD is largest caliber of the three and is responsible for draining the common hepatic duct and the cystic duct into the second part of the duodenum (Hadžić & Strazzabosco, 2018; Shanbhogue, Tirumani, Prasad, Fasih, & McInnes, 2011).

TABLE 48.1 ■ **Patient's Lab Test Values Prior to Presentation**

	ALT (U/L)	AST (U/L)	ALP (U/L)	BR (mg/dL)
1/2016	35	29	162	1.0
3/2016	19	23	248	1.0
8/2019	142	31	522	1.8
9/2019	77	63	672	5.0
10/2019	68	70	692	20.0
11/2019	61	56	593	22.3

ALP, Alkaline phosphatase; *ALT*, alanine aminotransferase; *AST*, aspartate aminotransferase; *BR*, total bilirubin.

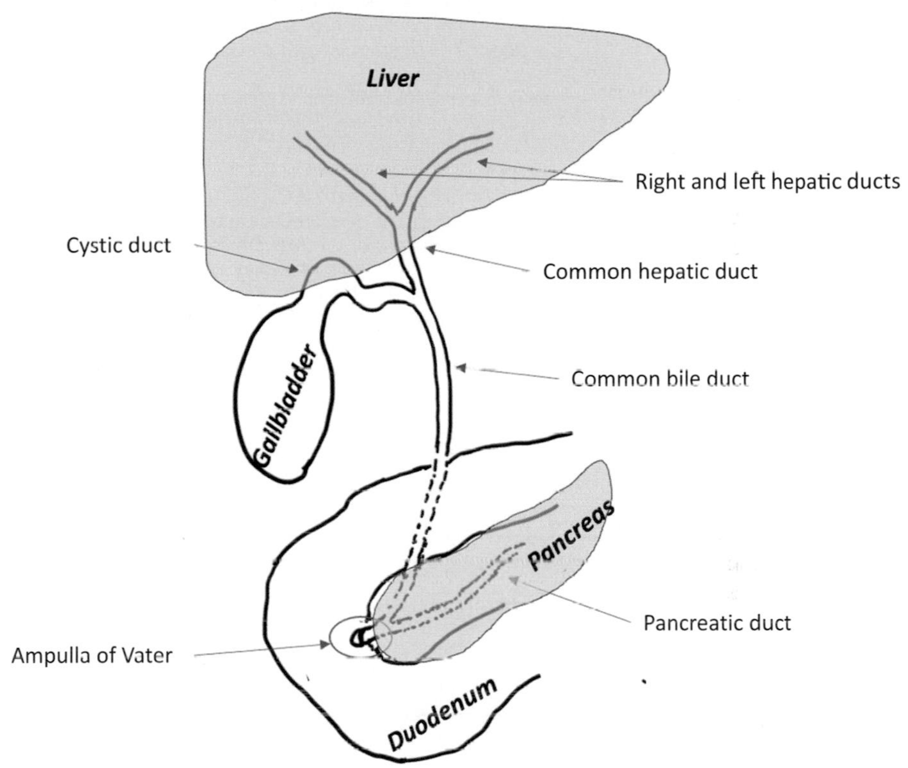

Fig. 48.1 Anatomy of the biliary system.

CLINICAL PEARL **STEP 2**

Biliary systems need to be carefully evaluated when a patient presents obstructive jaundice or cholestatic hepatic injury.

What is the differential diagnosis for biliary obstruction?

Numerous benign and malignant conditions result in strictures within the biliary tree. Most present with similar symptoms of obstructive jaundice. Chronic and recurrent obstruction may lead to frequent episodes of cholangitis and/or cirrhosis (Table 48.2).

TABLE 48.2 ■ **Differential Diagnoses of Strictures**

Causes of Biliary Obstrcutions	Pathophysiology
Choledocholithiasis	The presence of gallstones in the common bile duct obstructs bile flow.
Benign biliary strictures	Injury to bile ducts leads to isolated strictures in the common hepatic duct or the common bile duct.
Malignancy Cholangiocarcinoma Pancreatic adenocarcinoma Invasive hepatocellular carcinoma	Malignancy directly involves or externally compresses the bile ducts.
Primary sclerosing cholangitis (PSC)	An autoimmune condition causing inflammation and fibrosis in the intrahepatic and extrahepatic bile ducts resulting in diffuse strictures and dilations within the biliary tree.
Recurrent pyogenic cholangitis	Chronic biliary infection characterized by recurrent bouts of cholangitis with primary hepatolithiasis causing inflammation and scarring.
Congenital biliary cysts	Isolated segmental dilations and narrowing of the intrahepatic biliary ducts, which are formed from failure of proper development of the biliary tree.

From Hadžić, N., & Strazzabosco, M. (2018) Fibropolycystic liver diseases and congenital biliary abnormalities (pp. 308–327); Dooley, J.S., Gurusamy K.S., & Davidson B.R. Gallstones and benign biliary disease. (pp. 256–293); and Koti, R.S., & Bridgewater, J. Malignant biliary diseases (pp. 294–307). In J. S. Dooley, A. S. F. Lock, G. Garcia-Tsao, & M. Pinzani (Eds.), *Sherlock's diseases of the liver and biliary system* (13th ed.) Oxford: Wiley; and Pereira, S. P., Goodchild, G., & Webster, G. J. M. (2018). The endoscopist and malignant and non-malignant biliary obstruction. *Biochimica et Biophysica Acta Molecular Basis of Disease 1864*(4 Pt B), 1478–1483).

The patient's abdominal ultrasound is significant for increased liver echogenicity, evidence of prior cholecystectomy, and a patent portal vein with no ductal dilation. It was not possible to obtain a magnetic resonance cholangiopancreatography (MRCP) because of his pacemaker being MRI incompatible. Instead, he underwent multiphase contrast-enhanced computed tomography (CT) of his thorax, abdomen, and pelvis, which showed no obvious evidence of malignancy.

How is biliary obstruction diagnosed?

Imaging is key for the detection of biliary strictures and dilation. Abdominal ultrasound is often the initial test of choice due to its availability. Ultrasound is sensitive for detection of biliary obstruction but accuracy is highly operator dependent. Multiphase contrast-enhanced CT scan can help visualize thickening of the bile ducts, strictures, and dilations but are often nonspecific and require contrast for detail, which presents its own risks and limitations. CTs can also identify lymphadenopathy, which may be indicative of malignancy but may also be present in primary sclerosing cholangitis (PSC). MRCP allows a more detailed evaluation of the biliary tree and hepatic parenchyma without the use of contrast. MRCP has a superior sensitivity to ultrasound or CT scan for establishing a diagnosis of biliary obstruction. Therefore, MRCP is now recommended by all major professional societies as the diagnostic modality of choice. (Dooley, Gurusamy, & Davidson, 2018; Shanbhogue et al., 2011).

The gold standard for evaluation of stricture and source of obstruction remains endoscopic retrograde cholangiopancreatography (ERCP) or endoscopic ultrasound (EUS). These techniques offer the advantage of tissue sampling and interventions such as biliary balloon dilation/stenting, brush cytology and fine needle aspiration (FNA) (Table 48.3) (Pereira, Goodchild, & Webster, 2018).

TABLE 48.3 ■ **Pros and Cons of Various Imaging Modalities in the Diagnosis of Biliary Strictures**

	Pros	Cons
Ultrasound	• Readily available • Noninvasive • Easily can identify the level of intrahepatic obstruction	• Operator dependent • Not diagnostic
CT	• Can identify malignant characteristics • Noninvasive	• Requires contrast
MRCP	• 98% sensitive • Does not require contrast • Noninvasive • Able to assess hepatic parenchyma	• May not be able to visualize narrow strictures
ERCP/EUS	• Direct visualization of biliary tree • Can obtain tissues/cells • Intervention can relieve obstructions • EUS has 97% sensitivity and 88% specificity for differentiation between benign and malignant strictures	• Invasive, procedural risks

CT, Computed tomography; *ERCP*, endoscopic retrograde cholangiopancreatography; *EUS*, endoscopic ultrasound; *MRCP*, magnetic resonance cholangiopancreatography.

CLINICAL PEARL **STEP 2**

MRCP is the preferred imaging modality to evaluate biliary obstruction. However, ERCP remains the gold standard for establishing a diagnosis and offers the potential for tissue sampling and potential therapeutic intervention.

Given high suspicion for biliary obstructions, the patient underwent an ERCP. Cholangiogram showed a severe dominant stricture of the CBD. There were segmental biliary strictures alternating with biliary dilatation that were suggestive of PSC. Brushing was performed and a plastic 7 French stent was placed across the dominant CBD stricture (see Fig. 48.2).

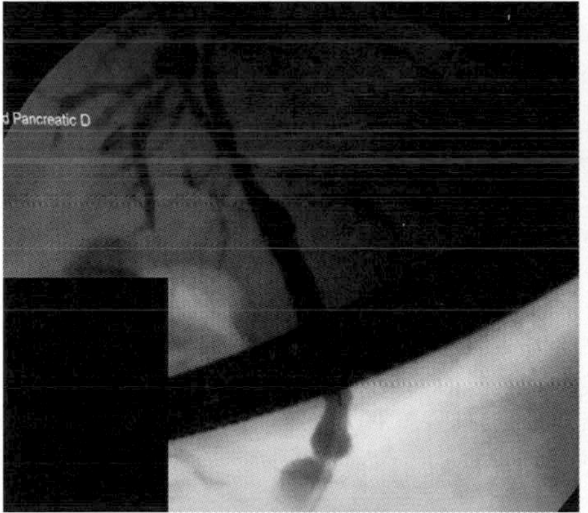

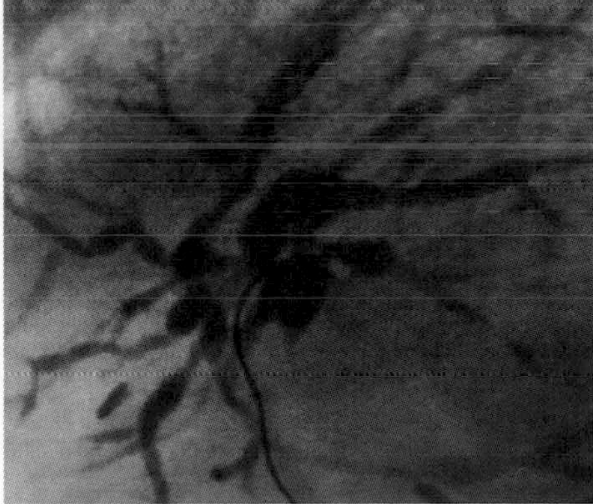

Fig. 48.2 The patient's cholangiogram was significant for a severe dominant stricture in the common bile duct and several other segmental biliary strictures alternating with areas of biliary dilation. These findings are suggestive of primary sclerosing cholangitis.

What is primary sclerosing cholangitis (PSC)? What is the risk for cholangiocarcinoma (CCA) in patients with PSC?

PSC is a chronic, progressive disease presenting with inflammation and fibrosis of both the intrahepatic and extrahepatic bile ducts. The diagosis of PSC is dependent on identification of a dominant stricture, which is defined as stenosis with diameter of <1.5 mm in the CBD or <1 mm in the hepatic duct. PSC often progresses to liver cirrhosis and carries a high risk of developing cholangiocarcinoma. In recent studies, the 10-year cumulative incidence of CCA is roughly 7%–9%. In approximately half of patients with PSC and superimposed CCA, malignancy is detected at the time of PSC diagnosis.

The diagnosis of CCA is dependent on brush cytology obtained via ERCP. Brush cytology has been found to have a limited sensitivity (18%–40%) but excellent specificity (95%–100%). Cytological evaluation for polysomy with fluorescent in situ hybridization (FISH) results in an improved sensitivity of 47% and a specificity of 100% for diagnosis of CCA in PSC. Unfortunately, distinguishing between benign versus malignant stricture remains and challenge and consensus does not currently exist on a standardized surveillance strategy.

CLINICAL PEARL **STEP 2**

Brush cytology and/or endoscopic biopsy should be obtained as part of endoscopic intervention to exclude superimposed malignancy in PSC.

There are no effective medical therapies for PSC. Liver transplantation (LT) remains the treatment option for patients with intractable pruritus, recurrent cholangitis, or decompensated cirrhosis. LT is highly successful with approximately 85% survival at 5 years. The early stage of hilar CCA is an indication for LT under a strict neoadjuvant chemoradiation protocol established in a few transplant centers. These patients must be carefully followed for recurrence of recurrence of PSC disease after transplantation. (Chapman, 2017; Chapman et al., 2010; Gochanour, Jayasekera, & Kowdley, 2020).

The patient underwent another ERCP with repeated brushing for cytology through the dominant stricture. Cytology returned as high-grade dysplasia. Because cholangiocarcinoma was suspected, he was referred for oncology consult. Unfortunately, the patient was a poor candidate for chemotherapy and due to his poor prognosis pursued palliative and hospice care.

Case Summary

- **Complaint/History:** A 77-year-old male referred for evaluation of abnormal liver enzymes and new onset jaundice and pruritus.
- **Lab Results/Tests:** Complete metabolic panel pertinent for an initial elevated alkaline phosphatase 672 U/L and total bilirubin 5.0 mg/dL. Total bilrubin had risen to 20 mg/L at the time of clinic evaluation. Cholangiogram identified common bile duct stricture. Endoscopic retrograde cholangiopancreatography (ERCP) was performed with brush cytology diagnosing cholangiocarcinoma.

Diagnosis: Primary sclerosing cholangitis (PSC) with development of cholangiocarcinoma.

- **Treatment:** There are no effective therapies for PSC. Patients with intractable pruritus, recurrent cholangitis, or decompensated cirrhosis are recommended for liver transplant.

Bibliography

Chapman, R., Fevery, J., Kalloo, A., Nagorney, D. M., Boberg, K. M., Shneider, B., ... Diseases AAftSoL, (2010). Diagnosis and management of primary sclerosing cholangitis. *Hepatology*, *51*(2), 660–678.

Chapman, R. W. (2017). Update on primary sclerosing cholangitis. *Clinical Liver Disease*, *9*(5), 107–110.

Dooley, J. S., Gurusamy, K. S., & Davidson, B. R. (2018). Gallstones and benign biliary disease. In J. S. Dooley, A. S. F. Lock, G. Garcia-Tsao, & M. Pinzani (Eds.). *Sherlock's diseases of the liver and biliary system* (13th ed.), pp. 256–293.

Gochanour, E., Jayasekera, C., & Kowdley, K. (2020). Primary sclerosing cholangitis: Epidemiology, genetics, diagnosis, and current management. *Clinical Liver Disease*, *15*(3), 125–128.

Hadžić, N., & Strazzabosco, M. (2018). Fibropolycystic liver diseases and congenital biliary abnormalities. In J. S. Dooley, A. S. F. Lock, G. Garcia-Tsao, M. Pinzani (Eds.). *Sherlock's diseases of the liver and biliary system* (13th ed.), pp. 308–327.

Koti, R. S., & Bridgewater, J. (2018). Malignant biliary diseases. In J. S. Dooley, A. S. F. Lock, G. Garcia-Tsao, & M. Pinzani (Eds.). *Sherlock's diseases of the liver and biliary system* (13th ed.), pp. 294–307.

Pereira, S. P., Goodchild, G., & Webster, G. J. M. (2018). The endoscopist and malignant and non-malignant biliary obstruction. *Biochimica et Biophysica Acta - Molecular Basis of Disease*, *1864*(4 Pt B), 1478–1483.

Schreiner, A. D., & Rockey, D. C. (2018). Evaluation of abnormal liver tests in the adult asymptomatic patient. *Current Opinion in Gastroenterology*, *34*(4), 272–279.

Shanbhogue, A. K., Tirumani, S. H., Prasad, S. R., Fasih, N., & McInnes, M. (2011). Benign biliary strictures: A current comprehensive clinical and imaging review. *American Journal of Roentgenology*, *197*(2), W295–306.

Woreta, T. A., & Alqahtani, S. A. (2014). Evaluation of abnormal liver tests. *The Medical Clinics of North America*, *98*(1), 1–16.

SECTION 11

Endocrine

CASE 49

A 49-Year-Old Male With Polyuria and Polydipsia

Maria Magar ■ Braden Barnett

A 49-year-old male with a history of obesity presents with 2 days of polyuria, polydipsia, abdominal pain, and nausea. He says that he has never had these symptoms before and has not seen a doctor in more than 10 years. He thinks that in his last clinic visit he was told he could develop diabetes in the future, but he was not prescribed anything at that time and is currently not taking any medications. On physical examination, his blood pressure is 112/75 mmHg, pulse rate is 108/min, respiratory rate is 26/min, oxygen saturation is 96% on room air, and weight is 97 kg (BMI 32.5 kg/m^2). The patient looks uncomfortable and has slight tenderness to palpation diffusely on abdominal exam. A fingerstick blood glucose (BG) reads >600 mg/dL.

What are some etiologies for hyperglycemia?

Various etiologies exist for hyperglycemia, including diabetes mellitus (type 1 or 2), other pathologic conditions, medications, acute illness, and stress. Table 49.1 lists a detailed differential diagnosis of hyperglycemia and its associated risk factors. In hospitalized patients, hyperglycemia is defined as any BG >180 mg/dL. Major endocrine societies recommend targeting glucoses of 140–180 mg/dL in critically ill patients, such as our patient. In the noncritically ill hospitalized patient, target glucoses should be <140 mg/dL in the fasting period or otherwise <180 mg/dL.

CLINICAL PEARL **STEP 3**

Serum glucose goals during hospitalization should be <140 mg/dL in noncritically ill patients and 140–180 mg/dL in critically ill patients.

The patient is given two boluses of normal saline. His serum lab results return as follows: venous blood gas (VBG) pH 7.1, basic metabolic panel with sodium 129 mEq/L, potassium 4.0 mEq/L, chloride 98 mEq/L, bicarbonate 15 mEq/L, glucose 636 mg/dL, and serum ketones 2.8 mmol/L (reference range <0.3 mmol/L). A urinalysis (UA) is positive for leukocytes and bacteria. The hemoglobin A1c (HbA1c) returns a few hours later at 11.6%.

What is your differential diagnosis?

This is a 49-year-old obese male with gastrointestinal symptoms, elevated serum glucose, and acidosis and ketosis with an elevated anion gap (16 mEq/L). At this point, diabetic ketoacidosis (DKA) is highest on our differential diagnosis.

TABLE 49.1 ■ **Hyperglycemia Risk Factors and Differential Diagnosis**

Risk Factors	Differential Diagnosis
Elevated BMI, hypertension, hyperlipidemia	Medications (glucocorticoids, phenytoin, estrogen)
Family history of diabetes	Reactive, e.g., acute illness
PCOS	Stress, e.g., surgery/procedure
Ethnicity (Hispanic, African American, Native American, Pacific Islander, Asian American)	Endocrine disorders (acromegaly, Cushing's syndrome, pheochromocytoma)
History of gestational diabetes	TPN, dextrose containing fluids
	DKA, HHS, MODY, LADA, gestational diabetes
	Pancreatic destruction (malignancy, chronic pancreatitis, cystic fibrosis, hemochromatosis)

BMI, Body mass index; *DKA*, diabetic ketoacidosis; *HHS*, hyperosmolar hyperglycemic state; *LADA*, latent autoimmune diabetes of adulthood; *MODY*, mature onset diabetes of the young; *PCOS*, polycystic ovarian syndrome; *TPN*, total parenteral nutrition.

Although the patient does not have a prior diagnosis of type 2 diabetes mellitus (T2DM), his age, BMI, HbA1c, and serum blood glucose all support T2DM. His ill-appearing state on physical examination and lab findings are consistent with ketoacidosis.

What is DKA?

DKA occurs when there is insufficient insulin in the body to suppress hepatic gluconeogenesis or to promote peripheral uptake of glucose. The rise in counterregulatory hormones, including catecholamines, cortisol, glucagon, and growth hormone, further exacerbates hyperglycemia and increases lipolysis. This process leads to increased catabolism and release of free fatty acids into circulation that undergo oxidation to ketone bodies. Decreased bicarbonate levels increase levels of beta-hydroxybutyrate, acetoacetate, and acetone, leading to an acidosis. Other electrolyte abnormalities such as phosphate and potassium depletion can lead to respiratory failure, and a compensatory hyperventilation may ensue to compensate for a concurrent metabolic acidosis.

CLINICAL PEARL **STEP 3**

DKA can be diagnosed in a patient such as this man with a serum glucose >250 mg/dL, pH <7.30, bicarbonate <15–18 mEq/L, ketones in the blood or urine, and an anion gap >10–12 mEq/L.

In the evaluation of DKA, it is important to discover and treat inciting factors, including decreased insulin use, infection, myocardial infarction or stroke, endocrinopathy (e.g., hyperthyroidism, Cushing's syndrome, or pheochromocytoma), excessive alcohol use, trauma, psychological stress, or pregnancy.

This patient's symptoms of polyuria and abdominal pain could be attributed to hyperglycemia and ketoacidosis, respectively. However, findings upon physical examination and UA supported the diagnosis of a concurrent urinary tract infection (UTI). The remainder of his workup, which included an electrocardiogram and chest X-ray examination, was within normal limits. His tachycardia, hyperpnea, relative hypotension, nausea, and abdominal pain are commonly seen in DKA. Other signs and symptoms of DKA include anorexia, vomiting, dry mucous membranes, poor skin turgor, myalgias, weakness, and altered mental status.

CLINICAL PEARL	STEP 1/2/3
Medication nonadherence and infection are common inciting factors for DKA occurrence.	

What are important management decisions for DKA?

Depending on the severity of DKA and hospital protocol, patients may need to be treated in the intensive care unit (ICU). Mainstays of treatment include adequate hydration (more cautiously in patients with chronic heart failure or renal disease), electrolyte repletion, glucose monitoring, insulin administration, and appropriate evaluation and management of underlying causes of DKA. Table 49.2 discusses management considerations.

CLINICAL PEARL	STEP 3
Bicarbonate administration is controversial in the management of DKA; it can be considered if arterial pH ≤7.0.	

Fluid and insulin infusions should be continued until the acidosis has cleared, BG <250 mg/dL, and the patient demonstrates an ability to tolerate an oral diet. DKA is considered resolved when venous pH >7.3, BG <200 mg/dL, and serum bicarbonate ≥18 mEq/L. At that point, the patient can be transitioned from insulin infusion to subcutaneous insulin with overlap occurring for at least 2 hours. If the patient suffers from diabetes that was previously well controlled, insulin can be restarted on similar doses prior to hospitalization. If the patient has newly diagnosed diabetes such as this case, basal insulin can be started at 0.2 units/kg and bolus insulin can be started at 0.1 units/kg/meal.

TABLE 49.2 ■ **Management of DKA**

Fluids: *typically TBW 4–6 L down*	• Resuscitation: NS 1 L/h • If repeat Na when corrected is normal or high, change fluids to 45% NS • If repeat Na when corrected is low, continue NS • Once BG ≤250 mg/dL, change to 5% dextrose with 45% NS at 150–250 mL/h (goal BG 150–200) • If DKA resolved but patient unable to eat, continue insulin drip and 5% dextrose with 45% NS at 100–200 mL/h
Electrolytes: *typically K+ deficit 3–5 mEq/kg, PO_4 deficit 5–7 mmol/kg*	• If K+ <3.3, hold insulin and give 40 mEq/h of K+ until ≥3.3 • If 3.3≤ K+ <5.0, give 20–30 mEq of K+ in each liter of IVF • If K+ ≥5.0, do not give K+ and check K+ level every 2 h • Replete PO_4 if <1.0 mg/dL or concomitant cardiorespiratory compromise
Insulin	• Can load with bolus of regular insulin 0.1–0.15 units/kg (not mandatory) • Start continuous infusion regular insulin 0.1 units/kg/h • BG should decline by 50–75 mg/dL in first hour; if it does not, double insulin infusion hourly until it does
Lab tests	• Obtain fingerstick BG every 1–2 h while on insulin infusion • Obtain venous pH, electrolytes, BUN, and creatinine levels every 2–4 h until K+ stabilized and anion gap normalized

BUN, Blood urea nitrogen; *IVF*, intravenous fluids; *K+*, potassium; *NS*, normal saline; PO_4, phosphate; *TBW*, total body water.

CLINICAL PEARL **STEP 2/3**

The mainstays of DKA management are intravenous fluids, electrolyte repletion, insulin, and frequent blood tests to monitor glucose, pH, creatinine, sodium, potassium, magnesium, phosphorus, bicarbonate, and the anion gap.

The patient shows clinical improvement upon targeted antibiotics for UTI and DKA management per ICU protocol. Subsequently, he is transferred to general medicine wards. Prior to being discharged home the next day, his primary team ensures that he receives counseling on diabetes management and insulin administration. He is also informed that he has probably developed early-stage, chronic kidney disease based on lab trends on kidney function (creatinine on admission of 2.01 mg/dL improved to 1.4 mg/dL upon fluid hydration, with no further change during this hospitalization).

How is subcutaneous insulin started?

If an oral agent and basal insulin will be used, a dose of basal insulin 0.1–0.2 units/kg can be initiated in the hospital then uptitrated as appropriate in the outpatient setting. If a patient will need multiple daily injections (MDI), a total insulin dose of 0.5 units/kg/day or more should be used (the total dose chosen depends on the degree of insulin resistance present based on BMI and past insulin usage, if any): 50% of this dose should be given as basal insulin and the remaining 50% as premeal doses. A sliding scale with or without carbohydrate counting for mealtime insulin dosing can also be used. Careful insulin titration should be performed upon changes in activity, diet, weight, and renal/hepatic function, as well as with illness/infection, other stressors, and certain medications such as glucocorticoids.

The patient is sent home on metformin 500 mg twice a day (with instructions to uptitrate to 1000 mg twice a day after 1 week if he does not experience side effects), glargine 10 units daily, and lispro 3 units prior to each meal. Before leaving the hospital, he tells you he is very motivated to change his lifestyle and lose weight, and he hopes to stop taking insulin in the future.

Three months later, the patient visits his primary care doctor (PMD) for follow-up on his diabetes. He has been running 1 mile every day and has been careful about what he eats. His measured weight in the office is now 86 kg, down from 97 kg previously. His kidney function remains unchanged and his A1c is significantly improved to 7.4%. However, he describes symptoms of sweating and shakiness when his blood glucoses are "low." He says he stopped taking his mealtime insulin when these symptoms began but they still occur occasionally. The PMD decides to stop his glargine insulin.

What is hypoglycemia, and what are its associated symptoms?

Hypoglycemia is defined as low blood glucose, classified into three levels. Level 1 hypoglycemia is 54≤ BG <70 mg/dL. Level 2 hypoglycemia is BG <54 mg/dL. Level 3 hypoglycemia is defined as a severe event secondary to a low blood glucose requiring assistance (e.g., a change in mental or physical status). Common symptoms include hunger, shakiness, tachycardia, irritability, confusion, and when very severe, seizure, loss of consciousness, coma, and death. To treat hypoglycemia, 15–20 g of oral glucose should be taken with a repeat BG check after 15 minutes. Glucose administration should be continued until BG are consistently >100 mg/dL. Once the BG has normalized, a meal or snack should be consumed.

CLINICAL PEARL **STEP 3**

Hypoglycemia can be defined in three levels. Level 3 hypoglycemia is defined by a severe event (a change in mental or physical status) secondary to a low blood glucose, which requires urgent intervention.

What are noninsulin medications that can be started on a patient with type 2 diabetes?

There are several, noninsulin antidiabetic medications. These drug classes include biguanides, sulfonylureas (SUs), a thiazolidinedione (TZD), sodium glucose cotransporter-2 (SGLT2) inhibitors, glucagon-like peptide 1 receptor agonists (GLP1 RAs), dipeptidyl peptidase 4 (DPP4) inhibitors, meglitinides, alpha glucosidase inhibitors, a bile acid sequestrant, and an amylin analog. Table 49.3 lists the various medications within each class as well as their mechanisms of action. In general,

TABLE 49.3 ■ **Noninsulin Antidiabetic Drugs—Mechanisms of Action and Side Effects**

Drug Class	Drug Names	Mechanism of Action	Side Effects
Biguanide	Metformin	Decreases hepatic glucose production and intestinal glucose absorption, increases peripheral glucose uptake	Lactic acidosis, interferes with vitamin B_{12} absorption
Sulfonylureas	Glipizide Glyburide Glimepiride	Directly stimulates pancreatic beta cells to secrete insulin	Weight gain, hypoglycemia
Thiazolidinedione	Pioglitazone	Peroxisome proliferator-activator receptor (PPAR) gamma modulator; increases the insulin sensitivity of liver, muscle, and fat	Weight gain, fluid retention, fractures in women
SGLT2 inhibitors	Dapagliflozin Canagliflozin Empagliflozin Ertugliflozin	Blocks glucose reabsorption transporter in the proximal tubule of the kidney, thereby increasing glucose excretion in urine	BP reduction, weight loss, UTIs, genital mycotic infections, euglycemic DKA, limb amputation
GLP1 receptor agonists	Dulaglutide Exenatide Lixisenatide Liraglutide Semaglutide	Increases glucose-mediated insulin secretion, slows down gastric motility, suppresses glucagon secretion	GI symptoms, weight loss, ?pancreatitis, ?pancreatic cancer; contraindicated if patient has C cell tumor of thyroid (MTC)
DPPIV inhibitors	Alogliptin Linagliptin Saxagliptin Sitagliptin	Enhances the effects of GLP1 and GIP, increases glucose-mediated insulin secretion, slows down gastric motility, suppresses glucagon secretion	Polyarticular arthralgia, ?pancreatitis, ?pancreatic cancer, ?hospitalization for heart failure
Meglitinides	Nateglinide Repaglinide	Stimulates pancreatic beta cells to secrete insulin	Hypoglycemia
Alpha glucosidase inhibitors	Acarbose Miglitol	Reduces rate of polysaccharide digestion in the proximal small intestine	GI symptoms, increased intestinal gas production

(Continued)

TABLE 49.3 ■ **Noninsulin Antidiabetic Drugs—Mechanisms of Action and Side Effects—cont'd**

Drug Class	Drug Names	Mechanism of Action	Side Effects
Bile acid sequestrant	Colesevelam	Resin; binds bile acids in the intestine, preventing their reabsorption	Contraindicated if history of small bowel obstruction, HTG induced pancreatitis, or TG >500 mg/dL
Amylin analog	Pramlintide	Synthetic analog of beta cell amylin hormone; inhibits glucose-dependent glucagon production, slows stomach emptying, increases satiety	GI symptoms, modest weight loss

Note: Not all SUs are listed, only the most common. Medications noted here are those available or most common in the United States. *BP*, Blood pressure; *GI*, gastrointestinal; *GIP*, gastric inhibitory polypeptide; *MTC*, medullary thyroid cancer; TG, hypertriglyceridemia/triglycerides.

prandial insulin should be discontinued if a sulfonylurea or meglitinide is started. It is unclear whether GLP1 RAs and DPP4 inhibitors, which have similar mechanisms of action, should be prescribed together, because there is no increased benefit nor FDA approval for concomitant use. If a patient's eGFR is >30 mL/min/1.73m^2 and no other contraindication exists, the first noninsulin antidiabetic medication initiated should be metformin. Initiation of second- or third-line agents depends on characteristics of the patient as well as the drug profile of the medication, for example, if the patient has a history of cardiovascular (CV) or renal disease and would benefit from a drug that has shown improved CV or renal outcomes. Of the medications listed in Table 49.3, all are administered orally except the GLP1 RAs and amylin analog (which are administered subcutaneously). There is only one GLP1 RA that is not administered subcutaneously, which is a novel oral version of semaglutide.

The patient and his PMD discuss various noninsulin diabetes medications. He is strongly opposed to sulfonylureas and thiazolidinediones because of the potential for weight gain. The patient expresses his desire to start canagliflozin. He knows that he had a UTI recently and is at higher risk of recurrent genitourinary infections in the future but insists he recalls a friend told him that canagliflozin can help his diabetic kidney disease. He also understands that he is stopping all insulin.

Which diabetes medications have proven benefits in patients with diabetic kidney disease?

Both GLP1 RAs and SGLT2 inhibitors have been shown to improve chronic kidney disease secondary to diabetes. In a trial specifically looking at canagliflozin's effect on kidney disease in patients with type 2 diabetes, kidney failure and cardiovascular events after 2.5 years were lower in those taking canagliflozin compared with placebo. Thus, this particular SGLT2 inhibitor has FDA approval for improving diabetic kidney disease and is indicated in CKD stage 3 with albuminuria. DPP4 inhibitors may also be effective in reducing albuminuria.

CLINICAL PEARL **STEP 3**

GLP1 RAs and SGLT2 inhibitors have shown benefit in diabetic kidney disease (DKD). Specifically, canagliflozin is FDA approved for DKD.

Three weeks later the patient calls his PMD telling her that he has not had any more hypoglycemia but has experienced a burning sensation with urination and foul-smelling urine. She tells him to stop the canagliflozin.

What are potential side effects of the noninsulin diabetes medications?

There are several side effects of antidiabetic medications, listed in Table 49.3. Notably, SGLT2 inhibitors can increase the risk of various genitourinary infections. In this case, the patient was not the ideal candidate for starting an SGLT2 inhibitor given his prior UTI history when he presented with DKA. Certain side effects such as weight loss and blood pressure (BP) reduction with SGLT2 inhibitors can be used for the patient's benefit. Clinicians need to be aware of certain diabetes medications that require adjustment or discontinuation upon worsening renal function.

The patient also mentions a family history of heart disease. In fact, his older brother had a heart attack recently and his father had a heart attack a few years ago. He is understandably very concerned. He asks whether there are any medications that might help reduce his risk of heart disease.

What are the cardiovascular benefits of different diabetes medications?

The SGLT2 inhibitors have been shown to prevent hospitalizations associated with heart failure (HF) and to decrease cardiovascular mortality and/or major adverse cardiovascular events (MACE) as seen in Table 49.4. The GLP1 RAs have not shown benefit in HF but do lower MACE. TZDs may reduce risk of stroke.

CLINICAL PEARL **STEP 3**

SGLT2 inhibitors have CV and heart failure benefits, whereas the GLP1 RAs have CV benefits.

The patient and his PMD together decide to start a trial with liraglutide, a GLP1 receptor agonist. The patient returns for follow-up after 3 months and says that he is very happy with his diabetes medications. However, he expresses some concern after reading online that semaglutide, a drug in the same class as liraglutide, can cause worsening of diabetic eye disease. He is also wondering what his A1c should be.

What is the association of GLP1 receptor agonists and diabetic retinopathy?

In a trial examining semaglutide's long-term outcomes compared with placebo over 2 years, patients taking semaglutide had worse retinopathy but nearly 30% had reduced risk of primary cardiovascular outcomes. Retinopathy complications included blindness and vitreous hemorrhage and/or a complication requiring treatment with an intravitreal agent or photocoagulation. However, this effect was thought to be a result of a rapid lowering of the HbA1c, as similar effects have been seen in patients who undergo intensive HbA1c lowering with insulin. In another study, liraglutide was found to be associated with increased retinopathy risk, although not statistically significant.

BASIC SCIENCE PEARL **STEP 3**

Diabetic retinopathy may be seen in GLP1 RAs most likely as a result of rapid lowering of the HbA1c. Similar effects have been seen in patients who undergo intensive HbA1c lowering with insulin: exogenous insulin can act concurrently with vascular endothelial growth factors (secreted from an ischemic retina) to trigger vascular proliferation and cause vision changes.

TABLE 49.4 ■ **Cardiovascular and Renal Benefits in SGLT2 Inhibitors and GLP1 RAs**

Drug Class	Drug Name	HFrEF	ASCVD	Renal Benefit
SGLT2 inhibitors	Dapagliflozin	x – *demonstrated efficacy in HFrEF, prevents HF hospitalization*		x
	Canagliflozin	x – *prevents HF hospitalization*	x – *FDA approved to reduce MACE*	x – *FDA approved for DKD*
	Empagliflozin	x – *prevents HF hospitalization*	x – *FDA approved to reduce CV mortality*	x
GLP1 receptor agonists	Dulaglutide		x – *reduces MACE*	x
	Exenatide		x	x
	Liraglutide		x – *reduces MACE*	x
	Semaglutide		x – *reduces MACE*	x

ASCVD, Atherosclerotic cardiovascular disease; CV, cardiovascular; *DKD*, diabetic kidney disease; *HFrEF*, heart failure with reduced ejection fraction; *MACE*, major adverse cardiovascular events.

What are various A1c target goals that can be considered for this patient?

For most nonpregnant adults, a target HbA1c <7% is a good starting point, although treatment goals should be individualized. Higher goals (e.g., <8%) can be made for patients who have a limited life expectancy, several comorbid conditions, advanced micro/macrovascular complications, history of severe hypoglycemia, or otherwise very difficult to control diabetes. Lower goals (e.g., <6.5%) can be made in certain individuals who have long life expectancy, short duration of diabetes, ability to control their T2DM with lifestyle modifications or metformin alone, and do not have significant cardiovascular disease.

It is reasonable to tell this patient that his A1c goal for now can be <7.0% while he is on metformin and liraglutide.

Case Summary

- **Complaint/History:** A 49-year-old man with a history of obesity comes in after 2 days of polyuria, polydipsia, abdominal pain, and nausea.
- **Findings:** The patient has tachycardia, tachypnea, hypotension, and diffuse abdominal tenderness.
- **Lab Results/Tests:** Lab tests show a widened anion gap, a metabolic acidosis, ketonemia, and an elevated serum glucose. In the workup of inciting factors for DKA, his physical examination and a positive UA pointed toward a UTI.

Diagnosis: T2DM complicated by DKA.

- **Treatment:** The patient was initially started on metformin and long-acting and short-acting insulin. After lifestyle modifications he was able to stop all insulin. He was started on an SGLT2 inhibitor but had a UTI recurrence; therefore, he was switched to a GLP1 RA with continued control of his diabetes.

BEYOND THE PEARLS

- The serum anion gap (AG) is sometimes reported in lab data but committing its formula to memory is useful: serum sodium – (serum chloride + serum bicarbonate).
- Hyperosmolar hyperglycemic state (HHS) differs from DKA in that plasma glucose will be markedly elevated (often >600 mg/dL), arterial pH >7.3, serum bicarbonate >18 mEq/L, anion gap normal or slightly elevated, and little to no ketones are present in the serum or urine. The serum osmolality will be >320 mOsm/kg and patients often present with stupor or coma. The management of HHS is very similar to DKA.
- The total body deficit of potassium at the time of DKA presentation is about 3–5 mEq/kg, although patients often present with mild to moderate hyperkalemia. Because volume expansion, insulin therapy, and overall correction of acidosis decrease serum potassium levels, it is imperative to replete potassium stores adequately during DKA.
- Treatment with bicarbonate in DKA can be considered if serum pH is 6.9–7.0 (50 mmol of $NaHCO_3$ dilute in 200 mL H_2O; 200 mL/h can be given) or pH <6.9 (100 mmol of $NaHCO_3$ dilute in 200 mL H_2O; 200 mL/h). Repeat administrations can be done every 2 hours until the pH >7.0.
- Of the sulfonylureas, glipizide does not need renal dose adjustment. Among the GLP1 RAs, dulaglutide, liraglutide, and semaglutide can be continued regardless of renal function. Linagliptin is the DPP4 inhibitor that also does not need renal dose adjustment.
- The dopamine receptor agonist bromocriptine mesylate is not often used as an antidiabetic but is FDA approved for the treatment of T2DM in a quick release tablet form.
- Metformin and GLP1 RAs are the two classes of noninsulin antidiabetics that lower HbA1c the most, by 1.0–2.0% and 0.5–2.5%, respectively.

Bibliography

Baranski, T., McGill, J., & Silverstein, J. (2020). *Washington manual endocrinology subspecialty consult* (4th ed.). Philadelphia, PA: Wolters Kluwer.

Consensus Statement by the American Association of Clinical Endocrinologists and American College of Endocrinology on the Comprehensive Type 2 Diabetes Management Algorithm – 2020 Executive Summary. AACE. https://www.aace.com/pdfs/diabetes/algorithm-exec-summary.pdf. Published January 2020.

Dhatariya, K. (2017). Blood ketones: Measurement, interpretation, limitations, and utility in the management of diabetic ketoacidosis. *The Review of Diabetic Studies: RDS*, *13*(4), 217–225.

For healthcare professionals: Invokana. *Invokana.com*. https://www.invokanahcp.com/?gclid=Cj0KCQjw_j1BRDkARIsAJcfmTFFxsA85YdL9ULcHHkaJufUu8nxUUm3NiP8hVZiuw31AM1YwyHRa_MaAsp3EALw_wcB&gclsrc=aw.ds. Updated 2020.

Glycemic targets: Standards of medical care in diabetes – 2019. (2019). *Diabetes Care*, *42*(1), S61–S70.

Kernan, W., Viscoli, C., Furie, K., et al. (2016). Pioglitazone after ischemic stroke or transient ischemic attack. *NEJM*, *374*, 1321–1331.

Marso, S., Bain, S., Consoli, A., et al. (2016). Semaglutide and cardiovascular outcomes in patients with type 2 diabetes. *NEJM*, *375*, 1834–1844.

Mouri M, Badireddy M. Hyperglycemia. StatPearls. https://www.ncbi.nlm.nih.gov/books/NBK430900/#article-23176.r1. Updated February 25, 2020.

Nauck, M. A., Kahle, M., Baranov, O., et al. (2017). Addition of a dipeptidyl peptidase-4 inhibitor, sitagliptin to ongoing therapy with the glucagon like peptide-1 receptor agonist liraglutide: A randomized controlled trial in patients with type 2 diabetes. *Diabetes, Obesity & Metabolism*, *19*(2), 200–207.

Perkovic, V., Jardine, M. J., Neal, B., et al. (2019). Canagliflozin and renal outcomes in type 2 diabetes and nephropathy. *NEJM*, *380*, 2295–2306.

Umpierrez, G., Murphy, M. B., & Kitabchi, A. E. (2002). Diabetic ketoacidosis and hyperglycemic hyperosmolar syndrome. *Diabetes Spectrum*, *15*(1), 28–36.

CASE 50

A 48-Year-Old Male With Bitemporal Hemianopsia

Chih-Han Lee ■ John David Carmichael

A 48-year-old male with past medical history of hypertension and type 2 diabetes mellitus presents to the neuro-ophthalmologist with 1 week of double vision. A visual field plot shows dense bitemporal hemianopsia suggesting a lesion compressing the optic chiasm.

An urgent magnetic resonance imaging (MRI) of the brain with and without contrast (Fig. 50.1) reveals a sellar mass most consistent with a pituitary macroadenoma extending superiorly with compression of the optic chiasm. The patient also reports feeling more fatigued over the past 3 months. On physical examination, blood pressure is 132/94 mmHg, pulse rate is 72 beats/min, respiration rate is 16 breaths/min, oxygen saturation is 100% on room air, and temperature is 97.2 °F. Examination is significant for bitemporal hemianopsia (Fig. 50.2). The remainder of the physical examination is normal with no evidence of round facies, dorsocervical fat pad, abdominal striae, central obesity, petechiae, or purpura. There is no acral enlargement, coarse facial features, or frontal bossing.

What is a sellar mass?

A sellar mass is a lesion located within or near the sella turcica, which is a saddle-like bony compartment in the skull. The pituitary gland is located within the sella turcica. Nearby structures include the cavernous sinuses, which are located laterally to the pituitary gland, forming the lateral boundary of the sella turcica and the optic chiasm and optic tracts, which are located superiorly. The diaphragma sellae is a thin membrane of dura mater separating the superior aspect of the sella turcica from the optic chiasm.

What is the differential diagnosis for a mass in the sellar region?

The types of lesions in the sellar region and the frequencies of these masses are summarized in Table 50.1. The vast majority of masses in the sellar region are pituitary adenomas. Other less common sellar lesions include Rathke's cleft cyst, craniopharyngioma, and meningioma. Therefore, a pituitary adenoma should be ruled out before considering the presence of other rare sellar lesions. Imaging characteristics of these lesions help refine the differential diagnosis as there are characteristic findings of craniopharyngiomas, meningiomas, and Rathke's cleft cysts that may favor these entities.

Pituitary adenomas are best shown on contrast-enhanced MRI and usually enhance later and/or to a lesser degree than normal pituitary tissue but enhance more than the surrounding central nervous system (CNS) tissue. Fig. 50.1 shows the classic appearance of a pituitary macroadenoma on contrast-enhanced MRI with enhancement to a lesser degree than normal pituitary tissue but more than CNS tissue. Based on the imaging features and location of the sellar mass, the sellar lesion shown on this patient's MRI is most likely to be a pituitary adenoma.

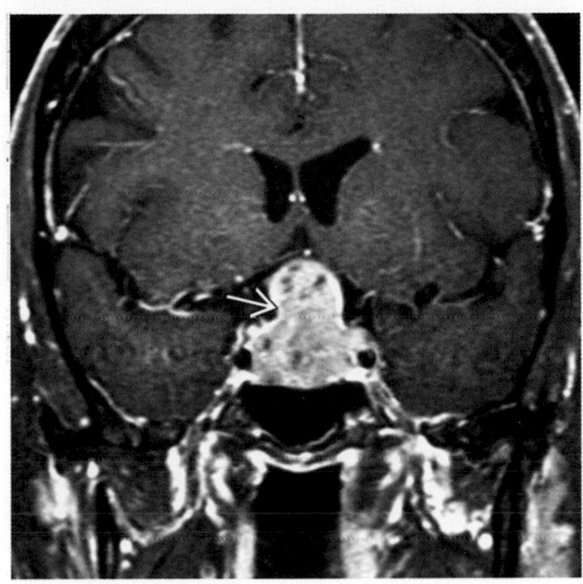

Fig. 50.1 Brain MRI with and without contrast. Coronal T1 postgadolinium (C+) fat-suppressed (FS) MR shows a heterogeneously enhancing pituitary macroadenoma with suprasellar extension and compression of the optic chiasm. (From Osborn, A. G. & Digre, K. B. (2016). *Imaging in neurology* (p. 268). Elsevier.)

TABLE 50.1 ■ **Frequency of Pituitary Adenomas and Other Lesions of the Sellar Region**

Lesion	Frequency (%)
Pituitary adenoma	74
Rathke's cleft cyst	5
Craniopharyngioma	4
Pituitary apoplexy	2
Cysts	2
Inflammatory lesions	1
Metastases	1
Meningiomas	1
Miscellaneous	1
Normal pituitary	9

From Lopes, M.B. (2013). Tumors of the pituitary gland. In C. D. M. Fletcher (Ed.) *Diagnostic histopathology of tumors* (4th ed., Vol. 2, pp. 1211–1243). Philadelphia: Livingstone.

What is the clinical significance of pituitary tumor size?

Pituitary microadenomas are tumors less than 1 cm. Microadenomas almost always remain confined to the sellar region but may compress on the anterior pituitary gland, causing some degree of hypofunction of the normal anterior pituitary. Microadenomas rarely compress the posterior pituitary gland, and function of the posterior pituitary is therefore typically preserved. In fact, diabetes insipidus is quite uncommon with pituitary adenomas of any size.

Pituitary macroadenomas are tumors measuring 1 cm or more. This patient has a pituitary macroadenoma. Unlike microadenomas, macroadenomas tend to exert pressure on or remodel adjacent bony structures and invade the meninges, possibly causing headaches. Macroadenomas also have the potential to extend superiorly, compressing the nearby optic chiasm and causing the classic symptom of bitemporal hemianopsia, which is seen in this patient as shown in Fig 50.2.

BASIC SCIENCE PEARL **STEP 1**

Information from the temporal visual field falls on the nasal (medial) retina. The nasal retina fibers, which carry information to the nasal retina, cross at the optic chiasm. Therefore, lesions of the optic chiasm typically cause impaired peripheral vision in the outer temporal halves of the visual field in each eye. This visual field defect is known as bitemporal hemianopsia. Bitemporal hemianopsia is the most common visual field defect in patients with pituitary macroadenoma.

What are the subtypes of pituitary adenoma?

Pituitary adenomas are monoclonal masses that arise from differentiated cells in the anterior pituitary. Pituitary adenomas may be clinically silent or secrete trophic hormones. These hormones include growth hormone (GH), prolactin (PRL), adrenocorticotrophic hormone (ACTH), thyroid-stimulating hormone (TSH), follicle-stimulating hormone (FSH), and luteinizing hormone (LH). The tumors are considered functional if they secrete in excess one or more of these hormones and are considered nonfunctional if they are not hormone secreting.

How to tell whether a pituitary adenoma is functional or nonfunctional?

The disorders associated with functional pituitary adenoma include acromegaly, prolactinoma, Cushing's disease, and, rarely, TSH-secreting and functional gonadotroph tumors. The functional pituitary adenomas and associated diagnostic workup are summarized in Table 50.2. It is important to keep in mind that the overall incidence of functional hormone-secreting tumors in asymptomatic subjects with incidentally discovered pituitary masses is low. Therefore, in the absence of

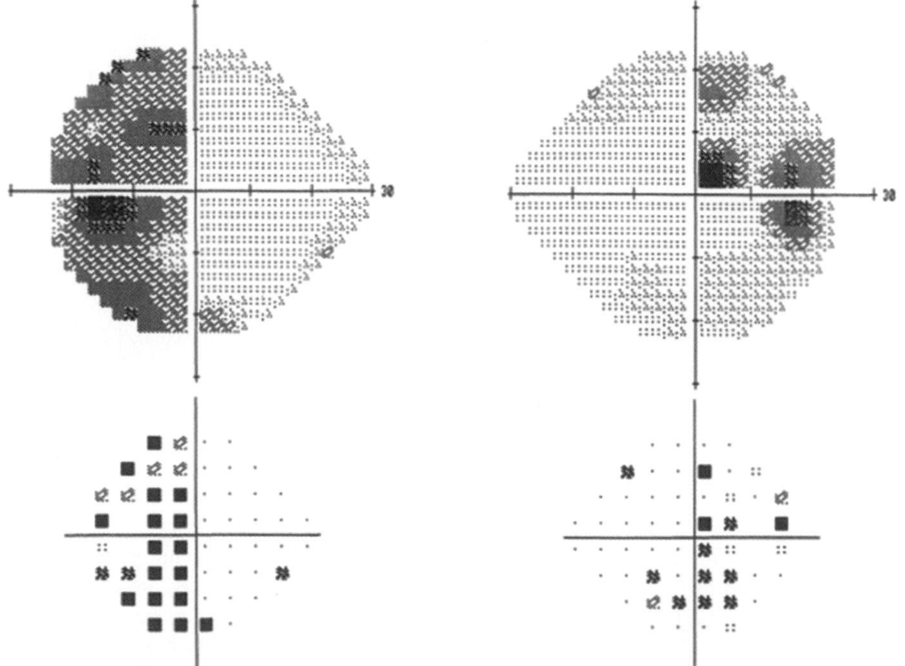

Fig. 50.2 Visual field plot demonstrating bitemporal hemianopsia. This is a common visual field deficit observed with growth of pituitary adenoma. (From Bi, W. L., Smith, T. R., Nery, B., Dunn, I. F. & Laws, E. R. (2011). Pituitary tumors: functioning and nonfunctioning, In H. R. Winn (Ed.), *Youmans and Winn neurological surgery* (pp. 1155–1182.e7). Philadelphia: Saunders.)

TABLE 50.2 ■ **Screening Tests for Functional Pituitary Adenomas**

Disorder	Test	Comments
Acromegaly	IGF-1	Interpret IGF-1 relative to age- and gender-matched controls.
	OGTT with GH obtained at 0, 30, and 60 min	Normal subjects should suppress GH to <1 µg/dL.
Prolactinoma	Serum PRL level	A level >500 µg/dL is pathognomonic for prolactinoma. If >200 µg/dL, prolactinoma is likely.*
Cushing's disease	24-h UFC	Ensure that urine collection is total and accurate by measuring urinary creatinine.
	Night-time salivary cortisol	Free salivary cortisol reflects circadian rhythm, and elevated levels may indicate Cushing's disease.
	Dexamethasone (1 mg) at 11 p.m. and fasting plasma cortisol measured at 8 a.m.	Normal subjects suppress to <5 µg/dL.
	ACTH assay	Distinguishes adrenal adenoma from ectopic ACTH or Cushing's disease.
TSH-secreting tumor	TSH measurement, free T4 by dialysis, total T3	If T4 or T3 is elevated and TSH is measurable or elevated, a TSH-secreting tumor is present.

From Melmed, S., Polonsky, K. S., Larsen, P. R., & Kronenberg, H. M. (2011). *Williams textbook of endocrinology* (12th ed.). Philadelphia: WB Saunders.
*Risperidone may result in prolactin levels >200 µg/dL.
ACTH, Adrenocorticotropic hormone; *GH*, growth hormone; *IGF-1*, insulin-like growth factor type 1; *OGTT*, oral glucose tolerance test; *PRL*, prolactin; *T3*, triiodothyronine; *T4*, thyroxine; *TSH*, thyroid-stimulating hormone; *UFC*, urinary free cortisol.

clinical features of a disorder associated with functional pituitary adenoma, cost-effective laboratory screening should be performed.

An insulin like growth factor 1 (IGF 1) or oral glucose tolerance test (OGTT) with GH obtained at 0, 30, and 60 minutes are the two screening tests that can be used to evaluate for acromegaly. IGF-1 should be interpreted relative to age-matched and gender-matched control groups. Normal subjects should suppress GH to less than 1 µg/L (or less than 0.4 µg/L using sensitive assays) after OGTT.

CLINICAL PEARL **STEP 2/3**

Acromegaly is caused by hypersecretion of GH and IGF-1. Clinical manifestations of acromegaly may not come to medical attention until 10 years or more after the onset of symptoms. Features of acromegaly include frontal bossing, increased hand and foot size, mandibular enlargement with protrusion of the lower jaw, hyperhidrosis, a deep and hollow-sounding voice, oily skin, arthropathy, proximal muscle weakness and fatigue, acanthosis nigricans, and skin tags.

Serum PRL above 200 ng/mL is suggestive of prolactinoma and any level above 500 ng/mL is considered strongly suggestive for prolactinoma. A minimal to moderate elevation can indicate stalk effect by a pituitary mass that is usually nonfunctional. Significant elevation in PRL can also be caused by psychiatric medications such as antipsychotics and antidepressants and part of the history should therefore include a thorough review of these medications.

BASIC SCIENCE/CLINICAL PEARL **STEP 1/2/3**

Pituitary stalk effect is caused by compression of portal vessels by a sellar mass. Compression of the portal vessels disrupts access of hypothalamic hormones and dopamine to the anterior pituitary. Dopamine holds a predominant role in the regulation of prolactin secretion by directly inhibiting the secretion of prolactin by anterior pituitary lactotrophs. Therefore, compression of the portal vessels can result in moderate hyperprolactinemia. Pituitary stalk effect can also contribute to hypopituitarism by impairing the secretion of pituitary hormones that are regulated by the hypothalamus.

Cushing's disease can be screened by measurement of urinary free cortisol over a 24-hour collection, night-time salivary cortisol, or the 1-mg dexamethasone suppression test, which is performed by administering dexamethasone 1 mg at 11 p.m. and then measuring fasting plasma cortisol at 8 a.m. A normal response to the dexamethasone suppression test is a plasma cortisol level of less than 5 μg/dL the following morning between 8 a.m. and 9 a.m. Selection of these tests depends on a variety of factors, with multiple tests required for diagnosis.

CLINICAL PEARL **STEP 2/3**

Clinical features of Cushing's syndrome include obesity, thin skin, round facies, hypertension, purple skin striae, hirsutism, acne, menstrual disorders, proximal muscle weakness, easy bruising, glucose intolerance or diabetes mellitus, and central redistribution of fat.

A TSH-secreting tumor may be present if free thyroxine (T_4) and total triiodothyronine (T_3) are elevated with a normal or elevated TSH.

The list of the patient's medications is shown in Table 50.3. The results of laboratory testing are shown in Table 50.4.

TABLE 50.3 ■ **Patient Medication List**

- Amlodipine 10 mg once a day
- Metformin 1000 mg twice a day

TABLE 50.4 ■ **Patient Laboratory Tests**

Laboratory Tests	
FSH	5.2 mIU/mL (ref 1.5–12.4 mIU/mL)
LH	1.8 mIU/mL (ref 1.7–8.6 mIU/mL)
Total testosterone	162 (ref 250–1100 ng/dL)
Prolactin	21.3 ng/mL (ref 4.0–15.2 ng/mL)
IGF-1	108 ng/mL (ref 41–279 ng/mL)
TSH	1.94 mIU/L (ref 0.3–4.0 mIU/L)
Free T4	0.57 ng/dL (ref 0.93–1.70 ng/dL)
ACTH Stimulation Test	
8 a.m. Cortisol (time 0)	19.1 μg/dL
Cortisol (time 30 min)	24.2 μg/dL
Cortisol (time 60 min)	23.6 μg/dL

What is your differential diagnosis based on these laboratory results?

This is a 48-year-old male who presents with 3 months of fatigue, 1 week of double vision, bitemporal hemianopsia on visual field plot, MRI showing a sellar mass with compression of the optic chiasm, mildly elevated serum prolactin low total testosterone after serum prolactin, and low free T4.

The patient has a pituitary macroadenoma. The next step in the diagnostic workup is to determine whether or not the pituitary tumor is functional or nonfunctional and to evaluate the patient for hypopituitarism. The common clinical manifestations of a nonfunctional pituitary tumor are shown in Table 50.5.

TABLE 50.5 ■ **Manifestations of Nonfunctional Pituitary Adenomas**

Organ	Manifestation
Nervous system	Visual field deficits, extraocular muscle palsy, headache
Endocrine	Amenorrhea, decreased libido, apoplexy

From Mayson, S. E. & Snyder, P. J. (2015). Silent pituitary adenomas. *Endocrinology and Metabolism Clinics of North America, 44,* 79–87.

How can ACTH deficiency be diagnosed?

Cortisol should be measured between 8 a.m. and 9 a.m. A serum cortisol value less than or equal to 3 µg/dL confirmed by repeat testing is strong evidence of cortisol deficiency. On the other hand, a serum cortisol value greater than or equal to 18 µg/dL indirectly indicates sufficient basal ACTH secretion. Because adrenal insufficiency caused by hypopituitarism is a result of ACTH deficiency, dynamic testing with ACTH stimulation can also be used as a surrogate. Although the ACTH stimulation test is a test of adrenal reserve rather than pituitary reserve, it can provide valuable information because the adrenal cortex atrophies when it lacks stimulation from pituitary ACTH. Adrenal atrophy takes time to develop and this test cannot therefore diagnose acute ACTH deficiency. The time it takes for adrenal atrophy to take place is variable but is usually greater than 4 weeks. An ACTH stimulation test is performed by drawing a baseline cortisol and then administering 250 µg of cosyntropin (a commercially available ACTH analog) intravenously or intramuscularly. Serum cortisol is again collected at 30 and 60 minutes postcosyntropin. A normal response is a cortisol level greater than 18–20 µg/dL at either time point.

This patient has a normal response to cosyntropin with cortisol 24.2 µg/dL and 23.6 µg/dL at 30 and 60 minutes postcosyntropin. Given these findings, hormone replacement with glucocorticoid is not indicated. Additionally, in the absence of signs and symptoms suggestive of Cushing's disease, screening for Cushing's disease is also not indicated.

How can secondary hypothyroidism be diagnosed?

Unlike patients with primary hypothyroidism, an elevated serum TSH cannot be used to make a diagnosis of secondary hypothyroidism. In fact, TSH is typically normal in patients with secondary hypothyroidism. Therefore, screening for hypothyroidism in patients with pituitary adenoma should be performed by measuring total T4 and T3 uptake or free T4. This patient has a low serum free T4 with inappropriately normal TSH, which is consistent with secondary hypothyroidism.

How can secondary hypogonadism be diagnosed?

In a man with pituitary adenoma, gonadotropin deficiency can be detected by measuring the serum testosterone and serum LH. This patient has a low total testosterone with inappropriately normal serum LH. The patient has secondary hypogonadism based on these findings. In women, testing for secondary hypogonadism depends on whether the patient is premenopausal and whether she has oligomenorrhea or amenorrhea. If the woman has a pituitary mass but normal menstrual menses, there is no need to check FSH or LH because the presence of a normal menstrual cycle is a more sensitive indicator of an intact hypothalamic-pituitary-gonadal axis. In a woman with oligomenorrhea or amenorrhea, serum LH and FSH should be measured. Low LH and FSH are suggestive of secondary hypogonadism.

How can growth hormone deficiency be diagnosed?

A serum IGF-1 test is helpful to exclude acromegaly and can rule out the disease in most cases when the result is in the normal range. Serum IGF-1 levels less than the lower limit of normal for age suggests but does not confirm the diagnosis of growth hormone deficiency. It is rarely necessary to diagnose GH deficiency prior to treating pituitary tumors. In adults, diagnosis relies on the presence of multiple pituitary deficiencies or the use of GH secretagogue testing to stimulate GH secretion. This patient has a serum IGF-1 normal for his age, making acromegaly unlikely. Further testing for GH deficiency may be required after other hormonal deficiencies and the tumor mass are treated.

BASIC SCIENCE/CLINICAL PEARL **STEP 1/2/3**

The order of pituitary dysfunction is usually as follows: GH > FSH > LH > TSH > ACTH. The corticotroph cell is particularly resistant to hypothalamic or pituitary destruction and is usually the last lineage to lose function.

How do you explain the hyperprolactinemia in this patient?

The minimal PRL elevation in this patient is most likely a result of stalk effect rather than a prolactinoma. The patient is also not taking medications known to cause elevation in PRL such as antidepressants and antipsychotics.

CLINICAL PEARL **STEP 2/3**

Symptoms of hyperprolactinemia in women include amenorrhea, galactorrhea, and infertility. Diminished libido, infertility, and visual loss are the usual presenting symptoms of hyperprolactinemia in men.

Based on these laboratory findings, the patient most probably has a nonfunctioning pituitary macroadenoma with secondary hypothyroidism, secondary hypogonadism, and mildly elevated prolactin, probably caused by stalk effect.

What are the treatment options for a nonfunctioning pituitary macroadenoma?

The patient has a nonfunctioning pituitary macroadenoma. Surgical resection of nonfunctioning adenoma is recommended if vision is threatened or if the size of the mass threatens vital structures. The macroadenoma has caused significant visual impairment in this patient and treatment must therefore be directed at reducing the size of the mass and restoring visual defects as soon as possible. Transsphenoidal surgery is the treatment of choice. Radiation therapy is used to prevent growth of residual adenoma tissue following surgery, especially when a considerable amount of tissue remains and/or risk for growth appears high.

CLINICAL PEARL **STEP 2/3**

Oral dopamine agonists (cabergoline and bromocriptine) are the first-line therapy for patients with micro- and macroprolactinomas. For patients with macroadenoma, a baseline visual field test should be performed prior to initiation of therapy. MRI and visual field tests should be assessed at 6- to 12-month intervals until the mass shrinks and annually thereafter until maximum size reduction has been achieved.

Treatment for functional pituitary adenoma is highly specific and depends on the tumor type. Medical therapy with a dopamine agonist (e.g., cabergoline and bromocriptine) is the initial step in treatment of prolactinoma. Except for prolactinomas, surgical resection using a transsphenoidal approach is the preferred primary treatment for acromegaly, Cushing's disease, and TSH-secreting adenomas. For persistent or recurrent acromegaly, somatostatin receptor ligands such as octreotide can be used as primary treatment for nonsurgical candidates or adjuvant therapy after transsphenoidal surgery. Postsurgical treatment of persistent disease or recurrence includes dopamine agonists, the GH receptor antagonist pegvisomant, or somatostatin receptor antagonists.

The patient is recommended for surgical resection of the pituitary macroadenoma by the transsphenoidal approach. Risks and benefits of the procedure are explained to the patient, and he agrees to proceed with surgery scheduled in 2 weeks. He is started on weight-based dosing of levothyroxine (1.6 μg /kg) daily prior to surgery given laboratory findings suggestive of secondary hypothyroidism. Testosterone replacement is not necessary prior to surgery. Recovery of the hypothalamic-pituitary-gonadal axis should be reassessed 4 to 6 weeks after surgical resection.

What are the common postoperative endocrine complications that can occur after surgical resection of pituitary macroadenoma?

Common endocrine complications that can occur in patients after surgical resection of a pituitary mass are transient diabetes insipidus (up to 30%) and new hypopituitarism (usually <5%) . Permanent diabetes insipidus may occur in up to 10% of patients, with most centers reporting frequencies less than 5%. In patients treated for microadenoma, permanent side effects are rare.

What are the postoperative considerations after pituitary surgery?

For patients who had a functional adenoma prior to surgery, any hormones that were produced in excess should be measured again. Screening for adrenal insufficiency should be performed in all patients the following day with a serum cortisol drawn between 8 a.m. and 9 a.m. Additional evaluation for hypopituitarism should be done 4 to 6 weeks after surgical resection.

Patients should also be monitored closely for fluid balance and serum sodium level after pituitary surgery. Isolated excess polyuria or hyponatremia are commonly encountered complications. When water balance disturbances occur in the postoperative period, they commonly appear in a triphasic response. In the early postoperative period, transient diabetes insipidus (DI) is more frequently encountered than syndrome of inappropriate secretion of antidiuretic hormone (SIADH). DI presents clinically with large volumes of dilute urine and increased thirst in patients with an intact thirst mechanism. Therefore, in the absence of hyperglycemia, a low urine specific gravity (<1.005) combined with a high urine volume greater than 300 mL/h for 2 consecutive hours is highly suggestive of DI. This typically resolves within 48 hours of surgery. Subsequently, hyponatremia may present later in the postoperative period, typically appearing around postoperative day 7. Because of the risk of delayed hyponatremia, patients are commonly scheduled for a serum sodium check about 1 week following surgery. The third and least common phase of water balance disturbance is diabetes insipidus, which may be permanent.

CLINICAL PEARL **STEP 2/3**

The full classic triphasic response of diabetes insipidus, syndrome of inappropriate secretion of ADH, and diabetes insipidus that has been described in the literature is only seen in a small percentage of patients after pituitary surgery. The pathophysiology of the triphasic response appears to be a result of early hypothalamic dysfunction followed by release of ADH from degenerating pituitary and, finally, depletion of ADH stores.

An uncomplicated endoscopic transsphenoidal craniotomy for resection of the pituitary macroadenoma is performed with rapid improvement in the patient's visual symptoms. He has a repeat 8 a.m. cortisol the next morning, which is 15.9 μg/dL. The patient is discharged on postoperative day 2 in stable condition with normal vital signs and no lethargy, polydipsia, polyuria, or electrolyte abnormalities.

The patient returns to the hospital 5 days later with symptoms of extreme fatigue, weakness, and poor appetite. He is found to be hypotensive with blood pressure of 76/48 mmHg. The rest of the vitals are normal with pulse rate of 79 beats/min, respiration rate of 18 breaths/min, oxygen saturation of 98% on room air, and temperature of 97.9 °F. Laboratory findings are significant for serum sodium of 132 mmol/L, serum osmolality of 278 mOsm/kg, urine sodium of 41 mmol/L, urine osmolality of 311 mOsm/kg, random cortisol of 1.3 μg/dL, and free T4 of 1.2 ng/dL.

What is the differential diagnosis based on these findings?

The patient is now presenting with symptoms of fatigue, weakness, and poor appetite with vital signs significant for hypotension and laboratory findings significant for hyponatremia. The differential diagnosis includes SIADH, cerebral salt wasting (CSW), adrenal insufficiency, and hypothyroidism (see Table 50.6).

CSW is a rare cause of postoperative hyponatremia. Although CSW can lead to hypovolemia, it is unlikely to contribute to this patient's hypotension. In addition, it is unlikely for hyponatremia to cause the degree of lethargy experienced by this patient. Both CSW and SIADH present with low plasma osmolality (<280 mOsm/kg), inappropriately high urine osmolality (urine osmolality >100 mOsm/kg), and natriuresis with urinary sodium that is typically >40 mmol/L. Adrenal insufficiency and hypothyroidism can also cause hyponatremia. Cortisol and thyroid hormone are both known to regulate ADH secretion. Thus, hypocortisolism and hypothyroidism can produce the SIADH-like clinical picture seen in this patient with delayed post-transsphenoidal hyponatremia. However, hypothyroidism is unlikely to be contributing to this patient's presentation given the normal free T4 of 1.2 ng/dL. Instead, the patient has signs and symptoms and a random cortisol of <2 μg/dL that are all more suggestive of adrenal insufficiency.

A day 1 postoperative early morning cortisol test has been shown by clinical studies to be a useful tool to predict ACTH deficiency postpituitary surgery. There is no consensus regarding the cutoff for the morning serum cortisol levels that points to ACTH-cortisol insufficiency or sufficiency. Some propose a cutoff of <3.6 μg/dL or <6 μg/dL for ACTH deficiency and a cutoff of >10.9 μg/dL or >18 μg/dL to correlate with ACTH sufficiency. These authors recommend further testing such as the ACTH stimulation test to assess pituitary-adrenal function in patients with morning serum cortisol levels between these cutoff values. This patient's day 1 postoperative early morning cortisol level is 15.9 μg/dL. This level of cortisol secretion correlates with ACTH sufficiency if using the cutoff of >10.9 μg/dL but indeterminate if using a cutoff of >18 μg/dL. A potential screening method for assessing cortisol stress response

TABLE 50.6 ■ **Etiologies of Hyponatremia After Pituitary Surgery**

Etiologies

- Syndrome of inappropriate antidiuretic hormone secretion (SIADH)
- Cerebral salt wasting (CSW)
- Desmopressin acetate overdose
- Adrenal insufficiency
- Hypothyroidism
- Excessive intake of hypotonic fluids

following pituitary surgery is the change (Δ) in cortisol index. The Δ cortisol index is defined as the difference between the postoperative day (POD) 1 morning cortisol level and the preoperative morning cortisol level. In the published study, the mean Δ cortisol index in patients who required postoperative glucocorticoids was −2.8 μg/dL and +14.4 μg/dL in patients without evidence of adrenal insufficiency. Thus, in patients with uncertain early morning cortisol values such as in this patient, alternative screening methods such as the Δ cortisol index or empiric treatment followed by further testing with an ACTH stimulation test can be considered.

The patient is admitted to the hospital. He receives 2 L of normal saline bolus and one dose of hydrocortisone 100 mg intravenous (IV) followed by hydrocortisone 50 mg IV every 6 hours with improvement in symptoms within the first 6 hours. He is discharged the next day with instructions to continue a twice per day oral regimen of hydrocortisone.

How do you monitor patients after surgical resection of pituitary adenoma?

Patients who have evidence of hormone deficiency before and after surgical resection should continue hormone treatment. In one study, improvement in preoperative hormonal dysfunction was noted in 49% of patients after removal of pituitary adenoma (Fatemi et al., 2008). Evaluation for hypopituitarism can be repeated 4 to 6 weeks after surgical resection. Because this patient is being treated with hydrocortisone and levothyroxine, he will need to be tapered off both medications before being evaluated for improvement in ACTH and TSH hormone deficiencies.

An MRI should be performed 6 months postoperatively and then annually to monitor for tumor regrowth. The patient should also have at least an annual follow-up with neuro-ophthalmology.

The patient remains on a twice per day oral regimen of hydrocortisone and once a day weight-based dosing of levothyroxine on follow-up in 6 weeks. Because his repeat free T4 in 6 weeks is elevated, the levothyroxine dose is reduced. Total testosterone is in the normal range on follow-up. Over the course of 6 months, he is tapered off both hydrocortisone and levothyroxine with no clinical evidence of adrenal insufficiency or hypothyroidism. Repeat free T4 on 6-month follow-up is normal. A follow up MRI 6 months postoperative demonstrates no recurrence of pituitary adenoma.

Case Summary

- **Complaint/History:** A 48-year-old-male presents with 3 months of fatigue and 1 week of double vision.
- **Findings:** Bitemporal hemianopsia on physical examination.
- **Lab Results/Tests:** Lab tests reveal mildly elevated prolactin, low total testosterone, and low free thyroxine (T_4) and bitemporal hemianopsia on visual field plot; magnetic resonance imaging of the brain with and without contrast reveals a pituitary macroadenoma with suprasellar extension and compression of the optic chiasm.

Diagnosis: Nonfunctioning pituitary macroadenoma with secondary hypothyroidism, secondary hypogonadism and mildly elevated prolactin likely from stalk effect.

- **Treatment:** The patient underwent pituitary macroadenoma resection by the transsphenoidal approach and was then discharged on a weight-based dose of levothyroxine. The patient then presented to the hospital 5 days later with signs, symptoms, and laboratory findings concerning for adrenal insufficiency. He was started on stress-dose hydrocortisone and then discharged on a twice per day oral regimen of hydrocortisone and continued taking weight-based levothyroxine. The patient was tapered off hydrocortisone and levothyroxine 6 months later without signs or symptoms of adrenal insufficiency or hypothyroidism. Free T_4 and total testosterone were normal on 6-month follow-up and repeat MRI in 6 months showed no evidence of recurrence.

BEYOND THE PEARLS

- Approximately 30% of surgically resected adenomas have persistent or progressive postoperative growth for up to four decades or longer.
- Pituitary carcinomas are extremely rare, accounting for less than 0.5% of pituitary tumors.
- Radiation therapy is typically reserved for tumors that are resistant to medical therapy or tumors that are not controlled by surgery. In most patients treated with radiation therapy, hypopituitarism develops within 10 years and lifelong hormone replacement is often required.
- Pituitary adenomas may occur in association with rare genetic syndromes. Multiple endocrine neoplasia type 1 is associated with pituitary adenomas and parathyroid and pancreatic islet tumors. McCune-Albright syndrome, which is characterized by polyostotic fibrous dysplasia, cutaneous pigmentation, and sexual precocity, is associated with hyperthyroidism, hypercortisolism, hyperprolactinemia, and acromegaly. Rare cases of familial pituitary adenomas have been reported in families with history of somatotroph tumors in childhood or young adulthood. The Carney complex is associated with pituitary adenomas, benign cardiac myxomas, schwannomas, thyroid adenomas, and pigmented skin spots.
- For patients with acromegaly, management of coexisting conditions, such as cardiac dysfunction, hypertension, sleep apnea, and elevated blood glucose levels, is important to reduce the risk of mortality.
- Because approximately 40% of ACTH-secreting corticotroph tumors are not visible on imaging and at least 10% of people in the general population have small, clinically silent microadenomas, accurate diagnosis of Cushing's disease can be difficult. This disorder may be overdiagnosed, especially because clinical features of Cushing's disease often overlap with other more common disorders such as obesity, hypertension, glucose intolerance, and osteoporosis.

Bibliography

Andy, A., Dixon, A. K., Grainger, R., & Allison, D. J. (2008). *Grainger & Allison's diagnostic radiology: a textbook of medical imaging* (pp. 1411–1440). Philadelphia, PA: Churchill Livingstone/Elsevier. Chapter 55.

Arraez. M. A. (2013). Assessment of postoperative hypercortisolism after pituitary surgery: when and how? *World Neurosurg*, *80*(5), 495–497.

Bi WL, Smith TR, Nery B, Dunn IF, Laws ER. (2011). *Youmans and Winn neurological surgery*. Philadelphia, PA: Saunders, Chapter 150, 1155–1182.67.

Bondugulapati, L. N., Campbell, C., Chowdhury, S. R., Goetz, P., Davies, J. S., Rees, D. A., & Hayhurst, C. (2016). Use of day 1 early morning cortisol to predict the need for glucocorticoid replacement after pituitary surgery. *British Journal of Neurosurgery*, *30*(1), 76–79.

Burke, W. T., Cote, D. J., Penn, D. L., Iuliano, S., McMillen, K., & Laws, E. R. (2020). Diabetes insipidus after endoscopic transsphenoidal surgery. *Neurosurgery*, *87*(5), 949–955. 15.

Carmichael, J. D. (2017). *Anterior Pituitary Failure. The pituitary, by S. Melmed* (pp. 329–364) (4th ed.). Elsevier/Academic Press.

Fatemi, N., Dusick, J. R., Mattozo, C., et al. (2008). Pituitary hormonal loss and recovery after transsphenoidal adenoma removal. *Neurosurgery*, *63*, 709–718.

Hensen, J., Henig, A., Fahlbusch, R., et al. (1999). Prevalence, predictors and patterns of postoperative polyuria and hyponatraemia in the immediate course after transsphenoidal surgery for pituitary adenomas. *Clinical Endocrinology*, *50*, 431–439.

Lopes M.B. (2013). Tumors of the pituitary gland. In C. D. M. Fletcher (Ed.) *Diagnostic histopathology of tumors*) (vol. 2.) (pp.1211–1243) (4th ed.). Philadelphia, PA: Livingstone.

Little, A. S., Gardner, P. A., Fernandez-Miranda, J. C., Chicoine, M. R., Barkhoudarian, G., Prevedello, D. M., Yuen KCJ, Kelly, D. F. (2019). Pituitary gland recovery following fully endoscopic transsphenoidal surgery for nonfunctioning pituitary adenoma: results of a prospective multicenter study TRANSSPHER Study Group.. *Journal of Neurosurgery*, *15*, 1–7.

Mayson, S. E., & Snyder, P. J. (2015). Silent pituitary adenomas. *Endocrinology and Metabolism Clinics of North America*, *44*, 79–87.

Melmed, S., Polonsky, K. S., Larsen, P. R., & Kronenberg, H. M. (2011). *Williams textbook of endocrinology* (12th ed.). Philadelphia: WB Saunders.

Melmed. S. (2020). Pituitary-Tumor Endocrinopathies. *The New England Journal of Medicine*, *382*(10), 937–950. 5.

Osborn, A. G., & Digre, K. B. (2016). *Imaging in neurology*. Elsevier.

Schreckinger, M., Walker, B., Knepper, J., Hornyak, M., Hong, D., Kim, J. M., Folbe A, Guthikonda M, Mittal S, Szerlip, N. J. (2013). Post-operative diabetes insipidus after endoscopic transsphenoidal surgery. *Pituitary*, *16*(4), 445–451.

Yuen, K. C. J., Ajmal, A., Correa, R., & Little, A. S. (2019). Sodium perturbations after pituitary surgery. *Neurosurgery Clinics of North America*, *30*(4), 515–524.

Zada, G., Tirosh, A., Huang, A. P., Laws, E. R., & Woodmansee, W. W. (2013). The postoperative cortisol stress response following transsphenoidal pituitary surgery: a potential screening method for assessing preserved pituitary function. *Pituitary*, *16*(3), 319–325.

CASE 51

A 32-Year-Old Female With Recurrent Pregnancy Loss

Reshma Patel ■ Caroline T. Nguyen

A 32-year-old female is referred to your office for outpatient evaluation of infertility. She has previously suffered several spontaneous miscarriages. She reports that her periods usually come every other month and are heavy when they happen. The first date of her last menstrual period was 7 days prior to this appointment. She also reports a 10-pound weight gain over the past 5 years as well as hair loss and dry skin. She also reports feeling cold, even in warm weather, and a history of constipation, for which she takes OTC psyllium husk as needed. She denies any recent fevers, chills, or neck pain. She denies heat intolerance, palpitations, tremors, or excessive sweating.

Her medical history is nonsignificant other than her mother having a history of Graves' disease. Gynecologic history is remarkable for menarche at the age of 13 years. She reports that her periods were regular for the first 10 years but have been irregular since then. She lives with her husband of 7 years. She denies tobacco, alcohol, or drug use. She works as a schoolteacher. She reports that she is currently sexually active with her spouse, not using contraception. She has had three partners since becoming sexually active and reports a history of chlamydia at the age of 17 years, which was treated with azithromycin.

On physical examination her temperature is 97.6°F, pulse rate is 68 beats per minute, blood pressure is 120/90 mm Hg, respiratory rate is 12 respirations per minute, and oxygen saturation is 99% on room air. Patient is 162 cm tall and weighs 72 kg with BMI of 27.4 kg/m^2.

Physical examination is significant for a thyroid that was two times enlarged, symmetric, and soft, with no discrete nodules when palpated. No thyroid bruit was heard upon auscultation. The patient's skin was cool to touch and dry, with hypertrophy/darkening on the extensor surfaces. Neurology exam was remarkable for delayed relaxation phase of the bilateral patellar and brachial reflexes. The patient was also found to have trace pitting edema at the ankles. Genitourinary exam was remarkable for appropriate Tanner stage of breast and pubic hair (Tanner 5) and no clitoromegaly.

What is the differential diagnosis at this time?

The differential diagnosis for this patient's difficulty conceiving is broad. There are multiple endocrinologic etiologies that could explain this patient's infertility. The first is hypothyroidism. This should be the first diagnosis on the differential given the patient's complaints of cold intolerance, weight gain, dry skin, hair loss, and menorrhagia. Thyroid stimulating hormone (TSH) and free thyroxine (T4) tests should be obtained to evaluate for either primary or central hypothyroidism. If the TSH is low in the setting of a low free T4, it may suggest central hypothyroidism and additional workup would be warranted to make sure the patient did not have a pituitary lesion. If the TSH was elevated and the free T4 was low, it would suggest primary hypothyroidism. The most common etiology of primary hypothyroidism is Hashimoto's thyroiditis or autoimmune thyroiditis. Additionally, given that the patient wishes to conceive, a thyroid peroxidase antibody (TPO-Ab), which is an antibody to the enzyme in the thyroid gland that is involved in organification of thyroid hormone, should also be ordered to assess whether thyroid autoimmunity is contributing to her infertility. Polycystic ovary syndrome (PCOS) should also be considered given the patient's irregular menstrual periods and weight gain. Although this patient lacks a hair growth pattern suggestive of PCOS (hair growth on face, more coarse hair in axillary and inguinal distribution), hair loss, weight gain, and oligomenorrhea are key features of PCOS. It is also important to consider Cushing's syndrome when diagnosing infertility because these patients can also have weight gain. However, this patient does not have typical features of Cushing's syndrome (dorsocervical adiposity, wide violaceous striae, central adiposity with thin extremities). An important endocrinologic etiology on the differential would be nonclassic congenital adrenal hyperplasia (CAH), which would present with oligomenorrhea, hirsutism, alopecia, and cliteromegaly. Another important consideration in this case should be physical barriers to embryological implantation; therefore, consultation with gynecology after workup of endocrinologic etiologies should be pursued and should include a hysterosalpingogram and a pelvic ultrasound.

Lab test results were remarkable for a TSH of 24 mIU/L (normal reference range 0.4–4.0 mIU/L) and a free T4 of 0.5 ng/dL (normal reference range 0.8–2.8 ng/dL), and TPO-Ab of 241 (normal reference range <9 IU/mL). Serum estradiol, total testosterone, DHEA-S, and OGTT are all normal.

What are the signs and symptoms of hypothyroidism?

Classically the symptoms of hypothyroidism are nonspecific and include but are not limited to dry skin, cold intolerance, psychomotor slowing, weight gain, constipation, and hoarseness of voice. On physical examination, patients tend to have a coarse, sallow appearance to the skin, slow cognition, cold extremities, and delayed relaxation phase of reflexes. Delayed relaxation phase of reflexes is specific for hypothyroidism and can be seen in severe cases, most notably in the Achilles tendon reflex. These findings may not necessarily be present with a TSH in the 4–10 mIU/L range. In the context of pregnancy, hypothyroidism is defined as a TSH elevated above the pregnancy specific reference range (Alexander et al., 2017). Table 51.1 differentiates the symptoms patients may report with mild hypothyroidism versus the symptoms and clinical findings that may appear in severe hypothyroidism (TSH >10 mIU/L).

CLINICAL PEARL **STEP 2**

Classic symptoms of hypothyroidism are nonspecific and may not necessarily be present in mild cases of hypothyroidism.

TABLE 51.1 ■ **Signs and Symptoms of Hypothyroidism**

TSH: 4.5–10 mIU/L	TSH >10 mIU/L
Cold intolerance	Bradycardia
Weight gain	Psychomotor slowing/delayed cognition
Leg swelling	Coarse skin
Constipation	Puffiness
	Delayed relation of ankle reflexes

From Jonklaas et al., 2014.

What is the incidence of hypothyroidism/thyroid autoimmunity in pregnancy?

Because of differences in normal reference ranges for the thyroid stimulating hormone (TSH) value between various regions of the world as well as recent revision of multiple society guidelines on the definition of an elevated TSH in the first trimester of pregnancy, the prevalence of both hypothyroidism and subclinical hypothyroidism have varied greatly, from 0%–13.1% for hypothyroidism and 1.5%–42.9% for subclinical hypothyroidism. A meta-analysis done by Dong and Stagnaro-Green in 2019 looked at 63 different studies and found that all studies had a pooled incidence of 2.09% of hypothyroidism and 5.1% of subclinical hypothyroidism (Dong & Stagnaro-Green, 2019). With regard to thyroid autoimmunity in pregnancy, a recent meta-analysis published by Korevaar and colleagues (2019) found that 7.5% of pregnant women were thyroid peroxidase antibody (TPO-Ab) positive.

What are the normal changes in thyroid function tests during pregnancy and how are thyroid function tests measured during pregnancy?

During pregnancy, thyroid hormone requirements increase by 30%–50%. This is a result of an increase in iodine excretion at the level of the kidney and an increase in thyroid-binding globulin (TBG) resulting from the effect of estrogen on hepatic TBG synthesis (Okosieme, Khan, & Taylor, 2018). A normal thyroid gland is able to meet this demand by increasing thyroid hormone production. Total thyroid hormone levels increase because of the stimulatory effect of human chorionic gonadotropin (HCG) on the thyroid gland. Free thyroid hormone levels (free T4 and free T3) are maintained in women with adequate iodine intake.

The above physiologic changes result in a decreased TSH level during the first trimester of pregnancy, with a TSH less than 0.4 mIU/L observed in as many as 15% of women (Soldin et al., 2004). The TSH rises during the second and third trimester of pregnancy, but can still remain lower than the normal level in nonpregnant women. Because of the increase in TBG during pregnancy, immunoassays commonly used to measure free T4 may not be an accurate measure of a pregnant woman's true free T4 concentration in the later part of pregnancy. Therefore, laboratory measurements that consider the increase in TBG such as the total T4 and free T4 index may be used as an alternative to measuring free T4, either directly or indirectly, during pregnancy. Fig. 51.1 illustrates the changes in thyroid hormone physiology by trimester. In the first

	TSH	Free T4	Total T4	Thyroxine Binding Globulin (TBG)
First trimester	↓	↑	↑	↑
Second trimester	↔	↓	↑	↑
Third trimester	↔	↓	↑	↑

Fig. 51.1 Changes in thyroid physiology during pregnancy.

trimester, there is an increased output of thyroid hormone because of metabolic demands of the fetus and increased stimulation of the thyroid gland by HCG. Increased estrogen also increases TBG, which leads to an increase in total T4 and decrease in free T4 by the second trimester. In the third trimester, total T4 and a TBG remain high, whereas free T4 starts to fall and TSH normalizes.

CLINICAL PEARL **STEP 1**

In pregnant women without thyroid dysfunction, there is an overall increase in thyroid hormone production and a decrease in TSH in the first trimester of pregnancy extending to the mid-second trimester of pregnancy, with an eventual return to baseline toward the second half of pregnancy.

What are the risks of hypothyroidism in pregnancy?

Multiple studies have demonstrated that overt hypothyroidism in pregnancy is associated with an increased risk of premature birth, low birth weight, pregnancy loss, and risk of lower offspring IQ. Gestational hypertension has also been described in women who are hypothyroid during pregnancy (Leung, Millar et al., 1993). Thyroid autoimmunity in particular carries a risk of pregnancy loss in clinically euthyroid women, although the exact mechanism of how this happens remains unclear (Korevaar et al., 2013).

CLINICAL PEARL **STEP 2**

Complications of overt hypothyroidism in pregnancy include premature birth, low birth weight, pregnancy loss, low offspring IQ, and gestational hypertension.

Who should be considered for hypothyroidism testing in pregnancy?

Populations of women who should be considered for testing of hypothyroidism and thyroid autoimmunity in pregnancy include those women who have had a previous history of hypothyroidism or thyroid autoimmunity and especially those women who are currently on thyroid hormone supplementation or antithyroid medications. Another high-risk population in whom screening for hypothyroidism and thyroid autoimmunity would be warranted would be women who have a history of miscarriage or women who are planning on having reproductive assistance in conceiving. The American Thyroid Association (ATA) and American College of Obstetricians and Gynecologists (ACOG) currently recommend testing of thyroid function in high-risk populations (see Alexander et al., 2017)..

CLINICAL PEARL **STEP 3**

Women who should have their thyroid function checked during pregnancy include those with previous history of recurrent miscarriage, those currently on thyroid hormone supplementation or antithyroid medication, or those with a history of head or neck radiation, a history of type 1 diabetes or other autoimmune disorders, family history of thyroid disease, prior use of amiodarone or lithium, or recent use of iodinated contrast, as well as living in an iodine deficient region.

How would you advise this patient prior to conception?

This patient clearly has evidence of overt hypothyroidism and a compromised thyroid gland. The patient is young and otherwise healthy and should be started on replacement dose thyroid hormone (1.6 μg for every kg of body weight) with a goal TSH level defined by the most recent ATA guidelines as <2.5 mIU/L.

If the patient had subclinical hypothyroidism in which TSH level was elevated in the setting of a normal free T4 level, the decision to treat is often complex and would require referral to an endocrinologist. Patients should be aware that levothyroxine should be taken after waking in the morning and patients should wait 30–60 minutes before taking other medications or supplements. Supplements that interfere with levothyroxine absorption in particular include calcium supplements, antacids such as proton pump inhibitors, H2 blockers, and iron supplements.

The patient is started on weight-based levothyroxine supplementation. The patient is seen again after 6 weeks when she reports better energy and some improvement in her hair and skin as well as some weight loss. She reports that her periods are regular, with her LMP occurring 1 week prior to this appointment. You order lab tests and find that her TSH is 1.3 mIU/L and her free T4 is 1.09 ng/dL. You advise her that should she become pregnant, she should immediately increase her levothyroxine dosage by 2 tablets/week, a 20%–30% dose increase, and to request an appointment to be seen immediately by you.

The patient calls you 6 weeks later and informs you that she is pregnant. She increased the dosage of her levothyroxine according to the instructions provided. You order lab tests and find that her TSH is 1.5 mIU/L and her free T4 is 1.40 ng/dL.

CLINICAL PEARL **STEP 3**

Patients who are overtly hypothyroid prior to pregnancy should be started on thyroid hormone supplementation with a goal TSH of <2.5 mIU/L if pregnancy is desired and should be counseled to use contraception until thyroid levels are normalized.

How would you manage this patient throughout pregnancy?

It is recommended that patients who have had overt hypothyroidism should be started on thyroid hormone replacement prior to conception and should use contraception until thyroid hormone levels have normalized. If patients are noted to be hypothyroid during pregnancy, the levothyroxine dosage should be titrated to the pregnancy specific reference range for TSH. If population specific pregnancy reference ranges are not available, the ATA recommends using a pregnancy specific reference range where the lower limit of normal for TSH is decreased by 0.1–0.2 mIU/L, and the upper limit of normal of TSH is decreased by 0.5–1.0 mIU/L (Alexander et al., 2017). TSH should be maintained within the normal pregnancy specific reference range and should be checked frequently during pregnancy, usually every 4 weeks or as clinically indicated. The dose requirement may increase until the mid-second trimester after which the dose may stabilize for the remainder of pregnancy.

The patient's TSH stays in pregnancy trimester specific reference ranges during her entire pregnancy and she gives birth to a healthy child at term.

CLINICAL PEARL **STEP 3**

Patients who successfully conceive and are on thyroid hormone should have their dosage checked throughout pregnancy and have their dose adjusted to stay in their pregnancy specific reference range.

How would you manage this patient's hypothyroidism postpartum?

The patient's levothyroxine dose should be reduced by 30%–50% to prepregnancy levels and TSH with reflex to free T4 should be checked 6–8 weeks thereafter.

Case Summary

- **Complaint/History:** A 32-year-old female presents with 5 years of several spontaneous miscarriages, menorrhagia, 10 pound weight gain, hair loss, cold intolerance, dry skin, and constipation.
- **Findings:** Physical exam is significant for a heart rate of 68 beats per minute, a thyroid that is two times enlarged, symmetric, soft, no discrete nodules when palpated, delayed relaxation phase of the bilateral patellar and brachial reflexes and trace pitting edema at the ankles.
- **Lab Results/Tests:** Lab test results were remarkable for a TSH of 24 mIU/L, free T4 of 0.5 ng/dL, and TPO-Ab of 241 IU/mL.

Diagnosis: Hypothyroidism as a cause of recurrent miscarriage.

- **Treatment:** Weight based levothyroxine.

Bibliography

Alexander, E. K., Pearce, E. N., Brent, G. A., Brown, R. S., Chen, H., Dosiou, C., Grobman, W. A., Laurberg, P., Lazarus, J. H., Mandel, S. J., Peeters, R. P., & Sullivan, S. (2017). 2017 Guidelines of the American Thyroid Association for the Diagnosis and Management of Thyroid Disease During Pregnancy and the Postpartum. *Thyroid*, *27*(3), 315–389. https://doi.org/10.1089/thy.2016.0457.

Dong, A. C., & Stagnaro-Green, A. (2019). Differences in diagnostic criteria mask the true prevalence of thyroid disease in pregnancy: A systematic review and meta-analysis. *Thyroid*, *29*(2), 278–289. https://doi.org/10.1089/thy.2018.0475.

Jonklaas, J., Bianco, A. C., Bauer, A. J., Burman, K. D., Cappola, A. R., Celi, F. S., Cooper, D. S., Kim, B. W., Peeters, R. P., Rosenthal, M. S., Sawka, A. M., & American Thyroid Association Task Force on Thyroid Hormone Replacement, (2014). Guidelines for the treatment of hypothyroidism: prepared by the american thyroid association task force on thyroid hormone replacement. *Thyroid*, *24*(12), 1670–1751. https://doi.org/10.1089/thy.2014.0028.

Korevaar, T. I., Schalekamp-Timmermans, S., de Rijke, Y. B., Visser, W. E., Visser, W., de Muinck Keizer-Schrama, S. M., Hofman, A., Ross, H. A., Hooijkaas, H., Tiemeier, H., Bongers-Schokking, J. J., Jaddoe, V. W., Visser, T. J., Steegers, E. A., Medici, M., & Peeters, R. P. (2013]). Hypothyroxinemia and TPO-antibody positivity are risk factors for premature delivery: the generation R study. *J Clin Endocrinol Metab*, *98*(11), 4382–4390. https://doi.org/10.1210/jc.2013-2855.

Korevaar, T. I. M., Derakhshan, A., Taylor, P. N., Meima, M., Chen, L., Bliddal, S., Carty, D. M., Meems, M., Vaidya, B., Shields, B., Ghafoor, F., Popova, P. V., Mosso, L., Oken, E., Suvanto, E., Hisada, A., Yoshinaga, J., Brown, S. J., Bassols, J., Auvinen, J., Bramer, W. M., López-Bermejo, A., Dayan, C., Boucai, L., Vafeiadi, M., Grineva, E. N., Tkachuck, A. S., Pop, V. J. M., Vrijkotte, T. G., Guxens, M., Chatzi, L., Sunyer, J., Jiménez-Zabala, A., Riaño, I., Murcia, M., Lu, X., Mukhtar, S., Delles, C., Feldt-Rasmussen, U., Nelson, S. M., Alexander, E. K., Chaker, L., Männistö, T., Walsh, J. P., Pearce, E. N., Steegers, E. A. P., Peeters, R. P., & Consortium on Thyroid and Pregnancy—Study Group on Preterm Birth, (2019). Association of Thyroid Function Test Abnormalities and Thyroid Autoimmunity With Preterm Birth: A Systematic Review and Meta-analysis. *JAMA*, *322*(7), 632–641. https://doi.org/10.1001/jama.2019.10931.

Leung, A. S., Millar, L. K., Koonings, P. P., Montoro, M., & Mestman, J. H. (1993). Perinatal outcome in hypothyroid pregnancies. *Obstet Gynecol*, *81*(3), 349–353.

Okosieme, O. E., Khan, I., & Taylor, P. N. (2018). Preconception management of thyroid dysfunction. *Clin Endocrinol (Oxf)*, *89*(3), 269–279. https://doi.org/10.1111/cen.13731.

Soldin, O. P., Tractenberg, R. E., Hollowell, J. G., Jonklaas, J., Janicic, N., & Soldin, S. J. (2004). Trimester-specific changes in maternal thyroid hormone, thyrotropin, and thyroglobulin concentrations during gestation: trends and associations across trimesters in iodine sufficiency. *Thyroid*, *14*(12), 1084–1090. https://doi.org/10.1089/thy.2004.14.1084.

CASE 52

A 60-Year-Old Female Presents for Wellness Visit

Diego Tabares ■ Braden Barnett

A 60-year-old asymptomatic female presents to her primary care doctor for a wellness visit. She asks the doctor if she has osteoporosis and whether she needs a "DXA scan." The patient is postmenopausal, denies family history of osteoporosis, and denies prior history of smoking, alcohol consumption, or fractures.

How is osteoporosis diagnosed?

Osteoporosis is the most common bone disease in humans, characterized as a skeletal disorder consisting of deteriorated bone tissue, altered bone architecture, compromised bone strength, reflecting bone density and bone quality, leading to an increased fracture risk. The World Health Organization (WHO) has defined the diagnosis of osteoporosis based on bone mineral density (BMD) T-scores less than or equal to –2.5 at the lumbar spine, femoral neck, hip, and/or distal third of the radius.

When evaluating patients for osteoporosis, start with a comprehensive history and physical examination to detect risk factors that alter skeletal function. Obtaining measurements of BMD (commonly via a dual-energy X-ray absorptiometry [correctly abbreviated DXA, *not* DEXA] scan), along with vertebral imaging, can further demonstrate the patient's fracture risk. As previously mentioned, if the T-score value based on the BMD test is less than or equal to –2.5 at any one of the specified sites, along with the clinical picture suggesting an increased risk of fracture, a patient can be diagnosed as having osteoporosis. However, osteoporosis may also be diagnosed clinically, without bone density measurements, in the setting of a new fracture occurring with little or no trauma and no predisposing metabolic bone disease (also known as fragility fractures).

Vertebral fractures may be confirmed via a lateral vertebral fracture assessment on a DXA machine or a standard lateral plain film X-ray of the thoracic and lumbar spine (Fig. 52.1).

What are the recommended screening guidelines for osteoporosis?

The United States Preventive Services Task Force (USPSTF) recommends BMD screening for osteoporosis in all women over the age of 65 years and younger women whose future fracture risk is greater than or equal to a 65-year-old Caucasian woman with no additional risk factors. Screening for osteoporosis, particularly in women, is essential because bone density significantly declines with menopause as a result of diminishing estrogen levels. The FRAX tool may also be used to estimate fracture risk if a DXA scan is not available or when a patient refuses imaging. Although there are no clear osteoporosis screening guidelines set by the USPSTF for men, the National Osteoporosis Foundation recommends testing all men over the age of 70 years.

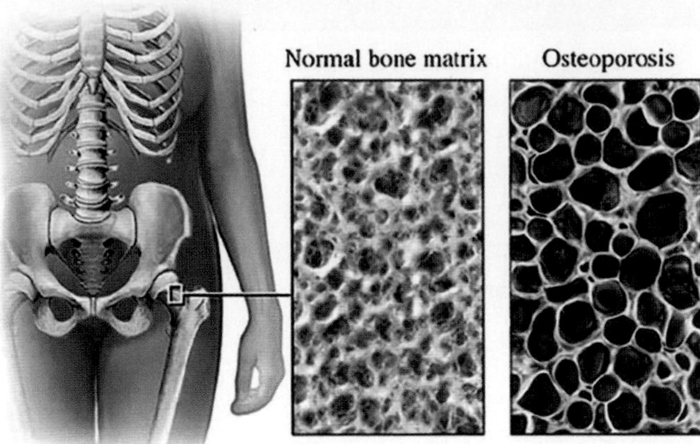

Fig. 52.1 Depiction of normal bone and osteoporotic bone architecture. (From Larsen, S., Bendtzen, K., & Nielsen, O. H. (2010). Extraintestinal manifestations of inflammatory bowel disease: epidemiology, diagnosis, and management. *Annals of Medicine, 42*(2), 97–114.)

TABLE 52.1 ■ **Additional Indications for BMD Testing**

Postmenopausal women	• Starting or on glucocorticoid therapy for at least 3 months • Radiographic evidence of osteopenia • History of fracture(s) with minimal or no trauma
Peri- or postmenopausal women with risk factors for osteoporosis and willing to consider pharmacologic interventions	• BMI <20 kg/m^2 or body weight <127 lb (57.6 kg) • At least 3 months' use of long-term systemic glucocorticoid regimen • Excess alcohol use • Current smoker • Menopause before age 40 years • Family history of osteoporotic fracture
All ages and genders	• Significant fracture history or specific risk factors for bone loss • Secondary osteoporosis

BMD, Bone mineral density; *BMI*, body mass index.

Other indications for BMD testing are described in Table 52.1.

The patient asks if there is any pharmaceutical therapy that may help her prevent osteoporosis.

All types of menopausal hormone therapy (MHT) contain an estrogen, which may provide beneficial effects to bone health because of its effect on bone resorption and bone formation. Although MHT is recommended for certain postmenopausal women with vasomotor symptoms, it is avoided in women with a history of breast cancer, myocardial infarction, stroke, unexplained vaginal bleeding, or active liver disease, or those at high risk of endometrial cancer. If MHT is prescribed, a progestin must be added to estrogen therapy for women who have not had a hysterectomy, and unopposed estrogen therapy is preferable for women who have undergone a hysterectomy. MHT is contraindicated in patients with a history of myocardial infarction or stroke. Another possible therapy for osteoporosis prevention is bazedoxifene, which is a selective estrogen receptor modulator (SERM) with conjugated equine estrogen (CEE), available as a combination pill. The SERM portion of the medication acts as an estrogen receptor antagonist in uterine and breast tissue and as an estrogen receptor agonist in bone tissue. The CEE is added to help alleviate vasomotor symptoms expected to occur from the SERM antagonism of vasomotor estrogen receptors. It has contraindications similar to those of MHT.

The patient asks which risk factors for osteoporosis might apply to her and whether there is a way to quantify that risk.

What are common risk factors for osteoporosis?

The high prevalence of osteoporosis in the general population means that it is essential for clinicians to identify risk factors and help the patient take appropriate steps to reduce the risk of fractures.

Risk factors:

- Prior fracture after the age of 50 years in the setting of low-level trauma (e.g., falling from ground height), excluding skull, fingers, and toes.
- Clinical risk factors: Age 65 years or older, low body weight <57.6 kg, family history of osteoporosis, smoking, early menopause, excessive alcohol use (three or more drinks daily)
- Secondary osteoporosis: hyperthyroidism, hypoparathyroidism
- Height loss or kyphosis
- Fall risk factors
  - Environmental factors
  - Impaired vision and/or hearing
  - Medications (e.g., sedatives, narcotics, antihypertensives, anticholinergics, first-generation antipsychotics)
  - Muscular disorders
  - Neurological disorders
- Patient's comprehension, willingness, and adherence to interventions
- Medications: glucocorticoid use (equivalent to at least 5 mg of prednisone daily for 3 months or more)

CLINICAL PEARL **STEP 2**

The FRAX score (Fracture Risk Assessment Tool) utilizes multiple clinical risk factors (country of residency, ethnicity, age, sex, weight in kg, height in cm, prior fracture, parental history of hip fracture, current smoking, glucocorticoid use, rheumatoid arthritis, secondary osteoporosis, three or more alcohol drinks per day), and femoral neck BMD value or T-score (if not available, the FRAX tool may be used without the femoral neck BMD/T-score) to predict the 10-year probability of major osteoporotic fracture (hip, spine, humerus, or forearm) and 10-year probability of a hip fracture for postmenopausal women and men aged 40 years and older. Although it plays a useful role in determining whether to initiate therapy, it has several limitations. First, the predictive probability calculated for future fracture risk in postmenopausal women with low bone mass reports those of major osteoporotic fractures and hip fractures, which only accounts for ~50% of all fragility fractures. Second, it underestimates fracture risk in patients with recent fractures, secondary osteoporosis, increased fall risk, or multiple osteoporotic fractures and those with a lumbar spine BMD less than femoral neck BMD. Secondary to the latter circumstance, the FRAX tool is therefore validated for hip BMD but not lumbar spine BMD. Third, it can also overestimate the risk of fractures as age increases in the setting of a stable BMD. The FRAX tool has not been validated for patients currently on or prior to osteoporosis medication. If obtained for patients with those circumstances, it is critical to use clinical judgment to interpret scores appropriately.

The FRAX tool is applied to this patient (without BMD measurements because they are not yet available) and her risk of osteoporotic fracture is not elevated. After serious consideration, the patient declines both MHT and bazedoxifene/CEE. Because of low risk factors, a DXA is not performed and she is told that she will undergo testing at the age of 65 years unless she develops new risk factors earlier. She returns 5 years later, a DXA scan is performed, and she asks you to help her interpret the various numbers on the report.

CLINICAL PEARL **STEP 2**

When measuring BMD, the local skeletal area is scanned and measured in units of grams of mineral per centimeter squared (g/cm²). The results are converted into T- and Z-scores. T-score values represent the number of standard deviations (SD) from the normal young-adult mean values of the same sex; however, the International Society for Clinical Densitometry (ISCD) recommends utilizing a uniform Caucasian (nonrace adjusted) female reference for males of all ethnic groups. The Z-score values are the number of SDs from the normal mean value of individuals matched for age, race/ethnicity, and sex. T-score criteria via BMD measurement of the lumbar spine and femoral neck are utilized to diagnose osteoporosis primarily in postmenopausal women and men over the age of 50 years, with BMD measurement of the distal radius used as an alternative option if the hip and lumbar spine cannot be measured or interpreted appropriately. Z-scores are utilized for premenopausal women, men younger than 50 years of age, and children. The former suggests the diagnosis of osteoporosis when the value is less than or equal to –2.5 SDs and a T-score between –1 and –2.5 SDs indicates low bone mass. A Z-score is considered "below the expected range for age" if less than –2.0 SDs and a Z-score above –2.0 is "within the expected range for age."

CLINICAL PEARL **STEP 3**

Patients considered low risk are those with no history of spine or hip fractures, a BMD T-score above –1.0 for both hip and spine, or a 10-year risk of hip fracture <3% and a 10-year risk of major osteoporotic fractures <20%. Moderate risk includes no history of spine or hip fractures, a BMD T-score above –2.5 for both hip and spine, or a 10-year risk of hip fracture <3% and a 10-year risk of major osteoporotic fractures <20%. High-risk patients have a history of spine or hip fracture, T-score at or below –2.5 for hip or spine, or a 10-year risk of hip fracture ≥3% and a 10-year risk of major osteoporotic fractures ≥20%. A very high-risk patient is someone with multiple spine fractures and a T-score at or below –2.5 for hip or spine.

The patient's DXA scan results meet densitometric criteria for a diagnosis of osteoporosis. After discussing the results, she asks about nonpharmacological interventions, such as exercise, calcium, and vitamin D.

Which medical conditions involve bone loss and present in a similar way?

Although no underlying etiology is found for most cases of osteoporosis (besides being postmenopausal in women), it is important to look for secondary and most importantly potentially reversible causes of bone loss once osteoporosis is diagnosed, based either on BMD measurements or the presence of a fragility fracture. A complete history, physical examination, and appropriate lab studies will aid in differentiating between the different secondary etiologies. Some of these causes have particular therapies that are treatable and therefore require diligent workup (see Table 52.2).

What are the complications of osteoporosis and the prognosis of those complications?

Clinically, having a low BMD and/or bone loss is asymptomatic until a fracture occurs. Common complaints of musculoskeletal pain in the absence of a fracture are more likely to be due to another

TABLE 52.2 ■ **Causes of Secondary Osteoporosis**

Endocrine	Genetic	Gastrointestinal	Medications	Miscellaneous
Cushing's syndrome Diabetes mellitus (type 1 or type 2) Early menopause Hyperparathyroidism Hyperthyroidism Osteomalacia	Cystic fibrosis Osteogenesis imperfecta	Celiac disease GI surgery IBD Malabsorption	Antacids Anticoagulants Chemotherapy Glucocorticoids Proton-pump inhibitors SSRIs Thyroid hormone excess	AIDS/HIV Amyloidosis COPD ESRD Sarcoidosis Weight loss (BMI <23 kg/m^2)

BMI, Body mass index; *COPD*, chronic obstructive pulmonary disease; *ESRD*, end-stage renal disease; *IBD*, inflammatory bowel disease; *SSRIs*, selective serotonin reuptake inhibitors.

cause such as osteoarthritis and may require further evaluation. However, once a fracture does occur, pain, disability, and deformity may follow. The sequelae of osteoporosis-related fractures are substantial: a mortality of 12%–20% in postmenopausal women with hip fractures is seen in the 2 years following the incident and ~50% of hip fracture survivors will not return to their baseline independent living, requiring long-term nursing home care.

What is the goal of therapy once a patient has been diagnosed with osteoporosis?

The goal of therapy is to decrease the risk of osteoporosis-related fractures, which can be accomplished with a balanced diet (incorporating adequate consumption of calcium and vitamin D), cessation of drug use and smoking, limiting alcohol consumption, regular exercise (implementing balance and resistance exercises), adequately treating comorbid conditions (particularly the conditions that negatively affect bone health), and appropriate osteoporosis medications for those at high risk. Patients may also be treated for osteoporosis if they are diagnosed with low bone mass (osteopenia) and the FRAX tool yields a major osteoporotic fracture 10-year probability greater than 20% or 10-year probability of a hip fracture greater than 3%.

The patient asks about pharmaceutical therapies.

What are a patient's treatment options?

There is a range of different therapies available for osteoporosis of which a patient may be a good candidate. However, some of the options have been shown to be more effective in reducing the risk of different fracture types. Table 52.3 gives a summary of those available.

Which of the treatment options is considered first-line therapy?

A number of factors should be accounted for when recommending therapies, including patient preference, out-of-pocket costs, side-effect profile, and availability. Oral bisphosphonates (BPs) are the most common initial therapy, given the extensive studies performed, tolerability, relatively low costs, and uncommon occasions of severe side effects, as well as the possibility of a drug holiday. The latter concept refers to temporary BP therapy discontinuation in patients on oral BPs for 3–5 years who are considered low risk after BMD reassessment, preferably with a DXA scan.

If a patient refuses BPs, denosumab or raloxifene may be considered as an alternative first-line treatment. Anabolic therapy may be used as first-line therapy in more severe cases. Calcitonin may also be considered, although studies have shown that the benefits occur to a smaller extent.

TABLE 52.3 ■ **Available Therapy Options for Osteoporosis**

Therapy	Dosing	Duration	Statistically Significant Risk Reduction of Fracture Types[a]
Bisphosphonates: Alendronate Ibandronate Risedronate Zoledronic acid	Alendronate: Prevention: 5 mg PO daily or 35 mg PO weekly Treatment: 10 mg PO daily, 70 mg PO weekly, 70 mg weekly with 2800 or 5600 IU of vitamin D_3, or 70 mg effervescent tablet Ibandronate: Prevention or treatment: 150 mg PO monthly or 3 mg IV every 3 months Risedronate: Prevention or treatment: 5 mg PO daily, 35 mg PO weekly, 75 mg PO for 2 consecutive days every month or 150 mg PO monthly Zoledronic acid: Prevention: 5 mg IV over 15 min every 2 years Treatment: 5 mg IV over 15 min once every year	For alendronate, risedronate, or ibandronate, up to 10 years, with reassessment every 2–4 years and potential drug holiday after 5 years. For zoledronic acid, up to 6 years, with reassessment after 3 years with potential drug holiday at 3 years.	Vertebral Hip[1] Nonvertebral[1]
Denosumab	60 mg subcutaneous injection every 6 months	Indefinitely or until switched to other antiresorptive therapy	Vertebral Hip Nonvertebral
Teriparatide Abaloparatide	Teriparatide: 20 µg subcutaneous injection daily Abaloparatide: 80 µg subcutaneous injection daily	2 years	Vertebral Nonvertebral
Romosozumab	210 mg subcutaneous injection every month	12 months	Vertebral Hip Nonvertebral
Selective estrogen receptor modulators (SERMs)[2]: Raloxifene	60 mg PO daily	Indefinitely, or switch to an alternative antiresorptive agent, or discontinue completely if risk of any treatment outweighs benefit	Vertebral
Hormone therapy[3] (HT)	Variable, depending on estrogen and hormone therapy selected	Many providers discontinue no later than 60 years of age, although others continue indefinitely	Vertebral Hip Nonvertebral
Calcitonin	200 IU intranasal spray daily, SQ injection also available	Optimal duration unknown	Vertebral
Calcium and vitamin D (combination)	Dietary and supplemental combined: Vitamin D: 800–1000 IU daily for ages 50+ Calcium: 1000 mg daily for men 50–70, 1200 mg for women 50+ and men 71+	Indefinitely	Hip[4] Nonvertebral[4]

[a]Risk reduction of drugs in trials compared with placebo.

[1] All bisphosphonates except ibandronate.

[2] Bazedoxifene is a SERM available in the US only as a combination with conjugated equine estrogen. FDA approved for osteoporosis prevention.

[3] Tibolone not included with hormone therapy because it is discontinued in the United States secondary to its association with cardiovascular side effects and increased recurrence of breast cancer in women with prior breast cancer history (LIBERATE study).

[4] The greatest risk reduction from calcium and vitamin D supplementation is observed in elderly patients living in residential care.

What are some side effects to monitor while using bisphosphonates?

The most common side effects with oral BP use are esophageal irritation and gastrointestinal intolerance. However, there are other side effects that have garnered more attention.

Osteonecrosis of the jaw (ONJ) has occurred as a side effect of bisphosphonates. It was first reported in cancer patients receiving zoledronic acid at a dose 10 times greater than the typically prescribed annual dose for osteoporosis, with an incidence ranging from 1% to 2%. However, the incidence rate of ONJ for oral bisphosphonates at the dosage mentioned in Table 52.3 is between 1 in 10,000 and 1 in 100,000 every year. Patients at highest risk are those with pathological dental conditions or poor oral hygiene, or those undergoing invasive dental procedures. If the patient is scheduled for an invasive dental procedure and bisphosphonates have not been started, it is recommended to delay therapy. However, when patients are already on bisphosphonates, there is no evidence that shows reduced ONJ risk or changes in outcome when therapy is discontinued prior to an invasive dental procedure.

Atypical femur fractures (AFFs) is a rare sequela that has been noted in patients on BP therapy for prolonged periods, typically at least 5 years, occurring with little or no trauma. Nearly 70% of AFFs will present with prodromal groin or thigh pain. If pain persists, stop therapy and obtain radiographs. However, subtrochanteric femur fractures can present in patients with low BMD while on other therapies, not only bisphosphonates.

Oral bisphosphonates may also increase the risk of atrial fibrillation and acute kidney injury; therefore, it is recommended to check creatinine clearance prior to administration (avoid if creatinine clearance is less than 30 mL/min).

CLINICAL PEARL **STEP 3**

Short-term discontinuation prior to a dental procedure has not shown to improve dental outcomes because BPs have shown to accumulate and reside in bone for months or years after discontinuation. If BP therapy is discontinued for an extensive period, the osteoporotic risk of fracture may increase. However, many providers will elect to delay initiating new BP therapy if the patient has dental procedures planned for the near future. Once the patient has completely healed from their dental procedures, BP therapy is initiated.

The patient decides to begin with an oral bisphosphonate. After 1 year of use, she returns to the clinic and undergoes a follow-up DXA scan.

Once a patient is started on therapy, how often should they be evaluated?

Patients who are started on therapy for osteoporosis should be reassessed with a DXA scan or bone turnover markers (BTMs) to identify whether the disease is progressing (defined as a lower BMD than baseline or new or worsening fractures), stable, or improving. Reassessment while on bisphosphonates should occur after 3–5 years (5 years when using oral BPs weekly). Therapy continuation is recommended if still high risk, and those at low or moderate risk can be considered for a bisphosphonate holiday. Treatment success is defined as someone who experiences stable or improving BMD measurements, no fractures, and no new clinical risk factors while on therapy. Treatment failure is considered when a patient has progressive disease or new clinical risk factors. Failure may occur as a result of improper use of medication (such as not taking medication as prescribed) or the medication is not at the potency level necessary to help create a beneficial effect.

If patients are placed on a bisphosphonate holiday, evaluate within 2–4 years and restart therapy if BMD shows significant decline, a recent fracture occurs, or a patient has new or worsening clinical risk factors. Extension studies with alendronate demonstrated that fracture risk was reduced in high-risk postmenopausal women when taken for 10 years (versus 5 years). The group of high-risk postmenopausal women who stopped after 5 years experienced twice as many nonvertebral fractures, although there was no difference in fracture rates in the first 2 years. This suggests that bisphosphonates have a residual beneficial effect.

For all other medications, patients should be regularly asked about any side effects, worsening clinical risk factors, or new fractures. Any of those findings may warrant a new BMD test and indicate switching to new medications.

CLINICAL PEARL **STEP 1**

Bone turnover markers (BTMs) are molecular markers involved in the dynamic process of bone remodeling, with different markers released during separate stages of bone resorption and formation. Postmenopausal women with low BMD and increased fracture risks usually present with an associated elevation in certain BTMs.

Prior studies focused on BTM level changes demonstrated that when these levels are elevated prior to bisphosphonate (BP) therapy and significantly decrease secondary to BP therapy, persistence of low BTM levels may be an indicator of residual beneficial effects, which may be explained by the mechanism of action of bisphosphonates—binding to bone hydroxyapatite and being taken up by osteoclasts, the latter action leading to osteoclast activity inhibition.

Serum C-terminal telopeptide (CTX) and serum carboxyterminal propeptide of type I collagen (PINP) are reference analytes that are elevated when there is high bone resorption or increased bone formation, respectively. If bone resorption markers are obtained before and after starting antiresorptive therapy, the marker levels may decrease 30%–50% with oral or intravenous (IV) bisphosphonates and 40%–80% with denosumab.

Nonetheless, their use is limited by high variability in vivo and assay, poor predictive ability in individual patients, and the lack of evidence-based thresholds to guide clinical decision-making. In an extension trial (FLEX trial) where alendronate (oral BP) was given to two groups of postmenopausal women for either 10 years or 5 years, followed by 5 years of placebo, the previously mentioned BTMs did not predict bone loss at the lumbar spine, total hip, or femoral neck during the 5-year treatment-free period for the group that discontinued alendronate after an average of 5 years. In the HORIZON extension trial, where postmenopausal women either took IV zoledronic acid for 3 years plus 3 years of placebo or 6 total years of zoledronic acid, PINP did not predict nonvertebral or morphometric fractures during the 3-year treatment-free period in the former group.

Given the findings of these trials, BTMs are currently not used for the diagnosis of osteoporosis, but some experts consider their measurements useful after BP therapy discontinuation to monitor residual effects of therapy and to resume treatment when levels exceed the lower half of premenopausal range (see Table 52.4).

The patient's follow-up DXA scan shows a decrease in BMD; therefore, it is considered treatment failure. She asks about denosumab.

TABLE 52.4 ■ **Common Bone Markers Used to Assess Bone Resorption and Formation**

Bone Marker Function	Bone Markers
Resorption	CTX, N-terminal telopeptide of type 1 collagen (NTX)
Formation	P1NP, bone-specific alkaline phosphatase (B-ALP), osteocalcin, procollagen I carboxyterminal propeptide (PICP)

What are the risks and benefits of denosumab and which side effects should clinicians monitor for?
Denosumab, which may be considered as an alternative first-line therapy, has a mechanism of action that involves a monoclonal antibody binding to receptor activator of nuclear factor kappa-B ligand (RANKL) leading to inhibition of osteoclast function and survival, which will result in decreased resorption and increased bone mass. Although trials have demonstrated risk reduction in vertebral, nonvertebral, and hip fractures, it is highly recommended not to discontinue denosumab unless switching the patient to another therapy, typically a bisphosphonate. Prior studies show that BMD decreases more than 5% in the lumbar spine and the total hip within the first 12 months of discontinuation, which creates rebound fractures that are probably secondary to loss of bone protection. However, after denosumab therapy for 1 year, alendronate appears to retain the anabolic effects of denosumab for at least 12 months, with similar retention of benefits also seen with zoledronic acid following denosumab therapy. As a result of denosumab's role, prescribing it to the elderly or patients who have failed BP therapy should be strongly considered.

Adverse events related to denosumab do not correspond with duration of treatment. There are a few reported cases of ONJ and the risk of hypocalcemia is approximately 0.05%, with underlying chronic kidney disease being a prominent risk factor. Increased bone resorption and vitamin D deficiency may also increase hypocalcemia risk. Serious skin infections (including cellulitis and erysipelas) are rare, with the most common skin condition associated with denosumab use being eczema.

The patient does not like the idea of indefinite therapy and is concerned about the risk of rebound fractures after discontinuation. She asks about other options.

What are some advantages and disadvantages of IV bisphosphonate therapy?
Ibandronate and zoledronic acid are the two IV BP options currently available and, similarly to the oral BPs, patients who experience beneficial effects may undergo a drug holiday with reassessment in 2–4 years. Extension studies with zoledronic acid demonstrated that prolonged use (6 years versus 3 years) further reduced the fracture risk for high-risk postmenopausal women.

Patient studies suggest that IV bisphosphonates work better than oral bisphosphonates, probably a result of increased absorption and compliance (because of the relative decreased frequency of taking the medication). If patients are unable to tolerate oral BPs due to GI intolerance or other contraindications, IV BPs can be used as an alternative, cost-effective therapy.

Although IV BPs share similar side effects to oral BPs and similar frequencies (ONJ, AFF, acute kidney injury), one common side effect in IV users is an acute phase reaction, with the majority of incidences occurring during or after the first administration. Rates of acute phase reactions diminish with subsequent infusions. Another possible side effect is atrial fibrillation, especially in elderly patients with a history of cardiovascular disease.

The patient is terrified of the acute phase reaction since she has a friend who had side effects while on zoledronic acid; therefore, she declines this. She has another friend who takes raloxifene and asks if she would be a good candidate.

Who are the best candidates to receive SERM therapy as osteoporosis treatment?
Raloxifene, a SERM known for its estrogenic activity in bone and antiestrogenic activity in breast and uterine tissues, is considered beneficial for postmenopausal women at high risk of breast cancer. It has been shown to reduce the incidence of invasive estrogen receptor-positive breast cancer during the course of therapy and for at least 5 years after completion. Raloxifene, like denosumab, should be continued indefinitely or, if it is to be discontinued, the patient should be switched to an antiresorptive medication. One factor to consider is that there are insufficient data

regarding the beneficial effects on nonvertebral fractures. Currently, the significant risk reduction while on raloxifene is seen with vertebral fractures. Another group of women who may benefit are younger women with osteoporosis and absent vasomotor symptoms due to potential decreased risk of atypical femur fractures. More data are needed to support recommending SERMs for this subpopulation; at this moment, BP therapy is preferred because of better efficacy for nonspinal fracture risk reduction. Contraindications include hot flushes, venous thromboembolism, malignancies, thrombophilia, or being a current smoker.

The patient declines changing therapy, stating that what may be contributing to her current situation is her nonadherence and promises to take her oral bisphosphonate as prescribed. Unfortunately, she develops a vertebral fracture 3 months later. She visits the office and reports that she is serious about intensifying her therapy.

Which medications should be considered if a patient fails a first-line therapy or is at a very high risk of fractures?

According to the Endocrine Society Guidelines, switching medications should be considered in postmenopausal women if they are not able to tolerate medications, are not appropriate for first-line medications, or have worsening osteoporosis. Typically, calcium and vitamin D are given as adjunct therapy and should be maintained regardless of the primary therapy because of the low side-effect profile.

When patients experience unsuccessful initial therapy with an antiresorptive medication such as an oral BP, either because of a new fracture or progressive disease, it is appropriate to consider an anabolic second-line therapy. Three anabolic agents are currently available: teriparatide, abaloparatide, and romosozumab. Teriparatide is a shorter peptide version of parathyroid hormone (PTH); abaloparatide is a PTH-related protein analog; and romosozumab is a monoclonal antibody. All three medications augment bone strength by increasing bone formation, but only romosozumab also appears to decrease bone resorption.

A 24-month trial of teriparatide comparing the fracture efficacy in patients with and without prior use of bisphosphonates demonstrated similar fracture risk reductions, suggesting that anabolic therapy after bisphosphonate use is effective in fracture risk reduction. In an extended study comparing 2 years of romosozumab with 2 years of alendronate, those in the former group had lower rates of vertebral, nonvertebral, and hip fractures at the end of the study period. Teriparatide and abaloparatide are daily injections and romosozumab is given as monthly injections. These anabolic agents, as mentioned in Table 52.3, may only be given for a limited amount of time because of limited study data and potential side effects.

Teriparatide and abaloparatide contain a black box warning for osteosarcoma, given the increase in incidence noted in rats that underwent lifelong treatment. However, teriparatide was introduced in 2002 and up to this point only three cases of osteosarcoma have been reported in humans who have used teriparatide. Causality could not be clearly established in any of the cases.

Both teriparatide and abaloparatide may also cause hypercalcemia; therefore, it is recommended to obtain a serum calcium level prior to use and to avoid use in patients with preexisting hypercalcemia.

For romosozumab, there is a black box warning for patients at risk of myocardial infarction, stroke, and cardiovascular death because of the number of major adverse cardiovascular events (MACEs). In a randomized controlled trial of 4093 patients comparing romosozumab with alendronate, a total of 16 patients (0.8%) in the romosozumab group and 6 (0.3%) in the alendronate group reported cardiac ischemic events (odds ratio, 2.65; 95% CI, 1.03 to 6.77). Cerebrovascular events were similarly more common but not to a statistically significant extent. The potential mechanism of this possibly increased risk is unclear. However, for this reason, romosozumab

TABLE 52.5 ■ **Summary of Serious Side Effects from Osteoporosis Therapy**

Medication	Serious Side Effects
All bisphosphonates	ONJ, AFF, new onset atrial fibrillation
Oral bisphosphonates	Esophageal irritation, GI intolerance
IV bisphosphonates	Acute phase reaction
Denosumab	ONJ, AFF, hypocalcemia, infections, eczema
Teriparatide (T)	Osteosarcoma[a]
Abaloparatide (A)	Dizziness and leg cramps (T) Postural hypotension, dizziness, palpitations, headache (A)
Romosozumab	ONJ, AFF, injection-site reactions, major adverse cardiovascular events
SERM	Venous thromboembolism, hot flushes, leg cramps
MHT[b]	Venous thromboembolism, stroke, MI, dementia, cancer (breast, endometrial, ovary), gallbladder pathology, and urinary incontinence
Calcitonin (nasal spray)	Increased risk of prostate and liver cancer
Vitamin D and calcium	When given in combination, may be a greater risk of kidney stones. High doses of intermittent vitamin D can lead to greater risk of falls and fractures.

[a]As mentioned previously, only one case of osteosarcoma has been reported in more than 1 million humans who have taken these medications as of 2016.
[b]Although included in this table, this medication is preferably given for prevention rather than therapy of osteoporosis.
AFF, Atypical femur fractures; *MHT*, menopausal hormone therapy; *MI*, myocardial infarction; *ONJ*, osteonecrosis of the jaw.

should not be initiated in patients who have had a myocardial infarction or stroke within the preceding year. Consider whether the benefits outweigh the risks in patients with other cardiovascular risk factors. If a patient experiences a myocardial infarction or stroke during therapy, romosozumab should be discontinued.

There have been a few cases of both ONJ and AFF in patients using romosozumab, but the majority have occurred in trials when the patient had been transitioned to either a bisphosphonate or denosumab after an initial 12-month period with romosozumab. Injection site reactions were also noted. As a result of its effect on the WNT pathway, which results in bone formation, the development of tumors was assessed and was not found to be contributory.

Other side effects from anabolic agents and those described previously have been included in Table 52.5.

The patient reports having a family history of heart disease, and for this reason she declines romosozumab, despite being told a family history of heart disease is not a contraindication. She is placed on teriparatide for 2 years and returns with 1 month left on her therapy regimen. A follow-up DXA scan shows improvement in her T-score and no new fractures. The patient asks what the next steps are.

Which medical therapy options are appropriate after anabolic agent use for osteoporosis?

The benefits achieved with anabolic therapy can quickly be lost after discontinuation, with BMD changes occurring as soon as 1 year posttherapy. Studies analyzing the durability of anabolic effects have demonstrated that subsequent use of bisphosphonates can sustain, and in some cases enhance, the effects created by prior use of anabolic agents. Therefore, it is essential to switch patients to antiresorptive therapy after anabolic agent use is completed, with bisphosphonates, denosumab, or raloxifene as adequate options.

The patient is fearful of the acute phase reaction from intravenous zoledronic acid, but eventually agrees after reflecting on her prior vertebral fracture. She starts zoledronic acid infusions, once every 12 months, with plans to follow her BMD with DXA testing to ensure efficacy.

Case Summary

- **Complaint/History:** A 60-year-old woman asks about screening for osteoporosis with a bone density DXA study.
- **Findings:** No high risk features for osteoporosis in her history or physical examination.
- **Labs/Test:** DXA performed at age 65 as per screening guidelines. DXA revealed a lowest T-score of -2.5 or lower, meeting densitometric criteria for a diagnosis of osteoporosis. Lab testing did not reveal a secondary reversible cause of bone loss/osteoporosis.

Diagnosis: Postmenopausal osteoporosis.

- **Treatment:** She initiates therapy with an oral bisphosphonate, but after one year, her bone density significantly worsens. She declines therapy with zoledronic acid or denosumab. She initially desires to stay on the oral bisphosphonate thinking the therapy has not been effective because she has not been adherent to therapy, but she develops a vertebral fracture three months later. She takes teriparatide for two years (24 months). Her bone density improves. After finishing the teriparatide therapy, she begins treatment with the intravenous bisphosphonate zoledronic acid once every 12 months.

Bibliography

Adler, R. A., El-Hajj Fuleihan, G., Bauer, D. C., Camacho, P. M., Clarke, B. L., Clines, G. A., Compston, J. E, Drake, M. T., Edwards, B. J., Favus, M. J., Greenspan, S. L., McKinney, R., Jr, Pignolo, R. J. & Sellmeyer, D. E. (2016). Managing Osteoporosis in Patients on Long-Term Bisphosphonate Treatment: Report of a Task Force of the American Society for Bone and Mineral Research. *Journal of bone and mineral research: the official journal of the American Society for Bone and Mineral Research*, *31*(1), 16-35.

Camacho, P. M., Petak, S. M., Binkley, N., Diab, D. L., Eldeiry, L. S., Farooki, A., Harris, S. T., Hurley, D. L., Kelly, J., Farooki, A., Harris, S. T., Hurley, D. L., Kelly, J., Lewiecki, E. M., Pessah-Pollack, R., McClung, M., Wimalawansa, S. J. & Watts, N. B., et al. (2020). AMERICAN ASSOCIATION OF CLINICAL ENDOCRINOLOGISTS/AMERICAN COLLEGE OF ENDOCRINOLOGY CLINICAL PRACTICE GUIDELINES FOR THE DIAGNOSIS AND TREATMENT OF POSTMENOPAUSAL OSTEOPOROSIS-2020 UPDATE. *Endocrine practice: official journal of the American College of Endocrinology and the American Association of Clinical Endocrinologists*, *26*(Suppl 1), 1–46.

Cosman, F., de Beur, S. J., LeBoff, M. S., Lewiecki, E. M., Tanner, B., Randall, S., Lindsay, R. & National Osteoporosis Foundation (2014). Clinician's Guide to Prevention and Treatment of Osteoporosis. *Osteoporosis international: a journal established as result of cooperation between the European Foundation for Osteoporosis and the National Osteoporosis Foundation of the USA*, *25*(10), 2359–2381.

Eastell, R., Rosen, C. J., Black, D. M., Cheung, A. M., Murad, M. H., & Shoback, D. (2019). Pharmacological Management of Osteoporosis in Postmenopausal Women: An Endocrine Society* Clinical Practice Guideline. *The Journal of clinical endocrinology and metabolism*, *104*(5), 1595–1622.

Larsen, S., Bendtzen, K., & Nielsen, O. H. (2010). Extraintestinal manifestations of inflammatory bowel disease: epidemiology, diagnosis, and management. *Annals of medicine*, *42*(2), 97–114.

Shoback, D., Rosen, C. J., Black, D. M., Cheung, A. M., Murad, M. H. & Eastell, R. (2020). Pharmacological Management of Osteoporosis in Postmenopausal Women: An Endocrine Society Guideline Update. *The Journal of clinical endocrinology and metabolism*, *105*(3), dgaa048.

CASE 53

A 19-Year-Old Female With Oligomenorrhea and Facial Hair Growth

Alyssa Lampe Dominguez ■ Caroline T. Nguyen

A 19-year-old female presents to her primary care physician complaining of oligomenorrhea and progressive facial hair growth over the past year. She reports irregular menses since menarche at the age of 13 years. She is not currently sexually active and has never been pregnant. She has noted dark hairs on her upper lip and chin. She has also noticed increase in hair growth on her abdomen and inner thighs. Additionally, she has noted worsening acne and a 20-lb weight gain over the past year.

Which diagnoses should be considered in the workup of oligomenorrhea?

When evaluating amenorrhea in a woman with previously normal menstrual cycles, it is important to consider a wide range of etiologies in the hypothalamic-pituitary-gonadal axis. Significant weight loss, increased exercise activity, or increased stress can lead to decreased production of gonadotropin-releasing hormone (GnRH), leading to decreased downstream production of estradiol and progesterone and functional hypothalamic oligomenorrhea.

Hyperprolactinemia also inhibits GnRH secretion and can be caused by prolactinoma, medication (particularly dopamine antagonists), and stalk effect from other pituitary tumors. The absence of galactorrhea does not rule out hyperprolactinemia.

Classic congenital adrenal hyperplasia (CAH) is caused by enzymatic defects in adrenal steroidogenesis that result in inadequate production of cortisol. As a result, there is an adrenocorticotropic hormone (ACTH)-driven excess adrenal production of androgens. Nonclassic CAH is a less severe form of the disease, which does not present with cortisol deficiency, but rather presents later (in childhood or adolescence) with signs of androgen excess such as hirsutism and acne.

Premature ovarian failure is defined by loss of ovarian function prior to age 40 and can present with menopausal symptoms such as oligomenorrhea or amenorrhea and vasomotor symptoms such as hot flashes.

Although rare, hypercortisolemia (Cushing's syndrome) can cause oligomenorrhea and hirsutism. Patients should be questioned about glucocorticoid use, central weight gain, proximal muscle weakness, thin skin, and easy bruising.

Acromegaly, or excess growth hormone, is a rare cause of oligomenorrhea that can present with changes in shoe or glove size and increased spacing between teeth. See Table 53.1.

CLINICAL PEARL **STEP 2/3**

Polycystic ovary syndrome (PCOS) is a diagnosis of exclusion. Pregnancy, thyroid disease, nonclassic CAH, and hyperprolactinemia should be ruled out in all patients. Additional testing should be considered based on the patient's clinical presentation.

TABLE 53.1 ■ **Diagnoses to Consider With Oligomenorrhea**

Pregnancy
Functional hypothalamic amenorrhea
Hyperprolactinemia
Hypothyroidism
Polycystic ovary syndrome
Nonclassic congenital adrenal hyperplasia
Premature ovarian failure
Acromegaly
Androgen-secreting tumor

TABLE 53.2 ■ **Diagnostic Criteria for PCOS**

Rotterdam (two of three required)	US National Institutes of Health	Androgen Excess/PCOS Society
Oligo- or anovulation	Oligo- or anovulation	Ovarian dysfunction (oligo- or anovulation and/or polycystic ovaries)
Clinical or biochemical hyperandrogenism	Clinical or biochemical hyperandrogenism	Clinical or biochemical hyperandrogenism
Polycystic ovaries on ultrasound		

PCOS, Polycystic ovary syndrome.

What is PCOS? What are the diagnostic criteria for PCOS?

PCOS is a disorder characterized by androgen excess and ovulatory dysfunction, which typically presents with abnormal hair growth in androgen-dependent areas, increased acne, oligomenorrhea, and sometimes infertility. Insulin resistance is also frequently present.

There are three sets of diagnostic criteria for PCOS: the Rotterdam criteria, US National Institutes of Health (NIH) criteria, and Androgen Excess/PCOS Society criteria. The Rotterdam criteria is the most widely accepted. Because PCOS is a diagnosis of exclusion, all three sets of criteria require the exclusion of other disorders that can mimic PCOS (see Table 53.2).

CLINICAL PEARL **STEP 2/3**

PCOS is the most common endocrinopathy affecting reproductive-aged women and affects 5%–15% of women of reproductive age.

CLINICAL PEARL **STEP 2/3**

PCOS typically presents in women of reproductive age with oligomenorrhea/amenorrhea and signs of androgen excess including increased hair growth in androgen-dependent areas such as the face, chest, and back.

On physical examination, body mass index (BMI) is 31, heart rate is 82 bpm, and blood pressure is 118/63 mmHg. She has dark hairs on her upper lip and chin, acanthosis in her axillae and behind her neck (see Fig. 53.1), and dark hair. Thyroid is nonpalpable. Pelvic exam reveals normal internal and external genitalia with no clitoromegaly (see Fig. 53.2).

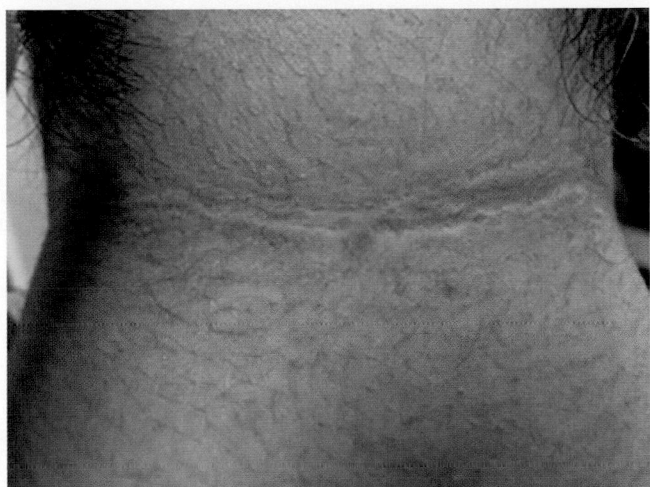

Fig. 53.1 Acanthosis nigricans on the posterior neck. (From Liu, K., Motan, T., & Claman, P. (2017). Hirsutism: Evaluation and treatment. *Journal of Obstetrics and Gynecology Canada*, *39* (11), 1054–1068.)

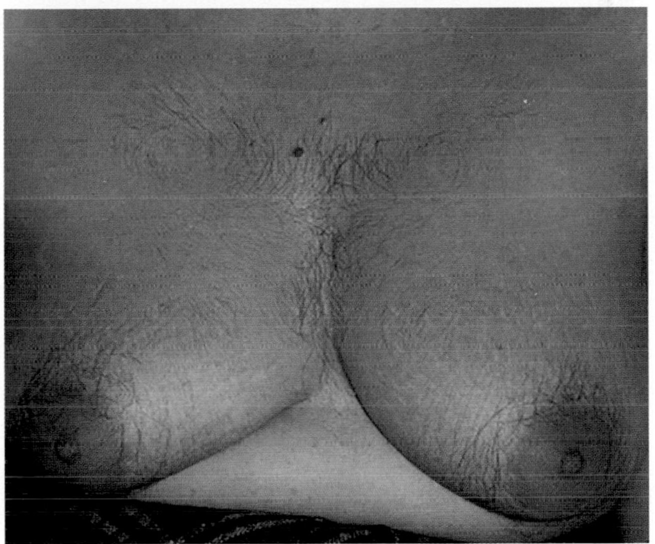

Fig. 53.2 Terminal hair growth on the chest and around the areolae. (From James, W. D., Elston, D. M., & McMahon, P. J. (2016). *Andrews' diseases of the skin* (12th ed.). Philadelphia: Saunders.)

How does the physical examination help you with your diagnostic evaluation?

The constellation of physical examination findings including obesity, signs of hyperandrogenism, and findings concerning for insulin resistance should raise concern for PCOS. This patient displays several signs of hyperandrogenism including hirsutism and acne. She has increased terminal hair growth in androgen-dependent areas. Terminal hairs are thick and pigmented, as opposed to vellus hairs, which are soft, thin, and skin colored. Another notable physical examination finding in this patient is the presence of acanthosis nigricans (hyperpigmentation of skin in the intertriginous areas) in the posterior neck and in the axillae, which might indicate insulin resistance.

BASIC SCIENCE PEARL **STEP 1**

Acanthosis nigricans is caused by hyperinsulinemia (a common feature in PCOS as a result of insulin resistance), which binds to insulin-like growth factor-1 receptors and causes epidermal keratinocyte and dermal fibroblast proliferation.

Cushing's syndrome (hypercortisolemia) would more likely reveal abdominal obesity with thin extremities, proximal muscle weakness, and striae. Although the patient does not have obvious clitoromegaly, a 17-hydroxyprogesterone level test should still be made to rule out nonclassic CAH because clitoromegaly can be subtle or absent.

Findings such as androgenetic alopecia (see Fig. 53.3), clitoromegaly, or voice deepening might be indicative of an androgen-secreting tumor.

What characterizes abnormal hair growth in a female?

Abnormal hair growth in a female, or hirsutism, is characterized by excess hair growth on the upper lip, chin, chest, abdomen, arms, upper thighs, and upper and lower back. The prevalence of hirsutism in the general population is 5%–15% depending on ethnicity. The most common method of assessing hirsutism is the modified Ferriman-Gallwey score (see Fig. 53.4), which numerically grades hair growth over nine androgen-sensitive areas based on a visual assessment. All scores are summed to obtain a final score. A score of 8 or more is typically considered abnormal, although thresholds vary depending on ethnicity. Certain medications are associated with hirsutism and patients presenting with this complaint should have a full review of current prescriptions (see Table 53.3).

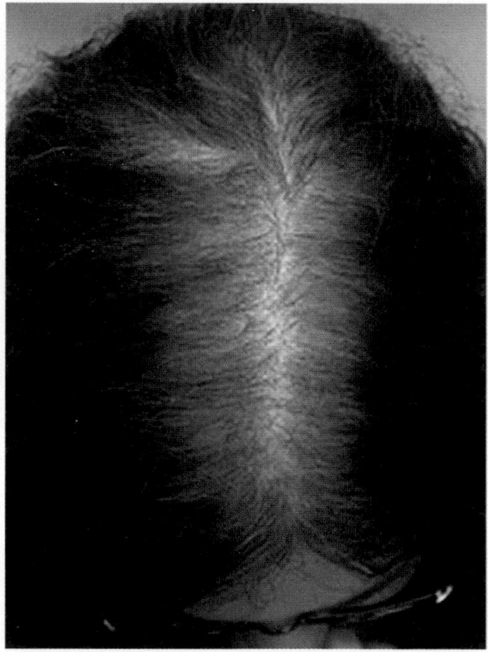

Fig. 53.3 Androgenetic alopecia. (From Hawryluk, E. B. & English, J. C. (2009). Female adolescent hair disorders. *Journal of Pediatric and Adolescent Gynecology*, *22* (4), 271–281.)

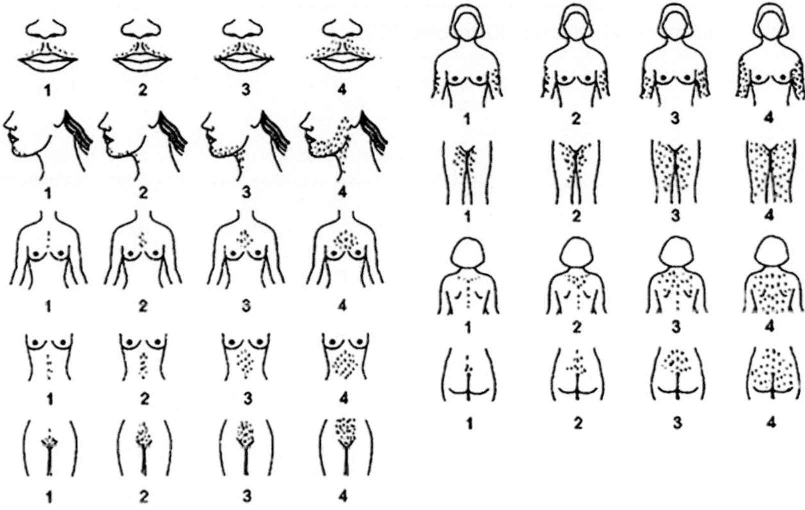

Fig. 53.4 Ferriman-Gallwey scoring system.

TABLE 53.3 ■ **Medications Associated With Hirsutism**

Danazol
Phenytoin
Valproic acid
Androgenic progestins
Cyclosporine
Minoxidil
Metoclopramide
Phenothiazines
Methyldopa
Diazoxide
Penicillamine

Which laboratory tests should be considered for this patient?

See Table 53.4.

Laboratory test results are as follows: thyroid stimulating hormone (TSH) 2.0 μIU/mL (normal range 0.27–4.20 μIU/mL); prolactin 5.0 ng/mL (normal range 4.0–15.2 ng/mL) 17-hydroxyprogesterone 70 ng/dL (normal range 23–431 ng/dL); urine pregnancy test negative; follicle stimulating hormone (FSH) 6.5 mIU/mL (normal range 4.5–21.5 mIU/mL); testosterone 60 ng/dL (normal <48 ng/dL); dehydroepiandrosterone (DHEA)-S 400 μg/dL (normal range 37–307 μg/dL).

The patient returns to the clinic after laboratory testing and is diagnosed with PCOS based on the presenting features of hyperandrogenism and anovulation, with the exclusion of pregnancy, hypothyroidism, nonclassic CAH, premature ovarian failure, and hyperprolactinemia. She asks whether any further testing needs to be done.

TABLE 53.4 ■ **Biochemical Testing in Suspected PCOS**

Pregnancy test	A pregnancy test should be performed in any reproductive-aged female with irregular menses.
Thyroid stimulating hormone (TSH) and free T4	Underlying thyroid disease can cause irregular menses. Free T4 should be sent in addition to TSH if pituitary dysfunction is suspected, in which case TSH may be inappropriately normal in the setting of hypothyroidism.
Prolactin	Hyperprolactinemia can inhibit GnRH secretion and decrease downstream production of estradiol and progesterone.
17-hydroxyprogesterone	Deficient activity of 21-hydroxylase causes accumulation of the substrate, 17-hydroxyprogesterone. 17-hydroxyprogesterone should be tested in all patients if PCOS is suspected to rule out nonclassic CAH. The sample should be taken in the early morning in the early follicular phase of the menstrual cycle. A level greater than 200 ng/dL is indicative of nonclassic CAH.
Testosterone and dehydroepiandrosterone sulfate (DHEA-S)	DHEA-S is an androgen produced in the adrenal gland. Elevation in DHEA-S would raise concern for an adrenal tumor although it may be mildly elevated in PCOS. Testosterone is produced in the ovary and adrenal gland. A marked elevation in testosterone could be indicative of a testosterone-secreting tumor.
Cushing's screening test	If the patient shows signs of hypercortisolemia, screen for Cushing's with an overnight 1 mg dexamethasone suppression test, 24-hour urine free cortisol and/or late-night salivary cortisol.
Insulin growth factor-1 (IGF-1)	Elevated IGF-1 raises concern for acromegaly (growth hormone excess). GH is secreted in a pulsatile manner and it would therefore not be appropriate to measure GH directly.
Follicle stimulating hormone (FSH)	In patients with premature ovarian failure, an elevated FSH level would be expected given lack of ovarian production, which provides negative feedback on pituitary production of FSH.

CAH, Congenital adrenal hyperplasia; *GH*, growth hormone; *GnRH*, gonadotropin-releasing hormone; *PCOS*, polycystic ovary syndrome.

What is the significance of the elevation in testosterone and DHEA-S levels? Does this patient need to undergo further evaluation for an androgen-secreting tumor?

Mild elevations in testosterone and DHEA-S are not unexpected in cases of PCOS. Testosterone is produced both by the ovary and adrenal gland and is one of the androgens that cause increased hair growth and acne as seen in PCOS. Markedly elevated levels of testosterone or signs of virilization should prompt evaluation for an androgen-secreting tumor.

DHEA-S is an androgen produced in the adrenal gland and is elevated in about 30%–35% of patients with PCOS. Mild elevation in DHEA-S is consistent with PCOS but marked elevation should prompt evaluation for an adrenal tumor.

Of note, if the patient has clinical hyperandrogenism, evidence of biochemical hyperandrogenism with elevated testosterone and/or DHEA-S levels is not required to make the diagnosis of PCOS.

Does this patient need a pelvic ultrasound?

No. If the diagnosis of PCOS is unclear, pelvic ultrasound can be considered, but it is not necessary to make the diagnosis.

CLINICAL PEARL **STEP 2/3**

PCOS is primarily a clinical diagnosis and if a patient has evidence of hyperandrogenism and ovulatory dysfunction, a pelvic ultrasound is not necessary. Ultrasound should not be used in the diagnosis of PCOS until at least 8 years after menarche given the high prevalence of multifollicular ovaries in younger women.

What are the appropriate treatment options for this patient's oligomenorrhea?

Although anovulation and resultant amenorrhea or oligomenorrhea may not be the most bothersome symptom to women with PCOS, a review completed by Chittenden et al. in 2009 showed that the risk of endometrial cancer is 2.7 times higher in women with PCOS than in women without PCOS. Prolonged estrogen-mediated stimulation of the endometrium coupled with inadequate progesterone exposure for endometrial differentiation increases the risk of endometrial hyperplasia and eventual endometrial cancer.

CLINICAL PEARL **STEP 2/3**

Although women with PCOS are at a higher risk of endometrial cancer, the overall incidence of endometrial cancer in the general population is very low; therefore, routine screening for endometrial cancer in women with PCOS is not recommended.

CLINICAL PEARL **STEP 2/3**

The cornerstone of treatment for the underlying hormonal imbalances in PCOS is weight loss. No specific diet or exercise plan has been shown to be superior. Weight loss of 5%–10% can reduce androgen levels and improve menstrual function.

In addition to weight loss, hormonal contraceptives are the first-line treatment option for oligomenorrhea in cases of PCOS. They act in several ways to decrease androgen levels:

- Decreasing ovarian androgen production
- Increasing hepatic production of sex-hormone binding globulin (SHBG), which decreases androgen bioavailability

If a patient does not want to take oral hormonal contraceptives, a levonorgestrel releasing intrauterine device also provides endometrial protection and reliable contraception, although it would not necessarily result in regular menstrual bleeding and may result in amenorrhea. Another option for patients with PCOS who do not want to take hormonal contraceptives but need endometrial protection is the use of episodic progestin for withdrawal bleeding. Oral micronized progestin or oral medroxyprogesterone is administered for 10–14 days every 1–3 months, which results in several days of menstrual bleeding similar to a regular menstrual cycle. This progesterone promotes endometrial differentiation and decreases the risk of endometrial cancer from prolonged hyperstimulation as a result of estrogen excess from anovulation.

It is important to screen patients considering hormonal contraceptive treatment for contraindications including cigarette smoking, hypertension, hyperlipidemia, and diabetes with vascular complications.

For women who cannot take or do not tolerate hormonal contraceptives, metformin is a second-line option for improving menstrual regularity. Metformin has been shown to regulate oocyte maturation, and some studies have shown that it modulates adrenal and ovarian androgen output. It does not directly provide endometrial protection, but decreases the risk of endometrial hyperstimulation indirectly if ovulatory function is restored. Patients on metformin alone should be counseled on adequate contraception because restoration of ovulatory function increases fertility and metformin does not provide contraception.

What are the appropriate treatment options for this patient's hirsutism?

Mechanical hair removal such as shaving and plucking may be adequate treatment for hirsutism for some patients. In patients who require medical therapy, hormonal contraceptives are the first-line treatment for hirsutism because they reduce androgen levels through decreasing ovarian production of androgens and reduce bioavailable androgens through increased SHBG. In addition, some progestins contained in hormonal contraceptives are antiandrogenic.

Oral spironolactone is an androgen-receptor antagonist that can be used to treat hirsutism, although it is not FDA approved for this condition. It is typically used in addition to hormonal contraceptives if symptoms do not improve after 6 months. Patients interested in treating hirsutism with spironolactone should be counseled on the necessity of adequate contraception. Spironolactone can disrupt androgen-dependent processes such as formation of external genitalia in a male fetus. Because spironolactone is also a mineralocorticoid-receptor antagonist, patients should be monitored for hyperkalemia after initiation.

Finally, metformin may reduce androgen levels but has minimal effect on terminal hair growth and should therefore not be used for this purpose.

Patients should be counseled that changes in the quality of terminal hair begin at the root and visible changes might therefore not be apparent for up to 6 months.

Given the new diagnosis of PCOS, which other conditions should this patient be screened for?

All women and adolescents with PCOS should be screened for depression and anxiety. Studies have shown an increased prevalence of depression in women with PCOS, which appears to be independent of obesity, androgen levels, acne, and infertility. A simple screening test such as a PHQ-2 would be appropriate.

Women with PCOS who are overweight or obese should also be screened for obstructive sleep apnea (OSA). Women with PCOS are 30 times more likely to have sleep-disordered breathing than BMI-matched controls. Patients should be asked about daytime sleepiness, snoring, or observed cessation of breathing. A screening questionnaire such as the STOP-BANG questionnaire could be used to evaluate the need for polysomnography. Interestingly, it appears that treating OSA in women with PCOS improves insulin sensitivity.

A diagnosis of PCOS confers a 5- to 10-fold increased risk of developing type 2 diabetes and impaired glucose tolerance is reported in 30%–35% of women with PCOS. Women and adolescents with PCOS should be screened for impaired glucose tolerance. The 2-hour oral glucose tolerance test (OGTT) is preferred to a hemoglobin A1c (HbA1c) because of limited sensitivity of HbA1c in detecting impaired glucose tolerance. The OGTT should be repeated every 1–5 years. Impaired glucose tolerance, when recognized, should be treated with diet and exercise plus medication such as metformin as needed.

BASIC SCIENCE/CLINICAL PEARL **STEP 1/2/3**

Women with PCOS who have insulin resistance have a primary dysfunction in postprandial glucose uptake. Commonly, fasting hyperglycemia is not present. Two-hour OGTT is a more sensitive screening test for insulin resistance, which tends to be predominantly postprandial in patients with PCOS because it mimics the response to a glucose load from a meal. Fasting plasma glucose may be normal and A1c normal or only slightly elevated in patients with PCOS and significant postprandial hyperglycemia.

Women and adolescents with PCOS should also be screened for cardiovascular risk factors including obesity, cigarette smoking, hypertension, dyslipidemia, vascular disease, and family history of premature cardiovascular disease. Screening includes measurement of BMI, waist circumference, and blood pressure at each visit. A fasting lipid panel should be checked at least once every 2 years.

CLINICAL PEARL **STEP 2/3**

All patients with PCOS should be screened for insulin resistance, depression, anxiety, OSA, and cardiovascular risk factors.

An oral glucose tolerance test is performed with a result of 2-hour postglucose blood glucose 215 mg/dL (normal ≤200 mg/dL).

What is the appropriate treatment for this patient's obesity and insulin resistance?

The first-line treatment for obesity and insulin resistance is diet and exercise. There is no evidence that one type of diet is superior to others, but starting with a calorie-restricted diet is suggested.

As metformin has not been shown to increase weight loss in patients using diet and exercise programs, it should be used primarily in women who have PCOS and impaired glucose tolerance or type 2 diabetes who have not lost weight as a result of diet and exercise.

CLINICAL PEARL **STEP 2/3**

The cornerstone of treatment for PCOS is lifestyle changes such as diet and exercise. OCPs are first line for oligomenorrhea and hirsutism. Metformin can be added if diet and exercise do not lead to weight loss in patients with impaired glucose tolerance.

The patient is counseled on diet and exercise and started on treatment with oral contraceptive pills, then started on spironolactone 6 months later given inadequate reduction in hair growth. She returns 6 months later and is started on metformin given minimal weight loss. She returns 2 years later and would like to become pregnant.

How do you counsel her?

PCOS is the most common cause of anovulatory infertility. The primary etiology of infertility appears to be oligo- or anovulation, although endometrial changes discouraging implantation may also play a role. All women with PCOS desiring fertility should be questioned regarding menstrual history to determine ovulatory status.

Because this patient wishes to become pregnant, oral contraceptive pills and spironolactone should be discontinued. Weight loss may improve fertility. Metformin should be continued because it may assist with weight loss, may be associated with monofollicular ovulation, and may decrease multiple pregnancy rates.

The patient should be counseled that women with PCOS are at increased risk of gestational diabetes, preeclampsia, small for gestational age infants, and perinatal mortality. All women with PCOS should have a preconceptual assessment of BMI, blood pressure, and OGTT.

The patient returns 6 months after stopping oral contraceptive pills and spironolactone. She has lost 3 kg with diet and exercise but is not having regular menses. She would like to become pregnant soon and is requesting additional treatment.

What additional treatment can be offered?

According to the 2013 Endocrine Society guidelines for PCOS, clomiphene, a selective estrogen receptor modulator, is the first-line treatment for infertility in PCOS, although the use of the aromatase inhibitor, letrozole, is becoming more prevalent. In several trials, clomiphene showed increased pregnancy rates compared with metformin alone, although in clomiphene-resistant women, the addition of metformin to clomiphene has led to higher birth rates than clomiphene alone. Metformin has shown higher pregnancy rates but not higher live-birth rates and it should therefore not be used as first-line therapy alone for infertility. Letrozole, an aromatase inhibitor, has also shown promise in increasing birth rates compared with clomiphene and may become first-line treatment for infertility in women with PCOS wishing to become pregnant, although it is not currently FDA approved for this condition. In some cases, ovarian stimulation with exogenous gonadotropins or in vitro fertilization may be required.

The patient returns 6 months later and reports that she recently found out that she is 8 weeks pregnant. She is currently taking metformin.

How should the patient be counseled?

In women with PCOS, the routine use of metformin during pregnancy is not recommended because it has not shown a significant difference in the prevalence of preeclampsia, preterm delivery, or gestational diabetes. If the indication for metformin is to treat PCOS (and not type 2 diabetes mellitus), it should be discontinued after a positive pregnancy test. Metformin has been shown to cross the placenta and is present in therapeutic concentrations in umbilical cord blood. There have been no reports of teratogenicity associated with the use of metformin during pregnancy, but a recent study has shown that children exposed to metformin in utero had a higher BMI and increased prevalence of overweight/obesity at 4 years of age.

Case Summary

- **Complaint/History:** A 19-year-old female with history of irregular menses since menarche presents with abnormal hair growth for 1 year.
- **Findings:** The patient is obese with excess hair growth in androgen-dependent areas and acanthosis nigricans.
- **Lab Results/Tests:** Lab tests reveal mild elevation in testosterone and DHEA-S levels with normal thyroid function tests, prolactin level, and 17-hydroxyprogesterone level.

Diagnosis: Polycystic ovarian syndrome.

- **Treatment:** The patient was counseled on weight loss through diet and exercise. The patient was started on oral contraceptives for regulation of menses and to decrease androgen-dependent hair growth. Spironolactone was later added because of insufficient reduction in hair growth with oral contraceptives alone. Metformin was prescribed and resulted in minimal weight loss. When the patient later wished to become pregnant, oral contraceptives and spironolactone were discontinued. Following confirmation of pregnancy, metformin was discontinued.

BEYOND THE PEARLS

- Daughters born to mothers with PCOS have a fivefold risk of developing PCOS themselves.
- Bariatric surgery has been shown to be effective in alleviating symptoms of PCOS in obese women, probably as a result of the ensuing weight loss.
- Thiazolidinediones have been shown to decrease androgen levels in women with PCOS but are not currently recommended by Endocrine Society guidelines because of safety concerns such as cardiovascular risk and fetal loss.
- In women with PCOS in whom hirsutism cannot be adequately controlled with oral contraceptives and spironolactone, finasteride, which inhibits the conversion of testosterone to dihydrotestosterone, can be considered.
- Women with PCOS who become pregnant are at higher risk of gestational diabetes, preeclampsia, fetal macrosomia, small for gestational age infants, and perinatal mortality.

- When checking testosterone levels in women being evaluated for hyperandrogenism, free testosterone is the most sensitive test for hyperandrogenism. Equilibrium dialysis is the gold standard for measuring free testosterone because other types of assays are relatively inaccurate at the low levels seen in women.
- Clomiphene and letrozole are the most commonly used medications for ovulation induction for patients with PCOS struggling with infertility.

Bibliography

Azziz, R., Carmina, E., Chen, Z., Dunaif, A., Laven, J. S. E., Legro, R. S., Lizneva, D., Natterson-Horowitz, B., Teede, H. J., & Yildiz, B. O. (2016). Polycystic ovary syndrome. *Nat. Rev.*, *2*(1), 1–18.

Chittenden, B.G., Fullerton, G., Maheshwari, A., Bhattacharya, S. (2009). Polycystic ovary syndrome and the risk of gynaecological cancer: a systematic review. *Reprod. Biomed. Online*, 19(3), 398–405.

Faure, M., Bertoldo, M. J., Khoueiry, R., Bongrani, A., Brion, F., Giulivi, C., Dupont, J., & Froment, P. (2018). Metformin in reproductive biology. *Frontiers in Endocrinology*, 9. https://doi.org/10.3389/fendo.2018.00675.

Ferriman, D., & Gallwey, J. D. (1961). Clinical assessment of body hair growth in women. *The Journal of Clinical Endocrinology and Metabolism*, *21*, 1440–1447.

Hanem, L. G. E., Stridsklev, S., Júlíusson P. B., Salvesen, Ø., Roelants, M., Carlsen, S. M., Ødegard, R., & Vanky, E. (2018). Metformin use in PCOS pregnancies increases the risk of offspring overweight at 4 years of age: follow-up of two RCTs. *The Journal of Clinical Endocrinology and Metabolism*, *103*(4), 1612–1621.

Legro, R. S., Arslanian, S. A., Ehrmann, D. A., Hoeger, K. M., Murad, M. H., Pasquali, R., & Welt, C. K. (2013). Diagnosis and treatment of polycystic ovary syndrome: an Endocrine Society Clinical Practice Guideline. *The Journal of Clinical Endocrinology and Metabolism*, *98*(12), 4565–4592.

Lizneva, D., Suturina, L., Walker, W., Brakta, S., Gavrilova-Jordan, L., & Azziz, R. (2016). Criteria, prevalence, and phenotypes of polycystic ovary syndrome. *Fertility and Sterility*, *106*(1), 6–15.

McCartney, C. R., & Marshall, J. C. (2016). Polycystic ovary syndrome. *The New England Journal of Medicine*, *375*, 54–64.

Rosenfeld, R., & Ehrmann, D. (2016). The pathogenesis of polycystic ovary syndrome (PCOS): The hypothesis of PCOS as functional ovarian hyperandrogenism revisited. *Endocrine Reviews*, *37*(5), 467–520.

Singh, D., Arumalla, K., Aggarwal, S., Singla V., Ganie, A., & Malhotra N. (2020). Impact of bariatric surgery on clinical, biochemical, and hormonal parameters in women with polycystic ovary syndrome (PCOS). *Obesity Surgery*, *30*(6), 2294–2300.

Teede, H. J., Misso, M. L., Costello, M. F., Dokras, A., Laven, J., Moran, L., Piltonen, T., Norman, R. J., & International PCOS Network. (2018). Recommendations from the international evidence-based guideline for the assessment and management of polycystic ovary syndrome. *Fertility and Sterility*, *110*(3), 364–379.

Witchel, S. F., Oberfield, S. E., & Peña, A. S. (2019). Polycystic ovary syndrome: pathophysiology, presentation, and treatment with emphasis on adolescent girls. *Journal of the Endocrine Society*, *3*(8), 1545–1573.

SECTION 12

Pulmonary

CASE 54

A 67-Year-Old Male With Sudden Onset of Dyspnea and Pleuritic Chest Pain

Anish R. Patel ■ Raj Dasgupta

A 67-year-old male presents to the emergency department with sudden onset of right sided chest pain while playing soccer with his grandchildren. He describes the pain as sharp in quality and has developed worsening shortness of breath. The patient is a shopkeeper by occupation; he is married with three healthy children and two grandchildren. He has a 30-pack per year smoking history but successfully quit 5 years ago. His past medical history is significant for hypertension and chronic obstructive pulmonary disease (COPD). His current medications include amlodipine, tiotropium/formoterol, albuterol, and budesonide inhaler. On physical examination, the patient is afebrile, blood pressure is 138/76 mmHg, pulse rate is 105 beats/min, respiration rate is 28 breaths/min, and oxygen saturation is 88% on room air. On lung examination, there are diminished breath sounds and hyperresonance with percussion on the right. There is no jugular vein distention (JVD) and the trachea is midline. The remainder of the examination is normal. Laboratory results are unremarkable.

Which causes of hypoxia should be considered in this patient?

There are two major causes of hypoxia at the tissue level, low blood flow to the tissue, or low oxygen content in the blood (hypoxemia); both of which our patient is at risk for. The cause of hypoxemia can be categorized into five categories, which are listed in Table 54.1. Two key clinical findings that help differentiate between the different causes of hypoxemia are the presence of an increased alveolar-arterial oxygen gradient and responsiveness to oxygen. Understanding the mechanism of hypoxia will provide clues to help determine the underlying diagnosis. Our patient appears to have an issue with his lungs preventing him from getting adequate oxygen to the blood.

Oxygen delivery is formally calculated using the degree of Hb oxygen saturation, and dissolved O_2 content in arterial blood and cardiac output (CO). The oxygen consumption (VO2) is a composite estimate of the global oxygen utilization (Fig. 54.1).

TABLE 54.1 ■ **Causes of Hypoxemia**

Hypoxemia Cause	O_2 Response	A-a Gradient
Reduced O_2 Tension(High Altitude)	Yes	Normal
Hypoventilation	Yes	Normal
Diffusion Impairment	Yes	Elevated
R to L Shunt	No	Elevated
V/Q mismatch	Yes	Elevated

$$DO_2 = CO \times \underbrace{[(1.38 \times Hb \times SaO_2) + (0.0031 \times SaO_2)]}_{\text{Arterial Oxygen Content}} \times 10$$

Fig. 54.1 Oxygen delivery equation. DO_2, oxygen delivery; CO, cardiac output L/min; Hb, hemoglobin concentration g/DL, SaO2 = arterial oxygen saturation. (From Cove, M. E., & Pinsky, M. R. (2012). Perioperative hemodynamic monitoring. *Best Practice & Research Clinical Anaesthesiology, 26*(4), 453–462.

The patient's pleuritic chest pain and persistent hypoxia may warrant urgent treatment. At this time, the emergency department physician decides to perform a bedside ultrasound. The results of the ultrasound (see Fig. 54.2) demonstrate key sonographic features highly suggestive of pneumothorax.

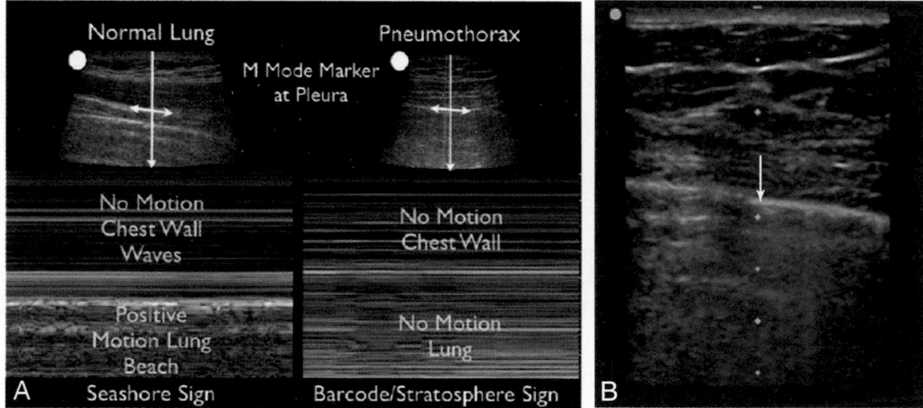

Fig. 54.2 (A) M-mode of normal lung US showing the seashore sign versus M-mode of PTX showing the barcode or stratosphere sign. (From Lobo, V et al: Thoracic ultrasonography. *Critical Care Clinics* 30(1), 93–117, 2014.). (B) Point-of-care lung sonogram of the left lung of a patient receiving high-frequency oscillatory ventilation (HFOV), confirming the presence of a pneumothorax by the presence of a lung point (arrow). (Republished with permission of the Journal of Ultrasound in Medicine: From Gillman, L. M., & Kirkpatrick, A. W. (2010). Lung sonography as a bedside tool for the diagnosis of a pneumothorax in a patient receiving high-frequency oscillatory ventilation. *Journal of Ultrasound in Medicine, 29*, 997–1000. Permission conveyed through the Copyright Clearance Center.)

CLINICAL PEARL **STEP 1/2/3**

Hypoxia and hypoxemia do not always coexist. Because they have similar spelling, these two conditions are often confused, or assumed to be the same. While they can co-occur, they're fairly different. Hypoxia historically refers to a problem with diffusion of oxygen from the atmosphere to the alveoli into the capillaries and eventually being utilized at the tissue level. This is in contrast to hypoxemia, which refers to the delivery of oxygen into the arterial circulation. Hypoxemia is primarily dependent on the cardiovascular system, particularly the cardiac output and amount of hemoglobin available. Patients can develop hypoxia without hypoxemia, if there is a compensatory increase in oxygen delivery through increased hemoglobin levels and cardiac output.

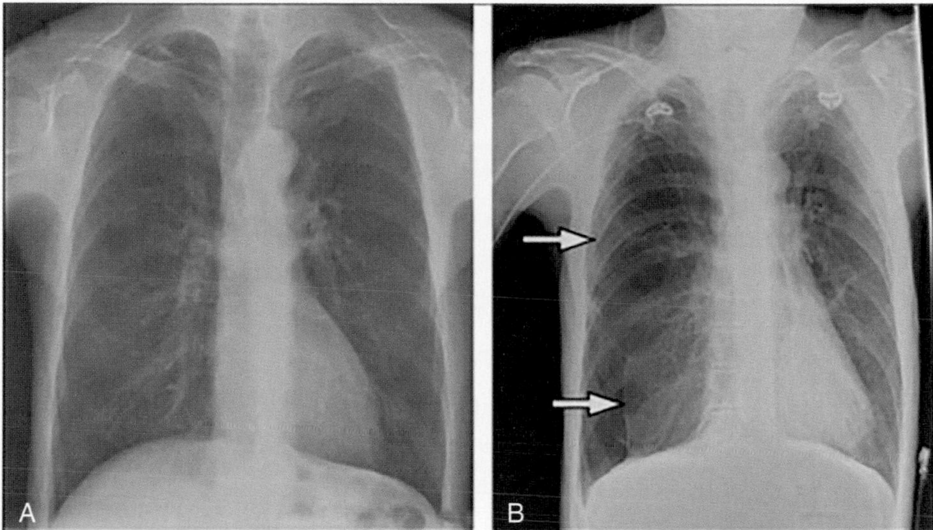

Fig. 54.3 A chest radiograph revealing spontaneous pneumothorax. The thin white line of the visceral pleura is outlined by a right-sided pneumothorax particularly in the right lower zone, with a shallower rim of pneumothorax in the upper zone *(arrows)*. (From Gupta, A., & Seely, J. M. (2019). *Muller's imaging of the chest.* pp. 942–962.)

A portable chest X-ray image confirms the diagnosis of a right-sided pneumothorax (see Fig. 54.3), with partial collapse in both the upper and lower portions of the right lung. Hyperinflation is consistent with the existing diagnosis of COPD.

BASIC SCIENCE/CLINICAL PEARL **STEP 1/2/3**

A pneumothorax is usually confirmed by upright CXR in the exhalation phase of the respiratory system. This results in reduction of lung volume, allowing the lung to become more dense making the pneumothorax easier to identify. If possible it is preferable to have patient in the upright or semi-upright position (Fig. 54.4).

CLINICAL PEARL **STEP 2/3**

Common classic radiographic signs of pneumothorax include:

- White visceral pleural line
- Absence of lung markings beyond the white line of visceral pleura
- Deep sulcus sign (supine radiograph)
- Prominent mediastinal fat tags

What are the different types of pneumothorax and how are they classified?

In the clinical setting, a pneumothorax is typically categorized as primary, secondary, iatrogenic, or traumatic, as demonstrated in Table 54.2. They may also be classified as simple versus tension, with the latter demonstrating a shift of the heart or mediastinal structures on imaging. Patients who suffer trauma to the chest or back can have an open or closed pneumothorax depending on whether the thoracic cage is intact and negative intrathoracic pressure is maintained. Open pneumothorax results from a penetrating thoracic injury than permits entry of air into the chest, while closed pneumothorax is the accumulation of air originating from the

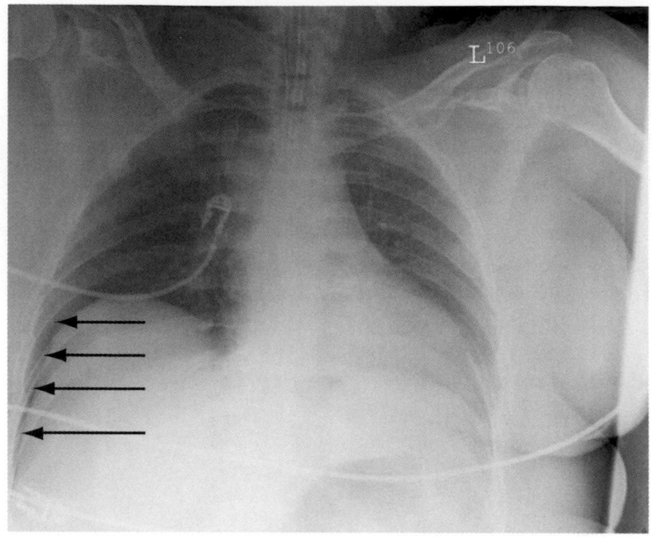

Fig. 54.4 Chest x-ray image of the patient with the indicated narrow, sharp, and black air line forward to the abdominal region at the right costophrenic angle, which represents the deep sulcus sign in pneumothorax. (From McQuillan KA, Makic MB, Trauma nursing, ed 5. St. Louis, Elsevier, 2020.)

TABLE 54.2 ■ **Types of Pneumothorax**

Spontaneous	Primary: No predisposing lung disease (tall, young, thin, male) Secondary: COPD, asthma, bronchiectasis
Traumatic	Open "sucking" chest wound (i.e., gunshot/stab wound) Closed (i.e., rib fracture)
Iatrogenic	Thoracentesis, Central Line placement, Bronchoscopy
Tension	Life-threatening. When a lung/chest wall injury allows air into pleural space but not out of it (a one-way valve)

COPD, Chronic obstructive pulmonary disease.

respiratory system within the pleural space. Any presence of fluid can result in a hydropneumothorax. Knowing the etiology of the lung injury will allow a timely response in deciding how to manage the condition.

BASIC SCIENCE PEARL **STEP 1**

Primary spontaneous pneumothorax is more common in smokers, men, and patients with tall and thin body habitus . It can be seen in patient's with Marfan's syndrome, which is a common inherited connective tissue disorder with several respiratory manifestations, spontaneous pneumothorax being the most frequently reported.

BASIC SCIENCE/CLINICAL PEARL **STEP 1/2/3**

Pneumocystitis jiroveci Pneumonia(PJP) is an atypical pulmonary infection and the most common opportunistic infection in patients with acquired immunodeficiency syndrome (AIDS). These fungal infections commonly result in pneumothorax.

What is your differential diagnosis?

Although this patient has an extensive smoking history, he is unlikely to have a primary spontaneous pneumothorax, which is typically a diagnosis of exclusion in patients who are young with no underlying lung disease. Because there is no trauma and no invasive medical procedures have been performed, the patient is most probably suffering from a secondary spontaneous pneumothorax. One of the most frequent underlying disorders causing secondary spontaneous pneumothorax is COPD. This patient is taking many medications and inhalers to manage his COPD, which suggests that the disease may be advanced. There are numerous other etiologies of secondary spontaneous pneumothorax that are listed in Table 54.3. It is hypothesized that the underlying lung injury caused a spontaneous rupture of a subpleural bleb or bullae resulting in a pneumothorax.

A CT chest from one of the patient's previous hospital visit was reviewed. The CT showed a large bleb/bullae in the setting of COPD and empysema. The likely etiology of this patient's pneumothorax is a rupture of a bleb (Fig. 54.5)

BASIC SCIENCE/CLINICAL PEARL **STEP 1/2/3**

The majority of secondary pneumothoraxes are iatrogenic. The most common causes are transthoracic needle aspiration, thoracentesis, subclavian venipuncture, and positive-pressure ventilation.

The patient continues to appear in respiratory distress. He is dyspneic with use of accessory respiratory muscles. SpO_2 remains below 92% despite supplemental oxygen.

What are the clinic considerations and treatment options for managing pneumothorax?

The major indications for immediate needle or tube thoracostomy are listed in Table 54.4. Irrespective of etiology, immediate management depends on the extent of cardiorespiratory

TABLE 54.3 ■ **Secondary Spontaneous Pneumothorax**

Disease	Manifestation
Pulmonary disease	COPD, asthma, emphysema, cystic fibrosis, sarcoidosis, IPF, idiopathic pulmonary hemorrhage, Langerhans cell histiocytosis, beryIliosis, silicosis, pulmonary alveolar proteinosis
Connective tissue disease	Marfan syndrome, Ehlers-Danlos syndrome, neurofibromatosis, tuberous sclerosis, lymphangioleiomyomatosis, mitral valve prolapse
Infection	Tuberculosis, pneumonia(bacterial/fungal), pericarditis, myocarditis
Drugs and toxins	Chemotherapy, radiation, hyperbaric oxygen therapy, aerosolized pentamidine
Immunologic disease	Rheumatoid arthritis, scleroderma, polymyositis, dermatomyositis, ankylosing spondylitis
Gastrointestinal disease	Boerhaave's syndrom, gastropleural fistula, colopleural fistula

COPD, Chronic obstructive pulmonary disease; *IPF*, idiopathic pulmonary fibrosis.

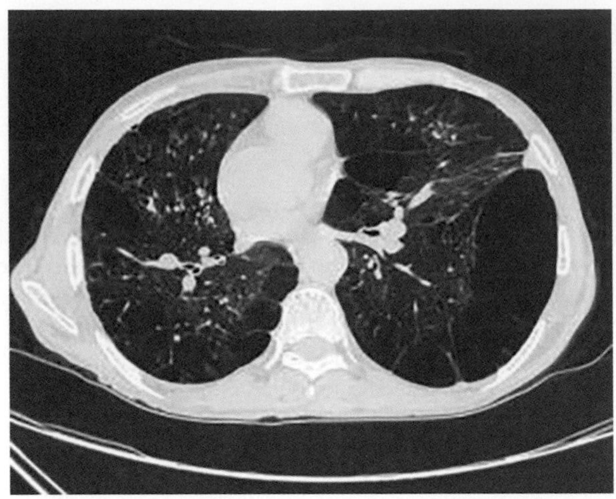

Fig. 54.5 Computed tomography thorax revealing large bullae. (From Dua, R., & Singhal, A. (2016). Localized hyperlucency in an acutely dyspneic patient: Always a pneumothorax? *Journal of Emergency Medicine*, *51*(2), e7–e9.)

TABLE 54.4 ■ **Indications for Thoracostomy**

- Traumatic cause of pneumothorax (except asymptomatic, apical)
- Moderate to large pneumothorax
- Respiratory symptoms regardless of size of pneumothorax
- Increasing size of pneumothorax after initial conservative therapy
- Recurrence of pneumothorax after removal of an initial chest tube
- Patient requires ventilator support
- Patient requires general anesthesia
- Associated hemothorax
- Bilateral pneumothorax regardless of size
- Tension pneumothorax

impairment, degree of symptoms, and size of pneumothorax. Guidelines have been produced that outline appropriate strategies in the care of patients with a pneumothorax and the emergence of video-assisted thoracoscopic surgery has created a more accessible and successful tool in order to prevent recurrence in select individuals. Medical optimization and management of secondary causes of pneumothorax are also critical in preventing recurrence.

CLINICAL PEARL **STEP 2/3**

Investigations or therapies may need to be targeted at suspected secondary causes to treat and prevent pneumothorax recurrence.

CLINICAL PEARL **STEP 1/2/3**

The different strategies available for treatment include observation, supplemental oxygen administration, needle aspiration, insertion of small-bore chest drains, and surgery. A chest tube is connected to a water seal device with or without suction and is kept until the pneumothorax resolves.

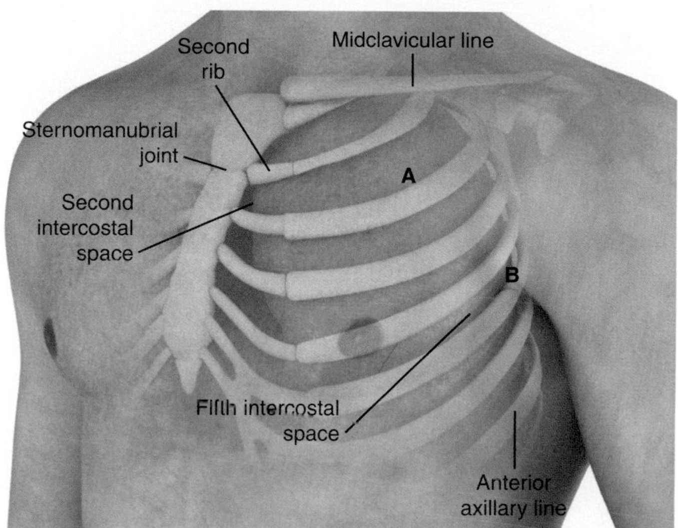

Fig. 54.6 Needle decompression is most often performed in the second intercostal space, midclavicular line. The chest wall is thick in this region and catheters shorter than 5 cm may fail to enter the pleural cavity. The subclavian vessels lay superior to the site and the internal mammary arteries lay medial to the site; both are at risk of being injured. (From Roberts, J. R. (2019). *Roberts and Hedges' clinical procedures in emergency medicine and acute care* (7th ed.). Elsevier.)

Needle aspiration was attempted in the second intercostal space, midclavicular line (see Fig. 54.6). Unfortunately, because of the incomplete resolution of the pneumothorax, it was decided to admit the patient for drainage via catheter. A pigtail catheter was placed (see Fig. 54.7) and the patient was observed over the next few days with subsequent improvement in his symptoms. Repeat X-ray image after pigtail catheter placement showed a marked improvement in the pneumothorax. The patient felt much better and he was scheduled for follow-up in the pulmonary clinic. Patient will also have follow-up with a CT surgeon in regards to possible blebectomy in the future.

What are possible complications of pneumothorax to look out for?

Many of the most common complications after a pneumothorax are included in Table 54.5. Issues such as effusion, hemorrhage, empyema, respiratory failure, or arrhythmias should be anticipated and treated accordingly in the days to weeks following a pneumothorax. Smoking cessation, persistent respiratory function exercise, proper breathing exercise, and proper expectoration are also means of reducing pneumothorax recurrence. Close follow-up and management of any other coexisting comorbidities are essential in preventing another occurrence.

Case Summary

- **Complaint/History:** A 67-year-old male presents with sudden onset of dyspnea and pleuritic chest pain.
- **Findings:** Oxygen saturation is 88% on room air; lung exam reveals diminished breath sounds and hyperresonance to percussion on right.
- **Lab Results/Tests:** Ultrasound demonstrates lung point sign and absence of lung sliding. Chest X-ray image confirms right-sided pneumothorax with white visceral line outlining border of collapsed lung.

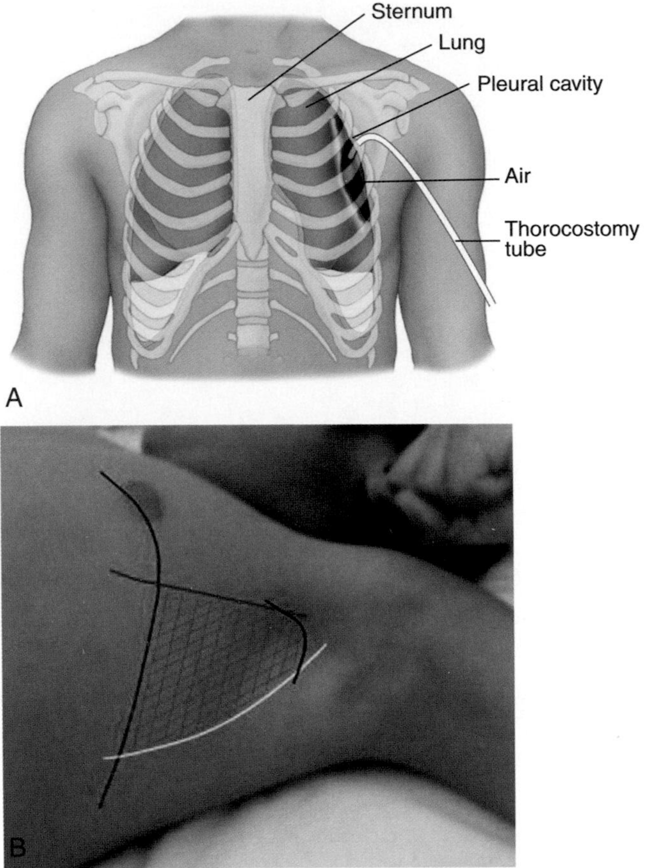

Fig. 54.7 (A) A chest tube place to relieve a pneumothorax. (B) The triangle of safety *(crosshatched area)* for insertion of a chest drain is typically within the third to fifth intercostal spaces. It is bordered by the anterior border of the latissimus dorsi *(yellow)*, lateral border of pectoralis major *(red)*, a line at the horizontal level of the nipple (in men) or base of the breast (in women) and the apex in the axilla. ((A) from Ehrlich, R. A., & Coakes, D. (2014). *Patient care in radiography: with an introduction to medical imaging* (10th ed.). Elsevier; (B) from Kirmani, B. H., & Page, R. D. (2014). Pneumothorax and insertion of a chest drain, *Surgery*, *32*(5), 272–275.)

TABLE 54.5 ■ **Posttreatment Complications**

- Intercostal vessel hemorrhage
- Lung parenchymal injury
- Tube malfunction
- Air leak
- Development of tension pneumothorax
- Reinflation pulmonary injury
- Infection of wound/puncture site

Diagnosis: Secondary spontaneous pneumothorax.

- **Treatment:** The patient received needle decompression and eventual pigtail catheter placement. Pleurodesis via VATS is planned for follow-up for recurrence prevention.

BEYOND THE PEARLS

- Primary spontaneous pneumothorax (PSP) presents in the absence of clinical lung disease, while secondary spontaneous pneumothorax (SSP) presents as a complication of underlying lung disease.
- Recurrence rates vary but, in general, the risk of recurrence is higher with SSP (30-50%) than with PSP (10-30%).
- Once patients have undergone initial management, clinicians should assess the risk of recurrence to evaluate whether definitive management is indicated.
- Indications include patients with PSP assessed to be at high risk of recurrence, patients with high risk professions or hobbies (eg. airplane pilot or deep sea diver), patients with a prolonged (persistent) air leak (typically >5 days), patients with SSP or recurrent pneumothorax, or patients with a concomitant indication for thorascopy (eg, hemothorax or lung biopsy).
- For most patients in whom a definitive procedure is indicated, surgical approaches are recommended rather than nonsurgical approaches. This preference is based upon the high efficacy of surgery in this population who are at a high risk of recurrence.
- For patients in whom a definitive procedure is indicated who are poor candidates for or are unwilling to undergo VATS, chemical pleurodesis is suggested via tube thoracostomy rather than tube thoracostomy drainage alone. This procedure reduces the recurrence rate.
- Choosing a sclerosing agent such a tetracycline or talc is individualized and clinicians should weigh the risks of adverse effects vs. efficacy.
- In the event that an air leak persists after the placement of chest tube, a multidisciplinary approach is advised where discussion of several options should be undertaken including catheter-directed pleurodesis, thorascopic revision, or conservative management.
- Pneumothorax ex vacuo results when the lung is trapped by thick fibrous pleural tissue, preventing full expansion. It is usually seen after pleural fluid removal. Instead of lung re-expansion, gas replaces the effusion.
- Avoid positive pressure therapy while draining a hydro- or pneumothorax as well as 1–2 weeks postdrain removal to avoid pleural fistula and risk of recurrence.
- Smoking cessation is always recommended to prevent recurrent pneumothoraces.
- Recurrence is greatest during the first month after presentation; patients should avoid air travel, scuba diving, and vigorous aerobic exercise for a limited period.

Bibliography

Alrajab, S., Youssef, A. M., Akkus, N. I., & Caldito, G. (2013, Sep 23). Pleural ultrasonography versus chest radiography for the diagnosis of pneumothorax: Review of the literature and meta-analysis. *Critical Care, 17*(5), R208.

Carr, J. J., Reed, J. C., Choplin, R. H., Pope, T. L., & Case, L. D. (1992). Plain and computed radiography for detecting experimentally induced pneumothorax in cadavers: Implications for detection in patients. *Radiology, 183*, 193.

Kosowsky, J., & Kimberly, H. (2018). Pleural disease. In R. Walls, R. Hockberger, & M. Gausche-Hill (Eds.), *Rosen's emergency medicine: Concepts and clinical practice* (9th ed., pp. 881–889). Philadelphia: Elsevier.

Nicks, B. A., & Manthey, D. (2016). Pneumothorax. In J. E. Tintinalli, J. Stapczynski, O. Ma, D. M. Yealy, G. D. Meckler, & D. M. Cline (Eds.), *Tintinalli's emergency medicine: A comprehensive study guide* (8th ed). New York, NY: McGraw-Hill. http://accessmedicine.mhmedical.com/content.aspx?bookid=1658§ionid=109429615.

Wong, A., Galiabovitch, E., & Bhagwat, K. (2019 Apr). Management of primary spontaneous pneumothorax: A review. *ANZ Journal of Surgery, 89*(4), 303–308.

CASE 55

A 27-Year-Old Male Who Experienced a Seizure

Chongiin Kim ■ Neha Mehta ■ Raj Dasgupta

A 27-year-old male presents to the emergency department after having his first seizure. He is intubated for airway protection and transferred to the medical intensive care unit for further care. He has no prior medical or surgical history. He takes no known medications and his only known allergy is to shellfish. His social history is significant for a 4-pack-year smoking history and alcohol abuse. While in the intensive care unit, he requires prolonged ventilation due to agitation and severe alcohol withdrawal. On day 7 of intubation, he is noted to have increasing oxygen requirements on the ventilator.

What are some causes of hypoxemia to consider in patients on mechanical ventilation in the ICU?
In the ICU, there are many acute causes of hypoxemia that can be separated into equipment failure versus development of a new disease process. Equipment failure includes displacement or obstruction of the endotracheal tube. Disease processes include but are not limited to pulmonary edema, atelectasis, pneumothorax, bronchospasm, pulmonary embolism, and pneumonia.

He developed a fever of 38.6°C and had increased thick secretions requiring frequent suctioning. A chest X-ray is performed, which demonstrates a new right lower lobe (RLL) consolidation.

What is the most likely cause of this RLL consolidation in this patient?
This patient demonstrates clinical changes consistent with the development of a new disease process. The fever in the setting of thick secretions and frequent suctioning with new RLL consolidation on chest X-ray examination indicates an infectious etiology, such as pneumonia. Pneumonia (lower respiratory tract infection) is the second most common cause of hospitalization and the most common infectious cause of death worldwide. In patients who are hospitalized, a new fever and clinical changes suggestive of a respiratory infection should immediately be investigated further.

How do we differentiate CAP, HAP, and VAP? Which type of pneumonia does this patient have?
There are three large categories of pneumonia that can be differentiated by their clinical onset of timing: community acquired, hospital acquired, and ventilator assisted. The first, community-acquired pneumonia (CAP), presents as an acute infection of the lung parenchyma that is acquired outside the hospitalized setting. Hospital-acquired pneumonia (HAP) is an infection of the lung parenchyma that begins at least 48 hours postadmission to a hospitalized setting. In order to qualify as an HAP, the patient's disease must not have been incubating during admission. Ventilator-associated pneumonia (VAP) presents in patients who have been intubated for at least 48 hours.

In our patient's case, he has been intubated for 7 days and the fever and lung consolidation are consistent with a new presentation of pneumonia, making this patient's disease process consistent with VAP.

CLINICAL PEARL **STEP 2/3**

Healthcare associated Pneumonia (HCAP) is no longer an entity. It was previously used to identify patients at risk for infection for Multidrug Resistant (MDR) pathogens. However, this designation was overly sensitive and increased antibiotic use in patients who did not necessarily require broad coverage.

What should be the next step in confirming our diagnosis?

Diagnosis of pneumonia is a clinical decision. In the outpatient setting, with patients presenting with CAP, they can be treated accordingly if the provider has a high clinical suspicion of pneumonia. In patients who have suspected VAP, noninvasive sampling for cultures is the preferred method. Antibiotics can then be narrowed accordingly once the results are available.

A serum procalcitonin is obtained and returns elevated at 4.2 ng/mL (normal < 0.25 ng/mL). A mini-bronchoalveolar lavage (BAL) is obtained from the intubated patient.

How can procalcitonin help with diagnosis and duration of treatment in this patient?

According to Infectious Diseases Society of America (IDSA) recommendations, procalcitonin and C-Reactive Protein (CRP) should not be used to diagnose pneumonia (as described previously, the diagnosis is clinical). However, procalcitonin can be utilized to guide duration of treatment for pneumonia. Utilizing quantitative measures of procalcitonin levels may not be as helpful as considering levels qualitatively (trending its rise, fall, peak, and/or trough) in conjunction with clinical parameters may help in the decision to discontinue antibiotic treatment.

CLINICAL PEARL **STEP 2/3**

Procalcitonin should not be used to diagnose pneumonia but can be used to help guide duration of treatment.

What is the role of sputum cultures in treating pneumonia?

The role of sputum cultures varies with the severity of illness. In patients with relatively straight forward CAP that can be treated on an outpatient basis, there is generally no utility in obtaining sputum cultures. However, in patients who have severe disease, especially those who are intubated, sputum cultures should be taken in order to guide narrowing of antibiotics. Patients who were previously infected with Methicillin-resistant Staphylococcus aureus (MRSA) or *Pseudomonas* or are being empirically treated for these organisms should also have cultures sampled.

The method of sampling recommended by agencies varies. The IDSA and American Thoracic Society (ATS) recommend noninvasive sampling in the form of sputum expectoration or endotracheal aspirates with semiquantitative culture reporting (i.e., reports of light, moderate, or abundant growth). They believe that these forms of sampling (as opposed to more invasive techniques, such as bronchoalveolar lavage and protected specimen brushing (PSB)) can be performed more rapidly, require fewer resources, and are associated with fewer complications.

The European guidelines differ slightly in that they recommend invasive sampling. Guidelines published by the European Respiratory Society (ERS) and European Society of Intensive Care Medicine (ESICM) recommend invasive sampling via BAL, bronchoscopy BAL, or PSB in order

TABLE 55.1 ■ **Invasive and Noninvasive Sampling Techniques**

Technique	Example
Invasive	Fiber-optic bronchoscopy with protected specimen brush Fiber-optic bronchoscopy with alveolar lavage Lung biopsy and tissue culture
Noninvasive	Simple culture of endotracheal aspirate (qualitative or quantitative) Blind protected specimen brush Blind alveolar lavage

Adapted from Torres, A., Niederman, M. S., Chastre, J., Ewig, S., Fernandez-Vandellos, P., Hanberger, H., Kollef, M. Bassi, G. L., Luna, C. M., Martin-Loeches, I., Paiva, J. A., Read, R. C., Rigau, D., Timsit, J. F., Welte, T. & Wunderink, R. (2018). Summary of the international clinical guidelines for the management of hospital-acquired and ventilator-acquired pneumonia. *European Respiratory Journal Open Research 26*, 4(2), 00028-2018.

to obtain quantitative cultures. A positive quantitative culture for endotracheal aspirates is generally >1,000,000 CFU/mL. For a bronchoscopic or mini-BAL a positive quantitative culture is >10,000 CFU/mL, and for a PSB >1000 CFU/mL is considered positive. (See Table 55.1 for other examples.)

CLINICAL PEARL **STEP 2/3**

Sputum cultures should not be obtained in uncomplicated CAP cases and patients may be treated empirically. However, if there is a concern for MRSA or *Pseudomonas*, a pretreatment sputum culture should be obtained in order to tailor antibiotics accordingly.

Which are the most common organisms that cause CAP, HAP, and VAP?

There are a variety of organisms that cause pneumonia, and they can be categorized into bacterial, viral, and fungal etiologies. In CAP, approximately one-third of cases have a viral etiology. The remaining two-thirds of pneumonia cases are attributed to bacterial etiologies including atypical species and *Streptococcus pneumoniae* (although the rate has decreased due to vaccination efforts).

In HAP or VAP, the most common etiologies include Gram-positive cocci, such as MRSA or *S. pneumoniae*, as well as Gram-negative rods (such as *Escherichia coli, Klebsiella pneumoniae*, or *Pseudomonas*). In 2009–2010, approximately 24% of VAP consisted of *Staphylococcus* species and *Pseudomonas* made up 16% of cases.

***When do we consider MRSA or* Pseudomonas?**

MRSA and pseudomonal coverage should be initiated in patients suspected of having HAP or VAP and antibiotics can then be narrowed based on resultant sputum culture speciation and local hospital antibiograms. Other patients in whom MRSA or *Pseudomonas* coverage should be considered is in those who have had prolonged antibiotic administration prior to the development of their pneumonia, because they are at higher risk of resistant organisms.

The patient is started on empiric treatment of vancomycin and cefepime while BAL cultures are still pending.

What are the therapies for CAP, HAP, and VAP?

In all cases clinicians should treat empirically based on the local antibiogram, local distribution of pathogens, and patient-specific risk factors (i.e., severity of illness, recent antimicrobial exposure, and history of resistant pathogens). See Fig. 55.1 for general guidelines.

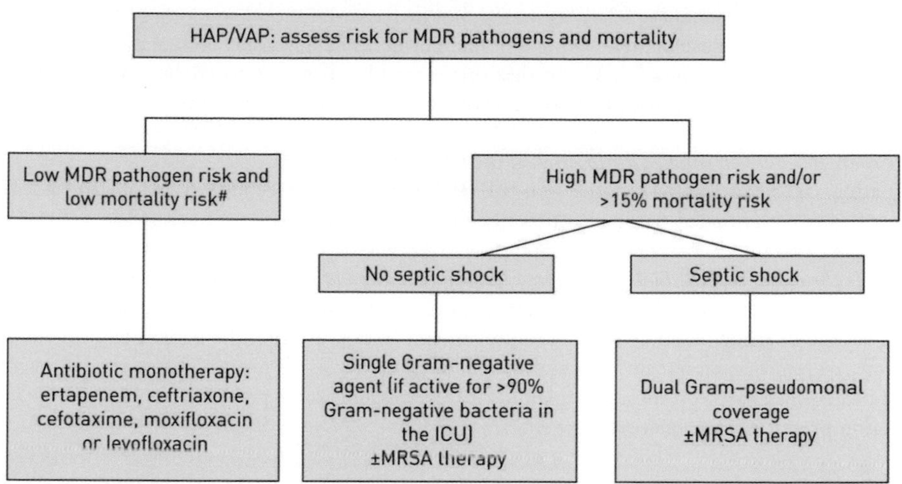

Fig. 55.1 Treatment guidelines. (From Torres, A., Niederman, M.S., Chastre, J., Ewig, S., Fernandez-Vandellos, P., Hanberger, H., Kollef, M. Bassi, G. L., Luna, C. M., Martin Loeches, I., Paiva, J. A., Read, R. C., Rigau, D., Timsit, J. F., Welte, T. & Wunderink, R. (2018). Summary of the international clinical guidelines for the management of hospital-acquired and ventilator-acquired pneumonia. *European Respiratory Journal Open Research 26*, 4(2), 00028-2018.).

In general, however, the IDSA recommends the following therapies for CAP, HAP, and VAP:

For CAP: in healthy patients, the IDSA recommends amoxicillin, doxycycline, or a macrolide. In patients who are high risk or have comorbid conditions, they recommend one of two options: amoxicillin/clavulanate or a cephalosporin AND a macrolide versus treatment with a respiratory fluoroquinolone.

For HAP: in patients who are not high risk, monotherapy with piperacillin-tazobactam, cefepime, levofloxacin, or meropenem is recommended. In those who are at higher risk of MRSA pneumonia based on the local prevalence of MRSA organisms, adding coverage for MRSA with linezolid or vancomycin is advised. If the patient was recently admitted and received IV antibiotics, the IDSA recommends treatment with two antipseudomonal agents in addition to MRSA coverage.

For VAP: the IDSA recommends two antipseudomonal agents as well as MRSA coverage.

There is not enough evidence to support routine use of steroids in patients who are diagnosed with CAP.

What is the duration of treatment recommended for CAP, HAP, and VAP?

CAP should be treated for a minimum of 5 days as long as the patient has been afebrile for 48 to 72 hours without oxygen requirements or signs of clinical instability. Longer durations may be needed for patients with parapneumonic effusions.

HAP and VAP should be treated for a minimum of 7 days. However, continued treatment after 7 days can and should be evaluated based on the clinical presentation of the patient.

Mini-BAL cultures return with 100,000 CFU of MRSA. The patient is continued on vancomycin monotherapy and cefepime is discontinued. Vancomycin is continued for a 7-day course. Patient's fever resolves and 11 days postintubation, he is successfully extubated.

What are some risk factors associated with development of pneumonia (CAP or HAP or VAP)?

There are several risk factors associated with development of pneumonia, including social/behavioral factors, underlying chronic illnesses, and demographic features.

In this case, our patient is relatively young, but he has a significant smoking history that predisposes him to the development of pneumonia. Furthermore, given his presentation of seizures, he is at higher risk of aspiration. Given that this patient has been intubated, he is also inherently at risk of ventilator-associated pneumonia secondary to aspiration of secretions.

Are there any data on inhaled antibiotics on ventilated patients?
In patients who have Gram-negative rods (GNRs) that are only susceptible to aminoglycosides or polymyxins, both inhaled systemic antibiotics should be considered.

What is the role of repeated imaging in monitoring resolution of pneumonia?
There is no role for repeat imaging in order to monitor resolution of pneumonia. Rather, the decision should be made based on clinical improvement. In the case that the patient clinically deteriorates or continues to remain with high suspicion of nonresolving pneumonia, repeated imaging may be obtained based on clinical suspicion. However, as long as the patient is improving, repeated imaging prior to discontinuing treatment is not useful.

CLINICAL PEARL **STEP 2/3**

Repeated imaging is not indicated unless there is lack of clinical improvement.

Case Summary

- **Complaint/History:** 27 year-old male who is intubated, presenting with fever and increasing oxygen requirements on the ventilator.
- **Findings:** Patient is found to have increased secretions seen while suctioning.
- **Lab Results/Tests:** Chest X-ray; Serum procalcitonin; Bronchoalveolar Lavage.

Diagnosis: Ventilator-associated pneumonia.

- **Treatment:** Vancomycin and Cefepime.

BEYOND THE PEARLS

- MRSA tends to cavitate and can be difficult to treat. Most common regimens for treatment include vancomycin and linezolid. Linezolid can be used as an outpatient regimen but monitor for myelosuppression that can be reversed once the agent is stopped. Daptomycin can cover MRSA but is inactivated by surfactant and is not an option for treatment of MRSA pneumonia.
- Always use your local antibiogram to make decisions about empiric coverage.
- Although aztreonam has a beta-lactam ring, it can be safely administered in a patient with a penicillin allergy for coverage of Gram-negative bacilli including *Pseudomonas*.
- Aminoglycosides have poor lung penetration and poor pleural fluid penetration, and thus are not recommended as monotherapy for Gram-negative pneumonias.
- VAP treatment can be extended to 14 days if the organism is a nonfermenting Gram-negative bacilli such as *Pseudomonas* because these organisms are associated with a higher reinfection rate when treated for only 7 days.
- The mnemonic SPICE-A (*Serratia, Pseudomonas*, Indole-positive *Proteus, Citrobacter, Enterobacter, Acinetobacter*) can be used to remember organisms that have inducible AmpC beta-lactamases rendering third-generation cephalosporins ineffective irrespective of in vitro susceptibility.
- The combination therapy of vancomycin and piperacillin-tazobactam has been shown to cause increased acute kidney injury in patients.

Bibliography

Guidelines for the management of adults with hospital-acquired, ventilator-associated, and healthcare-associated pneumonia. (2005). *American Journal of Respiratory and Critical Care Medicine*, *171*(4), 388–416.

Hill, A. T., Gold, P. M., El Solh, A. A., Metlay, J. P., Ireland, B., Irwin, R. S. (2019). Adult outpatients with acute cough due to suspected pneumonia or influenza: CHEST Guideline and Expert Panel Report. *Chest*, *155*(1), 155–167.

Kalil, A. C., Metersky, M. L., Klompas, M., Muscedere, J. Sweeney, D. A., Palmer, L. B., Napolitano, L. M., O'Grady, N. P., Bartlett, J. G., Carratalà, J., El Solh, A. A., Ewig, S., Fey, P. D., File, T. M. Jr., Restrepo, M. I., Roberts, J. A., Waterer, G. W., Cruse, P., Knight, S. L., & Brozek, J. L. (2016). Management of adults with hospital-acquired and ventilator-associated pneumonia: 2016 Clinical Practice Guidelines by the Infectious Diseases Society of America and the American Thoracic Society. *Clinical Infectious Diseases*, *63*(5), e61–e111.

Metlay, J. P., Waterer, G. W., Long, A. C., Anzueto, A., Brozek, J., Crothers, K., Cooley, L. A., Dean, N. C., Fine, M. J., Flanders, S. J., Griffin, M. R., Metersky, M. L. Musher, D. M., Restrepo, M. I., & Whitney, C. G. (2019). Diagnosis and treatment of adults with community-acquired pneumonia. *American Journal of Respiratory and Critical Care Medicine*, *200*(7), E45–E67.

Torres, A., Niederman, M. S., Chastre, J., Ewig, S., Fernandez-Vandellos, P., Hanberger, H., Kollef, M. Bassi, G. L., Luna, C. M., Martin-Loeches, I., Paiva, J. A., Read, R. C., Rigau, D., Timsit, J. F., Welte, T. & Wunderink, R. (2018). Summary of the international clinical guidelines for the management of hospital-acquired and ventilator-acquired pneumonia. *European Respiratory Journal Open Research 26*, *4*(2), 00028.

CASE 56

A 73-Year-Old Female With Dysphagia and Cough

Christine McElyea ■ Semi Han ■ Raj Dasgupta

A 73-year-old-woman presents to the emergency department from a skilled nursing facility with acute encephalopathy and hypoxia. She has a history of Parkinson's disease, dementia, type 2 diabetes mellitus, and coronary artery disease. Her medications are carbidopa-levodopa, memantine, metformin, aspirin, and atorvastatin. Her presenting vitals include a blood pressure of 140/80 mmHg, pulse rate of 102 beats/min, respiratory rate of 32 breaths/min, and temperature of 96.5 °F. Her oxygen saturation is 92% on 15 L non-rebreather mask. On physical examination, she is noticeably confused and responding minimally to questioning. She has a pill-rolling tremor and cogwheel rigidity worse in the right upper extremity. She has focal crackles in the left lower lobe.

What is the differential diagnosis for the hypoxemia in this patient?

Given the patient's history there is a broad differential diagnosis for her hypoxemia. Her history of diabetes and coronary artery disease puts her at risk of silent myocardial infarction. Fever and respiratory distress are suggestive of an infectious process in the lungs such as community-acquired pneumonia but not hospital-acquired pneumonia because this patient has not been in the hospital in the last 48 hours or within the last 90 days. Given her history of Parkinson's disease, the patient is at high risk of aspiration pneumonia or pneumonitis. Another cause of hypoxemia is pulmonary embolism causing ventilation and perfusion mismatch, which the patient may be at risk of if she lives a sedentary lifestyle. It is also important to investigate thoroughly for misuse of medications that can cause sedation or lower respiratory drive, such as opioid pain medications.

CLINICAL PEARL **STEP 2/3**

Healthcare-associated pneumonia is no longer a distinct type of pneumonia because the risk of infections with multidrug-resistant pathogens is low, and it is overly sensitive, leading to increased inappropriate use of antibiotics.

An electrocardiogram does not show any ischemic changes. A chest radiograph (CXR) (Fig. 56.1) is performed. You suspect a diagnosis of aspiration pneumonia or pneumonitis.

What is the difference between aspiration pneumonia and pneumonitis?

Aspiration pneumonitis is a noninfectious pulmonary inflammatory condition caused by aspiration of sterile gastric contents or other noninfectious materials such as blood or a foreign body. Low pH gastric content causes chemical burn in the airway and lung parenchyma, leading to tracheobronchitis and bilateral patchy infiltrates and may progress to acute respiratory distress syndrome. Sometimes bacterial superinfection occurs. Aspiration pneumonia is an infection caused

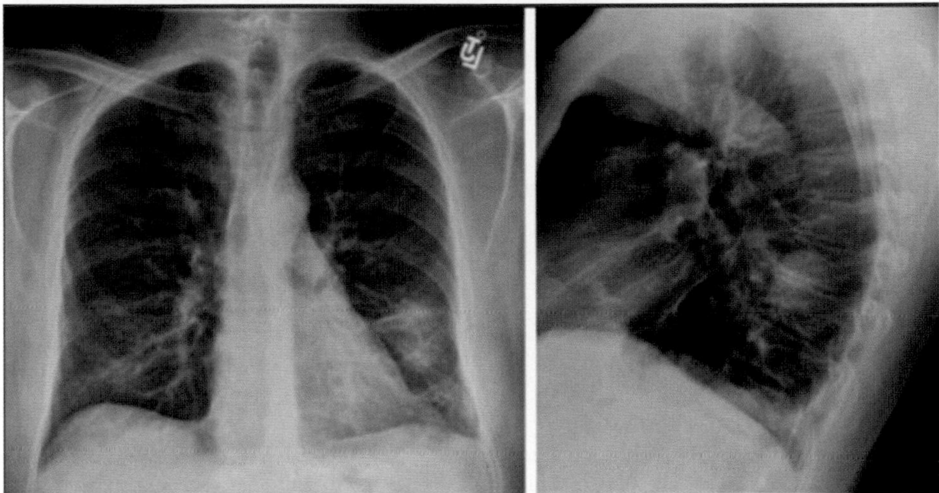

Fig. 56.1 Chest radiograph with frontal view demonstrating left lower lobe opacity and lateral view with round consolidation and blunted costophrenic angle. (From Goldman, L. (2008). *Cecil medicine* (23rd ed.). Elsevier.)

by specific pathogens in individuals with risk factors for aspiration. Both aspiration pneumonia and pneumonitis can cause coughing, wheezing, or shortness of breath. However, compared with bacterial aspiration pneumonia, chemical pneumonitis tends to improve more quickly, both clinically and radiographically.

Are there differences in diagnosis?

In both entities, aspiration should be suspected or witnessed. Pneumonitis is more acute in presentation, with abnormalities developing on chest X-ray within 2 hours of the aspiration event. The infiltrates associated with pneumonitis develop in the dependent portions of the lung, which are based on patient position during the aspiration event such that a supine patient may develop infiltrates in the superior segments of the lower lobes and the posterior segments of the upper lobes.

CLINICAL PEARL **STEP 2/3**

Although less subtle than macroaspiration, microaspiration is also a major cause of aspiration pneumonia.

The patient's bedside nurse at the nursing home reveals that the patient was eating and she may have had an aspiration event. Additionally, the nurse reports the patient has no history of *Pseudomonas* or methicillin-resistant *Staphylococcus aureus* infections.

What are the risk factors for aspiration?

Aspiration occurs when oropharyngeal or gastric contents enter the lungs. Risk factors include impaired swallowing from esophageal diseases such as oropharyngeal cancer or stricture, chronic obstructive pulmonary disease, mechanical ventilation, and general anesthesia. Impaired neurologic function from seizure, multiple sclerosis, stroke, or dementia are also common reasons for aspiration. Impaired consciousness such as that from intoxication or medications is also a common cause. These causes are summarized in Table 56.1.

TABLE 56.1 ■ **Risk Factors for Aspiration**

Altered Consciousness	Neurologic Disorder	Disruption of Barriers	Miscellaneous
Alcohol or drugs	Stroke	Nasogastric tube	Vomiting
Seizure	Multiple sclerosis	Endotracheal tube	Gastric outlet obstruction
Head trauma	Parkinson's disease	Bronchoscopy	Recumbent position
Anesthetic agents	Myasthenia gravis	Endoscopy	Ileus
	Amyotrophic lateral sclerosis		Vocal cord dysfunction

CLINICAL PEARL **STEP 2/3**

Aspiration may be silent (not associated with coughing) while eating or drinking.

What are common radiographic changes seen with aspiration pneumonia?

Radiographic findings include patchy infiltrates or dense opacity in gravity-dependent lung segments depending on the position of the patient at the time of the event. The basal segments of the lower lobe are commonly affected in patients who aspirate in an upright position. In patients who aspirate while in a supine position, the posterior segment of the upper lobe and apical segments of the lower lobe involvements are often observed. However, a chest radiograph may be negative early in the course of aspiration pneumonia; therefore, clinical history and assessment of the risk factors can be helpful in making the diagnosis.

CLINICAL PEARL **STEP 2/3**

Procalcitonin measurement is not useful for distinguishing between aspiration pneumonia and aspiration pneumonitis.

What are the common pathogens seen with aspiration pneumonia?

Overall bacteria that normally reside in the upper airways or stomach are often associated with aspiration pneumonia.

In the 1970s, anaerobes (particularly in normal oral flora) with or without aerobes were thought to be the predominant pathogens in aspiration pneumonia. More recently there has been a shift in dominant microbes toward bacteria associated with community and hospital acquired pneumonia. Community acquired pneumonia are commonly associated with *Streptococcus pneumoniae*, *Staphylococcus aureus*, *Haemophilus influenzae*, and *Enterobacteriaceae*, whereas *Pseudomonas aeruginosa* (Gram-negative bacilli) are dominant in hospital-acquired aspiration pneumonia. The Infectious Disease Society of America does not recommend routine addition of anaerobic coverage unless empyema or lung abscess is suspected in patients with aspiration pneumonia. However, oral anaerobes should be covered if the patient has significant dental or gingival diseases.

The patient develops a fever in the emergency department, and you decide to start an antibiotic.

Which antibiotics should be empirically started in a patient with suspected aspiration pneumonia?

Similar to the treatment approach for nonaspiration pneumonia, choice of antibiotic is dictated by the site of acquisition (community versus hospital), known exposure to multidrug resistance, and severity of illness (outpatient or inpatient). In patients who are clinically stable with mild symptoms, it is appropriate to withhold antibiotics initially and reassess in 48 hours even with abnormal CXR because those findings can be caused by chemical pneumonitis. If the patient is critically ill, it is reasonable to start antibiotics empirically. Choices of antibiotic treatment for aspiration pneumonia based on the risk factors are given in Table 56.2.

The patient is started on levofloxacin and she is admitted to the general medicine floor. The next day she is afebrile and her oxygen requirements improve. The nurse performs a bedside swallow evaluation and the patient coughs while swallowing pureed food.

CLINICAL PEARL **STEP 2/3**

The duration of antibiotics for aspiration pneumonia is not well studied. In general, they are administered for 7 days in patients with no evidence of necrotizing pneumonia.

What is dysphagia?

Dysphagia is the sensation of trouble swallowing and is manifested as difficulty moving food from the mouth into the pharynx and esophagus. The four stages of swallowing as described in Table 56.3 can be used to locate the disruption in the swallowing process and to determine the underlying cause of dysphagia. Oropharyngeal dysphagia is difficulty initiating swallow and transferring the food bolus into the esophagus. Neurologic or myogenic disorders such as Parkinson's disease increases the risk of dysphagia. Given this patient's advanced age, she may have cervical osteophytes rather than other structural abnormalities such as goiter, cricoid webs, or pharyngoesophageal (Zenker) diverticulum. Patients with esophageal dysphagia can trigger the swallowing process but have difficulty transporting from the esophagus to the stomach due to mechanical obstruction (i.e., strictures, neoplasm, esophageal ring) or a motility disorder (i.e., achalasia, esophageal spasm, systemic sclerosis).

Does placement of a nasogastric tube for enteral feeds prevent aspiration?

If possible, oral feeding is preferred over enteral feeding, which is preferred over parenteral feeding. However, if the patient cannot swallow safely, nasogastric tubes and postpyloric tubes are commonly placed for enteral feeding (Fig. 56.2). Table 56.4 summarizes the benefits and risks of each.

You decide to place a postpyloric feeding tube while the patient recovers her swallowing function.

TABLE 56.2 ■ **Aspiration Pneumonia Antibiotic Treatment**

Community-Acquired Pneumonia	Hospital-Acquired Pneumonia

• Outpatient
– Single
– Sulbactam
– Clavulanate[a]
  – fluroquinolone
  – amoxicillin-clavulanate
  – azithromycin
• Inpatient
– Nonsevere Medical ward:
  – Monotherapy with fluoroquinolone
  – A β-lactam[b] plus either macrolide[c] or doxycycline
– Severe Intensive care unit
  – A β-lactam plus either macrolide +/– fluoroquinolone
	• All should be treated empirically for *Pseudomonas aeruginosa* and other resistant Gram-negative bacilli with below agents:
	– Piperacillin-tazobactam
	– Cefepime
	– Fluoroquinolone
	– Carbapenem[d]
	• If patient is not at high risk of mortality but has risk factors for methicillin-resistant *Staphylococcus aureus* (MRSA) infection, give one of the agents listed above plus either vancomycin or linezolid.

[a]Suitable respiratory fluoroquinolones include levofloxacin or moxifloxacin
[b]β-lactams include ampicillin-sulbactam, cefotaxime, ceftriaxone, or ceftaroline
[c]Macrolide options include azithromycin or clarithromycin
[d]Carbapenem: imipenem, meropenem

TABLE 56.3 ■ **Four Stages of Swallowing and Symptoms of Dysphagia**

Stage	Description	Signs and Symptoms of Dysphagia
Oral preparatory	• Eating is anticipated, then food is brought to the mouth (i.e., bitten off or taken from the utensil) • Liquids are sipped or sucked through a straw • Food is chewed and mixed with saliva	Oropharyngeal dysphagia (transfer dysphagia) • Choking • Coughing • Nasal regurgitation of undigested food • Wet or gurgled voice after eating or drinking
Oral propulsive	• Food is collected and sealed between roof of the mouth and the tongue • Tongue moves the food back to the pharynx	
Pharyngeal	• Soft palate elevates in order to prevent from entering the nose • Tongue base moves back to contact the pharyngeal wall, then larynx moves up and forward • Food is moved toward the esophagus by muscles of the pharynx	
Esophageal	• Food moves through the esophagus by peristalsis • Lower esophageal sphincter relaxes	Esophageal dysphagia (transport dysphagia) • Frequent episodes of regurgitation • Discomfort in mid- to lower sternum as the food passes down • Refluxes/heartburn • Difficulty with solid food, sensation of food sticking in the throat or chest

What can be done to try and prevent aspiration in this patient?

In general, oral feeding is recommended rather than enteral tube feeding. Proper swallowing evaluation should be performed with the goal of discontinuing the feeding tube as soon as the patient is able to swallow safely. Once the feeding tube is removed, feeding in a semirecumbent position and use of a mechanical soft diet with thickened liquids rather than pureed food and thin liquids are some ways to prevent future aspiration pneumonia.

CLINICAL PEARL **STEP 2/3**

Routine monitoring of postfeeding residual volume is not necessary because of the lack of benefit in minimizing the risk of aspiration.

Case Summary

- **Complaint/History:** This is a 73 year old woman with history of Parkinson's disease and dementia who presents with shortness of breath.
- **Findings:** Respiratory rate of 32 breaths/min, oxygen saturation of 92% on 15L non-rebreather mask, altered mental status, left basilar focal crackles with lung auscultation.

- **Labs/Test:** ECG does not show ischemic changes, chest radiograph demonstrates left lower lobe opacity.

Diagnosis: Aspiration pneumonia.

- **Treatment:** supplemental oxygen, levofloxacin, swallowing evaluation, postpyloric feeding tube placement.

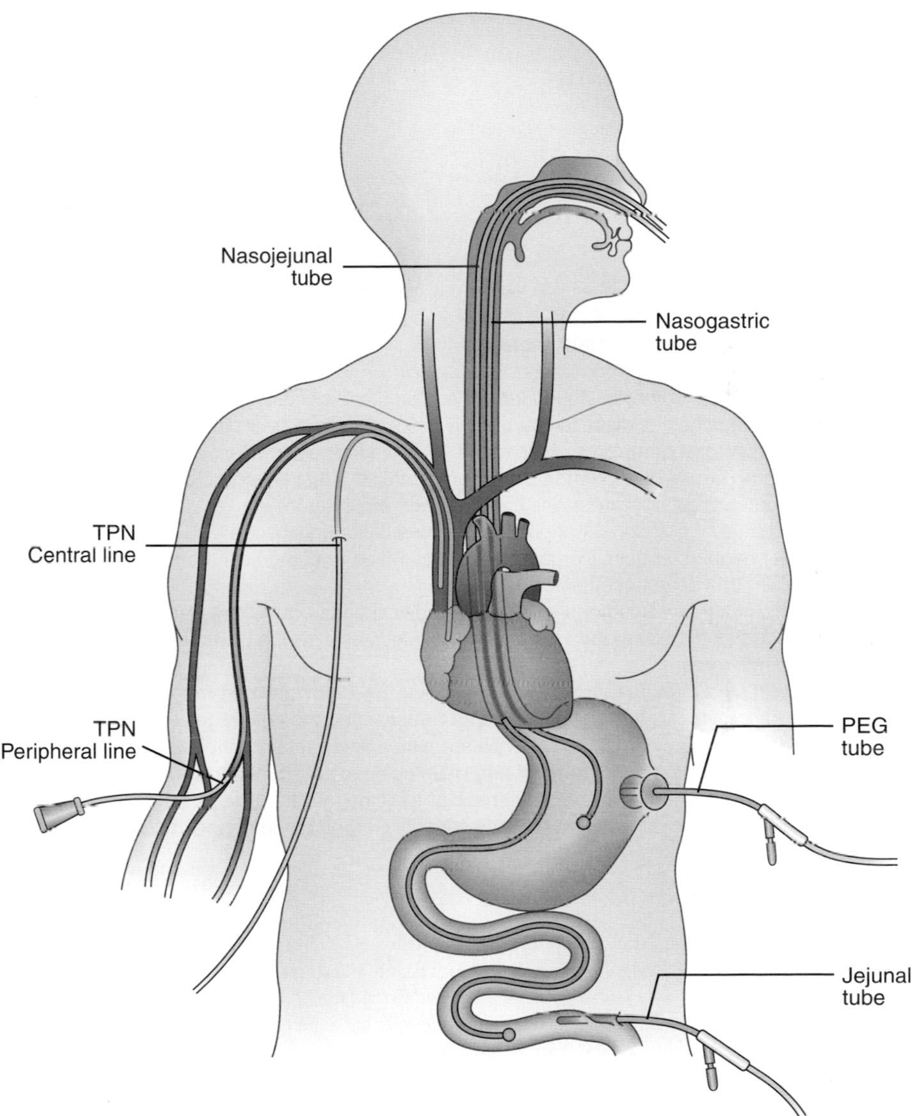

Fig. 56.2 Nasogastric tubes and postpyloric tubes are commonly placed for enteral feeding. (From Townsend, C. (2022). *Sabiston textbook of surgery* (21st ed.). Elsevier.)

TABLE 56.4 ■ **Advantages and Disadvantages of Nasogastric Versus Postpyloric Tubes**

	Nasogastric Tube	Postpyloric Tube
Advantage	• Replicates normal physiology • Easy to place • Safe procedure • Bolus or continuous feeds are available	• Minimizes aspiration risk • Delivers adequate nutrition in critically ill patients with impaired gastric emptying • Avoids gastric distension • Benefits in acute pancreatitis by minimizing stimulation of pancreatic secretions
Disadvantage	• Not helpful in patients with delayed gastric emptying • May cause/worsen gastroesophageal reflux and aspiration	• Difficulty with placement of the tubes and maintenance of the position • May cause dumping syndrome

BEYOND THE PEARLS

- Aspirated tube feeds or blood rarely causes aspiration pneumonia because the pH of the fluid is high and does not contain bacteria.
- A rare form of aspiration pneumonia is lipoid pneumonia, which can occur when aspirating mineral oil, which is commonly used for constipation and occasionally for bronchoscopy.
- Patients with Parkinson's disease can exhibit difficulty with all four phases of swallowing: oral preparatory, oral propulsive, pharyngeal, and esophageal phases.
- A less common cause of aspiration pneumonia cardiac arrest is aspiration of gastric contents during chest compressions and stomach ventilation.
- The composition of oral flora changes the longer a patient is hospitalized. Consider checking for hospital-acquired organisms for aspiration pneumonia if it occurs >5 days after a patient has been hospitalized.
- Moxifloxacin is a fluoroquinolone with activity against anaerobes; however, it is not recommended as monotherapy when anerobic infection is strongly suspected because of high resistance rates.
- "Clindamycin above the diaphragm and metronidazole below the diaphragm" has been proven to be a myth. Metronidazole contains better anaerobic coverage and has broader coverage than clindamycin alone when paired with a beta-lactam antibiotic.
- Dumping syndrome is a condition that can develop after surgery that removes all of, or part of, the stomach. It is due to rapid movement of food, especially sugar, from the stomach to the small bowel and can cause nausea, abdominal cramping and hypoglycemia.

Bibliography

Mandell, L. A., & Niederman, M. S. (2019). Aspiration pneumonia. *NEJM, 380*, 651–663.

Metlay, J. P., Waterer, G. W., Long, A. C., et al. (2019). Diagnosis and treatment of adults with community-acquired pneumonia. *American Journal of Respiratory and Critical Care Medicine, 200*(7), E45–E67.

Yerrabolu. S. R. (2012). Consideration of alternative designs for a percutaneous endoscopic gastrostomy feeding tube. State University of New York at Buffalo.

CASE 57

A 58-Year-Old Male With Occupational Lung Disease

Gregory Grandio ■ Drew Sheldon ■ Raj Dasgupta ■ Toby Maher

A 58-year-old male presents to the emergency department from his primary care physician's office after being found to have a blood pressure of 200/120 mmHg. At this time the patient is free of any symptoms. He denies chest pain, headache, visual changes, weakness, or dizziness. His past medical history is significant for poorly controlled hypertension. On physical examination he has a temperature of 37°C, blood pressure is 160/87 mmHg, pulse rate is 85 beats/min, respiration rate is 18 breaths/min, and oxygen saturation is 100% on room air. Bilateral lung fields are clear to auscultation and he has a 1/6 systolic murmur at the left lower sternal boarder. The remainder of the examination is normal. A chest radiograph shows innumerable small nodular opacities throughout both lungs with upper lobe predominance (Fig. 57.1).

How do you evaluate pulmonary nodules on imaging?

Pulmonary nodules are a very common finding seen on chest radiograph and computed tomography (CT) of the chest. The craniocaudal distribution, appearance, and location when compared to other structures can help narrow down the causes of pulmonary nodules. Certain diseases such as sarcoidosis and pneumoconioses can predominate the upper lobes and diseases such as hematogenous metastases may preferentially affect the lower zones of the lungs. Pulmonary nodules can vary in appearance from sharply marginated to ill defined, which helps differentiate an interstitial process from an alveolar process, respectively. Furthermore, high-resolution computed tomography can help narrow the distribution of pulmonary nodules to perilymphatic, random, and centrilobular, which can help further narrow the differential diagnosis (Fig. 57.2A–D).

What are some causes of multiple pulmonary nodules?

By definition, pulmonary nodules are less than 30 mm; those larger than this are considered pulmonary masses. The causes of pulmonary nodules can be broadly subdivided into infectious and noninfectious. A variety of infections can cause pulmonary nodules including viral, bacterial, and fungal infections as well as mycobacterial infections including miliary tuberculosis. Noninfectious causes of pulmonary nodules include malignancies (both primary and metastatic), airway diseases (hypersensitivity pneumonitis, interstitial lung diseases, and pneumoconioses), and vascular diseases (pulmonary edema, pulmonary hemorrhage, and pulmonary arterial hypertension).

What additional history is important to obtain for this case?

Even though the patient did not initially report any infectious symptoms, it would be important to identify symptoms of an indolent infection such as dyspnea on exertion, weight loss, night sweats, fever, and chills. Signs and symptoms of rheumatologic disease such as rashes and joint pain should also be included. Assessment of risk factors for tuberculosis (TB) such as originating from an area with high risk of TB transmission, history of incarceration or homelessness, and any known exposures

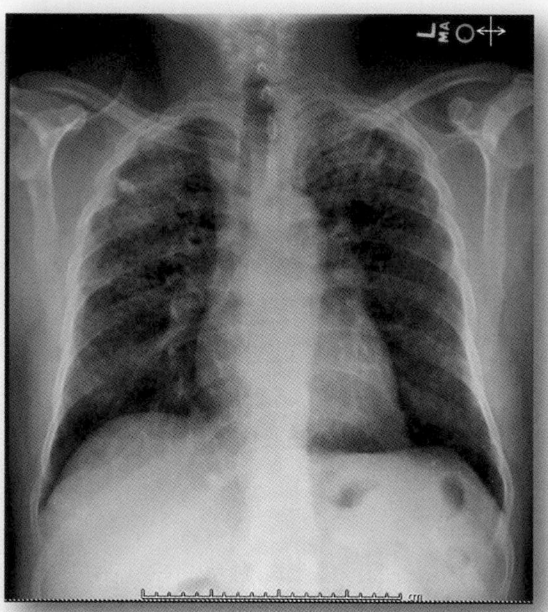

Fig. 57.1 Innumerable small nodular opacities throughout both lungs predominantly within upper lobes. (Courtesy of Dr. Gregory Grandio.)

to individuals with active TB infection is important. Social history is also crucial because a history of smoking could determine risk of malignancy as well as certain interstitial lung diseases such as respiratory bronchiolitis-interstitial lung disease (RB-ILD). Social history should include exposures to certain antigens such as bird feathers that would increase the risk of hypersensitivity pneumonitis. Finally, a detailed occupational history should be elicited when considering occupational lung diseases.

CLINICAL PEARL

Interstitial lung diseases strongly associated with smoking classically include pulmonary Langerhans cell histiocytosis (PLCH), RB-ILD, and desquamative interstitial pneumonia (DIP).

BASIC SCIENCE/CLINICAL PEARL **STEP 1/2/3**

Interferon-gamma release assays (IGRAs) are used to test for TB but cannot differentiate between active and latent TB. They work by assessing for the release of interferon-gamma by T-lymphocytes when exposed to a specific antigen. In the United States, there are two IGRAs available for testing for TB, the QuantiFERON Gold and the T-SPOT test.

Further history reveals an absence of shortness of breath, cough, fevers, chills, weight loss, or night sweats. He denies any known TB exposures and any recent travel. The patient has a 5-pack-year smoking history and quit 30 years ago. He is originally from Michoacán, Mexico, and moved to the United States 15 years ago. For the last 3 years he has been working as a landscaper, but former occupations include farming of beans and corn for 20 years, mining gold and silver for 10 years, and throughout his life he has also worked in construction, which includes excavation.

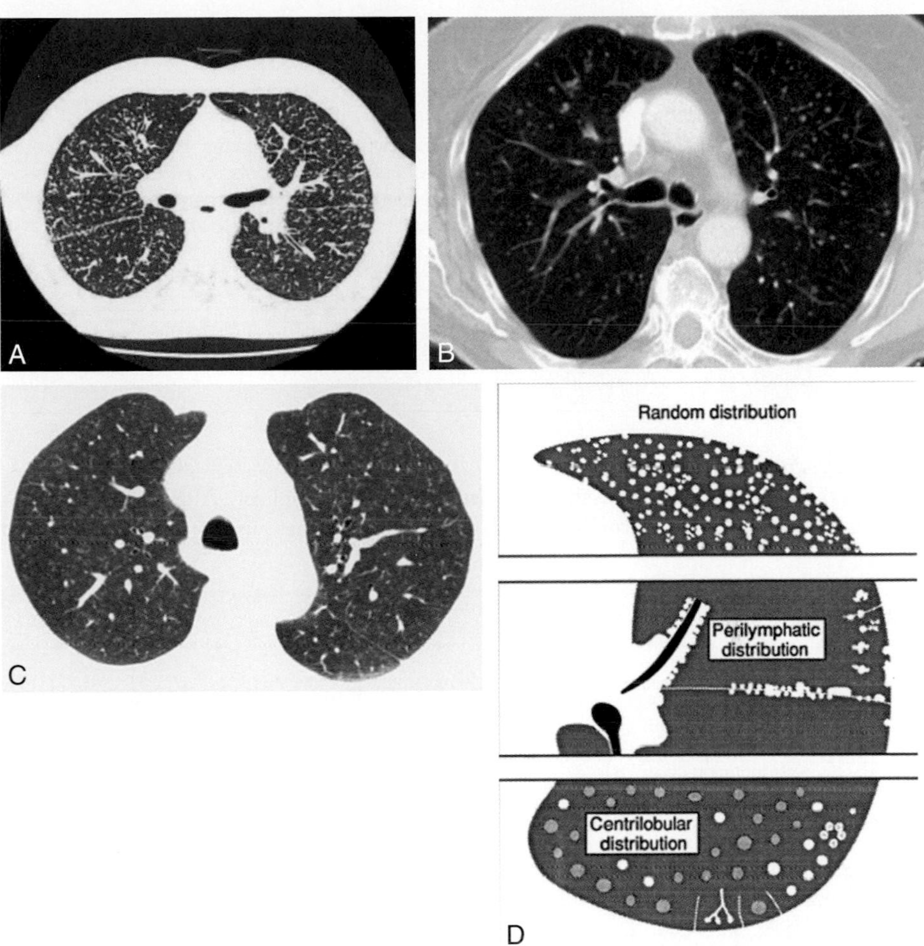

Fig. 57.2 (A) Axial high-resolution computed tomography (HRCT) of sarcoidosis with perilymphatic and subpleural nodules with "beading" of the fissures. (B) HRCT demonstrating multiple fine discreet nodules in random distribution representing miliary metastasis from thyroid cancer. (C) HRCT showing ill-defined centrilobular nodules in a heavy smoker with respiratory bronchiolitis. (D) Distribution of lung nodules. ((A) From Balan, A., Hoey, E., Sheerin, F., Lakkaraju, A., & Chowdhury, F. (2010). Multi-technique imaging of sarcoidosis. *Clinical Radiology*, *65* (9), 751, Figure 2; (B) from Nishino, M., Itoh H., & Hatabu, H. (2014). A practical approach to high-resolution CT of diffuse lung disease. *European Journal of Radiology, 83* (1) 12; (C) from Hobbs, S. B. (2018) Smoking-related interstitial lung disease. In C. M. Walker & J. H. Chung (Eds.), *Muller's imaging of the chest* (Figure 34.5, p. 505). Elsevier; (D) from Webb, W. R., Brant, W. E. & Major, N.M. (2019). *Fundamentals of body CT* (Fig. 6.46, p. 145). Elsevier.)

Which diagnostic studies help narrow your differential diagnosis?

Once an adequate history has been obtained, further workup should begin with laboratory testing. Lab tests if clinically indicated should include an initial workup for connective tissue disease–associated interstitial lung disease (CTD-ILD) including antinuclear, dsDNA, anti-Ro/SSA, anti-La/SSB, Scl-70, cyclic citrullinated peptide (CCP), rheumatoid factor, ribonucleoprotein (RNP), and anti-Jo-1 antibodies. Given the patient's risk factors for tuberculosis, an interferon-gamma release assay should be obtained. After obtaining lab test results, a chest CT scan should be performed. A high-resolution computed tomography (HRCT) is beneficial when interstitial lung disease is highly suspected, but based on the patient's history a standard chest CT scan should provide enough information. Finally, depending on the imaging characteristics, a bronchoscopy may be necessary to evaluate for infectious and malignant etiologies.

CLINICAL PEARL **STEP 2/3**

HRCT is often used for the diagnosis of diffuse parenchymal lung diseases. HRCT technique varies from standard computed tomography of the chest, and protocols for HRCT technique vary from institution to institution. Typical protocols consist of obtaining images with thin slices (<1.25 mm), obtaining images during both max inspiration and max expiration, and obtaining prone images of the lung bases.

The results of laboratory testing are shown in Table 57.1. A computed tomography (CT) scan of the chest showed upper lobe predominant perilymphatic nodules with calcified mediastinal and hilar lymph nodes (Fig. 57.3).

What is your differential diagnosis?

Based on the patient's history and laboratory data, CTD-ILD is unlikely. Although the patient's smoking history was brief, this combined with the imaging findings raise concern for a potential

TABLE 57.1 ■

Laboratory Tests	
Leukocyte count	7,800/μL (18 × 10^9/L)
Hematocrit	42.2%
Platelet count	258,000/μL (540 × 10^9/L)
Erythrocyte sedimentation rate	8 mm/h
CRP	1 mg/L
Antinuclear antibodies	Negative
Anti-myeloperoxidase antibodies	Negative
Anti-CCP antibodies	Negative
Antiproteinase-3 antibodies	Negative
Anti-Jo-1 antibodies	Negative
Anti-topoisomerase-1 antibodies	Negative
Rheumatoid factor	Negative

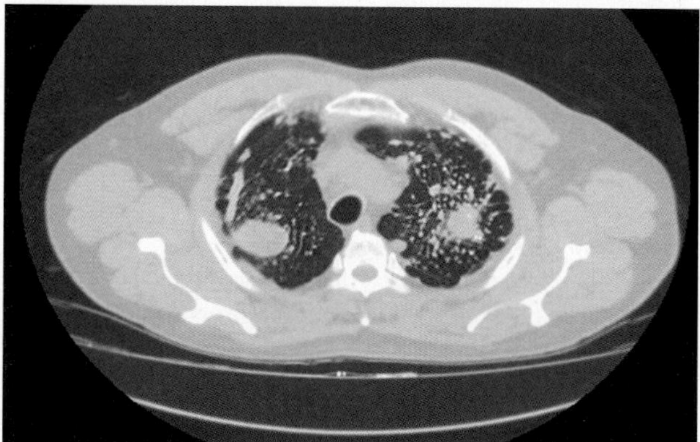

Fig. 57.3 Upper lobe predominant perilymphatic nodules with calcified mediastinal and hilar lymph nodes. Constellation of findings in this clinical context most consistent with silicosis.

malignancy. The lack of infectious signs and symptoms make a pulmonary infection unlikely, although fungal and mycobacterial infections can be indolent in nature. Finally, the patient's occupational history is very suggestive of a pneumoconiosis. In order to rule out a malignancy, a tissue diagnosis via bronchoscopy with transbronchial biopsy is required.

Which other occupational diseases affect the lungs?
See Table 57.2.

CLINICAL PEARL **STEP 2/3**

Patients with coal workers' pneumoconiosis can have melanoptysis, which is the expectoration of black sputum.

TABLE 57.2 ■ **Occupational Lung Diseases**

Type	Occupations	Presentation	Imaging Findings	Pathology
Coal workers' pneumoconiosis	Coal mining	Chronic bronchitis	Upper lobe predominant nodules a few mm in diameter	Focal collection of coal dust in pigment-laden macrophages; Caplan nodule
Berylliosis	Aerospace alloy production, automotive ceramics, dental prosthetics, electronics	Dyspnea, cough, fever, night sweats, fatigue, weight loss; 3- to 40-year latency before symptoms	CXR: upper lobe reticulonodular opacities with hilar and mediastinal LAD HRCT: septal thickening, parenchymal nodules, hilar and mediastinal LAD	Noncaseating granulomas, similar to sarcoidosis
Asbestosis	Insulation workers, pipefitters, boilermakers, shipbuilders, plastic and rubber manufacturing, textile manufacturing, brake lining manufacturing	Usually asymptomatic with incidental findings on imaging, dyspnea; 10- to 40-year latency	Pleural effusions, pleural thickening with calcifications, pleural plaques	Exudative effusion; asbestos bodies and fibers
Talcosis	Production of textiles, paper, and rubber; cosmetics and pharmaceutical industries	Cough and dyspnea	Nodular lung disease, fibrosis, and lower lobe emphysema similar to silicosis	Talc granulomas with multinucleated giant cells

HRCT, High-resolution computed tomography; *LAD*, lymphadenopathy.

CLINICAL PEARL **STEP 2/3**

Pneumoconioses typically affect the upper lobes as a result of the inhalational spread. The exception to this is asbestosis, which tends to affect the lower lobes.

CLINICAL PEARL **STEP 2/3**

Asbestos bodies are one type of ferruginous body that can be formed by iron encasement of inhaled inorganic dusts.

A bronchoscopy with transbronchial biopsy was performed, and the bronchoalveolar lavage was cultured and proved negative for bacterial, fungal, and AFB pathogens. Surgical pathology for the transbronchial biopsy showed alveolar tissue with abundant intra-alveolar dirty macrophages and abundant silica-like particles noted by polarization.

How do you establish a diagnosis of silicosis?

The most important part of establishing a diagnosis of silicosis is obtaining a good history and, in particular, a good occupational history. Identifying the onset of symptoms is important for determining whether the patient has acute or chronic silicosis. Silica is the most abundant mineral on earth and exists in crystalline and amorphous forms. Quartz is the most common type of crystalline silica and a major component of rocks such as granite, slate, and sandstone. Exposure to silica occurs in occupations that disrupt the earth's crust as well as those occupations that use silica containing rock or ores. Examples of these occupations include sandblasting, tunneling, drill operation, digging, glass manufacturing, hard rock mining, stone cutting, masonry, foundry work, and hydraulic fracturing.

There are no lab tests that can establish a diagnosis of silicosis. Lab tests should be targeted to rule out other potential etiologies for the patient's symptoms based on the patient's history. Because silicosis is often associated with mycobacterial infection, interferon-gamma release assay or a skin test can be used to identify latent tuberculosis. If the patient has any symptoms of an active infection, a sputum smear and culture for bacteria and acid-fast bacilli should be obtained. Pulmonary function testing (PFT) is not needed to diagnose silicosis but can be used to evaluate patients with respiratory symptoms and monitor progression of disease.

CLINICAL PEARL **STEP 2/3**

Silicosis classically on the USMLE shows a restrictive pattern with reduced forced vital capacity (FVC), reduced forced expiratory volume in 1 second (FEV1), normal to elevated FEV1/FVC ratio, reduced total lung capacity (TLC), and reduced diffusing capacity for carbon monoxide (DLCO) on PFTs.

What are the manifestations of acute and chronic silicosis?

After exposure to high concentrations of crystalline silica, symptoms of acute silicosis can develop within weeks to years of exposure. Symptoms include rapid onset of dyspnea, cough, weight loss, fatigue, and pleuritic pain with crackles usually present on physical examination. Symptoms can often precede imaging findings, but chest radiography of acute silicosis can demonstrate bilateral, diffuse, perihilar, or basilar opacities. High-resolution computed tomography may show numerous centrilobular nodular opacities, focal ground glass opacities, and patchy areas of consolidation. Hilar lymph node enlargement may also be seen.

In terms of chronic silicosis, symptoms often appear 10 to 30 years after exposure and usually include cough and dyspnea on exertion. On physical examination, chronic silicosis

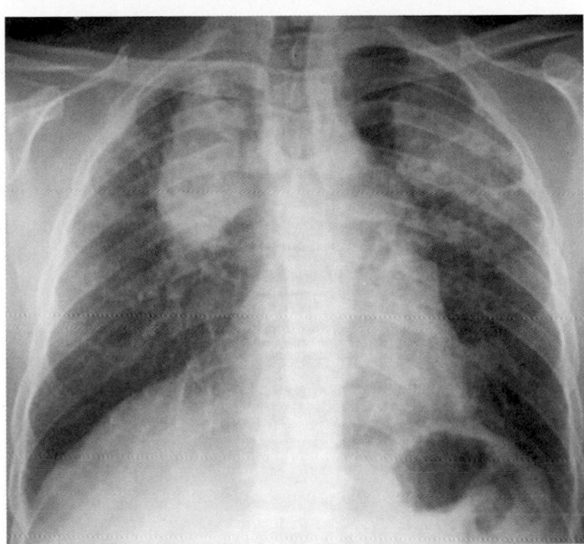

Fig. 57.4 Chest radiograph showing upper lung masses with background of small nodules and linear and reticular opacities consistent with progressive massive fibrosis from silicosis. (From Cowie, R. L. & Becklake, M. R. (2021). Pneumoconioses. In V. C. Broaddus (Ed.) *Murray and Nadel's textbook of respiratory medicine* (eFigure 73-5). Elsevier.)

can have a wide variety of findings including completely normal breath sounds to rhonchi, wheezing, and fine or coarse crackles. Clubbing is a physical examination finding that is seldom seen. When chronic silicosis advances to progressive massive fibrosis (PMF), symptoms are the same but worsened. However, on physical examination there are usually diminished breath sounds with inspiratory crackles. A chest radiograph will show innumerable, small, rounded opacities predominantly in the upper lung zones. When disease advances to PMF these small opacities enlarge and usually coalesce to form larger upper or mid-lung zone opacities representing confluent nodules and fibrosis. The hila also retract upward with the upper lobe fibrosis and lower lobe hyperinflation. In certain cases, these opacities may cavitate. A high-resolution CT scan is not necessary for the diagnosis of chronic silicosis and PMF in the right clinical setting. If obtained, bilateral, symmetric, centrilobular, and perilymphatic nodules with sharp margins may be seen reflecting the deposition of dust and fibrosis around small airways. Interlobular septal or subpleural nodules can be seen because of lymphatic clearance of silica dust (Fig. 57.4).

What are the major complications resulting from silicosis?

Patients with silicosis are at risk of several complications. The most well-established is mycobacterial infection; therefore, purified protein derivative (PPD) testing is recommended using ≥10 mm as a cutoff for positivity because silicosis can mask the radiographic findings of TB. Other infections include fungal infections such as chronic necrotizing aspergillosis, which can be seen in patients with progressive massive fibrosis where cavitation is present. Connective tissue diseases are also associated with silicosis with the most common being rheumatoid arthritis and scleroderma. Silicosis is also associated with an increased risk of lung cancers and the International Agency for Research on Cancer (IARC) classifies inhaled crystalline silica as a carcinogen. Finally, chronic bronchitis and airflow obstruction can result from narrowing of airways from nodules.

BASIC SCIENCE/CLINICAL PEARL **STEP 1/2**

A PPD test is an example of a type IV delayed hypersensitivity reaction.

BEYOND THE PEARLS

- Prevention is better than treatment for silicosis and can be achieved by limiting exposure and using respiratory protection during periods of exposure.
- Patients with accelerated silicosis are at highest risk of developing progressive massive fibrosis.
- "Eggshell calcification" is non-specific but most commonly occurs in silicosis and coal workers' pneumoconiosis. It can also be seen with post-irradiation lymphoma, sarcoidosis, scleroderma, amyloidosis, and infectious etiologies, such as blastomycosis and histoplasmosis.
- Rheumatoid pneumoconiosis (RP, also known as Caplan syndrome) is inflammation and scarring of the lungs. It occurs in people with rheumatoid arthritis who have breathed in dust, such as from coal (coal worker's pneumoconiosis) or silica (silicosis).
- Chronic beryllium disease is pathologically indistinguishable from sarcoidosis and therefore taking a good history is important. A beryllium lymphocyte proliferation test may also be performed on blood or bronchoalveolar lavage specimen to help in diagnosis.
- Pulmonary hypertension can be seen in patients with silicosis from parenchymal lung disease. A rare complication is pulmonary artery stenosis which may require invasive pulmonary artery stenting to alleviate symptoms.
- A lung transplant is an option for patients with advanced silicosis and is typically considered on a case-to-case basis.

Bibliography

Leung, Chi, Yu, I. T. S., & Chen, Weihong (2012). Silicosis. *The Lancet. 379*, 2008–2018.

Rice, F. (2000). Concise international chemical assessment document 24: Crystalline silica, quartz. IPCS Concise International Chemical Assessment Documents.

Czul, F., & Lascano, J. (2011). An uncommon hazard: Pulmonary talcosis as a result of recurrent aspiration of baby powder. *Respiratory Medicine CME, 4*, 109–111.

Elicker, B. M., & Webb, W. R. (2019). *Fundamentals of high-resolution CT: Common findings, common patterns, common diseases, and differential diagnosis* (2nd ed). Philadelphia, PA: Wolters Kluwer.

Puneet, S. G., Sachin, G., & Carlos, E. K. (2015). Diffuse parenchymal lung disease. In T. Le et al. (Ed.), *ATS review for the pulmonary boards* (pp. 276–287). New York, NY: ATS.

CASE 58

A 68-Year-Old Male With Progressively Worsening Dyspnea and Dry Cough

Drew Sheldon ■ Clay Wu ■ Raj Dasgupta ■ Toby Maher

A 68-year-old man presents to the outpatient clinic after 6 months of progressive exertional dyspnea and a persistent dry cough. He denies fevers, hemoptysis, or leg swelling. He has not traveled recently. He denies exposure to asbestos, molds, and chemicals. He does not have any pets including birds. He does not have any history of rheumatologic diseases. He has been prescribed an "inhaler" in the past, but this does not seem to help. He has a 15-pack-year smoking history but quit 20 years ago. He does not have any family history of lung disease.

On physical examination, blood pressure is 124/78 mmHg, pulse rate is 82 beats/min, respiratory rate is 18 breaths/min, and oxygen saturation is 94% on room air. There are Velcro-like crackles in the lung bases and clubbing of the fingers is noted. No wheezing or peripheral edema is noted. The remainder of the examination is normal. A chest radiograph (CXR) (Fig. 58.1) is obtained and reveals bilateral reticular infiltrates predominantly in the lower lung fields and the periphery with reduced inspiratory lung volumes.

CLINICAL PEARL **STEP 2/3**

Velcro crackles are predominantly heard during inspiration and mimic the sound made with separating Velcro. It is highly suggestive of interstitial lung disease.

CLINICAL PEARL **STEP 2/3**

Clubbing of the fingertips and toes is a symptom seen in pulmonary fibrosis and other heart and lung diseases that reduce the amount of oxygen in the blood. The sign is evident when fingertips are enlarged and rounded in contrast to the rest of the finger. A finger with clubbing at the tips resembles a drumstick-like shape.

The exact cause of clubbing is not fully understood, and has been associated as a marker of advanced-stage disease in some cases.

What is your differential diagnosis?

The patient's primary symptoms are cough and dyspnea. The causes of chronic cough are reviewed in a different chapter, but the presence of chronic dyspnea should increase the level of concern. Acute exacerbation of heart failure is a possibility. However, the presentation would not typically be as slow as in this patient. Given the slow progression of symptoms, there is a possibility of an indolent infection such as fungal etiologies. The other major category is interstitial lung disease (ILD), which can be related to rheumatologic diseases, drug toxicities, prolonged exposure to allergens, or idiopathic etiologies. Thus, it is very important to obtain a thorough history of potential exposures. Occasionally, these patients are misdiagnosed with chronic obstructive

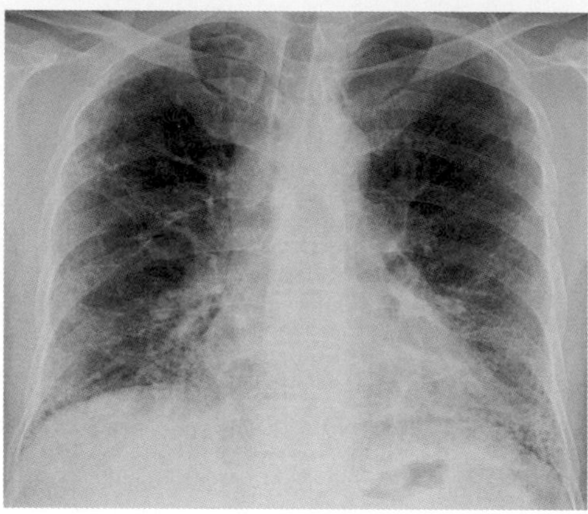

Fig. 58.1 Chest X-ray image showing bilateral reticular infiltrates with bibasilar predominance. (From Broaddus V. C. et al. (2022). *Murray & Nadal's textbook of respiratory medicine* (7th ed.), Elsevier.)

pulmonary disease (COPD) because of chronic dyspnea. However, COPD does not typically present with reticular infiltrates on CXR and the lungs are hyperinflated rather than showing low lung volumes. More evaluation needs to be done in this case.

CLINICAL PEARL **STEP 2/3**

Many patients with interstitial lung disease who present with chronic dyspnea are initially misdiagnosed with heart failure or chronic obstructive pulmonary disease; in some cases, there is an 18-month delay before interstitial lung disease is diagnosed. Therefore, it is important to include ILD in the differential for patients presenting with indolent progression of dyspnea.

What are the next steps that should be taken?

Further evaluation can be broken down into additional clinical, laboratory, and imaging assessments. Additional clinical history should be obtained, paying special attention to family history of lung disease, rheumatologic disease, or exposures (particularly to asbestos, silica, birds, etc.). A detailed medication history should also be obtained. Medications such as nitrofurantoin, amiodarone, and chemotherapy drugs such as bleomycin can cause pulmonary fibrosis. The patient needs additional evaluation with laboratory and pulmonary function tests, which can help identify other causes of cough and dyspnea. The lab tests that should be considered are antinuclear bodies (ANA), anticyclic citrullinated peptide (CCP) antibodies, and rheumatoid factor (RF). Other additional studies for rheumatologic diseases can be considered based on the patient's signs and symptoms. All patients should undergo complete pulmonary function tests (PFTs) to establish the pattern of lung involvement and assess the severity of the disease. Imaging will be discussed later in the chapter.

His lab results for autoimmune disease and connective tissue disease are negative. The patient underwent full PFTs with spirometry, lung volumes, and diffusing capacity for the lung of carbon monoxide (DLCO). Results are notable for a proportionately reduced forced vital capacity (FVC) and reduced forced expiratory volume in 1 second (FEV1) with a normal FEV1/FVC ratio, a reduced total lung capacity (TLC), and a reduced DLCO.

What pattern is reflected by these PFT results?

These PFT findings reflect a restrictive pattern of disease. A restrictive pattern of disease is defined by an FVC less than the lower limit of normal for adults and a preserved or elevated FEV1/FVC ratio. A low TLC clinches the diagnosis of restrictive disease and a low DLCO suggests an interstitial disease of the lung parenchyma rather than an extrinsic restrictive process.

BASIC SCIENCE/CLINICAL PEARL **STEP 1/2/3**

In patients who have a restrictive pattern on PFTs with a normal DLCO implies a "extrinsic restrictive" lung disease. Classic examples on the USMLE include neuromuscular disease, kyphoscoliosis, and obesity.

Which diseases can result in this pattern of PFTs?

The most common group of diseases that results in a restrictive pattern with a reduction in DLCO is the family of interstitial lung diseases (ILDs). These diseases are characterized by cellular proliferation, interstitial inflammation, fibrosis, or a combination of these findings within the alveolar wall that is not a result of infection or cancer. The most common phenotype is interstitial fibrosis with the most common diagnoses being chronic hypersensitivity pneumonitis, an underlying autoimmune disease, or idiopathic pulmonary fibrosis (IPF).

BASIC SCIENCE/CLINICAL PEARL **STEP 1/2/3**

In early ILD, a low DLCO may be the only PFT abnormality. However other causes of isolated low DLCO need to be evaluated, which include pulmonary hypertension, pulmonary embolism, and anemia.

These findings are concerning for interstitial lung disease and a high-resolution computed tomography (HRCT) of the chest is therefore obtained (Fig. 58.2).

Given the lower lobe predominance, presence of honeycombing, and subpleural fibrosis, the imaging pattern is most consistent with usual interstitial pneumonia (UIP).

CLINICAL PEARL **STEP 2/3**

Honeycombing refers to a cluster of cystic airspaces approximately 3 to 10 mm in diameter.

What is the difference between UIP and IPF?

UIP (usual interstitial pneumonia) is a terminology used histopathologically and radiographically, but they represent separate entities. The histopathologic pattern of UIP will be discussed later in this chapter. Radiographic UIP has a characteristic HRCT pattern that is summarized in Table 58.1. The pattern of radiographic UIP can be caused by many different etiologies such as connective tissue diseases, drug toxicities, asbestosis, and chronic hypersensitivity pneumonitis. When the cause is unknown or idiopathic, a diagnosis of IPF can be strongly considered.

HRCT and its patterns provide a clue into the etiology of the ILD. This patient's HRCT is characteristic of a definite UIP pattern because of the traction bronchiectasis, subpleural fibrosis, and bibasilar predominant honeycombing. If other etiologies have been ruled out, then IPF is the most likely diagnosis for this patient.

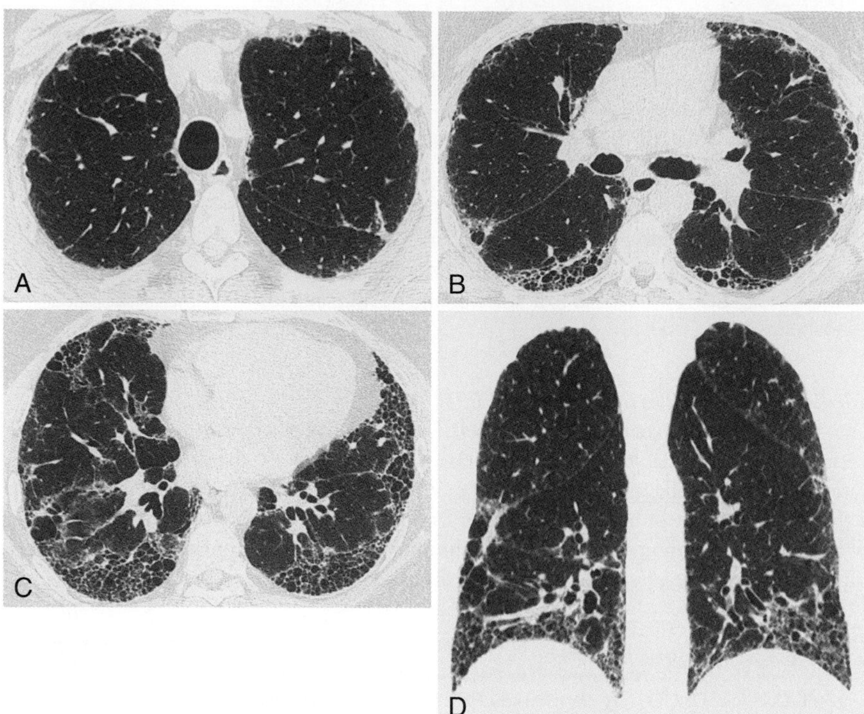

Fig. 58.2 High-resolution computed tomography of the chest. (From Walker, C. M. and Chung, J. H. (2019). *Müller's imaging of the chest* (2nd ed.). Elsevier.) A, B, and C: cranial to caudal (from A to C) axial cuts of an HRCT demonstrating typical UIP findings of subpleural and basal predominant fibrosis with traction bronchiectasis, architectural distortion, and honeycombing. D: coronal cut of HRCT again redemonstrating basilar predominant distribution of fibrosis and honeycombing.

TABLE 58.1 ■ **HRCT Patterns of ILD**

HRCT Patterns			
Typical UIP	**Probable UIP**	**Indeterminate for UIP**	**Alternative Diagnosis**
• Subpleural and basal predominant; distribution is often heterogeneous • Honeycombing with or without peripheral traction bronchiectasis or bronchiolectasis	• Subpleural and basal predominant; distribution is often heterogeneous • Reticular pattern with peripheral traction bronchiectasis or bronchiolectasis • May have mild GGO	• Subpleural and basal predominant • Subtle reticulation; may have mild GGO or distortion ("early UIP pattern") • CT features and/or distribution of lung fibrosis that do not suggest any specific etiology ("truly indeterminate for UIP")	Findings suggestive of another diagnosis, including cysts, predominant GGO, nodules, consolidation and non-basilar distribution.

CT, Computed tomography; *GGO*, ground glass opacity; *HRCT*, high-resolution computed tomography; *ILD*, interstitial lung disease; *UIP*, usual interstitial pneumonia.

BASIC SCIENCE/CLINICAL PEARL **STEP 1**

Medications commonly associated with pulmonary fibrosis are amiodarone, bleomycin, and nitrofurantoin.

How is IPF diagnosed?

IPF is diagnosed when there is a HRCT pattern of UIP best seen on HRCT with or without biopsy in the absence of any identifiable cause. This includes patients who meet the classic presentation (slow onset, age 60–70 years), imaging that shows a definite UIP pattern as discussed previously, and exclusion of other causes of UIP such as exposure, medications, and rheumatologic diseases. It is the preferred standard of care for these diagnoses and the decision whether a biopsy should be pursued to take place in a multidisciplinary setting with a pulmonologist, radiologist, rheumatologist, and pathologist.

A multidisciplinary panel of experts reviews the data and agrees the patient's HRCT is consistent with a definite UIP pattern and a surgical lung biopsy (SLB) is not needed. He is diagnosed with idiopathic pulmonary fibrosis (IPF).

When is a surgical lung biopsy needed to diagnose IPF?

In a patient with newly detected ILD of unknown cause with clinically suspected IPF and an HRCT pattern not consistent with Typical UIP (probable UIP, indeterminate for UIP, or alternative diagnosis to UIP, Table 58.1), a tissue diagnosis should be considered in consultation with a multidisciplinary panel of experts. This may include advanced bronchoscopic techniques or surgical lung biopsy. If the decision is made to pursue a surgical lung biopsy, the potential benefits should be weighed against the risks. Some of the potential benefits include more accurate estimates of prognosis, cessation of additional diagnostic testing, or the initiation of more specific treatment. However, in some cases invasive lung biopsy may not add any further significant information to the diagnostic work up.

CLINICAL PEARL **STEP 2/3**

The most notable risks of a surgical lung biopsy include procedural mortality (1.7%), perioperative infections (6.5%), and perioperative exacerbation of underlying lung disease (6.1%).

What is the classic histologic pattern of UIP?

The histopathologic pattern of UIP is a separate entity from the radiologic pattern of UIP. A biopsy may be needed if the diagnosis of IPF is in question. However, the positive predictive value of radiologic definite UIP for histopathologic UIP is between 90% and 100%. The histopathologic hallmark and chief diagnostic criterion of UIP is a low magnification appearance of patchy dense fibrosis that (1) is causing remodeling of lung architecture, (2) often results in honeycomb change, and (3) alternates with areas of less-affected parenchyma. Converse to the radiologic diagnosis of definite UIP, the histopathologic diagnosis of definite UIP does not require the presence of honeycombing if all other typical features above are present (Fig. 58.3) (Tables 58.2 and 58.3).

BASIC SCIENCE PEARL **STEP 1**

The proposed pathogenesis for IPF is recurrent, subclinical epithelial injury superimposed on accelerated epithelial aging in genetically susceptible individuals, which leads to aberrant repair of the injured alveolus and deposition of interstitial fibrosis by myofibroblasts.

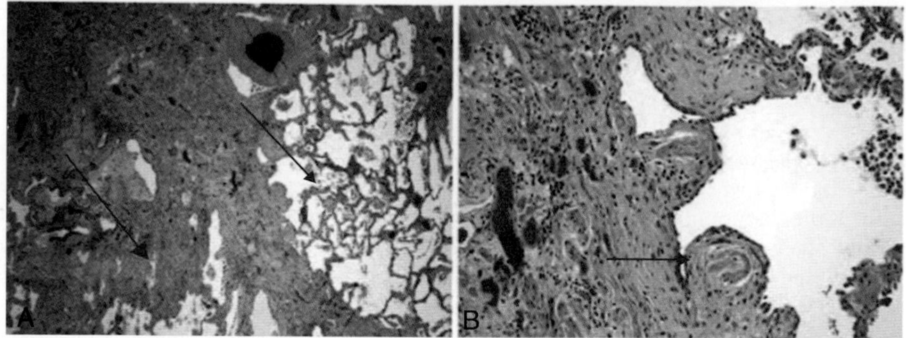

Fig. 58.3 (A) Low magnification view of hematoxylin and eosin stain demonstrating usual interstitial pneumonia/idiopathic pulmonary fibrosis pattern characterized by temporal heterogeneity. Marked interstitial fibrosis with subpleural microscopic honeycombing seen in the bottom left of the image (*large arrow head*) and relatively normal-appearing parenchyma is in the center and lower right of the image (*small arrow head*). (B) High magnification view of an area at the interface between fibrotic and less-involved parenchyma shows several fibroblast foci (*arrow*). (From Jones, K. D., & Urisman, A. (2012). Histopathologic approach to the surgical lung biopsy in interstitial lung disease. *Clinics in Chest Medicine*, *33* (1), 27–40.)

TABLE 58.2 ■ **Histopathology Patterns**

Histopathology Patterns and Features			
UIP	**Probable UIP**	**Indeterminate for UIP**	**Alternative Diagnosis**
• Dense fibrosis with architectural distortion (i.e., destructive scarring and/or honeycombing) • Predominant subpleural and/or paraseptal distribution of fibrosis • Patchy involvement of lung parenchyma by fibrosis • Fibroblast foci • Absence of features to suggest an alternate diagnosis	• Some histologic features from column 1 are present but to an extent that precludes a definite diagnosis of UIP/IPF AND • Absence of features to suggest an alternative diagnosis OR • Honeycombing only	• Fibrosis with or without architectural distortion, with features favoring either a pattern other than UIP or features favoring UIP secondary to another cause • Some histologic features from column 1, but with other features suggesting an alternative diagnosis	• Features of other histologic patterns of IIPs (e.g., absence of fibroblast foci or loose fibrosis) in all biopsies • Histologic findings indicative of other diseases (e.g., hypersensitivity pneumonitis, Langerhans cell histiocytosis, sarcoidosis, LAM)

IPF, Idiopathic pulmonary fibrosis; *UIP*, usual interstitial pneumonia.

The patient presents to the clinic and asks you what the risk factors for his condition are and if there is anything he can avoid.

Which risk factors are associated with IPF?

The incidence of IPF increases with older age with patients typically presenting in their 60s and 70s. Patients with IPF who are younger than 50 years old are rare. The prevalence and incidence is higher in men compared with women. Most patients have a history of past cigarette smoking. It is uncertain whether smoking cessation improves outcomes in patients with IPF; however, smoking

TABLE 58.3 ■ **Diagnostic Table for IPF Based on HRCT and Histopathology Patterns**

IPF Suspected		Histopathology Pattern: UIP	Probable UIP	Indeterminate for UIP	Alternative Diagnosis
HRCT pattern	UIP	IPF	IPF	IPF	Non-IPF diagnosis
	Probable UIP	IPF	IPF	IPF (likely)	Non-IPF diagnosis
	Indeterminate for UIP	IPF	IPF (likely)	Indeterminate for IPF	Non-IPF diagnosis
	Alternative diagnosis	IPF (likely)/non-IPF diagnosis	Non-IPF diagnosis	Non-IPF diagnosis	Non-IPF diagnosis

HRCT, High-resolution computed tomography; *IPF*, idiopathic pulmonary fibrosis; *UIP*, usual interstitial pneumonia.

cessation should be recommended independent of IPF. Other risk factors include gastroesophageal reflux, chronic viral infections such as Epstein-Barr virus, hepatitis C, and a family history of ILD. Exposure to stone, metal, wood, and organic dusts has also been suggested as a risk factor.

CLINICAL PEARL **STEP 2/3**

Smoking-related ILDs include respiratory bronchiolitis-interstitial lung disease (RB-ILD) and desquamative interstitial pneumonia (DIP), each with its own unique radiographic features.

The patient then asks if there are any therapies for his condition.

Which treatments are recommended for IPF?

One of the most important first steps in the approach to therapy for IPF is early recognition and accurate diagnosis. Supportive care is the foundation of treatment of IPF, particularly supplemental oxygen for resting or exertional hypoxemia, as well as pulmonary rehabilitation, which is used to help improve functional status. Antifibrotic agents such as nintedanib, a tyrosine kinase inhibitor, and pirfenidone, an antifibrotic with pleiotropic effects, are now being recommended to slow the progression of disease and potentially decrease mortality.

Other than antifibrotic agents, which other actions should be taken?

Clinically silent gastroesophageal reflux has been observed in up to 90% of patients with IPF. Because aspiration and microaspiration can cause pneumonitis, 2015 guidelines recommend to treat patients with proton pump inhibitors or histamine-2 blocker receptor antagonists. This treatment may decrease the risk for microaspiration-associated lung injury or damage. However, these recommendations are based on observational studies, and more recent data suggest that antacid therapy may increase the risk of respiratory infections in patients with IPF. Patients should be up-to-date on their vaccinations and be referred for pulmonary rehabilitation programs. Patients should also be evaluated for related comorbidities, particularly pulmonary hypertension.

CLINICAL PEARL **STEP 2/3**

Pulmonary rehabilitation can reduce dyspnea and improve 6-minute walk distance.

CLINICAL PEARL **STEP 2/3**

A recent clinical trial showed that inhaled treprostinil, a prostacyclin analogue which promotes pulmonary vasodilation, improved exercise capacity from baseline in patients with pulmonary hypertension due to interstitial lung disease.

What should be avoided in patients with chronic IPF?

Unlike other ILDs in managing these patients chronically, corticosteroids and other immunosuppressive agents such as azathioprine have not been proven to affect disease course. Steroids and azathioprine were shown to increase hospitalization and death. Other treatments that are not recommended include anticoagulation with warfarin (unless there is another indication for anticoagulation); imatinib, a selective tyrosine kinase inhibitor against platelet-derived growth factor (PDGF) receptors; the combination of prednisone, azathioprine, and N-acetylcysteine; and ambrisentan, a selective endothelin receptor antagonist.

The patient is started on nintedanib to slow the rate of disease progression and is followed routinely in the outpatient pulmonary clinic. Serial PFTs are performed and show stabilization of his disease after initiation of nintedanib. Over time, his lung function tests eventually show continued decline of lung function because of the natural progression of his disease. FVC is noted to decline by >10% over a period of 6 months. Moreover, he now requires supplemental oxygen with his most recent 6-minute walk test showing a pulse oximetry nadir below 88%. He is subsequently referred for lung transplant.

CLINICAL PEARL **STEP 2/3**

Patients with IPF have increased risk of other comorbidities such as pulmonary hypertension (WHO Group 3), cardiovascular disease, obstructive sleep apnea, and lung malignancy.

When should lung transplantation be considered for patients with IPF?

In general, lung transplantation should be considered for patients with progressive advanced lung disease with a suspected 50% survival less than 3 years despite maximal medical therapy. Lung transplant should be considered in patients with severe IPF and early referral to a transplant center is prudent. Patients with the criteria listed in Table 58.4 should be referred for transplant, and patients with the criteria listed in Table 58.5 should be placed on the transplant list.

The patient is referred for lung transplantation and successfully undergoes a double lung transplantation without significant complications.

TABLE 58.4 ■ **Criteria for Lung Transplant Referral**

DLCO <40%
FVC <80%
Any dyspnea or functional limitation attributable to lung disease
Decrease in pulse oximetry <89%[a]

[a]Even if decrease occurs during exertion only.
DLCO, Diffusing capacity of the lung for carbon monoxide; *FVC*, forced vital capacity.

TABLE 58.5 ■ **Criteria to List Patients for Lung Transplant**

(Any one of the following):
A decline in FVC ≥10%[a] during 6 months of follow-up
A decline in DLCO ≥15% during 6 months of follow-up
During 6MWT: oxygen desaturation to <88% or distance walked <250 m or >50 m decline in distance walked over 6 months
Pulmonary hypertension on right heart catheterization or transthoracic echocardiogram
Hospitalization because of respiratory decline, pneumothorax, or acute exacerbation

[a]A decline ≥5% may also warrant lung transplant listing.
DLCO, Diffusing capacity of the lung for carbon monoxide; *FVC*, forced vital capacity; *6MWT*, 6-minute walk test.

CLINICAL PEARL **STEP 2/3**

After undergoing lung transplantation, patients with IPF have a 53% survival rate after 5 years.

BEYOND THE PEARLS

- A bronchoscopy with BAL and cell count is not helpful in the diagnosis of IPF; however, it may help exclude other diagnoses.
- Hermansky-Pudlak syndrome is a very rare cause of the UIP pattern. It is an autosomal recessive disorder characterized by albinism, bleeding diathesis, and pulmonary fibrosis.
- An emerging technique for biopsy is transbronchial cryobiopsy (TBCB), which can obtain larger samples of tissue compared with traditional transbronchial lung biopsy (TBLB).
- There is a commercially available genomic test (Envisia) to improve the ability to differentiate UIP/IPF from non UIP/IPF interstitial lung diseases. Current testing is performed on less invasive transbronchial biopsy samples obtained during bronchoscopy.
- Both nintedanib and pirfenidone have been shown to slow annual FVC decline by 50%.
- IPF is the second most frequent disease for which lung transplantation is performed in the United States.
- A disease entity exists which manifests both pulmonary fibrosis and emphysema phenotypes called combined pulmonary fibrosis and emphysema (CPFE). CT Chest imaging typically shows apical emphysema with a bibasilar predominant typical UIP pattern with a severely low DLCO on PFTs. Patients with CPFE have a higher incidence of pulmonary hypertension and lung cancer suggesting the potential need for a more routine and thorough assessment for these complications in this population.

Bibliography

Raghu, G., Rochwerg, B., Zhang, Y., et al. (2015). An Official ATS/ERS/JRS/ALAT Clinical practice guideline: treatment of idiopathic pulmonary fibrosis. An update of the 2011 Clinical Practice Guideline. *American Journal of Respiratory and Critical Care Medicine*, *192*(2), e3–e19.

Diagnosis of idiopathic pulmonary fibrosis. (2018). An Official ATS/ERS/JRS/ALAT Clinical Practice Guideline. *American Journal of Respiratory and Critical Care Medicine*, *198*(5), e44–e68.

Hewson, T., & McKeever, T. M. (2017). Timing of onset of symptoms in people with idiopathic pulmonary fibrosis. *Thorax*, 11.

Lederer, D., & Martinez, F. (2018 May 10). Idiopathic pulmonary fibrosis. *The New England Journal of Medicine*, *378*(19), 1811–1823.

Weill, D., & Benden, C. (2015). A consensus document for the selection of lung transplant candidates: 2014 - An update from the Pulmonary Transplantation Council of the International Society for Heart and Lung Transplantation. *The Journal of Heart and Lung Transplantation*, *34*(1), 1.

Waxman, A., Restrepo-Jaramillo, R., Thenappan, T., et al. (2021). Inhaled treprostinil in pulmonary hypertension due to interstitial lung disease. *New England Journal of Medicine, 384*, 325–334.

CASE 59

A 47-Year-Old Female With Shortness of Breath

Samantha Quon ■ Yash Kothari ■ Clay Wu ■ Drew Sheldon ■ Raj Dasgupta ■ Sivagini Ganesh

A 47-year-old female presents to the emergency department with 6 months of shortness of breath and dyspnea on exertion, which became acutely worse for the past 2 weeks. She denies fever, chills, night sweats, cough, sputum production, unintentional weight loss, or sick contacts. She denies any known medical history; however, she does take bumetanide at home. She denies tobacco, alcohol, or recreational drug use. She denies recent travel or tuberculous (TB) risk factors. On physical examination, her temperature is 36.4°C, blood pressure is 94/62 mmHg, heart rate is 108 beats/min, respiratory rate is 28 breaths/min on oxygen saturation is 86% on 6 L nasal cannula, which improved to 95% on 60 L/min and 60% FiO_2, and high flow nasal cannula. A 5/6 holosystolic murmur is auscultated over the left lower sternal border. The jugular venous pressure is 13 cm of water with 3+ pitting edema to the knees. Notably, her lungs are clear to auscultation. The remainder of the examination is normal.

What are some causes of chronic shortness of breath?

The differential for chronic shortness of breath is broad and typically organized by the anatomy or organ system involved. Obstruction of the upper airways or head and neck region should be considered, as well as chronic weakness caused by stroke, neuromuscular disease, or rheumatologic diseases. Musculoskeletal causes such as scoliosis can impair respiratory function. Cardiovascular causes are further broken down into arrhythmias, valvular disease, and cardiomyopathies (i.e., dilated, restrictive, and/or ischemic). Pulmonary causes can be broken down into obstructive airway disease (i.e., bronchospasm or endobronchial lesions), restrictive disease (pleural-based diseases, interstitial lung disease), alveolar disease (i.e., indolent infections such as fungal pneumonias or tuberculosis), or vascular disease (i.e., pulmonary hypertension). A detailed history and physical examination will help narrow the differential diagnosis.

CLINICAL PEARL **STEP 2/3**

Jugular venous distention (JVD, >7 cm above the sternal angle) suggests right heart failure, pulmonary hypertension, volume overload, tricuspid regurgitation, or pericardial disease.

Which diagnostic tests would you order to diagnose this patient's shortness of breath?

Based on the history and physical examination, this patient's shortness of breath is probably cardiac or pulmonary in origin. There is evidence of fluid overload with pitting edema and notable jugular venous distention (JVD), and a 5/6 holosystolic murmur suggestive of tricuspid regurgitation. She has no notable TB risk factors and no history of upper airway/nasopharyngeal disease. The standard workup including complete blood count (CBC) and complete metabolic panel

(CMP) can be done to evaluate for anemia, kidney, or liver disease. A chest radiograph (CXR) and electrocardiogram (ECG) should also be ordered to assess for obvious pulmonary irregularities, arrhythmias, and clues regarding cardiac chamber size and heart strain. In this case, additional laboratory studies such as brain natriuretic peptide (BNP) and troponin help evaluate for evidence of ventricular distension, volume overload, and cardiac ischemia. Further imaging should include a transthoracic echocardiogram (TTE), which is valuable in assessing both right and left heart function, valvular abnormalities, and cardiac pressures.

CLINICAL PEARL **STEP 2/3**

In addition to a holosystolic murmur, another physical examination finding suggestive of elevated right heart pressure is a prominent S2 on cardiac auscultation (pronounced P2).

Her CBC and CMP are unremarkable. Her troponin is elevated mildly to 0.12 ng/mL. Her brain natriuretic peptide is elevated to 580 pg/mL. Her CXR and ECG are shown in Figs. 59.1 and 59.2.

Her CXR is notable for enlarged central pulmonary arteries. Her ECG is notable for right ventricular hypertrophy. Her transthoracic echocardiogram shows a normal left ventricular ejection fraction of 70% with no wall motion abnormalities. The right ventricle cavity size is mildly increased with a moderately reduced systolic function. The pulmonary artery systolic pressure (PASP) is estimated to be 74 mmHg. There is significant right atrial dilation and severe tricuspid regurgitation.

CLINICAL PEARL **STEP 2/3**

The most common ECG findings seen in pulmonary hypertension are right axis deviation, right bundle branch block, right ventricular hypertrophy, and right atrial enlargement.

When should a diagnosis of pulmonary hypertension be considered?

Pulmonary hypertension should be considered in patients with chronic dyspnea or fatigue. Signs or symptoms of right heart failure, such as lower extremity edema, JVD, congestive hepatopathy, and elevated estimated pulmonary arterial systolic pressure on echocardiography, especially with

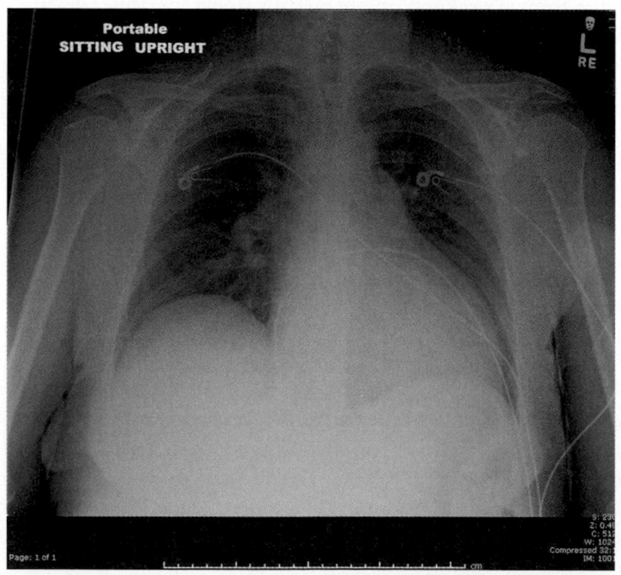

Fig. 59.1 Chest X-ray image showing enlarged pulmonary artery.

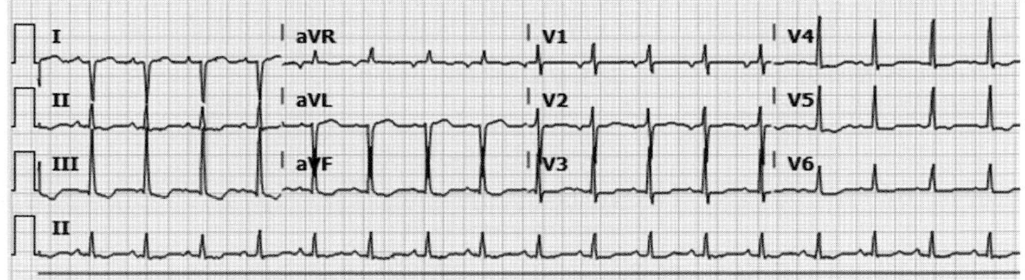

Fig. 59.2 Electrocardiogram showing right ventricular hypertrophy.

concomitant tricuspid valve regurgitation or right atrial or right ventricular dilation should prompt further evaluation. In addition, presence of comorbidities associated with pulmonary hypertension, such as connective tissue diseases, rheumatoid arthritis, obstructive sleep apnea, interstitial lung disease, cirrhosis, and scleroderma should also raise suspicion of pulmonary hypertension.

CLINICAL PEARL **STEP 2/3**

TTE estimation of PASP poorly correlates with values obtained by right heart catheterization and thus pulmonary hypertension cannot be definitively diagnosed.

What are the five groups of pulmonary hypertension?

There are five groups of pulmonary hypertension (PH) based on etiology and mechanism (see Table 59.1). Another way to classify PH anatomically includes precapillary (involving pulmonary arteries—i.e., Group I) and postcapillary (involving the pulmonary venous system—i.e., Group 2) or combined.

CLINICAL PEARL **STEP 2/3**

Drugs associated with PAH include weight loss drugs (aminorex, fenfluramine), amphetamines, and methamphetamines.

How do you make a diagnosis of pulmonary hypertension?

Diagnosis of pulmonary hypertension is made with a mean pulmonary artery pressure of greater than 20 mmHg at rest. An elevated pulmonary vascular resistance (PVR) of ≥3 Wood units and pulmonary capillary wedge pressure of <15 is needed to confirm a diagnosis of Group 1 pulmonary hypertension or pulmonary arterial hypertension. A right heart catheterization is not indicated in all patients. However, in this patient, because of her normal left heart function and lack of underlying lung disease, pulmonary vascular disease is strongly suspected.

BASIC SCIENCE/CLINICAL PEARL **STEP 1/2/3**

Pulmonary capillary wedge pressure is a surrogate for left atrial pressure, which is an indirect estimate of left ventricular end-diastolic pressure. This will be elevated in patients with Group 2 pulmonary hypertension.

The patient is admitted to the hospital and undergoes a right heart catheterization. The diagnosis of pulmonary hypertension is confirmed with a mean pulmonary artery pressure of 55 and a PVR of 8.

TABLE 59.1 ■ **Five Groups of Pulmonary Hypertension Based on Etiology and Mechanism**

Group 1: Pulmonary arterial hypertension	– Idiopathic (primary) – Familial – Drugs and toxins (methamphetamine, cocaine) – Connective tissue diseases – HIV infection – Schistosomiasis – Portal hypertension – Left to right intracardiac shunts
Group 2: Pulmonary venous hypertension	– Left sided atrial or ventricular disease – Left sided valvular disease
Group 3: Associated with hypoxemia	– Chronic obstructive pulmonary disease – Interstitial lung disease – Sleep-disordered breathing (obstructive sleep apnea, obesity hypoventilation syndrome) – Alveolar hypoventilation disorders – Chronic exposure to high altitude – Developmental abnormalities
Group 4: Chronic thromboembolic pulmonary hypertension (CTEPH)	– Thromboembolic obstruction – Pulmonary embolism (tumor, parasite)
Group 5: Miscellaneous	– Sarcoidosis – Pulmonary Langerhans cell histiocytosis – Lymphangiomatosis – Compression of pulmonary vessels (adenopathy, tumor, fibrosing mediastinitis)

From Rich S. Executive summary the World Symposium on primary pulmonary hypertension 1998. World Health Organization.

How do you identify the etiology of pulmonary hypertension?

The etiology of pulmonary hypertension, and therefore which group of pulmonary hypertension, has implications for treatment options. Elucidating which group this patient belongs to starts with a detailed history, including past medical history, use of recreational drugs, symptoms of rheumatic conditions such as joint pains or rashes, family history, night time snoring or day time fatigue (sleep disordered breathing), and prior travel (parasitic infections). Depending on clinical suspicion, additional diagnostic tests and laboratory workup should be ordered (Table 59.2).

CLINICAL PEARL **STEP 2/3**

Obstructive sleep apnea only leads to the development of pulmonary hypertension if there is significant nocturnal hypoxia. The other notable complication of sleep apnea is arrhythmias, typically atrial fibrillation or atrial flutter.

She is diagnosed with pulmonary arterial hypertension (Group 1).

What is the pathophysiology of pulmonary arterial hypertension?

Pulmonary arterial hypertension is caused by vasoconstriction, smooth-muscle cell and endothelial-cell proliferation, and thrombosis in small pulmonary arterioles, leading to increased pulmonary arterial resistance (see Fig. 59.3). Prostacyclin and nitric oxide are both potent vasodilators, inhibit platelet activation, and have antiproliferative properties. Decreased levels of prostacyclin and nitric

TABLE 59.2 ■ **Additional Diagnostic Tests and Laboratory Workup**

Sleep study	Obstructive sleep apnea, obesity hypoventilation syndrome
Pulmonary function test with DLCO	Obstructive lung disease, interstitial lung disease
High-resolution chest CT	Interstitial lung disease
Antibody titers	Connective tissue disease
Liver function test	Cirrhosis
Abdominal ultrasound	
V/Q scan	Chronic pulmonary thromboembolism
HIV screen	HIV

DLCO, Carbon monoxide diffusion capacity; *V/Q*, ventilation/perfusion.

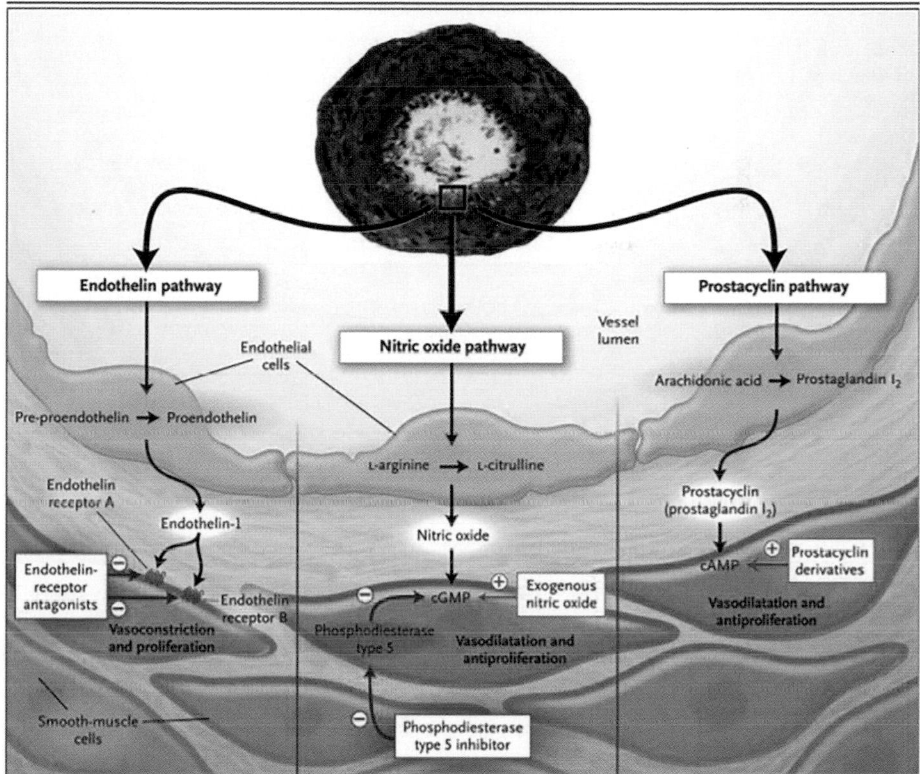

Fig. 59.3 Illustration of the three mechanisms of pulmonary arterial hypertension. (From Humbert, M., Sitbon, O., & Simonneau, G. (2004). Treatment of pulmonary arterial hypertension. *New England Journal of Medicine, 351* (14), 1425–1436.)

oxide are associated with pulmonary hypertension resulting from increased vasoconstriction, cell proliferation, and thrombosis. Endothelin-1 is a potent vasoconstrictor that, stimulates the proliferation of pulmonary-artery smooth-muscle cells. Increased levels of endothelin-1 are found in patients with pulmonary hypertension and lead to vasoconstriction and increased cell proliferation.

BASIC SCIENCE/CLINICAL PEARL **STEP 1/2/3**

Prostacyclin is in endothelial cells via the arachidonic acid pathway from prostaglandins. In addition to its direct vasodilatory effects, it also inhibits platelet aggregation.

What is the treatment for pulmonary arterial hypertension?

Current therapies target the mediators of increased pulmonary arterial resistance. A summary of the various therapies is listed in Table 59.3.

Initial therapy is based on the patient's World Health Organization (WHO) function class, as defined in Table 59.4.

For patients with WHO Class I pulmonary hypertension, management is aimed at treating the underlying cause and their symptoms observed (see Table 59.5). Patients with WHO Class II and III pulmonary hypertension are started on dual combination therapy with endothelin

TABLE 59.3 ■ **Current Therapies for Pulmonary Artery Hypertension**

Mediators of Vascular Response	Effect on Pulmonary Arterioles	Targeted Therapy	Mechanism of Action
Decreased prostacyclin	– Vasoconstriction – Cell proliferation – Thrombosis	Prostacyclin derivatives e.g., epoprostinil, treprostinil, selexipag	– Induces relaxation of vascular smooth muscle (stimulating the production of cyclic AMP (cAMP)) – Inhibits the growth of smooth-muscle cells
Decreased NO	– Vasoconstriction – Cell proliferation – Thrombosis	Phosphodiesterase 5 inhibitor (PDE-5 inhibitor) e.g., sildenafil, tadalafil	– Enhance nitric oxide–dependent, cGMP-mediated pulmonary vasodilatation through inhibition of the breakdown of cGMP
Increased endothelin-1	– Vasoconstriction – Cell proliferation	Endothelin receptor antagonist (ERA) e.g., bosentan, ambrisentan, macetentan	– Endothelin-1 receptor antagonist (ERA)

TABLE 59.4 ■ **WHO Functional Classification for Pulmonary Hypertension**

Class I	Patients with pulmonary hypertension but without resulting limitations of physical activity. Ordinary physical activity does not cause undue fatigue or dyspnea, chest pain, or heart syncope.
Class II	Patients with pulmonary hypertension resulting in slight limitation of physical activity. They are comfortable at rest. Ordinary physical activity results in undue fatigue or dyspnea, chest pain, or heart syncope.
Class III	Patients with pulmonary hypertension resulting in marked limitation of physical activity. They are comfortable at rest. Less than ordinary physical activity causes undue fatigue or dyspnea, chest pain, or heart syncope.
Class IV	Patients with pulmonary hypertension resulting in inability to carry on any physical activity without symptoms. These patients manifest signs of right heart failure. Dyspnea and/or fatigue may be present even at rest. Discomfort is increased by physical activity.

From Rich S. Primary pulmonary hypertension: executive summary. Evian, France. World Health Organization, 1998.

WHO, World Health Organization.

TABLE 59.5 ■ **Management of Pulmonary Hypertension**

WHO Class	Treatment
I	Observation Treatment of contributing factors/underlying conditions
II & III	Dual combination therapy: ERA plus PDE-5 inhibitor (e.g., ambrisentan + tadalafil)
IV	Add parenteral prostacyclin analogue to ERA plus PDE-5 inhibitor

ERA, Endothelin receptor antagonist; *PDE-5 inhibitor*, phosphodiesterase-5 inhibitor.

receptor antagonists plus a phosphodiesterase-5 (PDE-5) inhibitor, such as ambrisentan and tadalafil. When patients progress to WHO Class IV, a parenteral prostacyclin analog is added to the treatment regimen.

Calcium channel blockers can also be used if there is evidence of vasoreactivity. Vasoreactivity testing is performed during the right heart catheterization by administering a vasodilatory agent such as nitric oxide. If there is a decrease in mean pulmonary artery pressure by at least 10 mmHg and to a value less than or equal to 40 mmHg, this is consistent with positive vasoreactivity and predicts a favorable response to calcium channel blockers.

BASIC SCIENCE/CLINICAL PEARL **STEP 1/2/3**

PDE-5 inhibitors are also used for the treatment of erectile dysfunction and benign prostatic hyperplasia (BPH).

You ask the patient about her functional status and she reports she has no respiratory symptoms at rest but is becoming extremely short of breath just walking around the house. You decide to start her on combination endothelin receptor antagonist and phosphodiesterase type 5 inhibitor.

What are the major side effects from endothelin receptor antagonists and phosphodiesterase inhibitors?

Endothelin receptor antagonists are associated with hepatotoxicity and peripheral edema. They are also teratogenic, so the patient needs to be counseled on the importance of birth control. Phosphodiesterase inhibitors are associated with headache, gastrointestinal upset, flushing, and musculoskeletal pain, and can augment hypotensive effects of nitrates and alpha blockers.

She feels better over the next few days and is able to be weaned off oxygen therapy. She is subsequently discharged home with follow-up in the pulmonary hypertension clinic within 2 weeks.

Case Summary

- **Complaint/History:** A 47-year-old-woman presents to the emergency department with 6 months of shortness of breath.
- **Findings:** Oxygen saturation is 86% on 6 L nasal cannula, a 5/6 holosystolic murmur is auscultated over the left lower sternal border, jugular venous pressure is 13 cm of water and 3+ pitting edema to the knees, and lungs are clear to auscultation.
- **Lab Results/Tests:** Transthoracic echocardiogram shows a normal left ventricular ejection fraction of 70% and moderately reduced right systolic function; PASP is estimated to be 74 mmHg with significant right atrial dilation and severe tricuspid regurgitation. Right heart catheterization shows mean pulmonary artery pressure of 55 and a PVR of 8.

Diagnosis: Group 1 pulmonary hypertension.

- **Treatment:** Patient was started on dual combination therapy with endothelin receptor antagonist and phosphodiesterase type 5 inhibitor.

BEYOND THE PEARLS

- The most common genetic mutations associated with heritable pulmonary arterial hypertension are bone morphogenetic protein receptor type II (BMPR2 mutation) and activin receptor-like kinase (ALK-1).
- Transthoracic echo with agitated saline contrast or "bubble" study can be used to look for intracardiac shunts as a cause of pulmonary hypertension.
- Chronic thromboembolic pulmonary hypertension occurs in approximately 10%-15% of those patients with acute thromboemboli.
- A calcium channel blocker is used for patients with a positive vasoreactivity test; however, its effects are typically not sustained.
- Riociguat is a stimulator of soluble guanylate cyclase and is approved for treatment of Group 1 pulmonary arterial hypertension and Group 4 chronic thromboembolic pulmonary hypertension (CTEPH). The preferred treatment of choice for CTEPH is a surgical procedure called pulmonary thromboendarterectomy (PTA). Riociguat is used for the treatment of inoperable, persistent, or recurrent CTEPH.
- Lung transplantation should be offered to patients who are refractory to medical therapy.
- Concurrent heart transplant is typically not required because the heart can remodel with removal of the elevated pulmonary arterial pressures. In patients with pulmonary hypertension due to interstitial lung disease (Group 3), inhaled treprostinil improved exercise capacity from baseline, assessed with the use of a 6-minute walk test, as compared with placebo. Therefore treprostinil received FDA approval for Groups 1 and 3.

Bibliography

Humbert, M., Sitbon, O., & Simonneau, G. (2004). Treatment of pulmonary arterial hypertension. *The New England Journal of Medicine*, *351*(14), 1425–1436.

Farber, H. W., & Loscalzo, J. (2004). Pulmonary arterial hypertension. *The New England Journal of Medicine*, *351*(16), 1655–1665.

Rich S. Executive summary from the World Symposium on primary pulmonary hypertension 1998. World Health Organization website. Available at: www.who.int/ncd/cvd/pph.html.

Galiè N, Humbert M, Vachiery JL, et al. 2015 ESC/ERS Guidelines for the diagnosis and treatment of pulmonary hypertension: The Joint Task Force for the Diagnosis and Treatment of Pulmonary Hypertension of the European Society of Cardiology (ESC) and the European Respiratory Society

McLaughlin, V. V., Archer, S. L., Badesch, D. B., et al. (2009). ACCF/AHA 2009 expert consensus document on pulmonary hypertension: a report of the American College of Cardiology Foundation Task Force on Expert Consensus Documents and the American Heart Association: developed in collaboration with the American College of Chest Physicians, American Thoracic Society, Inc., and the Pulmonary Hypertension Association [published correction appears in Circulation. 2009 Jul 14;120(2):e13]. *Circulation*, *119*(16), 2250–2294.

CASE 60

A 64-Year-Old Male With a 3-Month History of Worsening Cough

Swathi Nallapa ■ Shiqian Li ■ Raj Dasgupta ■ Diana H. Yu

A 64-year-old male presents to the primary care clinic with a 3-month history of a gradually worsening cough. He describes a dry cough with occasional blood-tinged sputum and associated shortness of breath. He reports mild night sweats and approximately 10-lb unintentional weight loss in the past year. He denies fevers, chills, chest pain, sore throat, rhinorrhea, or recent travel. His past medical history is significant for chronic obstructive pulmonary disease (COPD), for which he uses an inhaler twice weekly. He previously worked in construction and smoked one pack of cigarettes per day for 30 years but quit 10 years ago. He was born in Mexico but moved to the United States at the age of 16. On physical examination, blood pressure is 124/78 mmHg, pulse rate is 92 beats/min, and oxygen saturation is 94% on room air. On auscultation, there are decreased breath sounds at bilateral lung bases without any focal wheezes, crackles, or rhonchi. Hyperresonance is diffusely noted on percussion. There is no palpable lymphadenopathy and the remainder of the examination is normal. A chest radiograph reveals a 3.3 cm right lung opacity with irregular borders and an enlarged right hilum.

What is your differential diagnosis?

This gentleman is presenting to your clinic with a constellation of gradually worsening physical symptoms that raise several red flags. Most notably, his progressive cough and shortness of breath with recent unintended weight loss and night sweats are concerning for underlying malignancy infection. He has several risk factors for pulmonary disease. His most significant risk factor is having a 1 pack-year smoking history for 30 years, which probably led to his COPD. Additionally, working in construction can lead to heightened environmental exposures to harmful dust, fumes, and gases. Other concerning symptoms include his blood-tinged sputum production, which can be seen in the setting of malignancy and COPD exacerbation but should also raise concern for pulmonary tuberculosis. Although the time course of his illness is relatively subacute, it is also important to evaluate for common illnesses such as bacterial pneumonia or other lung infections. Based on an initial evaluation of this patient's symptoms, our initial differential diagnosis includes:

- Malignancy
- Tuberculosis
- COPD exacerbation
- Viral or bacterial pneumonia

Which imaging studies would be useful in establishing the diagnosis?

The first imaging modality of choice is a chest radiograph. Chest X-rays use a very small amount of radiation and provide an initial evaluation of the heart, lungs, airways, and bones within the chest. It is almost always the first imaging study to obtain in this clinical setting because it is fast and, easy to obtain, and confers the least amount of risk and radiation to the patient. Fig. 60.1 shows the patient's chest X-ray image.

The chest X-ray image reveals a right lung opacity with irregular borders and an enlarged right hilum. The irregular borders make it less likely that this opacity represents a benign pulmonary nodule. Given the apical position of the lesion, it is possible that this represents pulmonary tuberculosis or an atypical infection. However, the presence of hilar lymphadenopathy with an irregular lung mass should be considered malignant until proven otherwise.

There are several options for diagnosing this lung opacity. A computed tomography (CT) scan functions like a series of X-ray images taken from all angles to provide a more detailed image than a plain film X-ray. Another option is a positron emission tomography/computed tomography (PET-CT), which is a nuclear medicine scan that appears similar to a CT image but also displays the metabolic or biochemical activity within the body. Both of these imaging modalities will expose the patient to more radiation than a plain film X-ray, but advanced imaging is often necessary to diagnose many illnesses accurately, including malignancies. Relatively speaking, PET-CTs are far more expensive and time consuming, and require advanced nuclear medicine trained radiologists for interpretation. In this case, it would be reasonable to obtain a CT thorax for visualization of the patient's lung opacity (Fig. 60.2). Often, CT images of the chest, abdomen, and pelvis are obtained when diagnosing a potential malignancy to evaluate for any sites of distant metastases.

The CT thorax reveals a peripheral right lung opacity that will require a biopsy to provide a pathological tissue diagnosis prior to initiating treatment for a suspected primary lung malignancy. Lung cancer is divided into two broad categories, small-cell lung cancer (approximately 15% of all lung cancers) and non-small-cell lung cancers (NSCLC, approximately 85% of all lung cancers). It is imperative that a tissue sample is obtained prior to any definitive surgical or medical management because all major treatment options are based on histopathology.

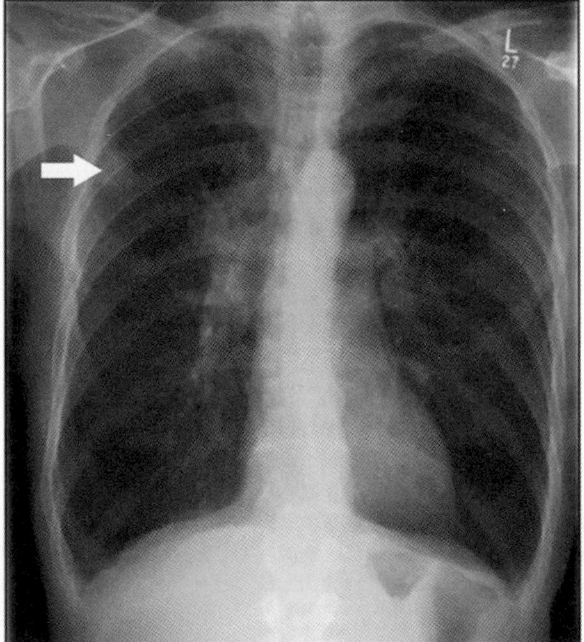

Fig. 60.1 Chest radiograph showing right lung opacity with irregular borders *(arrow)*.

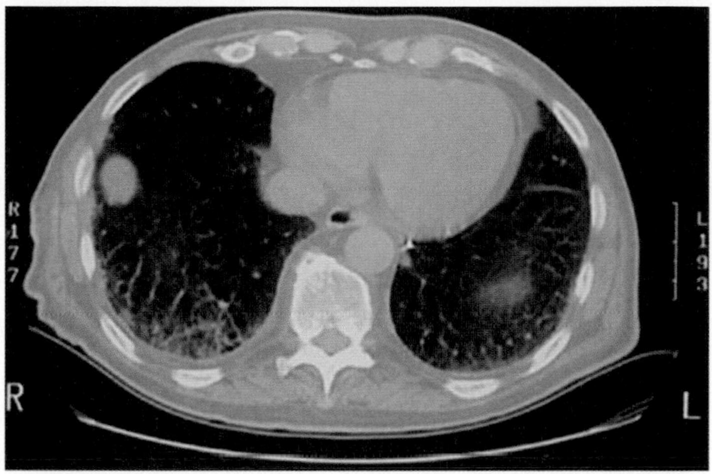

Fig. 60.2 Computed tomography scan of thorax showing right lung opacity *(red arrowhead).*

Which surgical and nonsurgical methods are used to perform a biopsy?

There are surgical and non-surgical approaches to obtaining a lung biopsy. Prior to advancement of non-invasive, non-surgical bronchoscopic biopsies and mediastinal / hilar cancer staging, many primary lung nodule tissue diagnosis was made via surgical biopsies by thoracic surgeons in an operating room with general anesthesia. Surgeons perform video-assisted thoracoscopic surgery (VATS) guided lung resections (some VATS are converted to open lung surgery) and lymph node dissection for diagnosis and staging. Surgical mediastinoscopies are also performed to biopsy lymph nodes. Given the high risks associated with a surgical approach, all non-surgical biopsy options should be considered prior to pursuing a surgical biopsy.

Non-surgical bronchoscopic biopsies are performed by advanced bronchoscopists or interventional pulmonologists. Bronchoscopic biopsy of the lung nodule and mediastinal/hilar staging (biopsy of lymph nodes to evaluate for metastasis) are performed at the same time in majority of cases. Endobronchial ultrasonography (EBUS) accesses the airways and is used for the transbronchial needle aspiration (TBNA) of mediastinal and hilar lymph nodes. EBUS can also reach centrally located lung nodules/masses for direct ultrasound visual guided biopsy.

Since the advancement of EBUS, which can access most mediastinal and hilar lymph nodes, practice of surgical mediastinoscopy guided biopsy of lymph nodes have declined.

After thorough mediastinal and hilar lymph nodes have been biopsied for complete staging, biopsy of the primary lung tumor can be pursued. Non-surgical bronchoscopic options for primary tumor biopsy include conventional bronchoscopy with transbronchial biopsy, electromagnetic navigational bronchoscopy or robotic bronchoscopy with transbronchial biopsy. Referral to interventional radiologist can be made for CT-guided percutaneous transthoracic biopsy. A conventional bronchoscopy accesses the airways and is followed by a transbronchial biopsy of the lung tumor often using fluoroscopic guidance (2D continuous plain x-ray). An electromagnetic navigational (EMN)bronchoscopy is relatively a novel technique similar to 'GPS for the lungs' that utilizes electromagnetic fields to track the instruments through the airways. Virtual bronchoscopic navigation utilizes an internal rendering of the airway from CT data to generate a 'virtual roadmap' to the target lung lesion. Most recently, developments in robotic assisted technologies have led to the introduction of robotic bronchoscopy (RB). These novel devices may allow bronchoscopist to more precisely maneuver into the periphery of lungs with greater stability and accuracy.

Finally, patients who have a solitary peripheral primary lesion may benefit from a referral to radiology for evaluation for a CT-guided percutaneous transthoracic needle biopsy. In this procedure, radiologists will use the patient's CT scan to guide a needle directly through the chest wall to access a peripheral lung mass for tissue diagnosis. The location of the mass relative to other vital structures and vasculature will determine whether or not it can be accessed by external needle aspiration.

After extensive evaluation of the patient's diagnostic imaging, we must determine the best method for biopsy. Given that the patient has imaging evidence of hilar lymph nodes involvement, an endobronchial approach (EBUS) with transbronchial needle aspiration of the lymph nodes is the most preferred method of obtaining a biopsy.

This patient's final histopathology confirms a diagnosis of NSCLC, specifically primary adenocarcinoma of the lung with contralateral hilar lymph node involvement. NSCLC is an umbrella term that encompasses many subtypes including adenocarcinoma, squamous cell carcinoma, and large cell carcinoma.

After diagnosis, management of all subtypes of NSCLC depends on the patient's clinical and pathologic stage, with a multidisciplinary approach involving medical oncology, radiation oncology, and thoracic surgery.

What are the stages of NSCLC?

After a biopsy sample has been obtained and the histopathology confirms a diagnosis, the next step is to classify the patient's disease burden based on a staging system. The most common staging system used in cancer is known as the TNM staging system. The T refers to size and extent of the primary tumor, the N refers to the number of regional lymph nodes affected, and the M refers to sites of distant metastases.

For lung cancers specifically, the primary tumor will be classified as T1 if the size is less than 3 cm. If the tumor is larger than 7 cm, it will be classified as T4, which is the highest value in the TNM staging system. Additionally, any direct invasion of vital structures such as the diaphragm, heart, and great vessels will automatically confer a T4 classification. Although there are more specific criteria that separate T1–T4, these general guidelines will help provide an overview for classification of the primary tumor.

Regional lymph nodes are assessed in terms of ipsilateral and contralateral involvement, relative to the primary lung tumor. For example, no regional lymph node involvement would be stage N0. Ipsilateral lymph node involvement, meaning lymph nodes draining the same lung as the primary tumor, can be classified as N1 or N2 based on the specific nodes involved. Any involvement of contralateral lymph nodes will result in stage N3.

Staging based on metastasis is relatively straightforward. If no metastatic disease is present, the patient is classified as M0. If any metastasis is present, the patient is classified as M1. Within the M1 classification, there are subgroups (M1a, M1b, and M1c) based on the extent and location of metastatic disease.

Typically, clinical staging is estimated based on imaging at the time of diagnosis to guide the initial treatment plans. Clinical staging is divided into stage I to stage IV disease based on the extent of disease as appreciated by pretreatment imaging. If a patient undergoes surgical resection (more on this later) with a lymph node dissection, patients may be restaged based on tissue pathology. Typically, restaging only occurs if surgery reveals a greater extent of tumor burden than initially predicted by imaging alone.

By definition, patients with NSCLC localized to one lung and with no mediastinal involvement will have clinical stage I or stage II disease. If technically feasible, surgical resection is the gold-standard approach in these patients. If there is evidence of mediastinal involvement, as shown by imaging or appreciated at the time of surgery, this is automatically indicative of stage III disease. The overall 5-year survival is 10%–15% in patients with NSCLC. This number is probably skewed by the fact that the vast majority (around 70%) of patients present with locally advanced (stage III) disease or distant metastatic (stage IV) disease.

In the case of our patient with biopsy-proven primary adenocarcinoma of the right lung and contralateral hilar lymph node involvement via EBUS biopsy, we know that clinically he has stage III disease with no evidence of distant metastasis. Based on his histopathology, he has a TNM stage score of T2N3M0. T2 is based on tumor size of 3.3 cm, N3 is based on contralateral lymph node involvement, and M0 is based on further diagnostic imaging, including abdomen and pelvis CT and brain MRI, with no evidence of distant metastasis.

What are the surgical options?

As discussed, patients with stage I or stage II disease should be evaluated for complete and total surgical resection, if technically feasible. After the tumor is removed, the final pathology report will determine whether the patient will require postoperative chemotherapy. Typically, if patients have pathologic stage IB or stage II disease, they will warrant consideration for postoperative chemotherapy.

In patients with NSCLC, stage I and stage II offer the most favorable long-term survival and potential for cure. In order to determine which patients qualify for surgery, an extensive preoperative evaluation must be performed. This involves risk stratification of medical comorbidities, assessment of the patient's functional status, and a measurement of pulmonary function tests (PFTs). Although it may be technically feasible to resect NSCLC, a surgeon may determine that a patient is not an ideal surgical candidate based on the patient's comorbidities, functional status, or PFTs. For example, if the resection of a large tumor will result in markedly reduced lung function postoperatively, the operation may leave the patient without sufficient residual lung function to maintain an adequate quality of life and thus surgery might not be a viable option.

The optimal technique for surgical resection is a lobectomy, which is the surgical resection of a single lobe of the lung. This procedure can be done as an open thoracotomy or with video-assisted thoracoscopic surgery (VATS), or more recently with robotic-assisted thoracoscopic surgery (RATS). If a patient is unable to tolerate a lobectomy, based on comorbidities or diminished overall pulmonary function, alternatives include a smaller segmentectomy or a nonanatomic wedge resection. These procedures are typically performed with VATS technique and can be considered in patients with smaller primary tumors (less than 3 cm). However, it is important to note that these patients will be at higher risk of local recurrence.

As discussed earlier, postoperative care is dictated by surgical margins and pathologic staging. Any patient with pathologic stage II disease or stage IB disease with high-risk features will require chemotherapy after surgery. Patients with positive surgical margins will also require postoperative radiation therapy. Finally, if mediastinal involvement is discovered during surgery, patients will require adjuvant chemotherapy followed by radiation therapy.

After surgery, there is always a risk of local recurrence postoperatively. The 5-year incidence of local recurrence is 23% with a median time to recurrence of 14 months. This risk is increased depending on the pathologic stage, and certain subtypes of NSCLC, such as squamous cell carcinoma or large cell carcinoma, confer a greater risk of local recurrence. In cases of local recurrence, options include repeat surgical resection, radiation therapy, or concurrent chemotherapy and radiation therapy, depending on the clinical circumstances.

How are nonsurgical cases managed?

As discussed, patients with stage I or stage II disease should undergo surgical resection with the goal of total resection and cure. However, if patients cannot or choose not to undergo surgery, patients with stage I or II disease can be evaluated for stereotactic body radiation therapy (SBRT). This form of radiation therapy is typically limited to patients with lesions less than 5 cm in size. For those with larger tumors who opt out of surgery, full-dose fractionation is required and SBRT will probably not be an option.

For patients with stage III (locally advanced, such as our patient) or stage IV disease (distant metastasis), the next steps in treatment are determined by molecular testing for driver mutations. Currently, most of these molecular tests can be performed on the initial biopsy or cytology samples obtained at the time of diagnosis and thus do not require additional diagnostic testing. Molecular testing, in this case, is performed with immunohistochemistry (IHC) or fluorescence in situ hybridization (FISH) to identify mutations in the genetic sequence. For patients with an identifiable driver mutation, targeted therapies are offered. If no driver mutations are present, patients can be considered for new immunotherapy. If neither option is applicable, patients will be offered a traditional platinum-based chemotherapy regimen.

Which driver mutations are found in NSCLC?

Molecular testing for driver mutations includes an evaluation for mutations in the genes encoding epidermal growth factor receptor (EGFR), anaplastic lymphoma kinase (ALK), rat osteosarcoma (ROS1), KRAS, RET, and MET, and BRAF V600E. Analysis of patients who have driver mutations and appropriately received targeted therapies shows an overall increased survival compared with both patients who do not have driver mutations and patients who have driver mutations but did not receive targeted therapy. The key driver mutations to be aware of include:

- EGFR
- ALK
- ROS1
- BRAF V600E

The presence of these driver mutations warrants consideration for targeted therapies such as erlotinib (EGFR mutation), crizotinib (ALK, ROS-1), erlotinib, gefitinib (EGFR mutation), crizotinib, ceritinib, lorlatinib (ALK, ROS-1), dabrafenib, trametinib (BRAF), sotorasib (KRAS), pralsetinib, selpercatinib (RET), crizotinib (MET), or trametinib (BRAF V600E) as a first-line therapy and possible continuation as maintenance therapy. If a patient was to relapse in the future, traditional platinum-based therapies can be considered as second-line therapy.

What is immunotherapy and which options are available?

For patients who lack driver mutations, the next step is to assess the possibility of immunotherapy. The role of immunotherapy is determined by the expression of programmed death 1 (PD-1) or programmed death ligand 1 (PD-L1) on molecular analysis. Recent studies have shown certain tumors have developed a mechanism to evade the body's natural immune defenses by suppressing natural immune checkpoints. In patients with a high degree of PD-1, immunotherapy drugs also known as checkpoint inhibitors can be given to block PD-1 and thus increase the ability of the patient's own immune system to attack cancerous cells. In patients with molecular evidence of >50% expression of PD-1, immunotherapy medications such as pembrolizumab can be administered instead of the traditional platinum-based therapy. Although immunotherapy has demonstrated some promising results, it is important to note that significant adverse effects have been noted involving the endocrine, gastrointestinal, and hepatic systems and patients often require close monitoring of symptoms and lab tests.

If targeted therapy and immunotherapy are not feasible based on molecular testing, traditional platinum-based therapy is offered to patients with stage III and stage IV disease.

Which palliative options are available?

As discussed, NSCLC carries a high risk of morbidity and mortality. Some patients will opt for more conservative management, focusing on alleviating symptoms and managing local complications rather than pursuing surgery, chemotherapy, and radiation in the face of a difficult prognosis. Other patients may have disease recurrence after trying various treatment options and may request more palliative interventions. For example, some patients may develop bothersome, recurrent pleural effusion that negatively impacts their quality of life and require frequent hospital admissions for thoracentesis. For these patients, VATS or indwelling pleural catheters may be an option for definitive, palliative management of recurrent malignant effusions. In patient with airway involvement of tumor with difficulty breathing or hemoptysis, therapeutic bronchoscopy with tumor debulking, debridement and excision with laser therapy or argon plasma coagulation (APC), or airway stents can be placed to alleviate symptoms. It is important to be aware of these palliative interventions because they can dramatically improve the quality of life for these patients, particularly in their final days. It is imperative to encourage an open and honest dialogue with patients about their goals and how our medical interventions can assist in achieving these goals.

Case Summary

- **Complaint/History:** A 64-year-old man with a worsening chronic cough presents to his primary care doctor.
- **Findings:** He is found to have some red flag symptoms such as unintentional weight loss and blood tinged cough in the setting of COPD secondary to a significant smoking history.
- **Lab Results/Tests:** He undergoes CT scans and found to have a pulmonary mass and subsequently undergoes EBUS given his lymphadenopathy.

Diagnosis: High stage non-small cell lung cancer.

- **Treatment:** Chemotherapy and radiation with possible immunotherapy.

BEYOND THE PEARLS

- EBUS has replaced mediastinoscopy as the modality of choice for intra-thoracic mediastinal staging for lung cancer.
- Pneumothoraces can occur in up to 25% of patients who undergo CT guided biopsy.
- Mutational drivers and immunotherapy have improved outcomes substantially in advanced staged lung cancers.
- Early palliative care has been shown to extend survival compared to those that do not receive palliative care.

Bibliography

Detterbeck F. C., Chansky, K., Groome, P., Bolejack, V., Crowley, J. Shemanski, L., Kennedy, C., Krasnik, M., Peake, M., Rami-Porta, R., Goldstraw, P., Asamura, H., Ball, D., Beer, D. G., Beyruti, R., Bolejack, V. Chansky, V., Crowley, J., … Travis, W. D. (2016). The IASLC lung cancer staging project: methodology and validation used in the development of proposals for revision of the stage classification of NSCLC in the forthcoming (eighth) edition of the TNM classification of lung cancer. *Journal of Thoracic Oncology, 11* (9), 1433–1446. ISSN 1556-0864. https://doi.org/10.1016/j.jtho.2016.06.028.

Reck, M., & Rabe, K. F. (2017). Precision diagnosis and treatment for advanced non-small-cell lung cancer. *The New England Journal of Medicine, 377*(9), 849–861. https://doi.org/10.1056/NEJMra1703413.

Temel, J. S., Greer, J. A., Muzikansky, A., Gallagher, E. R., Admane, S., Jackson, V. A., Dahlin, C. M., Blinderman, C. D., Jacobsen, J., Pirl, W. F., Billings, J. A., & Lynch, T. J. (2010). Early palliative care for patients with metastatic non-small-cell lung cancer. *The New England Journal of Medicine,* 363(8), 733–742. https://doi.org/10.1056/NEJMoa1000678.

CASE 61

A 58-Year-Old Female With Acute-on-Chronic Abdominal Pain

Justine Ko ■ Shiqian Li ■ Raj Dasgupta ■ Diana H. Yu

A 58-year-old female presents to the emergency department complaining of acute-on-chronic abdominal pain for the past 3 months associated with food intake. She also reported some mild chest pain and dyspnea on exertion. She had associated fevers, nausea, vomiting, and diarrhea, but denied weight loss or sick contacts. Her past medical history is significant for hypertension and allergic rhinitis. The patient has never smoked and is not exposed to environmental toxins or cigarette smoke. Her medications include amlodipine and loratadine. Her family history is significant for lung cancer as a result of her two brothers, both of whom passed away from related sequelae. On physical examination, temperature is 37.5°C, blood pressure is 110/74 mmHg, heart rate is 104 beats/min, respiratory rate is 20 breaths/min, and oxygen saturation is 98% on 2 L nasal cannula. The patient had tenderness to palpation over the epigastric region without rebound tenderness. She had swelling of her left lower extremity. The rest of her examination was normal. A computed tomography (CT) scan of her chest, abdomen, and pelvis performed to evaluate for pulmonary embolism and intra-abdominal pathologies was negative. However, the scan shows an 18-mm subsolid nodule within the left upper lobe (Fig. 61.1).

What is an "incidental lung nodule" and what is its clinical significance?

An "incidental lung nodule" refers to a pulmonary nodule (≤3 cm lesion) that is identified on a radiographic imaging study obtained for an unrelated reason. Although many incidental nodules are ultimately benign, the concern for malignancy can cause emotional distress to patients and possibly subject them to unnecessary imaging studies and biopsies. A lung mass is defined as a lesion that measures >3 cm and carries a much higher risk of malignancy.

What are the differential diagnoses for a solitary pulmonary lung nodule?

The differential diagnoses for a solitary pulmonary lung nodule are summarized in Table 61.1. The differentials are typically separated by malignancy and benign lesions. Malignant lesions are subcategorized into lung primary and metastatic lesions and benign lesions are subsequently subcategorized into infectious, inflammatory, and benign tumors.

Infectious granulomas caused by fungi, mycobacteria, and abscess-forming bacteria compose up to 80% of benign nodules. The remaining causes of benign nodules include inflammatory processes such as rheumatoid arthritis (Fig. 61.2) and granulomatosis with polyangiitis. Other causes of a benign nodule include but are not limited to sarcoidosis, amyloidosis, hamartoma, fibroma, chondroma, and leiomyoma.

Malignant etiologies of lung nodules include primary lung cancers, metastases (Fig. 61.3A,B), and hematologic and carcinoid tumors.

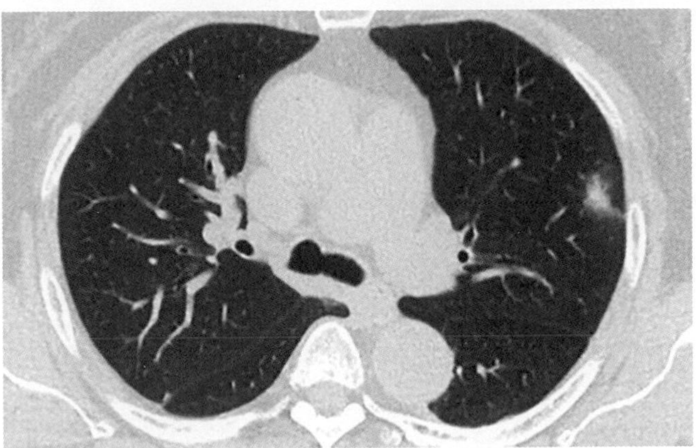

Fig. 61.1 Computed tomography scan of the chest demonstrates a subsolid nodule measuring 18 mm in the left upper lobe.

TABLE 61.1 ■ **Differential Diagnosis for a Lung Nodule**

Benign	Malignant
Infectious (80%): fungi, mycobacteria, abscess forming bacteria Inflammatory: rheumatoid arthritis, granulomatosis with polyangiitis Other: sarcoidosis, amyloidosis, hamartoma, fibroma, chondroma, leiomyoma	Primary lung cancers: small cell, non-small cell, large cell Metastases; Hematologic: lymphoma Carcinoid tumors

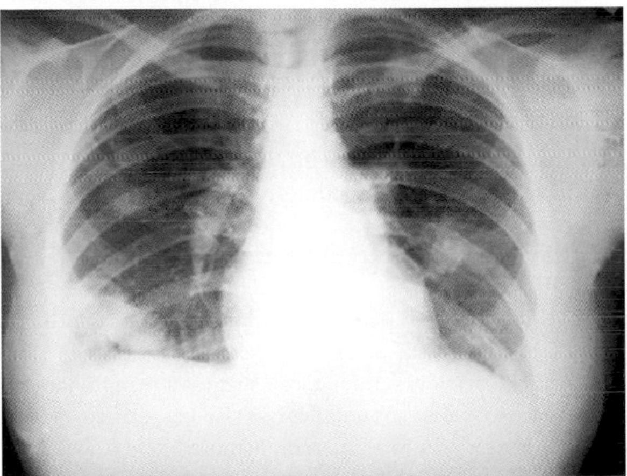

Fig. 61.2 Rheumatoid nodules in the lung.

She is discharged from the emergency room after a diagnosis with follow-up in the pulmonary clinic. Upon evaluation, the patient denies any symptoms of fevers, cough, hemoptysis, night sweats, sick contacts, and tuberculosis risk factors. She denies joint pain, skin rashes, and fatigue. She has never smoked, she worked in an office, and she denies history of lung disease or cancer. Unfortunately, she does not have any prior imaging.

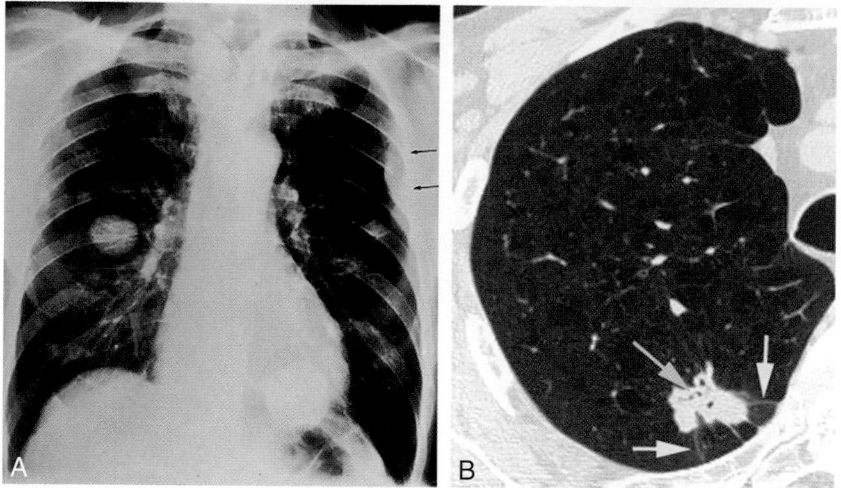

Fig. 61.3 (A) Metastases in the lung. Arrows are demonstraing pleural metastasis. (B) Spiculated invasive adenocarcinoma. Blue arrow demonstrating possible cavitation. Yellow arrows demonstrating outline of secondary pulmonary lobule.

What history should be obtained from patients to help estimate the malignant potential of lung nodules?

The relevant risk factors associated with malignancy include tobacco history, age, prior exposure to carcinogenic agents (such as asbestos, dusts, metals, and fumes), occupational history personal history of previous lung cancer, family history of lung cancer, and the presence of chronic lung disease.

CLINICAL PEARL **USMLE STEP 2 CLINICAL KNOWLEDGE AND USMLE STEP 3**

Tobacco smoking is by far the major cause of lung cancer. This includes exposure to secondhand smoke and electronic cigarettes.

Which characteristics of a lung nodule help diagnosis?

A lung nodule is characterized by size, attenuation, growth, or stability of the lesion on subsequent imaging over time, presence and pattern of calcification and fat, borders, and location. A CT scan is the best imaging modality to provide these characteristics.

Attenuation: Nodules can be either solid or subsolid in type. Subsolid nodules are pure ground-glass without solid components or part-solid with both ground-glass and solid components. Examples are noted in Fig. 61.4B.

Calcification and fat: Calcification of a nodule can suggest a benign nature, but it is important to see the pattern because malignant nodules can also be calcified. A laminated, central pattern, otherwise known as a "popcorn" pattern, is more likely to be a benign hamartoma as shown in Fig. 61.5. On the other hand, a stippled or eccentric calcification pattern suggests a malignant nodule.

Borders: A nodule can have a smooth, irregular, or spiculated border.

Location: The location of a nodule includes its central or peripheral position as well as the lung lobe that it occupies.

Which characteristics of a lung nodule suggest malignancy?

The concern for malignancy increases with a patient's age and known risk factors including smoking history, other known malignancies, family history, and environmental exposures.

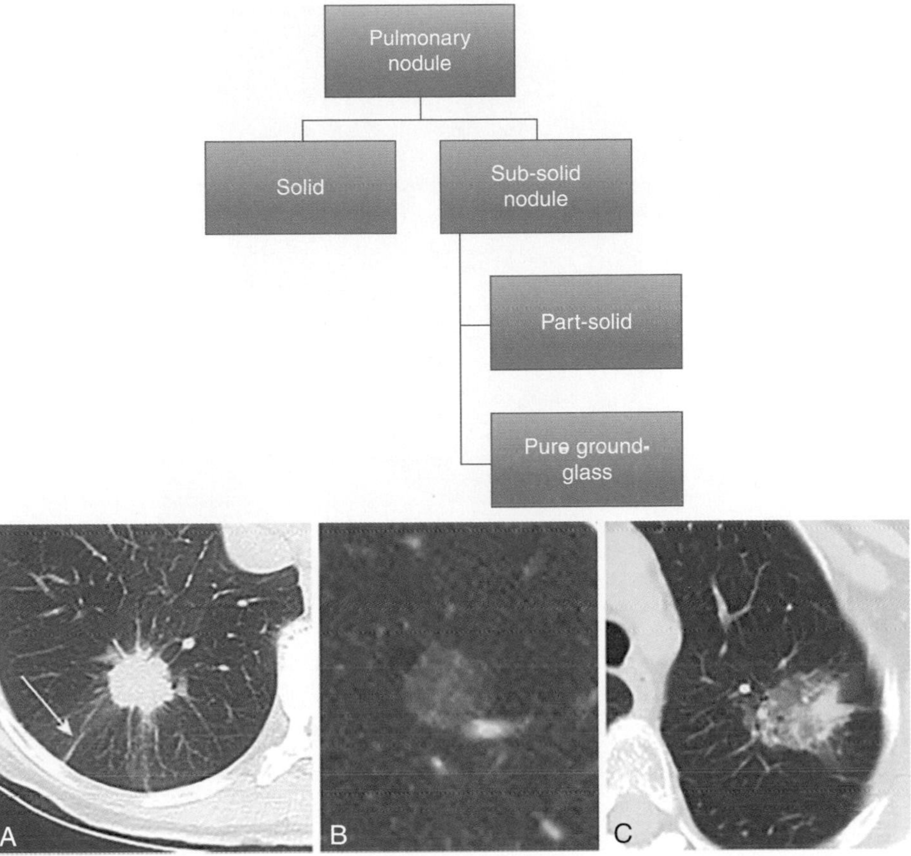

Fig. 61.4 (A) Types of attenuation in pulmonary nodules. (B) Examples of different nodule attenuations on computed tomography imaging: (a) solid, (b) pure ground glass, (c) part solid.

CT images are the most reliable in providing details suggestive of malignancy (summarized in Table 61.2).

Size: Solid lung nodules ≥8 mm, part-solid ≥6 mm, and subsolid nodules ≥6 mm are more concerning for malignancy than smaller lesions.

Borders: Malignant lesions often appear to have a spiculated or irregular border, although a smooth margin does not necessarily exclude neoplasm (Fig. 61.5).

Calcification and fat: Although calcifications are more commonly associated with benign lung nodules, pulmonary carcinoid tumors and some metastatic lesions from chondrosarcoma or osteosarcoma may have calcified nodules.

Location: Cancerous nodules are often located in the upper lobes.

Growth: Nodule growth can be measured as volume doubling time. Nodules that grow rapidly under 20 days or remain stable for more than 2 years are less suggestive of malignancy.

CLINICAL PEARL **USMLE STEP 2 CLINICAL KNOWLEDGE USMLE STEP 3**

Malignancies such as carcinoid tumors and adenocarcinoma in situ can appear stable on serial imaging over the course of 2 years because of their slow growing nature.

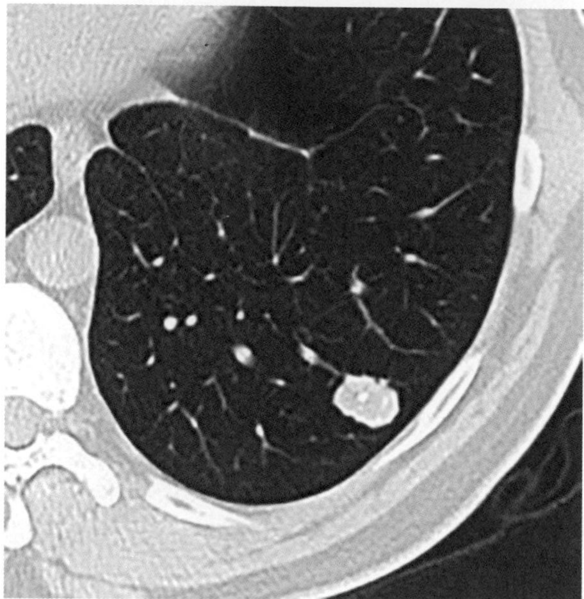

Fig. 61.5 Lobulated nodule with calcification characteristic of a hamartoma.

TABLE 61.2 ■ **Findings Suggestive of Malignancy on CT Imaging**
Size: solid nodule ≥8 mm, part-solid nodule ≥6 mm, subsolid nodule ≥6 mm
Spiculated or irregular border
Location in the upper lobes

The patient asks you whether it might be cancer and what should be done next.

What is the Fleischner Society? What is their approach to management of an incidental lung nodule?
The Fleischner Society is a multidisciplinary organization of radiologists. In 2017 the guidelines were updated regarding the management of solid and subsolid incidental nodules in individuals without a known primary malignancy, not immunosuppressed, and not undergoing lung cancer screening. The current recommendations are summarized in Tables 61.3 and 61.4.

Based on the Fleischner Society guidelines and after a discussion with the patient regarding repeat imaging or biopsy, the decision is taken to perform a repeat CT scan of the chest in 3 months. The nodule appears stable in size and without evidence of new nodules on subsequent imaging. The solid component of the scan remains >8 mm.

What are the advantages of performing a fluorodeoxyglucose (FDG)-position emission tomography (PET) scan over serial CT scans?
In a nodule of indeterminate character as described by a CT scan, a PET scan offers the benefit of measuring metabolic activity through increased uptake of FDG. PET is best used for solid

TABLE 61.3 ■ **Fleischner Society Guidelines for Management of Incidental Solid Nodules**

Solid Nodules			
Nodule type	<6 mm (<100 mm³)	6–8 mm (100–250 mm³)	>8 mm (>250 mm³)
Single			
Low risk	No routine follow-up	CT at 6–12 months, then consider CT at 18–24 months	Consider CT at 3 months, PET/CT, or tissue sampling
High risk	Optional CT at 12 months	CT at 6–12 months, then CT at 18–24 months	Consider CT at 3 months, PET/CT, or tissue sampling
Multiple			
Low risk	No routine follow-up	CT at 3–6 months, then consider CT at 18–24 months	CT at 3–6 months, then consider CT at 18–24 months
High risk	Optional CT at 12 months	CT at 3–6 months, then at 18–24 months	CT at 3–6 months, then at 18–24 months

From MacMahon, H., Naidich, D. P., Goo, J. M., Lee, K. S., Leung, A. N. C., Mayo, J. R., Mehta, A. C., Ohno, Y., Powell, C. A., Prokop, M., Rubin, G. D., Schaefer-Prokop, C. M., Travis, W. D., Van Schil, P. E., & Bankier, A. A. (2017). Guidelines for management of incidental pulmonary nodules detected on CT images: from the Fleischner Society. *Radiology*, 284(1), 228–243.

TABLE 61.4 ■ **Fleischner Society Guidelines for Management of Incidental Subsolid Nodules**

Subsolid Nodules		
Nodule type	<6 mm (<100 mm³)	≥6 mm (<100 mm³)
Single		
Ground glass	No routine follow-up	CT at 6–12 months to confirm persistence, then CT every 2 years until 5 years
Part solid	No routine follow-up	CT at 3–6 months to confirm persistence. If unchanged and solid component remains <6 mm, annual CT should be performed for 5 years.
Multiple	CT at 3–6 months. If stable, consider CT at 2 and 4 years.	CT at 3–6 months. Subsequent management based on the most suspicious nodules.

From MacMahon, H., Naidich, D. P., Goo, J. M., Lee, K. S., Leung, A. N. C., Mayo, J. R., Mehta, A. C., Ohno, Y., Powell, C. A., Prokop, M., Rubin, G. D., Schaefer-Prokop, C. M., Travis, W. D., Van Schil, P. E., & Bankier, A. A. (2017). Guidelines for management of incidental pulmonary nodules detected on CT images: from the Fleischner Society. *Radiology*, 284(1), 228–243.

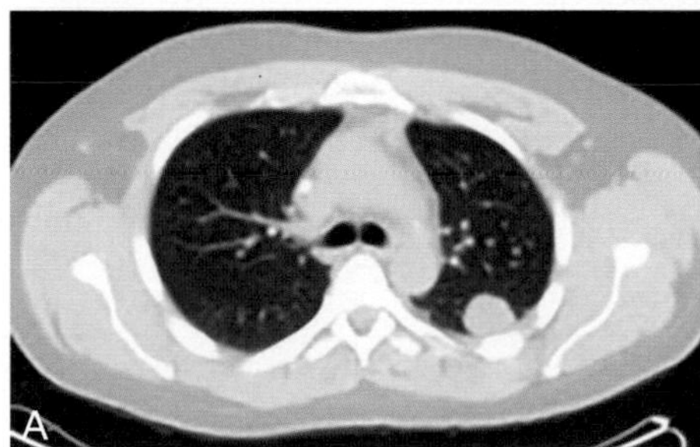

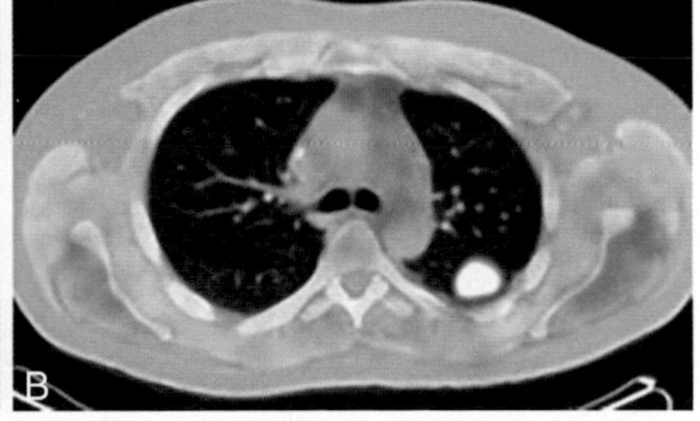

Fig. 61.6 Pulmonary metastasis noted on CT Scan (Image A) with uptake on fluorodeoxyglucose position emission tomography computed tomography (Image B). The high uptake is consistent with malignancy.

nodules or subsolid nodules with a large solid component (>8 mm). In nodules with intermediate suspicion for cancer on CT, a PET scan can help increase the likelihood of malignancy if the lesion is FDG avid. In highly suspicious lesions, a PET scan can provide information of metastases for staging as well as best targets for biopsy as shown in Fig. 61.6.

CLINICAL PEARL **USMLE STEP 2 CLINICAL KNOWLEDGE USMLE STEP 3**

False-positive PET results can be seen with infectious and inflammatory conditions. False-negative PET results can be seen with adenocarcinoma in situ, carcinoid tumors (i.e., slow growing malignancies), and patients with uncontrolled hyperglycemia.

The patient's nodule comes back PET avid without evidence of extrapulmonary spread, and you discuss biopsy options with her.

When should tissue biopsy be performed?

Biopsy should be performed on a low-risk nodule that has undergone growth in serial CT scans, a nodule with intermediate probability of malignancy that is FDG avid on PET scan, or a nodule with high probability of malignancy.

CLINICAL PEARL **USMLE STEP 3**

There are quantitative predictive models that seek to estimate the probability of malignancy of lung nodules. These include the Mayo, Gould (VA) and Brock Models among others that have all been externally validated.

What are the different ways to obtain a tissue biopsy?

Tissue biopsy can be obtained through nonsurgical and surgical approaches. Nonsurgical approaches for biopsy include use of bronchoscopy or a transthoracic needle biopsy. This less invasive approach is preferred in patients with an intermediate risk of malignancy, nonsurgical candidates with high-risk lesions, and low-risk lesions that require diagnosis for tailored therapy such as in fungal or mycobacterial diseases. The type of bronchoscopic procedure utilized depends on the size and location of the nodule. Endobronchial ultrasound (EBUS) is utilized in larger, centrally located lesions and a percutaneous needle biopsy can provide access to smaller, peripherally located lesions. Other bronchoscopic techniques include transbronchial biopsies and needle aspirations. Unfortunately, a nondiagnostic or negative result from a nonsurgical biopsy does not exclude malignancy, and the patient might require a surgical approach for a more definitive diagnosis.

More invasive surgical approaches offer the benefit of certain tissue acquisition and the potential for cure. An excisional biopsy is held as the gold standard. If a nonsurgical biopsy is nondiagnostic in a surgical candidate, a video-assisted thoracoscopic surgery (VATS) is preferred for nodules at intermediate or high risk of malignancy. This wedge-resection technique is best suited for lesions close to the pleural surface. VATS offers the benefit of being converted to a lobectomy if intraoperative frozen section analysis shows malignancy. It has been associated with shorter hospital stays and improved mortality when compared with conventional thoracotomies.

The patient was recommended to undergo surgical resection for diagnostic and therapeutic purposes. Given the size and location, a sublobar resection was planned.

Case Summary

- **Complaint/History:** A 58-year-old-woman presents to the emergency department with nonspecific complaints and was found to have a pulmonary nodule.
- **Findings:** The patient showed no significant personal risk factors for lung cancer; however, the family history of lung cancer and certain characteristics of the nodule were concerning for malignancy.
- **Lab Results/Tests:** Serial chest CTs showed persistence of the lung nodule with a large solid component. A PET scan showed avidity suggestive of malignancy without evidence of mediastinal/hilar adenopathy and extrapulmonary spread.

Diagnosis: Suspected primary lung malignancy.

- **Treatment:** Surgical resection.

BEYOND THE PEARLS

- When multiple pulmonary nodules are found, the most suspicious nodule should be used to direct further clinical decision-making.
- More than half of all lung cancers develop in those older than 70 years of age.
- Chronic obstructive pulmonary disease (particularly emphysema) is associated with a higher risk of lung cancer even when adjusted beyond smoking history.
- PET-CT is of minimal use in ground-glass nodules because of the high false-negative rate.
- FDG avidity is measured by the standard uptake value. A cutoff of >2.5 is typically used to distinguish nodules that have a higher probability of malignancy.
- Bronchoscopy with transbronchial biopsy yields higher accuracy with central lesions; however, radial endobronchial ultrasound and electromagnetic navigation can be used to increase the diagnostic yield of peripheral lesions.
- The most common complication with a CT-guided transthoracic needle biopsy is pneumothorax with rates up to 25%.

Bibliography

Godoy, M. C. B., Odisio, E. G. L. C., Truong, M. T., de Groot, P. M., Shroff, G. S., & Erasmus, J. J. (2018). Pulmonary nodule management in lung cancer screening: a pictorial review of lung-RADS Version 1.0. *Radiologic Clinics of North America*, *56*(3), 353–363.

Gould, M. K., Donington, J., Lynch, W. R., Mazzone, P. J., Midthun, D. E., Naidich, D. P., & Wiener, R. S. (2013). Evaluation of individuals with pulmonary nodules: when is it lung cancer? Diagnosis and management of lung cancer, 3rd ed: American College of Chest Physicians evidence-based clinical practice guidelines. *Chest*, *143*, e93S.

MacMahon, H., Naidich, D. P., Goo, J. M., Lee, K. S., Leung, A. N. C., Mayo, J. R., Mehta, A. C., Ohno, Y., Powell, C. A., Prokop, M., Rubin, G. D., Schaefer-Prokop, C. M., Travis, W. D., Van Schil, P. E., & Bankier, A. A. (2017). Guidelines for Management of Incidental Pulmonary Nodules Detected on CT Images: From the Fleischner Society 2017. *Radiology*, *284*(1), 228–243.

Ost, D., Fein, A. M., & Feinsilver, S. H. (2003). Clinical practice. The solitary pulmonary nodule. *The New England Journal of Medicine*, *348*(25), 2535–2542.

Webb, W. R., Brant, W. E., & Major, N. M. (2006). *Fundamentals of Body CT* (pp. 105–155) (5th Edition). St. Louis, Missouri: Elsevier.

CASE 62

A 55-Year-Old Female With Chronic Cough

Patrick Chan ■ Clay Wu ■ Raj Dasgupta

A 55-year-old female was a new referral to the pulmonary clinic with acute on chronic productive cough and dyspnea. She reports symptoms for the past 2 years, but they have worsened in the past 3 months. She denies hemoptysis, weight loss, or night sweats. Her medical history is significant for gastroesophageal reflux disease (GERD); tuberculosis (TB) treated several years ago with rifampin, isoniazid, pyrazinamide, and ethambutol; and scleroderma. The patient reports that her cough sometimes improves after a course of antibiotics, which her primary doctor occasionally prescribes for her. On physical examination, her blood pressure is 110/70 mmHg, pulse is 80 beats/min, respiratory rate is 28 breaths/min, and oxygen saturation is 92% on room air. The patient is visibly coughing throughout the examination and has mild wheezing at the end of expiration, but otherwise the remainder of the examination is normal. A chest radiograph (CXR) is obtained, which shows increased bronchovascular markings in the right lower base along with tram track opacities (Fig. 62.1).

What are some causes of chronic cough?

Chronic cough is one of the most common outpatient primary care chief complaints. The four main differential diagnoses that must be considered from a primary care perspective include GERD, upper airway cough syndrome, asthma, and medication induced such as angiotensin-converting enzyme (ACE) inhibitor use. Although these four diagnoses will encompass the majority of etiologies of chronic cough, there are other etiologies of cough that must also be considered. One approach is to use a top-down anatomical approach to build a differential, such as identifying etiologies associated with the nasopharynx, larynx, pulmonary, cardiac, esophagus, or diaphragm. For example, laryngeal etiologies of chronic cough include vocal cord dysfunction, pulmonary etiologies include infections, cardiac etiologies include heart failure, esophageal etiologies include GERD, and diaphragmatic etiologies include irritation caused by hepatic abscess, for example.

In this patient's case, given her history of GERD, likely from scleroderma, it is possible that her cough is caused by reflux; however, the positive CXR findings must be further evaluated.

CLINICAL PEARL **STEP 2/3**

A cough can sometimes be the only symptom present in asthma. This entity is known as cough-variant asthma.

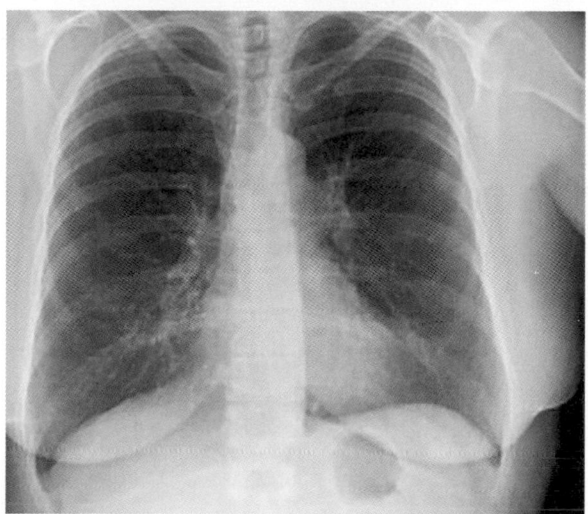

Fig. 62.1 Upright posteroanterior (PA) chest X-ray image with increased bronchovascular markings and tram track opacities.

What is the next step in the management of this patient?

Pulmonary function tests (PFTs) should be performed to evaluate functional impairment. A computed tomography (CT) scan of the chest should be obtained to further evaluate the abnormal CXR (Fig. 62.2).

PFTs showed an FEV1/FVC ratio of 66%, FEV1 58% estimated, FVC 92%. The CT scan of the chest is obtained and demonstrates focal bronchiectasis localized to the right middle lobe.

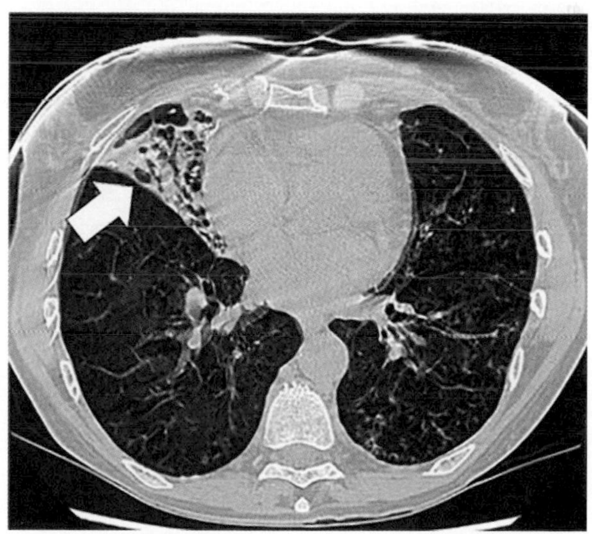

Fig. 62.2 Computed tomography chest scan without contrast showing bronchiectasis *(arrow)*.

CLINICAL PEARL **STEP 2/3**

Obstructive impairment is the most common PFT finding for patients with bronchiectasis.

What are the radiographic features of bronchiectasis?

Bronchiectasis can have four different macroscopic appearances: cylindrical, varicose, cystic, and traction. The tram track sign can be seen with cylindrical bronchiectasis, which demonstrates bronchi with a uniform caliber with lack of bronchial tapering. The signet ring sign can be seen in the axial view when the bronchi are dilated 1–1.5 times relative to the adjacent pulmonary vessel. The string of pearls sign has been used to describe varicose bronchiectasis resulting from intermittent narrow and dilated segments of affected bronchi (Figs. 62.3–62.5).

CLINICAL PEARL **STEP 2/3**

Traction bronchiectasis is seen in association with pulmonary fibrosis and is not associated with the classic symptoms of bronchiectasis.

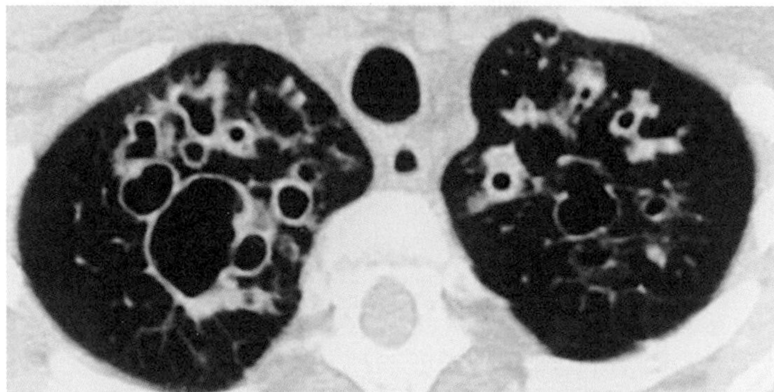

Fig. 62.3 Example of computed tomography chest scan showing cystic bronchiectasis.

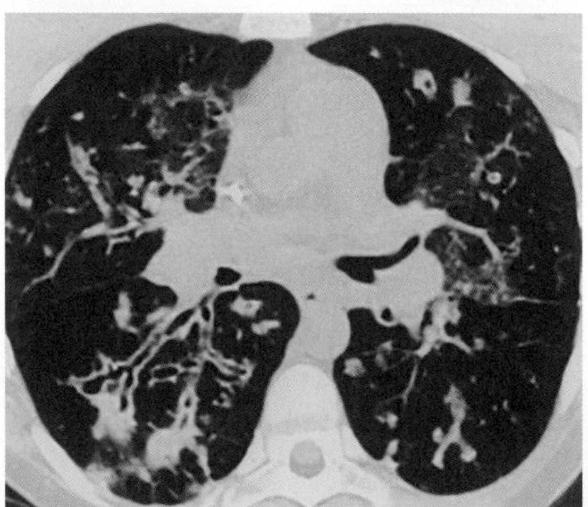

Fig. 62.4 Example of computed tomography chest scan showing cylindrical bronchiectasis.

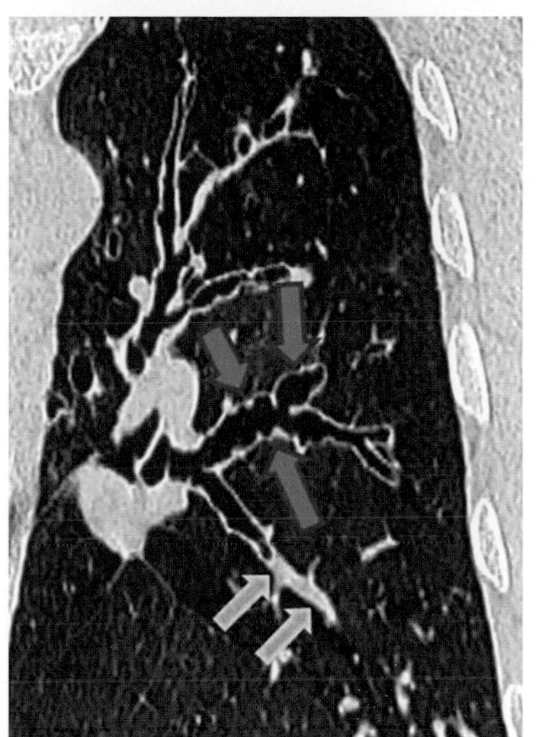

Fig. 62.5 Example of computed tomography chest scan showing varicose bronchiectasis (blue arrows). There are also areas of mucus plugging (yellow arrows).

What are the different etiologies of bronchiectasis?

Bronchiectasis in its simplest definition is a condition in which the airways are abnormally dilated. This can be the result of impaired drainage with subsequent infectious insult. The infection leads to neutrophils being attracted to the airways, which result in the release of elastase, causing the dilatation. There are many etiologies of bronchiectasis, but an easy way to organize the differential includes grouping via similar mechanisms. The major categories for the etiologies include airway obstruction, conditions predisposing to decreased airway clearance, infections, autoimmune disorders, and structural destruction. To expand on the differential diagnosis:

- Airway obstruction could be secondary to foreign body aspiration, obstructing tumor, or recurrent aspiration, most often secondary to GERD or esophageal pathology.
- Deficient airway clearance includes ciliary dysfunction such as Young's syndrome or primary ciliary dyskinesia or a result of ion transport such as cystic fibrosis.
- Infectious etiologies most commonly associated with bronchiectasis include chronic infections such as tuberculous and nontuberculous mycobacterium, allergic bronchopulmonary aspergillosis (ABPA), or recurrent infections caused by primary immunodeficiencies such as combined variable immunodeficiency or X-linked hypogammaglobulinemia.
- Autoimmune etiologies include rheumatoid arthritis, Sjogren's, or scleroderma.
- Structural etiologies include chronic obstructive pulmonary disease or alpha-1 antitrypsin deficiency.

The etiology can also be elucidated by disease location (Table 62.1).

TABLE 62.1 ■ **Etiologies of Bronchiectasis**

Disease Location	Possible Etiology
Focal bronchiectasis	Bronchiolithiasis Endobronchial neoplasm Foreign body Congenital bronchial atresia Mucus plugging
Upper lung	Cystic fibrosis Sarcoidosis Posttuberculosis bronchiectasis
Central lung	ABPA
Right middle lobe and lingula	Atypical mycobacterial infection Right middle lobe syndrome Primary ciliary dyskinesia
Lower lung	Chronic aspiration Usual interstitial pneumonia Hypogammaglobulinemia Alpha-1 antitrypsin deficiency

ABPA, Allergic bronchopulmonary aspergillosis.

TABLE 62.2 ■ **Causes of Bronchiectasis by Distribution**

Focal bronchiectasis	Bronchoscopy: tumor, foreign body Sputum for AFB
Diffuse bronchiectasis	Sputum for AFB CF genotyping, sweat chloride test Quantitative immunoglobulin testing IgG subclass level Alpha-1 antitrypsin level Ciliary testing Aspergillus Ab and total IgE levels Autoimmune workup HIV

AFB, Acid-fast bacilli.

CLINICAL PEARL **STEP 2/3**

Bronchiectasis can be a cause of massive hemoptysis which can be life threatening due to airway obstruction.

The patient reports she had a normal CXR after her TB treatment and denies any significant GERD symptoms currently. We decide to perform further testing.

Which tests should be taken?

All patients with bronchiectasis should undergo routine blood work, such as complete blood count with differential, sputum sample sent for bacterial culture, and acid-fast bacilli (AFB) stain and culture. In other patients with the appropriate clinical context, specific aspergillus IgE and IgG antibodies, total serum IgE level, rheumatoid factor (RF), anticyclic citrullinated peptide (anti-CCP), antinuclear antibodies (ANA), and antineutrophil cytoplasmic antibodies (ANCA) should be performed (Table 62.2).

CLINICAL PEARL **STEP 2/3**

Bronchoscopy can be considered in the workup of bronchiectasis to rule out endobronchial lesions or foreign bodies as the cause of bronchiectasis.

After these tests, the patient's two consecutive sputum AFB culture (AFB stain negative, TB polymerase chain reaction negative) returned positive for mycobacterium avium complex (MAC).

How should this patient be managed?

The management of bronchiectasis has three main parts: treatment of the underlying cause, prevention of exacerbations, and treatment of acute exacerbations.

This patient was started on MAC treatment with clarithromycin, rifampin, and ethambutol, which should be continued for at least 12 months. Repeat AFB sputum cultures would have to be obtained to demonstrate clearance, and antibiotics should be continued for at least 12 months after last negative sputum culture.

CLINICAL PEARL **STEP 2/3**

The diagnosis of non-tuberculous mycobacterial (NTM) infection requires the appropriate clinical setting with corresponding imaging findings <u>and</u> one of the following: two consecutive induced sputum cultures positive for NTM, one bronchoalveolar lavage sample positive for NTM, <u>or</u> one transbronchial biopsy positive for mycobacterial features

CLINICAL PEARL **STEP 2/3**

The decision to treat MAC should not be taken lightly as patients need to be on antibiotics for more than one year and there are considerable side effects from the drug regimen.

CLINICAL PEARL **STEP 2/3**

"Hot tub lung" is a disease associated with MAC thought to trigger a hypersensitivity reaction.

Which therapies are available to prevent exacerbations in patients with bronchiectasis?

Airway clearance therapy including chest physiotherapy, mechanical vest therapy, or a oscillatory positive expiratory pressure (PEP) device are the mainstays of prevention and are used to help mobilize tenacious secretions. An oscillatory PEP device, or flutter valve device, is a device that causes reverberations to be transmitted throughout the airway to loosen secretions, allowing better clearance. Mucolytic agents such as inhaled hypertonic saline are effective to help break up thick secretions. Other adjuncts include bronchodilators to dilate airways to assist in clearance, treatment of GERD, and vaccines such as influenza and pneumococcal vaccines are recommended to decrease risk factors for further exacerbations.

CLINICAL PEARL **STEP 2/3**

Neither inhaled glucocorticoids nor long-acting beta-adrenergic agonists are not routinely used in bronchiectasis unless there is another indication.

The patient was provided with an oscillatory PEP device, albuterol as needed, and appropriate vaccines. Her symptoms improve over the next couple of months, but she makes an urgent clinic follow-up with you because of worsening shortness of breath, cough, sputum production, and development of fever.

How should this patient be managed?

There should be high index of suspicion for an acute exacerbation of bronchiectasis. The diagnosis of acute exacerbation of bronchiectasis should be made upon symptoms rather than laboratory values. The patient may have symptoms of increased sputum production, increased cough, fevers, and worsening shortness of breath. Bronchiectasis patients are at significant risk of chronic colonization and development of antibiotic resistance, which would limit future therapies. In the work up of acute exacerbation, a sputum sample should be obtained to guide therapy and to allow the narrowest antibiotic to be prescribed, usually for a total of 7 to 14 days.

CLINICAL PEARL **STEP 2/3**

Old sputum cultures should be used to guide empiric treatment for bronchiectasis exacerbations. This is to prevent the development of multidrug resistant organisms, such as multidrug resistant pseudomonas or methicillin resistant staphylococcal aureus.

A sputum sample was obtained for this patient, which ended up growing *Streptococcus pneumoniae*. The patient was sent home with a prescription for amoxicillin for 14 days.

Although the patient improves over the next couple of days, she has several decompensations over the next year, requiring three hospitalizations for exacerbation for bronchiectasis, with her last hospitalization being a month ago where she was found to have *Pseudomonas aeruginosa*.

***Which other therapies can be used for recurrent exacerbations, particularly with* Pseudomonas aeruginosa?**

Pseudomonas is a pathogen seen commonly in bronchiectasis patients associated with increased risk of exacerbations, hospital admissions, and death.

Our patient should be started on azithromycin three times a week and an inhaled antibiotic with efficacy against *Pseudomonas aeruginosa*. Inhaled tobramycin has the most evidence in noncystic fibrosis bronchiectasis with several studies showing reduced sputum density, reduced hospitalizations, and improvement in lung function on pulmonary function tests.

After initiation of inhaled tobramycin in repeated cycles of 28 days followed by 28 days off, our patient's symptoms improve. She continues to be followed in the pulmonary clinic for routine management of her bronchiectasis.

If her symptoms recur, what other recommendations can be made?

Pulmonary rehabilitation has been shown to increase exercise capacity in patients with bronchiectasis. If the bronchiectasis is localized, patients can undergo resection of the bronchiectatic lung. Ultimately, a bilateral lung transplant can be considered.

Case Summary

- **Complaint/History:** 55 year-old female with history prior tuberculosis infection presenting with chronic cough.
- **Findings:** She was found to have bronchiectasis.
- **Lab Results/Test:** Her AFB cultures came back positive for Mycobactrium avium complex infection

Diagnosis: MAC infection

- **Treatment:** She completed a course of clarithromycin, rifampin, and ethambutol.

BEYOND THE PEARLS

- Clubbing is a physical examination finding that can be seen with bronchiectasis that is not seen in chronic obstructive lung disease or asthma.
- If a patient develops recurrent hemoptysis or uncontrolled hemorrhage, consider bronchoscopic intervention to tamponade or control bleeding, interventional radiology to embolize the bronchial artery, or surgery to resect the bronchiectatic lung.
- Patients with bronchiectasis have an accelerated decline in their PFTs compared with normal individuals.
- Aerosolized dornase alfa is a mainstay mucolytic in patients with cystic fibrosis; however, this should NOT be used in noncystic fibrosis bronchiectasis because of the potential harm.
- Prior to initiation of azithromycin for frequent exacerbations of bronchiectasis, a sputum culture for AFB should be used to rule out nontuberculous mycobacterium to avoid development of resistance.
- Pulmonary hypertension can be a complication of chronic bronchiectasis.

Bibliography

Hill, A. T., Sullivan, A. L., Chalmers, J. D., Soyza, A. D., Elborn, J. S., Floto, R. A., Grillo, L., Gruffydd-Jones, K., Harvey, A., Haworth, C. S., Hiscocks, E., Hurst, J. R., Johnson, C., Kelleher, W. P., Bedi, P., Payne, K., Saleh, H., Screaton, N. J., Smith, M., … Loebinger, M. R. (2018). British Thoracic Society Guideline for Bronchiectasis in Adults. *Thorax*, *74*(Suppl 1), 1–69.

Polverino, E., Goeminne, P. C., McDonnell, M. J., Aliberti, S., Marshall, S. E., Loebinger, M. R., Murris, M., Cantón, R., Torres, A., Dimakou, K., Soyza, A. D., Hill, A. T., Haworth, C. S., Vendrell, M., Ringshausen, F. C., Subotic, D., Wilson, R., Vilaró, J., Stallberg, B., … Chalmers, J. D. (2017). European Respiratory Society guidelines for the management of adult bronchiectasis. *The European Respiratory Journal*, *50*, 1700629.

Grant. L. A. (2019). *Grainger & Allison's diagnostic radiology essentials* (2nd ed.). Elsevier.

Cohen, M., & Sahn, S. A. (1999). Bronchiectasis in systemic diseases. *Chest*, *116*, 1063–1074.

Haworth, C. S., Banks, J., Capstick, T., Fisher, A. J., Gorsuch, T., Laurenson, I. F., Leitch, A., Loebinger, M.R., Milburn, H. J., Nightingale, M., Ormerod, P., Shingadia, D., Smith, D., Whitehead, N., Wilson, R., & Floto R. A. (2017). BTS Guidelines for the management of non-tuberculous mycobacterial pulmonary disease. *Thorax*, *72*, 1–64.

Barker. Alan F. (2008). Bronchiectasis. *Clinical Respiratory Medicine*, 425–431.

CASE 63

A 64-Year-Old Female With Fevers

Dafang Chen ■ Clay Wu ■ Raj Dasgupta

A 64-year-old female with history of hypertension, diabetes, and chronic kidney disease (CKD) stage III presents to the emergency department with 3 days of subjective fever, chills, lethargy, and dysuria. Family members report that the patient had dysuria, nausea, and vomiting for the last few days and on the day of admission became slightly confused. They deny any changes to her medications or, recent travel. She does not have headache, shortness of breath, cough, or neck pain. On physical examination, she has a temperature of 38.8°C, blood pressure is 90/60 mmHg, pulse is 119 beats/min, respiratory rate is 24 breaths/min, and oxygen saturation is 96% on room air. She is alert and oriented to person and place but not time. Her cardiopulmonary examination was within normal limits. There was no abdominal pain; however, the patient had costovertebral angle (CVA) tenderness. The rest of her examination is unremarkable. The chest X-ray is unremarkable. Computed tomography (CT) head scan was normal. Urinalysis showed positive nitrite and leukocyte esterase with 4+ white blood cells. The patient's blood pressure did not respond to 1L normal saline. A decision was made to admit the patient to the ICU for further workup.

What is the most likely diagnosis?

This patient has signs and symptoms concerning for infection and sepsis. She is febrile, tachycardic, and hypotensive, with dysuria. The clinical presentation of sepsis can vary based on the organ system involved. However, in this case, her symptoms are suggestive of a urinary tract infection or, even worse, pyelonephritis. Sepsis can be caused by any type of infection, including bacteria, viruses, and fungi.

How is sepsis defined?

The definition of sepsis has been evolving since the early 1990s and to this day remains without a "gold standard." The latest definition published by the Third International Consensus Definitions for Sepsis and Septic Shock (Sepsis-3) in 2016 defines sepsis as life-threatening organ dysfunction caused by a dysregulated host response to infection. This definition has widely been accepted in the medical community to date. Certain groups (e.g., Center for Medicare and Medicaid Services), however, still support the previous definitions of SIRS, sepsis, and severe sepsis. Regardless of which expert definition is followed, it is important to understand that sepsis exists on a continuum from mild infection to septic shock and a delayed response can lead to multiorgan dysfunction and even death.

CLINICAL PEARL **STEP 2/3**

Risk factors for sepsis include intensive care unit (ICU) admission, nosocomial infection, bacteremia, advanced age, immunosuppression, previous hospitalization and community-acquired pneumonia. Genetic defects have also been identified that may increase susceptibility to specific classes of microorganisms.

What can be used to help in the early identification of sepsis?

Prior to this, the systemic inflammatory response syndrome (SIRS) criteria was used to screen patients for sepsis in the emergency department. However, its limitations of being overly sensitive and nonspecific have resulted in it falling out of favor and it is no longer included in the current definition. Instead, the quick SOFA (qSOFA) was developed and validated in the Sepsis-3 guidelines for clinicians to quickly identify patients at risk of sepsis in the ED. The Sequential Organ Failure Assessment or SOFA score, on the other hand, is used to predict mortality in patients that are in the ICU. The benefit of qSOFA is that you do not need blood work! It can be obtained promptly at bedside for patients outside the ICU. Table 63.1 compares SIRS and qSOFA criteria. Box 63.1 lists SOFA parameters for patients in the ICU.

CLINICAL PEARL **STEP 2/3**

Supplemental oxygen should be applied to patients with sepsis, who have indications for oxygenation, and oxygenation should be monitored continuously with pulse oximetry. Ideal target values for peripheral saturation are not well defined but we typically target values >90%. Intubation and mechanical ventilation may be required to support the increased work of breathing that typically accompanies sepsis, or for airway protection since encephalopathy and a depressed level of consciousness frequently complicate sepsis.

The patient's initial presentation in the ED meets SIRS criteria for sepsis. More so, her change in mental status and respiratory rate of 24/min give her 2 points on the qSOFA score, which is associated with a 3- to 14-fold increase in hospital mortality. The next step in management would be to assess for evidence of end organ dysfunction with blood tests and calculation of the full SOFA score when she is admitted to the ICU. Box 63.2 lists initial lab tests that may help guide therapy.

TABLE 63.1 ■ **SIRS Versus qSOFA**

SIRS	qSOFA
• ≥2 meets SIRS criteria	• ≥2 identifies high risk patients for in-hospital mortality
• Temperature ≥38°C (100.4 °F) or <36°C (96.80 °F) • Heart rate >90/min • Respiratory rate >20 or $PaCO_2$ <32 mmHg • WBCs >12,000/mm³, <4,000/mm³, or >10% bands	• Altered mental status (GCS <15) • Respiratory rate ≥22 • Systolic blood pressure ≤100 mmHg
• ≥2 SIRS criteria and a suspected or confirmed infection should be assessed for severe sepsis based on previous sepsis definitions (lactate ≥4 mmol/L)	• qSOFA score ≥ 2 is associated with 3- to 14-fold increase in hospital mortality rate (outside of ICU)

SIRS, Systemic inflammatory response syndrome; *qSOFA*, quick sequential organ failure assessment; *GCS*, Glasgow coma scale; *WBCs*, white blood cells.

BOX 63.1 ■ **SOFA Score**

SOFA Parameters

- PaO²
- FiO²
- Use of mechanical ventilation
- Platelets
- Glasgow coma scale
- Bilirubin
- Hypotension or use of vasoactive agents
- Creatinine

SOFA score determines level of organ dysfunction and predicts ICU mortality.

SOFA, Sequential Organ Failure Assessment.

BOX 63.2 ■ Initial Sepsis Workup

- CBC with differential
- CMP
- Lactate
- ABG
- Procalcitonin
- Blood cultures ×2
- Imaging targeting suspected source of infection

ABG, Arterial Blood Gas; *CBC*, Complete Blood Count; *CMP*, Complete Metabolic Panel.

CLINICAL PEARL **STEP 2/3**

Procalcitonin's greatest use is to guide antibiotic discontinuation in patients with community acquired pneumonia.

What is the next step in management?

Early, empiric antibiotics should be given to patients with suspected sepsis. The choice of antibiotics should be based on the suspected source of infection (i.e., Gram negatives and anaerobes for intra-abdominal infections, Gram negatives for urinary sources, etc.). Antibiotics should be given within 1 hour of suspicion because it has been shown that mortality in sepsis increases by 7.6% per hour delay in the administration of antibiotics.

The patient's initial presentation was suggestive of a urinary tract infection with possible pyelonephritis. Lab tests including a complete blood count (CBC), complete metabolic panel (CMP), lactic acid, and two sets of peripheral blood cultures are made. Given patient's comorbidities and possible septic shock, vancomycin was initiated for enterococcus. A 4th generation cephalosporin, Cefepime was also initiated to cover gram negative bacteria such as Pseudomonas, E. coli, and Klebsiella. The nurse calls and reports that the patient's blood pressure is 85/50 mmHg.

What type of fluid resuscitation should be given?

The goal of initial resuscitation is tissue reperfusion within the first 3 hours. Deciding which crystalloid or colloid fluid to initiate requires an understanding of how these fluids distribute in plasma. Crystalloid fluids (i.e., 0.9% NaCl, Ringer's lactate) are electrolyte solutions with small molecules that can diffuse freely from intravascular to interstitial fluid compartments. Colloid fluids (i.e., 5% albumin), on the other hand, have larger solute molecules that are not readily diffusible. Because plasma volume is only about 25% of the extracellular fluid or ECF, only 25% of an infused crystalloid fluid will expand plasma volume and the remaining 75% will expand the interstitial compartment. Thus, the predominant effect of crystalloid fluid is to expand interstitial volume. Colloid fluids have molecules that create an osmotic or oncotic pressure, which can hold water in the vascular compartment. When compared with 0.9% NaCl, colloid fluid is at least three times more effective than in expanding the plasma volume. Despite this theoretical benefit, studies have not shown any benefit to giving colloid over crystalloid and therefore crystalloids are typically used. The goal of initial resuscitation is tissue reperfusion within the first 3 hours and is usually crystalloid given at 30 mL/kg. Table 63.2 compares content of 0.9% normal saline, lactated Ringer's solution, and plasma.

Despite giving the patient 30 mL/kg of fluid resuscitation, she continues to deteriorate. Her mean arterial pressure remains below 60 mmHg, and her lactate acid is 6 mmol/L.

TABLE 63.2 ■ **Content Comparison Between Plasma, NS, and LR**

	Plasma	0.9% Normal Saline (NS)	Lactated Ringer (LR)
pH	7.4	5.5	6.5
Osmolality (mOsm/L)	290	308	309
Sodium (Na^+)	140	154	130
Chloride (Cl^-)	103	154	109
Potassium (K^+)	4	–	4
Calcium (Ca^{2+})	4	–	3
Magnesium (Mg)	2	–	–
Buffer system	Bicarbonate	–	Lactate

What has occurred in this patient?.

This patient has developed septic shock. Clinically, septic shock is defined by those who meet criteria for sepsis and require vasopressors to maintain a mean arterial pressure (MAP) >= 65 mmHg despite adequate fluid resuscitation and have a lactate >=2 mmol/L. Septic shock is a type of distributive shock and a subset of sepsis in which there are profound circulatory, cellular, and metabolic abnormalities present. The primary hemodynamic issue is systemic vasodilatation of both arteries and veins, causing reduction in both ventricular preload and afterload. The typical hemodynamic pattern seen in septic shock includes low cardiac filling pressures (CVP or PCWP), a high cardiac output, and a low systemic vascular resistance.

CLINICAL PEARL **STEP 2/3**

Large volume infusion of 0.9% NaCl can lead to a hyperchloremic, metabolic acidosis, which can make the lactic acidosis seen in sepsis even worse. Not an absolute contraindication, but more of a consideration, is the administration of Ringer's lactate in patients with liver dysfunction. Most of the lactate is metabolized in the liver, and any hepatic dysfunction will result in an accumulation of lactate. This can confuse the interpretation of lactate levels.

A pressor is used because her blood pressure has not responded to fluid resuscitation. A central venous catheter is inserted in the right internal jugular vein under sterile conditions.

CLINICAL PEARL **STEP 2/3**

Venous access should be established as soon as possible in patients with suspected sepsis. While peripheral venous access may be sufficient in some patients, particularly for initial resuscitation, the majority will require central venous access at some point during their course. Insertion of a central line should not delay the administration of resuscitative fluids and antibiotics. A central venous catheter (CVC) can be used to infuse vasopressors and to draw blood for frequent laboratory studies. While a CVC can be used to monitor the therapeutic response by measuring the central venous pressure (CVP) and the central venous oxyhemoglobin saturation (ScvO2), evidence from randomized trials suggest that their value is limited.

CLINICAL PEARL **STEP 2/3**

The mean arterial pressure (MAP) goal in a patient with sepsis is >=65 mmHg.

What is the appropriate initial pressor for this patient?

Intravenous vasopressors are used in patients who remain hypotensive despite adequate fluid resuscitation. These agents should be administered through a central venous catheter. However, their use should not be delayed by waiting for a catheter. The first-line single agent used for septic shock is norepinephrine (Levophed). In fact, it is the initial vasopressor of choice for undifferentiated shock.

Additional agents may be required in refractory shock. Choosing the right agent is often determined by patient comorbidities contributing to shock (i.e., heart failure, arrhythmias). Vasopressin is often used as a second agent to supplement norepinephrine in refractory septic shock. It has been shown to augment the effect, to reduce norepinephrine requirements, and to decrease the progression to renal failure. Other vasopressors and their roles in septic shock are listed in Table 63.3.

CLINICAL PEARL **STEP 2/3**

MAP is the product of cardiac output and systemic vascular resistance, and cardiac output is the product of heart rate (HR) and stroke volume (SV). Thus, MAP = HR * SV * SVR. Agents that alter any of these factors will affect MAP.

Which other agents have been tried in sepsis?

Corticosteroids, particularly hydrocortisone, are used in patients with septic shock refractory to adequate fluid resuscitation and vasopressor administration. Steroids, thiamine, and vitamin C have also been studied; however, thus far they are not formally recommended because only small trials have shown their potential benefit. There is no role for blood transfusions in patients without active bleed and a hemoglobin >7 g/dL. Inotropes may be used in patients who have concurrent decrease in their cardiac output.

TABLE 63.3 ■ **Vasopressors in Septic Shock**

Vasopressor (US Trade Name)	
Norepinephrine (Levophed)	• First-line agent for septic, cardiogenic, and hypovolemic shock
Vasopressin (Vasostrict)	• Add-on to norepinephrine in septic shock to increase MAP and reduce norepinephrine requirements
Epinephrine (Adrenalin)	• First-line agent for anaphylactic shock • Add-on to norepinephrine in septic shock • May cause tachyarrhythmias
Dopamine (Inotropin)	• Can be considered in patient with bradycardia • Causes more arrhythmias and higher mortality compared to norepinephrine alone
Dobutamine (Dobutrex)	• First-line agent for cardiogenic shock • Add-on to norepinephrine in septic shock for augmentation of cardiac output • Increases cardiac contractility • May cause hypotension and tachyarrhythmias
Phenylephrine (Neo-Synephrine)	• Purely alpha-adrenergic vasoconstrictor • Can be considered when tachyarrhythmias preclude use of norepinephrine, epinephrine, or dopamine • Can reduce cardiac output and induce reflux bradycardia
Angiotensin II (Giapreza)	• Can be considered in patients refractory to septic shock despite multiple pressors • May not be readily available in all centers.

CLINICAL PEARL **STEP 2/3**

Following discharge from the hospital, sepsis carries an increased risk of death as well as an increased risk of further sepsis and recurrent hospital admissions. Poor prognostic factors include the inability to mount a fever, leukopenia, age >40 years, certain comorbidities (AIDS, cirrhosis, cancer, alcohol dependence, immunosuppression), a non-urinary source of infection, a nosocomial source of infection, and inappropriate or late antibiotic coverage.

Blood cultures and urine cultures from our patient were positive for *Escherichia coli* sensitive to ceftriaxone. The blood cultures were clear by day 2. She was able to come off pressors on day 3. Her mentation improved and rapidly returned to her baseline. She was transferred to the ward to complete her treatment of antibiotics and was sent home a few days later.

Case Summary

- **Complaint/History:** 64 - year- old female presents to the emergency department with fever, chills, and lethargy found to have severe urinary tract infection.
- **Findings:** Fever, tachycardia and hypotension without response to IV fluid resuscitation.
- **Lab Results/Test:** Urinalysis positive for nitrite, leukocyte esterase, and WBCs. Elevated lactic acid. Urine culture grew E. Coli.

Diagnosis: Septic shock.

- **Treatment:** Broad spectrum IV antibiotics, IV fluids and vasopressors. Antibiotics deescalated based on cultures and sensitivity.

BEYOND THE PEARLS

- Gram-negative sepsis is typically more severe than Gram-positive sepsis and warrants the use of multiple antibiotics from different classes covering the suspected pathogen (double coverage).
- A new pressor angiotensin II (Giapreza) was approved by the US Food and Drug Administration in 2017 for use in cases of septic shock. Angiotensin II raises blood pressure via vasoconstriction and increased aldosterone release.
- Critical illness induces a state of absolute or relative adrenal insufficiency that may contribute to shock. Corticosteroids may offset this condition.
- Common infections seen in the intensive care unit include catheter-related infections (Foley and central line).
- Deescalation of antibiotics should be done based on culture data and clinical improvement as prolonged broad-spectrum antibiotic use can lead to the development of *Clostridium difficile* colitis as well as developing drug resistance.

Bibliography

Singer, M., Deutschman, Clifford, S., et al. (2016). The Third International Consensus Definitions for Sepsis and Septic Shock (Sepsis-3). *The Journal of the American Medical Association*, *315*(8), 801–810.

Rhodes, A., Evan, L., et al. (2018). International guidelines for management of sepsis and septic shock: 2016. *Critical Care Medicine*, *45*(3), 486–552.

Mouncey, P. R., Osborn, T. M., Power, G. S., et al. (2015). Protocolised management in sepsis (ProMISe): a multicentre randomised controlled trial of the clinical effectiveness and cost-effectiveness of early, goal-directed, protocolised resuscitation for emerging septic shock. *Health Technology Assessment*, *19*(97), i–150.

ProCESS Investigators, Yealy, D. M., Kellum, J. A., et al. (2014). A randomized trial of protocol-based care for early septic shock. *The New England Journal of Medicine*, *370*(18), 1683–1693.

Marino, Paul L. *The ICU Book*. Baltimore: Wolters Kluwer Health/Lippincott Williams & Wilkins, 2014.

Peake, S. L., et al. (2014). ARISE Investigators; ANZICS Clinical Trials Group, Goal-directed resuscitation for patients with early septic shock. *The New England Journal of Medicine*, *371*(16), 1496–1506.

De Backer, D., Aldecoa, C., Njimi, H., & Vincent, J. L. (2012). Dopamine versus norepinephrine in the treatment of septic shock: a meta-analysis. *Critical Care Medicine*, *40*(3), 725–730.

Vasu, T. S., Cavallazzi, R., Hirani, A., Kaplan, G., Leiby, B., & Marik, P. E. (2012). Norepinephrine or dopamine for septic shock: systematic review of randomized clinical trials. *Journal of Intensive Care Medicine*, *27*(3), 172–178.

Venkatesh, B., Finfer, S., Cohen, J., et al. (2018). Adjunctive glucocorticoid therapy in patients with septic shock. *The New England Journal of Medicine*, *378*(9), 797–808.

CASE 64

A 53-Year-Old Male With Fever, Fatigue, and Myalgia

Sahar Rabiei-Samani ■ Raj Dasgupta ■ Soroush Rabiei-Samani ■ Rennie L. Rhee

A 53-year-old male presents to the emergency room with complaints of intermittent fever, fatigue, and myalgia for the past month, which has now progressed to new onset hemoptysis. He has a history of hypertension and sinusitis. He denies history of peptic ulcer disease or bleeding per rectum. He also denies any recent travels or exposure with known tuberculosis-infected individuals. He notes paresthesia and weakness of his left foot and right hand. His home medications include amlodipine.

How is hemoptysis classified?

Hemoptysis is defined as coughing up blood that originates from the lower respiratory tract (trachea, bronchi, and bronchioles). Blood expectorated from the upper respiratory tract (pseudohemoptysis) and upper gastrointestinal tract (hematemesis) can mimic lower respiratory tract bleeding. Hemoptysis is further classified as nonmassive, which is generally referred to production of less than 200 mL/day of blood, and massive hemoptysis, which is potentially life threatening and includes production of >100 cc/h or >600 cc/24 h of blood (Table 64.1 and Table 64.2).

CLINICAL PEARL **STEP 2/3**

A dedicated examination of the nose, mouth, and pharynx is an important first step to an obvious site of bleeding. Examination with rhinoscopy and laryngoscopy may be needed when an upper airway source cannot be reliably excluded.

TABLE 64.1 ■ **Differentiating between Hemoptysis and Hematemesis.**

Hemoptysis	Hematemesis
Absence of nausea/vomiting	Nausea/vomiting
Associated hypoxia	Hypoxia less common
History of lung disease	History of gastrointestinal and/or hepatic disease
Frothy or clotted sputum	Coffee ground sputum
Bright red or pink colored sputum	Dark red, brown, or black
Alkaline pH (>7)	Acidic pH (<7)

TABLE 64.2 ■ **Early Management Approaches for Massive Hemoptysis.**

Early Management Approaches
Massive Hemoptysis • Intubation for airway protection • Large-bore endotracheal tube (8 mm) to allow early bronchoscopic evaluation • Placing the patient in lateral decubitus position toward the site of bleeding • Interventional angiography if bronchoscopy intervention fails • Tranexamic acid (TXA) is a synthetic antifibrinolytic agent that has mainly been used in oral and cardiac surgeries to stop bleeding. It can also be used in aerosolized and intrapulmonary injection forms to stop bleeding. It has been associated with higher risk of seizures.

On physical examination, the patient appears pale and in moderate respiratory distress. His vitals are as follows: pulse rate 118 beats/min, blood pressure 152/93 mmHg, respiratory rate 27 breaths/min, oxygen saturation 90% on air, and body temperature of 38.5°C.

His oropharyngeal examination does not reveal stigmata of mucosal or gingival bleeding. Diffuse expiratory wheezing is heard over bilateral lungs. There is 2+ pitting edema of the legs. Multiple erythematous papules and purpura are found over the lower extremities. He has diminished sensation to light touch over the ulnar aspect of the right forearm and lateral aspect of the left lower leg along with difficulty walking on the left heel (foot drop). (Fig. 64.1).

What are the most common causes of hemoptysis?

In the United States, bronchitis, bronchiectasis, and neoplasm such as bronchogenic carcinoma are the most common etiologies. However, tuberculosis remains the most common cause worldwide. A good history and review of system can help in distinguishing the cause of hemoptysis. Isolated weight loss in a smoker with hemoptysis raises concern for carcinoma. The consistency of blood, such as red, frothy, and mixed with purulent sputum, along with fever supports an underlying pulmonary infection. Constitutional symptoms such as fatigue, night sweats, and fever in an immunocompromised individual with risk factors may require evaluation for active tuberculosis or

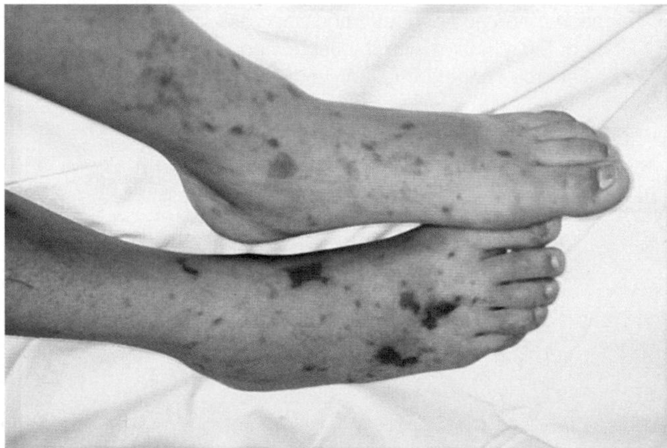

Fig. 64.1 Petechiae and purpuric macules on the lower extremity. Some of the lesions have central hemorrhagic crusts. (From Kessler, C. M. et al. (2019). *Consultative hemostasis and thrombosis* (4th ed.). Elsevier.)

lung abscess. History of nose and gum bleeds, easy bruising, or liver disease point to an underlying coagulopathy. Pattern of bleeding such as monthly with menses in women supports pulmonary endometriosis. Chest pain, dyspnea, leg swelling, and recent immobilization or surgery or use of oral contraceptives suggest pulmonary embolism.

Autoimmune diseases such as vasculitis, antiglomerular basement membrane disease (or Goodpasture's syndrome), antiphospholipid antibody syndrome, or systemic lupus erythematosus may often be accompanied by other organ involvement, such as neuropathy, rash, joint pain, or prior history of thromboembolism. Conditions that can lead to bronchiectasis (dilated airways on imaging studies) include undiagnosed cystic fibrosis, rheumatoid arthritis, chronic obstructive pulmonary disease (COPD), and recurrent aspiration. Taking past medical history will help to formulate a focused differential diagnosis. Review of medications and illicit drug use are also vital because the use of anticoagulants, antiplatelet drugs, and cocaine are important risk factors for hemoptysis.

CLINICAL PEARL **STEP 3**

The three predictors of primary pulmonary malignancy are:

- Male sex
- Age 50 years
- Smoking of 40-pack-years or more

What is the initial evaluation in this patient?

Chest radiography is useful for rapid evaluation of disease processes such as cavitary lesions, infiltrates, and tumors. The findings are termed "localizing" versus "nonlocalizing." Localization of the bleeding site is usually seen in about 40% of patients; that is a clear mass, cavity, or infiltrate is evident on the chest radiograph. The nonlocalizing category refers to chest radiograph findings that are either normal or demonstrate nonspecific findings such as interstitial fibrosis, emphysema, pleural thickening, peribronchial thickening, and increased bronchovascular markings. A normal chest radiograph does not obviate further workup. Computed tomography (CT) and fiberoptic bronchoscopy (FOB) have important roles in patients with hemoptysis and normal chest radiographs. CT may reveal endobronchial lesions or a parenchymal cavity/nodule or mass that is not apparent on chest X-ray image. This modality can further localize the site where a bronchoscopy and biopsy may be needed. CT is also helpful in providing additional details about an abnormality previously recognized on an X-ray image. CT angiography can also diagnose pulmonary emboli. Flexible FOB is important in the diagnostic evaluation for both identifying the site of pathology and confirming an alveolar source of hemorrhage (Figs. 64.2, 64.3, and 64.4).

CLINICAL PEARL **STEP 3**

- The major function of bronchoscopy is to 1) exclude bronchogenic carcinoma and other endobronchial neoplasms, 2) temporize any visible site of active bleeding using endobronchial balloon tamponade or application of localized Tranexamic acid; an antifibrinolytic agent or epinephrine or to perform Argon plasma coagulation for hemostasis.
- It is also used in embolization of vessels to control bleeding or application of fibrinogen-thrombin for treatment of massive hemoptysis.
- FOB is not indicated or effective at detecting other causes of hemoptysis when the chest X-ray is nonlocalizing. It can yield a nonneoplastic etiology of hemoptysis in 10% of cases. About 6% of patients with nonlocalizing chest X-ray images will have cancer; these patients usually have risk factors such as history of smoking and older age.

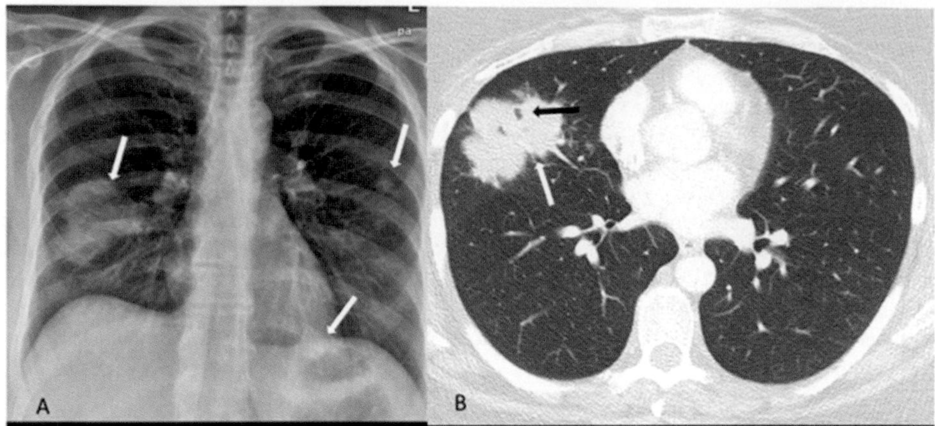

Fig. 64.2 (A) Chest radiograph (posteroanterior view) reveals right mid-lung zone mass *(arrow)* and multiple pulmonary nodules *(arrows)* in left lung. (B) Chest computed tomography scan in axial plane, in lung window, confirms presence of right middle lobe mass *(white arrow)*, with well-defined borders, lobulated outline, and cavitation *(black arrow)*. (From Shoki, A. et al. (2016). An important cause of non-resolving pneumonia. *Respiratory Medicine Case Reports*, *19*, 40–42.)

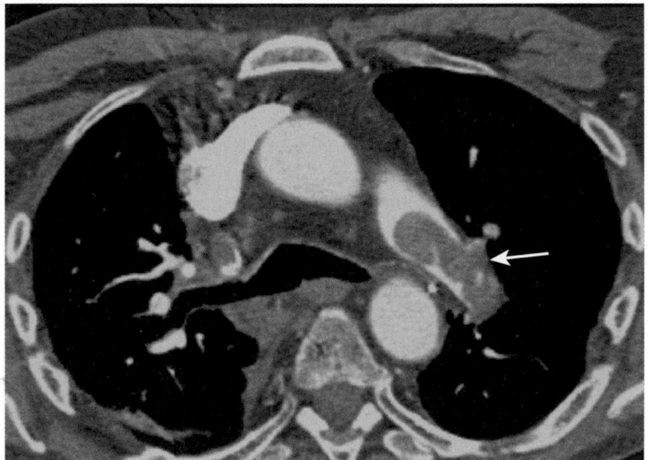

Fig. 64.3 Acute pulmonary embolism. An axial computed tomography image shows a massive clot in the left main pulmonary artery *(arrow)*. (From Soto, J. A., & Lucey, B. C. (2017). *Emergency radiology: the requisites*, (2nd ed.). Elsevier.)

Upon further questioning, the patient becomes dyspneic with increased difficulty in breathing. He is intubated for impending respiratory failure. Blood-tinged secretions are noted in the endotracheal tube.

Laboratory findings are significant for hemoglobin 12.7 mg/dL, total leukocyte count 12,400/μL (12.4 × 10^9/L) (neutrophils 62%, lymphocytes 15%, monocytes 1%, and eosinophils 22%), and platelet count 250,000/μL (250 × 109/L). Creatinine 2.1 mg/dL (185.6 μmol/L). INR 1.2. Normal C3, C4, and rheumatoid factor levels. Urinalysis reveals 3+ protein; 50 erythrocytes/hpf; 20 leukocytes/hpf; several granular casts. Blood and sputum cultures are negative.

A chest X-ray image is obtained. This is followed up by a chest CT examination (Fig. 64.5).

Given the patient's hemoptysis and alveolar infiltrate findings on imaging, he undergoes bronchoscopy with bronchoalveolar lavage (BAL) (Fig. 64.6).

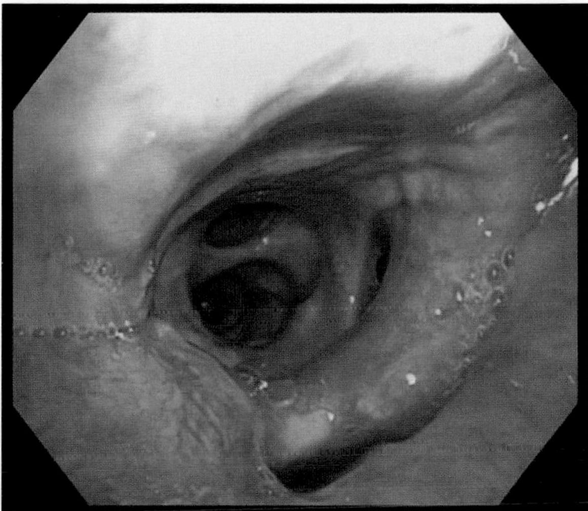

Fig. 64.4 Flexible bronchoscopy showing a mass lesion in right bronchus intermedius with areas of vascularity. This was identified as mucoepidermoid carcinoma of the bronchus on histopathology. (From Baldeyrou, P. (2019). *Normal and pathological bronchial semiology*. Elsevier.)

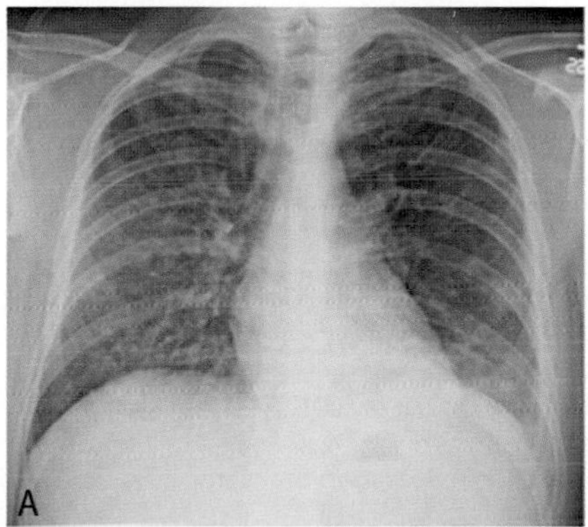

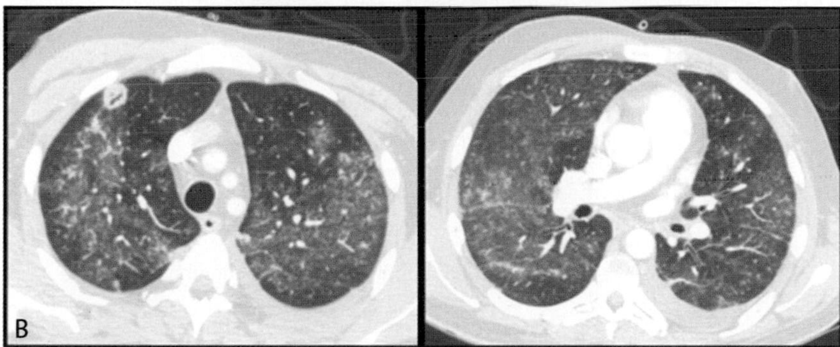

Fig. 64.5 (A) Chest radiograph shows bilateral patchy infiltrate. (B) Computed tomography images show bilateral ground-glass infiltrates with associated necrotizing nodule in right upper lobe. (From Krause, M. L. et Al. (2012). Update on diffuse alveolar hemorrhage and pulmonary vasculitis. *Immunology and Allergy Clinics of North America, 32*(4), 587–600.)

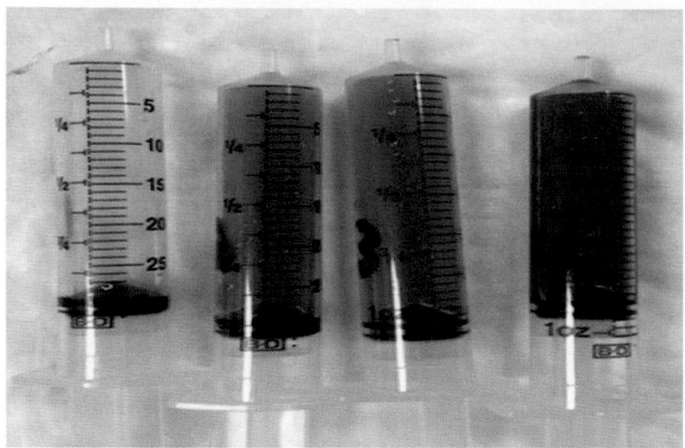

Fig. 64.6 Sequential bronchoalveolar lavage of the right middle lobe showing progressively increasing hemorrhagic fluid. (From Shafi, M. I., & Liaquat, S. (2018). Up in smoke: an unusual case of diffuse alveolar hemorrhage from marijuana. *Respiratory Medicine Case Reports*.)

What do the BAL findings indicate?

Diffuse alveolar hemorrhage (DAH) is not a specific disorder but, rather, a clinicopathologic syndrome; it may result from both immune (vasculitides and connective tissue disorders) and nonimmune disorders (heart failure, infection, trauma, clotting disorders, and drugs). Classically, DAH is characterized by the presence of hemoptysis, diffuse alveolar infiltrates on imaging, and a drop in hematocrit. Profound anemia or hemoptysis may not always be present; hence, DAH must be considered in those with unexplained alveolar infiltrates because it may lead to acute respiratory failure and death. DAH is diagnosed by obtaining serial BALs that progressively get bloodier on serially aspirated aliquots Table 64.3; (Fig. 64.7).

CLINICAL PEARL **STEP 1/2/3**

- Perls Prussian blue is used on BAL fluid to show hemosiderin-laden macrophages.

TABLE 64.3 ■ **Histopathological features of DAH**

The underlying etiology of DAH is reflected in the histopathologic pattern. DAH has three distinct histologic patterns:

1. Pulmonary capillaritis
   - Neutrophilic infiltration of the alveolar septa, which progresses to necrosis of alveolar and capillary walls. As the alveolar-capillary basement membrane is destroyed and red blood cells spill into the alveolar space and interstitium.
   - Commonly seen in systemic vasculitides and other rheumatic diseases.
2. Bland pulmonary hemorrhage
   - Accumulation of fibrin and erythrocytes within the alveolar spaces without alveolar destruction or inflammation.
   - Commonly seen in elevated left ventricular end diastolic pressure, anticoagulation therapy, and bleeding disorders.
3. Diffuse alveolar damage
   - Presence of alveolar septal edema with formation of hyaline membranes but no inflammation.
   - Commonly found in acute respiratory distress syndrome (ARDS).

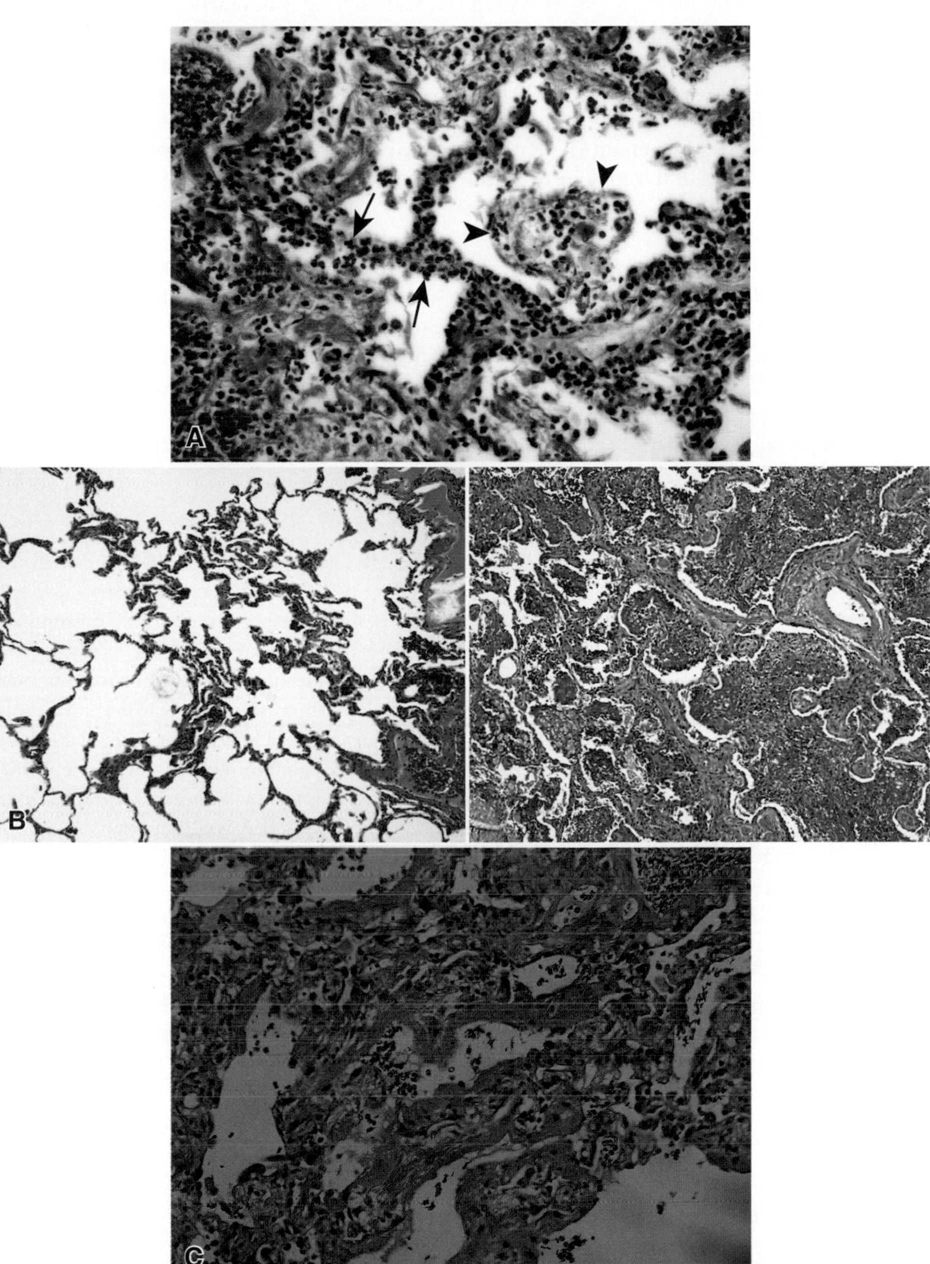

Fig. 64.7 (A) Pulmonary capillaritis identified by accumulation of neutrophils *(arrows)* within alveolar septa with accompanying fibrinoid necrosis and adherent alveolar fibrin within air spaces *(arrowheads)*. (B) Bland pulmonary hemorrhage identified by alveoli filling and distention by red blood cells admixed with fibrin. (C) Diffuse alveolar damage characterized by interstitial edema, prominent type II pneumocyte hyperplasia, and hyaline membranes lining the surfaces of alveoli. (From (A) Broaddus, V. C. et al. (2022). *Murray and Nadel's textbook of respiratory medicine*, (7th ed.). Elsevier; (B) Leslie, K. O., & Wick, M. R. (2018). *Practical pulmonary pathology: a diagnostic approach*, (3rd ed.). Elsevier; (C) Yung-Cheng, S. et al. (2011). Rituximab-induced acute eosinophilic pneumonia with diffuse alveolar damage: a case report. *Journal of Experimental and Clinical Medicine*, *3*(6), 314–317.)

Which other diagnostic tests are available in the evaluation of DAH?

Performing pulmonary function tests (PFT) in the acute setting is impractical. However, an elevated diffuse capacity of carbon monoxide (DLCO) of 30% over baseline or a value of >130% can be used as an adjunctive test to alert the clinician to the possibility of alveolar hemorrhage in those patients who are at risk of recurrence of DAH (i.e. systemic vasculitis). DAH causes an increase in DLCO due to the binding of carbon monoxide to the abundance of hemoglobin in the airspaces. A transthoracic echocardiography (TTE) is routinely performed to rule out valvular disease or myocardial dysfunction as the etiology of DAH.

What is vasculitis?

Vasculitis is a heterogeneous group of disorders with the common characteristic of vessel wall inflammation and necrosis with the potential for vascular destruction leading to end-organ dysfunction. These disorders can be confined to a single organ or occur as a systemic disorder affecting multiple organs. Currently, the vasculitides are classified based on size of the vessel affected (large, medium, small) (Table 64.4). The small-vessel vasculitides are further subdivided by the presence of antineutrophil cytoplasmic antibodies (ANCAs), which incite inflammation through the activation of neutrophils leading to endothelial damage.

Which diagnostic study should be performed next?

A blood test for ANCAs should be performed.

ANCA-associated vasculitis (AAV) is a group of small-vessel vasculitides associated with the presence of ANCA. ANCAs are autoantibodies that target two particular types of antigens found in neutrophil: myeloperoxidase (MPO), which causes a perinuclear pattern on indirect immunofluorescence staining, and proteinase-3 (PR3), which causes a cytoplasmic pattern.

The three main diseases of AAV are granulomatosis with polyangiitis (GPA: formerly known as Wegener's granulomatosis), eosinophilic granulomatosis with polyangiitis (EGPA: previously known as Churg-Strauss syndrome), and microscopic polyangiitis (MPA). These diseases share the manifestations of lung involvement (infiltrates or DAH), pauciimmune glomerulonephritis, mononeuritis multiplex, and constitutional symptoms (such as fever, malaise, and arthralgias).

There are several distinctions between the three types of AAV. GPA is differentiated by granulomatous inflammation and destructive sinonasal involvement (chronic sinusitis, bloody nasal crusts, and/or saddle nose deformity), which is seen at some point during the disease course in 90% of patients. GPA can also cause subglottic stenosis and multiple lung nodules with or without cavitation. GPA is more commonly associated with PR3-ANCA, although MPO-ANCA and negative ANCA can also occur. Almost all patients with EPGA have asthma, typically refractory adult-onset asthma, and peripheral blood eosinophilia. Nasal polyps, chronic sinusitis, and fleeting pulmonary infiltrates (eosinophilic pneumonia) are also common features of EGPA. Only 40% of patients with EGPA have positive ANCA, usually MPO-ANCA. MPA has the highest prevalence of renal involvement and, at times, this is the only manifestation of the disease. There is also an increasing awareness of MPO-ANCA associated interstitial lung disease (ILD), which can occur prior to, concurrent with, or after the onset of the vasculitic manifestations such as glomerulonephritis. MPO-ANCA ILD more often has features of usual interstitial pneumonia (UIP) and therefore has a poorer prognosis compared with other forms of ILD.

Additional workup reveals: ANCA, positive with perinuclear pattern; antimyeloperoxidase antibodies, positive; antiproteinase 3 antibodies, negative.

A renal biopsy is pursued and shows focal segmental necrotizing glomerulonephritis. Immunofluorescence is negative for deposition of immunoglobulins or immune complexes (Fig. 64.8).

TABLE 64.4 ■ **Classification of Vasculitides Based on Size of Affected Vessel**

Vessel Size	Distinguishing Features	Histopathology
Small		
ANCA-Associated		
Granulomatosis with polyangiitis (GPA)	Recurrent middle ear infection; sinusitis; pulmonary cavitary lesions; PR3-ANCA (+) in most cases	Necrotic vasculitis with granulomatous inflammation
Eosinophilic granulomatosis with polyangiitis (EGPA)	Asthma; cardiomyopathy; neuropathy; eosinophilia; MPO-ANCA (+) in about 40% of cases	Extravascular granulomas; eosinophilic infiltrates; necrotizing vascular infiltration
Microscopic polyangiitis (MPA)	Pauciimmune glomerulonephritis; MPO-ANCA (+) in most cases	Necrotizing vascular inflammation without granulomas
Immune Complex-Associated		
Anti-GBM	Lung and kidney involvement; rapidly progressive glomerulonephritis; DAH, tobacco abuse	Crescentic glomerulonephritis; linear IgG deposition along glomerular capillaries
Cryoglobulinemic vasculitis	Clinical triad of neuropathy, arthralgias, and purpura; low complement levels; can be secondary to infections (e.g., hepatitis C), lymphoproliferative disorder, or underlying rheumatic disease (e.g., lupus)	Varies by organ, but generally involves deposition of immune complexes in the vascular wall
IgA vasculitis (Henoch-Schönlein purpura)	Tetrad of palpable purpura, arthralgia, abdominal pain, and renal disease	Leukocytoclastic vasculitis in postcapillary venules with IgA deposition; IgA deposition in the mesangium of glomeruli
Medium		
Polyarteritis nodosa (PAN)	Dermatologic manifestations (nodules, purpura, livedo reticularis); nonglomerular renal disease; multiple microaneurysms on angiography; ischemic abdominal pain due to mesenteric arteritis; mononeuropathy multiplex; orchitis	Transmural inflammatory vasculitis in muscular arteries
Primary angiitis of the central nervous system	Recurrent headaches, CVA, TIA, progressive encephalopathy; systemic vasculitis absent	Granulomatous vasculitis affecting the leptomeningeal and cortical arteries
Large		
Takayasu's arteritis	Stenosis of large vessels (frequently aorta, subclavian and carotid arteries) leading to pain, hypertension, and ischemia; usually occurs before the age of 30 years	Granulomatous inflammation with giant cells, typically in vessel media
Giant cell	New headache, temporal artery tenderness, transient painless monocular vision loss, jaw claudication; often concurrent polymyalgia rheumatica and temporal arteritis; occurs in patients older than 50 years	Temporal artery biopsy with infiltration of lymphocytes and monocytes resulting in panarteritis
Variable-Vessel Vasculitis		
Behçet syndrome	Recurrent painful oral and/or genital aphthous ulcers; panuveitis; thrombosis and arterial aneurysms. Affects any sized vessel in both arteries and veins	No specific histopathological findings; relies on clinical criteria

ANCA, Antineutrophil cytoplasmic antibodies; *CVA*, cerebrovascular accident; *DAH*, diffuse alveolar hemorrhage; *GBM*, glioblastoma; *MPO*, myeloperoxidase; *TIA*, transient ischemic attack.

What is the most likely diagnosis?

Microscopic polyangiitis (MPA) is the most likely diagnosis. It is one of the most common causes of pulmonary-renal syndrome along with other autoimmune diseases such as GPA, antiglioblastoma (GBM) disease, and systemic lupus erythematosus. MPA is a type of ANCA-associated vasculitis characterized by pulmonary involvement and pauciimmune glomerulonephritis. MPA affects men more than women in a 2:1 ratio and tends to occur in the fourth to fifth decade of life.

What are the clinical features of MPA?

Renal involvement is seen in 90% of cases. Urine analysis is significant for proteinuria, red cells, and red cell casts, which indicate glomerular involvement. A total of 20% of cases rapidly progress to renal failure requiring dialysis. The pulmonary involvement occurs in 30% of cases and has a wide range of presentation from mild dyspnea to life-threatening pulmonary hemorrhage requiring intubation. Skin is another commonly affected organ with findings such as palpable purpura, nailbed infarcts, splinter hemorrhages, and ulceronodularity of the lower extremities. The presence of mononeuritis multiplex is a common peripheral neurologic involvement with findings of axonal pattern of conductive impairment on conduction studies. Unlike GPA, sinusitis and bloody nasal crusts are not typically seen in MPA and, unlike EGPA, adult-onset asthma and eosinophilia are also uncommon in MPA.

CLINICAL PEARL **STEP 3**

- The radiographic findings in MPA show bilateral patchy alveolar consolidations in a random distribution. Nodular or cavitary lesions are more typical of granulomatosis with polyangiitis.
- The CT chest findings in MPA show ground-glass attenuation with eventual honeycombing in the later stages when fibrosis occurs.

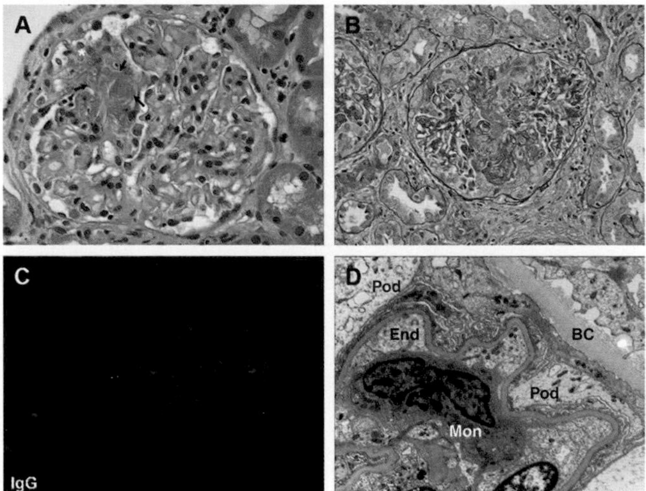

Fig. 64.8 Pauci-immune crescentic glomerulonephritis. Demonstration of classic histology with light microscopy, immunofluorescence, and electron microscopy from a kidney biopsy in a patient presenting with RPGN from AAV. (A) Focal necrotizing glomerulitis with early cellular crescent (hematoxylin-eosin, original magnification x 160). The glomerulus revels segmental fibrinoid necrosis of the tuft (arrows) and limited karyorrhexis (nuclear fragmentation), with formation of an early cellular crescent (white asterisk). (B) Focal necrotizing glomerulitis with early crescent formation (periodic acid-Schiff, original magnification x 135). There is also mild periglomerular interstitial inflammation. (C) ANCA-associated diseases are usually pauci-immune, and significant immunoglobulin or complement deposits are not seen in the glomeruli. The glomerulus depicted here shows background staining for IgG, similar in intensity to the staining with antialbumin reagents (not shown) (FITClabeled human IgG antibodies, original magnification x 120). (D) ANCA-associated glomerular lesions are usually pauci-immune, showing few or no deposits on electron microscopy (hematoxylin-eosin, original magnification X 3500). BC, Bowman capsule; End, endothelial cell; Mon, monocyte occupying. (Courtesy of Helmut Rennke, MD, Boston, MA.)

CLINICAL PEARL **STEP 2/3**

- The gold standard to diagnose MPA is histopathological evidence of vasculitis by obtaining a biopsy of the involved organ (commonly lung, kidney, or skin).
  - Lung: nongranulomatous necrotizing capillaritis.
  - Kidney: pauciimmune necrotizing crescentic glomerulonephritis.
  - Skin: acute or chronic leukocytoclastic vasculitis with neutrophilic infiltrate in the superficial dermis.

How is MPA differentiated from anti-GBM (Goodpasture) disease?

The presence of ANCA level and evidence of peripheral vasculitis lesion, MPA is a more suggestive diagnosis. In 70% of cases ANCA levels are negative in MPA. In that case, a kidney biopsy demonstrating no immune deposits in glomeruli is suggestive of MPA. However, presence of linear deposition of IgG is diagnostic of anti-GBM disease. About 10% of patients with AAV will also have concurrent anti-GBM disease, although the clinical course is more similar to AAV. The concurrent diagnosis of anti-GBM would necessitate the use of plasma exchange.

The patient was treated with pulse doses of glucocorticoids and cyclophosphamide over the next several days. His respiratory status started to improve, requiring a lower fraction of inspired oxygen (FiO_2) on assist controlled mode ventilation. The blood-tinged secretions from the endotracheal tube decreased and patient was subsequently extubated. He was ultimately discharged home on a prolonged taper course of steroids and cyclophosphamide over the next few months. A follow-up chest CT scan in the outpatient clinic also revealed that the diffuse, patchy consolidations in both lungs were significantly absorbed. Through this treatment, the renal function and hematuria improved.

How is MPA managed?

There are two parts to the treatment of MPA: induction and maintenance. Choice of induction therapy depends on severity of disease; for cases where there is risk of organ damage (e.g., renal failure, lung hemorrhage), a combination of high-dose glucocorticoids and either cyclophosphamide or rituximab is used. A clinical trial known as the RAVE trial found that rituximab was noninferior to cyclophosphamide for the induction of remission in AAV. Although no significant differences in short-term adverse events were seen between the two therapies, cyclophosphamide is associated with long-term risk of malignancy and infertility, which limits repeated use of cyclophosphamide for relapsing disease. Less severe manifestations of AAV such as arthritis or purpura can be managed with lower dose glucocorticoids and methotrexate. The induction phase usually lasts for 3 to 6 months.

The timing of initiation of maintenance depends on the agent used during the induction phase. If cyclophosphamide was used for induction, the maintenance therapy is usually started 2 to 4 weeks after the last dose of cyclophosphamide only if the white blood cell count is >4000 cells/μL and the absolute neutrophil count (ANC) is >1500 cells/μL. If rituximab was used for induction, the maintenance agent can be started 4 to 6 months after the last induction dose. The choice of maintenance agents include rituximab, azathioprine, methotrexate, and mycophenolate. Two clinical trials have shown that repeated infusions of rituximab every 4–6 months is superior to azathioprine in maintaining remission in AAV (Table 64.5).

CLINICAL PEARL **STEP 2/3**

- Rituximab is an effective induction therapy in AAV. Rituximab depletes B cells and is thought to be effective in AAV because of the decreased production of pathogenic antibodies (ANCAs) and effects on T cells.

CLINICAL PEARL **STEP 2/3**

- Avoid methotrexate in patients with renal impairment: eGFR <60 mL/min/1.73 m^2.
- Avoid rituximab in patients with hepatitis B virus because it can cause reactivation and fatal hepatitis.
- Choose azathioprine over methotrexate if pregnancy is desired. The safety profile of rituximab during pregnancy is unclear.

CLINICAL PEARL **STEP 2/3**

- Mesna (sodium-2-mercaptoethane sulfonate) is a detoxifying agent that inactivates acrolein (a urotoxic breakdown product of cyclophosphamide or ifosfamide that accumulates in the bladder) by forming a conjugate bond with it in the urine to prevent hemorrhagic cystitis in patients receiving alkylating agents such as cyclophosphamide or ifosfamide.

TABLE 64.5 ■ **The Adverse Effects of Medications Used in the Management of MPA.**

Side Effects of Management	
Glucocorticoids	• Osteoporosis • Cataract • Glaucoma • Diabetes mellitus • Electrolyte abnormalities • Avascular necrosis of bone
Cyclophosphamide	• Bone marrow suppression • Hemorrhagic cystitis • Bladder carcinoma • Myelodysplasia
Methotrexate	• Hepatotoxicity • Pneumonitis • Bone marrow suppression
Azathioprine	• Hepatotoxicity • Bone marrow suppression
Rituximab	• Progressive multifocal leukoencephalopathy • Opportunistic infections

Case Summary

- **Complaint/History:** 53-year-old male presents to the emergency room with complaints of intermittent fever, fatigue and new onset hemoptysis and was found to have bilateral patchy infiltrate on imaging.
- **Findings:** No significant personal risk factors for hemoptysis such as lung cancer or infection exposure. However, he had multiple erythematous papules and purpura over the lower extremities.
- **Lab Results/Tests:** Sequential bronchoalveolar lavage of the right middle lobe showed progressively increasing hemorrhagic fluid. On his blood work ANCA was positive. A renal biopsy showed focal segmental necrotizing glomerulonephritis with negative immunofluorescence deposition of immunoglobulins or immune complexes.

Diagnosis: Microscopic polyangiitis (MPA).

- **Treatment:** Pulse doses of glucocorticoids and cyclophosphamide.

BEYOND THE PEARLS

- The use of plasma exchange has been commonly used in cases of severe alveolar hemorrhage and/or renal insufficiency due to AAV (serum creatinine >4.0 mg/dL or who require dialysis) for the rapid removal of pathogenic autoantibodies (ANCAs) and other inflammatory mediators. However, routine use of plasma exchange is now being called into question after the results of a large randomized clinical trial. This trial, known as the PEXIVAS trial, found no difference in the outcome of end-stage renal disease or death among recipients of plasma exchange or not; in this trial, plasma exchange was adjunctive to high-dose glucocorticoids and either cyclophosphamide or rituximab.
- Important mimics of ANCA-associated vasculitides include:
  - Infective endocarditis, which can cause positive ANCA, skin vasculitis, and multisystem organ failure
  - Cocaine use. Intranasal cocaine use can lead to chronic nasal crusting and sinusitis as well as saddle nose deformity similar to GPA; levamisole is an antihelminthic agent often added to cocaine that can lead to ANCA production and necrotic skin lesions and digital ulceration.
- Hydralazine and propylthiouracil (PTU) can cause drug-induced AAV manifesting with DAH and pauciimmune glomerulonephritis. In addition to cessation of the offending agent, these patients will also need aggressive induction therapy.
- Healthy people can develop nonpathogenic ANCA. Therefore, the presence of positive ANCA on a blood test is not sufficient to diagnose AAV.

Bibliography

Callahan, Sean, J., Sturek, Jeffrey, M., Richard, Ryan, P., et al. (2019) Clinical Pulmonary Medicine. *Wolters Kluwer*, 26(8), 10–17. https://doi.org/10.1097/CPM.0000000000000290.

Frankel, S. K., & Schwarz, M. I. (2012). The pulmonary vasculitides. *Am J Respir Crit Care Med*, *186*, 216–224.

Gagnon, S., Quigley, N., Dutau, H., Delage, A., & Fortin, M. (2017). Approach to Hemoptysis in the Modern Era. *Can Respir J*, *2017*, 1565030. https://doi.org/10.1155/2017/1565030. Epub 2017 Dec 21. PMID: 29430203; PMCID: PMC5752991.

John W. Kreit, Clinical Respiratory Medicine (Third Edition), Chapter 24 – Hemoptysis. Pages 311–316, https://doi.org/10.1016/B978-032304825-5.10024-8.

Marvin I. Schwarz. Clinical Respiratory Medicine (Third Edition), Chapter 63 - Pulmonary Vasculitis and Hemorrhage. Pages 797–807. https://doi.org/10.1016/B978-032304825-5.10063-7.

INDEX

Page numbers followed by '*f*' indicate figures, '*t*' indicate tables, '*b*' indicate boxes.

A

AAV. *See* ANCA-associated vasculitis (AAV)
Abaloparatide
  for osteoporosis, 454*t*, 458
  side effects, 459*t*
Abdomen, quadrants of, 387*f*
Abdominal compartment syndrome, 16
Abdominal radiograph, toxic megacolon, 347*t*, 348*f*
ABI. *See* Arterial-brachial index (ABI)
Abnormal hair growth, in female, 464, 464*f*
Abnormal liver tests, evaluation of, 405–410
Absolute neutrophil count (ANC), 369*b*, 563–565
Acanthosis nigricans, 463–464, 463*f*, 464*b*
Acetaminophen
  drug-induced liver injury, 329*t*
  hepatocellular liver injury, 407*t*
Achalasia
  clinical symptoms in, 338–339
  diseases associated with, 338
  Eckhardt score, 338–339, 339*t*
  esophageal manometry, 336–338
  nonpharmacologic treatments for, 340, 342*t*–343*t*
  pathophysiology, 338
  pharmacologic treatments for, 340
  primary, 338, 344*b*
  secondary, 338, 339*b*
  symptoms, 338
  type I, 339
  type II, 339
  type III, 339
Acid fast bacilli (AFB) stain, 542–543, 543*b*
Acidosis, 383
Acquired hypocomplementemia, 267*b*
Acromegaly, 433*b*, 433*t*, 461
ACS. *See* Acute coronary syndrome (ACS)
Activin receptor-like kinase (ALK-1), 522*b*
Acute abdominal pain
  appendicitis, 388–391
  causes, 307–315, 308*t*
  differential diagnosis, 307–315, 308*t*, 386, 386*b*
  laboratory testing, 307*b*, 308*t*, 387
  physical examination, 386
Acute coronary syndrome (ACS), 196–198, 206, 212
  diagnostic workup, 198–199
  management, 201–204
  troponin levels, 201
Acute decompensated heart failure (ADHF) exacerbation, 158
Acute interstitial nephritis, 8*f*, 34, 36
Acute kidney injury (AKI)
  causes, 15–16, 15*f*
  vs. chronic kidney disease (CKD), 4
  differential diagnosis, 4–6, 5*t*, 32–33, 33*t*
Acute monoarticular arthritis
  calcium pyrophosphate disease (CPPD)
    conditions commonly associated with, 277
    management, 279
    recurrence of flares, prevention, 279–280
  crystal arthritis, radiologic findings, 277–279, 278*f*
  differential diagnosis, 275–280
  physical examination findings, 275
  pseudogout, 276
  synovial fluid analysis, 275–276, 277*t*
Acute myeloid leukemia (AML), 372*b*
Acute myocardial infarction (AMI), 206
Acute pancreatitis, 307
  causes, 310, 310*t*
  complications, 313–315
  diagnosis, 309–310
  incidence, 314*b*
  management, 311
  recurrent, 314*b*
  severity assessment, 310–311
Acute promyelocytic leukemia (APL), 53–55
  bone marrow biopsy, 54, 55*f*
  management, 56–57
Acute pulmonary embolism, 556*f*
Acute renal papillary necrosis, 6, 6*f*
Acute tubular necrosis (ATN), 7–8
AD. *See* Atopic dermatitis (AD)
ADPKD. *See* Autosomal dominant polycystic kidney disease (ADPKD)
Adrenal atrophy, 435
Adrenal insufficiency, 435, 438
Adrenocorticotrophic hormone (ACTH), 461
  deficiency, evaluation of, 435
  stimulation test, 435
AIN. *See* Allergic interstitial nephritis (AIN)
Airway clearance therapy, for bronchiectasis, 543
Airway obstruction, 541
AKI. *See* Acute kidney injury (AKI)

Alanine aminotransferase (ALT), 260, 317–320, 324, 324*b*, 405
elevated, causes of, 325*t*
upper limit of normal for, 319*b*
Alberta Stroke Program Early Computed Tomography Score (ASPECTS), 147*b*
Alcohol, in acute pancreatitis, 310
Alendronate, for osteoporosis, 454*t*, 458
Alkaline phosphatase (ALP), 405, 412
Allergic interstitial nephritis (AIN), 8
causes, 8–10, 9*t*
clinical presentation, 10
All-trans retinoic acid (ATRA), 53–54, 56–57
Alpha-fetoprotein (AFP), 321–323
Alpha glucosidase inhibitors, 425–426, 425*t*–426*t*
ALT. *See* Alanine aminotransferase (ALT)
Alvarado's Scoring system, 388, 389*t*
American Association for the Study of Liver Diseases (AASLD), 317–320
American Cancer Society, 103
American College of Cardiology/American Heart Association (ACC/AHA) staging system, 172
American College of Obstetricians and Gynecologists (ACOG), 445
American College of Rheumatology (ACR) classification criteria
for giant cell arteritis (GCA), 298, 298*t*
for polymyalgia rheumatica (PMR), 295, 298*t*
American Thyroid Association (ATA), 445
5-Aminosalicylates (5-ASA), for inflammatory bowel disease (IBD), 349
Aminotransferases, 405
Amiodarone, for pulmonary fibrosis, 509*b*
Amlodipine, 434*t*
Amoxicillin
for *C. difficile* infection, 365
for community-acquired pneumonia (CAP), 487
Amphotericin and fluconazole, for cryptococcal meningoencephalitis, 356
Amphotericin and flucytosine, for cryptococcal meningoencephalitis, 356
Amylase, 309*b*
Amylin analog
side effects, 425*t*–426*t*
for type 2 diabetes, 425–426
Anabolic therapy, for osteoporosis, 459–460
ANCA-associated vasculitis (AAV), 560
mimics of, 565
types, 560
Androgenetic alopecia, 464, 465*f*
Androgen Excess/PCOS Society criteria, 462
Androgenic progestins, associated with hirsutism, 465*t*
Anemia, 383
history, 41–42
laboratory results, 43–44, 43*t*
signs and symptoms, 42
Anginal pain
beta blocker therapy, 193–194
diagnosis, 188
differential diagnosis, 188
risk factors, 188
stress modality, 189
types, 187–188
typical and atypical, 186–187
Angiotensin-converting enzyme (ACE) inhibitor, 538
Angiotensin II, in septic shock, 550*t*
Anion gap (AG), 429*b*
Ankylosing spondylitis (AS), 295
Ankylosis human (ANKH) gene, 280
Antibiotics, 329*t*
for appendicitis, 390
for aspiration pneumonia, 492–493, 493*t*
for cholangitis, 314*b*
de-escalation, 551
for infected necrosis, 314*b*
for sepsis, 548
Anticoagulant therapy, 201–202
Anticyclic citrullinated peptide antibodies (anti-CCP), 295
Antifungal prophylaxis, 373–374
Anti-GBM (Goodpasture) disease, 563
Antimalarial therapy, 384
Antimicrobials, for neutropenic fever, 373–375
Antimicrobial stewardship programs, 365*b*
Antineutrophil cytoplasmic antibodies (ANCA), 560
Antineutrophil cytoplasmic antibody (ANCA)-associated vasculitis, 269–271, 274
cytoplasmic (c-ANCA) pattern, 269*b*, 271*f*
perinuclear (p-ANCA) pattern, 269*b*, 271*f*
Antiphospholipid syndrome (APS)
clinical manifestations, 235
diagnosis, 238
laboratory findings, 235–238
management, 238–239
pathogenesis, 239*f*
pregnancy, 239–241
scenarios, 234
Antipseudomonal agents, for ventilator-associated pneumonia (VAP), 487
Anti-retroviral therapy (ART)
for elevated intracranial pressure (ICP), 357
HIV diagnosis, 399–400
Antismooth muscle antibody (SMA), 327
APACHE II score, 310–311
APL. *See* Acute promyelocytic leukemia (APL)

Apolipoprotein 1, 33
Appendicitis
  Alvarado's Scoring system, 388, 389*t*
  computed tomography, 388–390, 389*f*
  diagnosis, 388–390
  history and presentation, 388
  incidence, 388
  Infectious Diseases Society of America Practice guidelines, 390, 390*t*
  physical examination findings, 388, 388*t*
  treatment, 390–391, 390*t*
  ultrasound, 388–390, 389*f*
APS. *See* Antiphospholipid syndrome (APS)
Arboviruses, 379*t*
Argon plasma coagulation (APC), 528–529
Artemisinin-based combination therapy (ACT), for malaria, 384, 384*b*
Arterial-brachial index (ABI), 177–178, 178*t*, 180*f*
Artesunate, for malaria, 384
Arthralgia, 266, 269–273
Arthritis
  gonococcal, 362*b*
  infectious, 360
  monoarticular, 358
  septic, 358–362, 358*b*
Arthrocentesis, 359*b*
Asbestosis, 501*t*
Ascites, 18*b*
Aspartate aminotransferase (AST), 260, 324, 324*b*, 325*t*, 405
Aspiration pneumonia, 490–491
  antibiotics for, 492–493, 493*t*
  nasogastric and postpyloric tubes placement, 493–494, 495*f*, 496*t*
  pathogens, 492
  prevention, 494–496
  radiographic changes, 492
  risk factors, 491–492, 492*t*
Aspirin, 191
Assessment of Spondyloarthritis International Society (ASAS), 251–252
AST. *See* Aspartate aminotransferase (AST)
Asterixis, 326*b*, 327*f*
Astrocytomas, 133
Atopic dermatitis (AD)
  complications, 122–123
  diagnosis, 119–120
  differential diagnosis, 120*t*
  epidemiology, 118
  histologic features, 120, 121*f*
  pathogenesis, 118–119
  treatment, 121–122, 122*t*
  variants, 120
Atovaquone, for *Pneumocystis jirovecci* pneumonia (PCP) prophylaxis, 302*b*
Atovaquone-proguanil, for malaria, 384
ATRA. *See* All-trans retinoic acid (ATRA)
Atypical femur fractures (AFFs), 455
Auerbach's plexus, 338, 339*b*
Autoantibodies, 263, 263*t*
Autoimmune hepatitis (AIH), 326–328
Autoimmune thyroiditis, 442–443
Autosomal dominant polycystic kidney disease (ADPKD)
  diagnosis, 21, 22*f*, 24*t*
  hypertension, 24
  kidney imaging studies, 21, 22*f*
  management, 24
  renal and extrarenal manifestations, 24
  treatment, 25–26
Azathioprine, 512
  for microscopic polyangiitis (MPA), 563–565
  side effects, 564*t*
Azotemia, 5

B

Bacteria, 381
Bacterial pneumonia, 379*t*
BAL. *See* Bronchoalveolar lavage (BAL)
Barium esophagram swallowing study, 333, 334*f*, 336, 336*f*, 337*f*
Barium sulfate, 333
Basal insulin, 424
Bazedoxifene, for osteoporosis prevention, 450–451, 454*t*
Bedside Index of Severity in Acute Pancreatitis (BISAP) score, 310–311, 310*b*, 311*t*
Beevor's sign, 128
Beighton score, 291
  defined, 282
  joint hypermobility, 282, 283*f*, 283*t*, 284*f*
Berylliosis, 501*t*
Beta blocker therapy, 193–194, 201
Bezlotoxumab, for recurrent *C. difficile* infection, 367*b*
Biguanides, 425–426, 425*t*–426*t*
Bilateral hilar lymphadenopathy, 96*f*
Bilateral lower extremity pain, 177, 178*t*
Bilateral mammography, 88
Bilateral shoulder pain, 293
  differential diagnosis, 293–295, 294*t*
  location and distribution, 293
  morning stiffness, 294
Bile acid sequestrant, 425–426, 425*t*–426*t*
Bile cast nephropathy, 17, 17*f*
Biliary decompression, 312, 312*b*
Biliary obstruction
  differential diagnosis, 413–414, 414*t*
  imaging, 414–416, 415*t*

Biliary systems, anatomy of, 412–413, 413*f*
Bilirubin (BR), 405, 412
BinaxNOW test, 382*b*
Bisphosphonates (BPs), for osteoporosis, 454*t*
  advantages and disadvantages, 457
  side effects, 455, 459*t*
Bitemporal hemianopsia, 430, 432*f*
Bland pulmonary hemorrhage, 558*b*
Blastomyces, 393*b*
Bleomycin, for pulmonary fibrosis, 509*b*
Blood culture, 370, 370*b*
Blood urea nitrogen (BUN), 5, 311
BMD. *See* Bone mineral density (BMD)
Bone architecture, 449, 450*f*
Bone loss, 452
Bone markers, 456*t*
Bone mineral density (BMD), 449, 455–456
  femoral neck, 451
  lumbar spine, 451
  T- and Z-scores, 452*b*
  testing, indications for, 450*t*
Bone morphogenetic protein receptor type II (*BMPR2* mutation), 522*b*
Bone turnover markers (BTMs), 455–456, 457*b*
Botulinum toxin injections, for achalasia, 340
Brachial plexopathy, 140
Brain natriuretic peptide (BNP), 515–516
Bromocriptine, for micro- and macroprolactinomas, 436*b*
Bronchiectasis
  bronchoscopy, 543*b*
  causes, 542*t*
  computed tomography (CT), 539–540, 539*f*, 540*f*, 541*f*
  cylindrical, 540*f*
  cystic, 540*f*
  diffuse, 542*t*
  etiology, 541–542, 542*t*
  focal, 542*t*
  management, 544
  radiography, 540–541
  recurrent exacerbations, 544
  tests, 542–543
  therapy, 543–544
  traction, 540*b*
  tram-track sign, 540
  varicose, 541*f*
Bronchoalveolar lavage (BAL), 398, 556, 558–560, 558*f*
Bronchoscopy, 502*b*, 543*b*
B symptoms, 392, 393*t*
BTMs. *See* Bone turnover markers (BTMs)
Budesonide, for hepatic sarcoidosis, 410
BUN. *See* Blood urea nitrogen (BUN)

C

Cabergoline, for micro- and macroprolactinomas, 436*b*
Calcification, of nodule, 532
Calcitonin
  for osteoporosis, 453, 454*t*
  side effects, 459*t*
Calcium
  for osteoporosis, 454*t*, 458
  side effects, 459*t*
Calcium channel blockers, 193, 340, 521
Calcium pyrophosphate disease (CPPD) arthritis
  conditions commonly associated with, 277
  crystals, 276, 276*f*
  management, 279
  recurrence of flares, prevention, 279–280
Candida glabrata, 375
Candida krusei, 375
Candida overgrowth, 394–395
CAP. *See* Community-acquired pneumonia (CAP)
Capillaritis, 77, 79*f*
Cardiac filling pressures (CVP), 549
Cardiac syndrome X. *See* Microvascular angina
Cardiogenic shock (CS), 158–159
  causes, 159, 159*t*
  criteria, 158, 159*t*
  diagnosis, 159–163
  symptoms and laboratory data, 159
  treatment, 164–166
Carney complex, 440
Carpal tunnel syndrome, 140
  diagnosis, 141, 141*f*, 142*f*
  evaluation, 142–143
  symptoms, 142
  treatments, 143–144
CD. *See* Crohn's disease (CD)
Cefepime, for hospital-acquired pneumonia (HAP), 487
Cellulitis, 77
Centers for Disease Control and Prevention's (CDC) 2019 Antibiotic Resistant Threats report, 363–364
Cerebral aneurysm, 25
Cerebral angiogram, 150*f*
Cerebral malaria, 384
Cerebral salt wasting (CSW), 438
Cerebral vascular accident (CVA) syndromes, 146–147, 147*t*
Cerebrospinal fluid (CSF) analysis, 354, 354*t*
Cervical radiculopathy, 140
Charcot's triad, 326*b*
CHB. *See* Chronic hepatitis B (CHB)

Chest pain
  differential diagnosis, 186, 187*t*, 196, 198*t*, 206, 207*t*, 208–209
  laboratory tests, 207*t*
  ST-segment elevation, 206*b*, 207–208, 208*t*
Chest physiotherapy, for bronchiectasis, 543
Chest radiograph (CXR)
  aspiration pneumonia, 490*b*, 491*f*
  bilateral patchy infiltrate, 557*f*
  bilateral reticular infiltrates, 505, 506*f*
  bronchovascular markings and tram track opacities, 538, 539*f*
  enlarged pulmonary artery, 516, 516*f*
  innumerable small nodular opacities, 497, 498*f*
  Mycobacterium tuberculosis (MTB), 395–396, 395*f*
  pneumothorax, 477*b*, 477*f*
  retrocardiac air-fluid level in mediastinum at level of aortic arch, 331, 332*f*
  right lung opacity, 523–524, 524*f*
Chicago Classification of Motility Disorders, 339, 341*f*
Chikungunya, 379*t*
Cholangiocarcinoma (CCA), 416
Cholangitis, 312*b*, 326*b*
Choledocholithiasis
  endoscopic retrograde cholangiopancreatography (ERCP), 311–313, 313*f*
  magnetic resonance cholangiopancreatography (MRCP), 311–313, 313*f*
Cholelithiasis, 307*b*, 308*b*, 309*b*, 309*f*
Cholestasis, 326*b*–327*b*, 328*f*
Cholestatic liver injury, 406, 406*t*
Chondrocalcinosis, 277–279, 278*f*
Chronic beryllium disease, 504*b*
Chronic bilateral leg edema
  differential diagnosis, 27
  management, 30–31
Chronic cluster headache, 136
Chronic cough
  bronchiectasis, 540–545
  causes, 538–545
  management, 539–540
Chronic diarrhea
  causes, 345–350
  defined, 345–350
  differential diagnosis, 345–350, 346*t*
  evaluation, 345–346
  laboratory tests, 346*b*, 346*t*
Chronic hepatitis B (CHB)
  antiviral therapy, 317–320
  definitions, 319*t*
  hepatocellular carcinoma (HCC) screening in, 321–323
  perinatal transmission, 316–317
    prevention, 321
  during pregnancy, 320–321, 321*b*
Chronic hepatitis B (CHB) *(Continued)*
  prevalence, 316–317, 317*t*
  subgroups, 321*t*
  treatment, 320
Chronic kidney disease (CKD) *vs.* acute kidney injury (AKI), 4
Chronic obstructive pulmonary disease (COPD), 475, 505–506, 523
Ciprofloxacin, for neutropenic fever, 373*b*, 376–377
Clindamycin, for aspiration pneumonia, 496
Clomiphene, for polycystic ovary syndrome (PCOS), 469–471
Clopidogrel, 191
Clostridium difficile, 345–350, 363–364
  colonization, 363
  hypervirulent strain, 364*b*
  infection
    control measures, 365
    diagnostics tests, 366–367
    pathogenesis, 364–365
    prognosis, 367–368
    risk factors, 364*b*, 365–366
    symptoms, 365
    transmission, 364–365
    treatment, 367
Clubbing, 502–503, 545
Cluster headaches, 136
  autonomic symptoms, 136–137, 136*f*
  diagnostic tests, 137
  differential diagnosis, 134–136
  signs and symptoms, 134
  treatment, 137
Coal workers' pneumoconiosis, 501*t*
Coccidioides immitis, 393*b*
Coccidioides posadasii, 393*b*
Cognitive behavioral therapy (CBT), 287–291
Colchicine
  for CPPD arthritis, 275
Colloid fluids, 548
Colonoscopy, 346*b*, 347*f*
Common bile duct (CBD), 412–413, 415*b*, 415*f*
Community-acquired pneumonia (CAP), 484–485
  duration of treatment recommended for, 487
  etiologies, 486
  HIV, 397
  risk factors, 487–488
  therapies for, 486–487
Complete blood count (CBC), 295, 387
Comprehensive metabolic panel (CMP), 387
Computed tomography (CT)
  abdomen, 314*b*
  appendicitis, 388–390, 389*f*
  biliary obstruction, 414

Computed tomography (CT) *(Continued)*
hemoptysis, 555–556, 556*f*
septic arthritis, 359
thorax, 524, 524*b*, 525*f*
Confusion, 61
Confusion assessment method (CAM), 63–64, 63*b*
Congenital adrenal hyperplasia (CAH), 442–443, 461
Conjugated equine estrogen (CEE), 450–451
Connective tissue disease-associated interstitial lung disease (CTD-ILD), 499–500
Conventional manometry, 336–338
Coronary artery bypass graft surgery (CABG), 191
Cortisol, 435, 438–439
Cough
differential diagnosis, 394–395, 523–529
imaging studies, 523–525
Cough-variant asthma, 538*b*
COVID-19, 397–398
CPPD. *See* Calcium pyrophosphate disease (CPPD) arthritis
Craniopharyngioma, 430
C-reactive protein (CRP), 266, 269*f*, 295, 345–346
Creatinine, 16
Crohn's disease (CD), 346–347, 347*t*, 349–350, 349*t*
CRP. *See* C-reactive protein (CRP)
Cryoglobulinemia, 267*b*
Cryoglobulinemic vasculitis
clinical and laboratory features of, 271–273, 272*t*
prednisone for, 272*b*
rituximab for, 272*b*
sofosbuvir-velpatasvir for, 272*b*
treatment, 273–274
Cryoglobulins, 271, 271*b*, 272*t*
Cryptococcal antigen (CrAg), 355
Cryptococcal meningoencephalitis
diagnosis, 355–356
treatment, 356
Cryptococcosis, 354–355, 354*b*
Cryptococcus gattii, 353*b*
Cryptococcus neoformans, 353*b*, 356–357
Crystal arthritis
fever in, 275*b*
radiologic findings, 277–279, 278*f*
Crystal arthropathies, 360*b*
CS. *See* Cardiogenic shock (CS)
CT. *See* Computed tomography (CT)
C-terminal telopeptide (CTX), 456
Cushing disease, 432–434, 433*t*, 434*b*, 442–443, 465
Cutaneous ecthyma gangrenosum, 374*b*
Cutaneous leukocytoclastic vasculitis, 83–84. *See also* Leukocytoclastic vasculitis
Cutaneous purpuric eruptions, 83
Cutaneous Sarcoidosis Activity and Morphology Instrument (CSAMI), 98
CXR. *See* Chest radiograph (CXR)
Cyclophosphamide
for cryoglobulinemic vasculitis, 273–274, 273*b*
for microscopic polyangiitis (MPA), 563–565
side effects, 564*t*
Cyclosporine, associated with hirsutism, 465*t*
Cytomegalovirus (CMV) retinitis, 400

D

DAH. *See* Diffuse alveolar hemorrhage (DAH)
Danazol, associated with hirsutism, 465*t*
Decompensated cirrhosis
differential diagnosis, 16–17
medical history and physical examination, 14–15
portal hypertension, 13–14, 14*f*
signs and symptoms, 13, 14*f*
Degeneration, of myenteric plexus, 338, 339*b*
Dehydroepiandrosterone sulfate (DHEA)-S, 465*b*, 466
Delirium, 61–67
causes, 62
diagnosis, 62–64
DSM-5 criteria, 63*b*
history and physical examination, 63*b*
initial workup, 64
management, 64–66, 65*t*
medications, 63*b*, 66*t*
prevention, 66–67
risk factors, 62*t*
Denosumab, for osteoporosis, 454*t*
risks and benefits of, 457
side effects, 459*t*
Dermatomyositis (DM), 260
Desquamative interstitial pneumonia (DIP), 511*b*
Dexamethasone suppression test, 434
DEXA scan, for osteoporosis, 449, 452*b*, 455
β-(1-3)-D-glucan, 375
Diabetes insipidus (DI), 437–438
Diabetes medications
cardiovascular benefits, 427
for diabetic ketoacidosis (DKA), 425*t*–426*t*, 426–427, 426*b*
Diabetic ketoacidosis (DKA), 421–423
basal insulin, 424
bicarbonate administration, 423*b*
diabetes medications, 426–427
diagnosis, 422–423, 422*b*
fluid and insulin infusions, 423–424
glucagon-like peptide 1 receptor agonists (GLP1 RAs) for, 425*t*–426*t*, 426–427, 426*b*
management, 423–424, 423*t*
signs and symptoms, 422*b*
sodium glucose cotransporter-2 (SGLT2) inhibitors for, 425*t*–426*t*, 426–427, 426*b*

Diabetic nephropathy
histology, 28, 29*f*
management, 29–31, 30*f*
pathophysiology, 28, 29*f*
Diabetic retinopathy, 427–428, 427*b*
Diarrhea
causes, 363, 364*t*
C. difficile infection, 363–368
defined, 363
Diazoxide, associated with hirsutism, 465*t*
DIC. *See* Disseminated intravascular coagulation (DIC)
Diclofenac, 326–327, 329*b*
Diffuse alveolar damage, 558*b*
Diffuse alveolar hemorrhage (DAH)
bronchoalveolar lavage (BAL), 558–560, 559*f*
pulmonary function test (PFTs), 560
Diffusing capacity for lung of carbon monoxide (DLCO), 506*b*, 507, 560
Digital subtraction angiography (DSA), 182, 184*f*
DILI. *See* Drug-induced liver injury (DILI)
Dipeptidyl peptidase 4 (DPP4) inhibitors, 425–426, 425*t*–426*t*
Direct fluorescence antibody (DFA), for PJP pneumonia, 398
Direct immunofluorescence, 266–268
Disease-modifying antirheumatic drugs (DMARDs), 256
Disseminated candidiasis, 375*b*
Disseminated intravascular coagulation (DIC)
causes, 50–51, 52*t*
management, 52–53
Distal interphalangeal (DIP) joints, 252
DKA. *See* Diabetic ketoacidosis (DKA)
DLCO. *See* Diffusing capacity for lung of carbon monoxide (DLCO)
Dobutamine, in septic shock, 550*t*
Dopamine, in septic shock, 550*t*
Doxycycline
for community-acquired pneumonia (CAP), 487
for malaria, 384
Drug-induced liver injury (DILI), 326–328
causes, 329*b*, 329*t*
diclofenac-associated, 328–330
Dry eyes. *See* Keratoconjunctivitis sicca
Dry mouth. *See* Xerostomia
Duloxetine, for Ehlers-Danlos Syndromes (EDS), 291
Dysphagia, 259–260, 493
causes, 331–344, 333*t*
defined, 331
diagnosis, 333–338
differential flowchart, 332*f*
esophageal, 331
evaluation, 333–336
Dysphagia *(Continued)*
oropharyngeal, 331
stages of swallowing and symptoms of, 494*t*
symptoms, 333*t*
types, 331–332
Dyspnea, 505–506

E

Eckhardt score, 338–339, 339*t*
E. coli, 381
EDS. *See* Ehlers-Danlos Syndromes (EDS)
EGD. *See* Esophagogastroduodenoscopy (EGD)
Eggshell calcification, of lymph nodes, 504*b*
Ehlers-Danlos Syndromes (EDS), 282, 283*f*, 286*b*
arthrochalasia type VIIa or VIIb, 286
dermatosparaxis type VIIc, 286
diagnosis, 285–286
hypermobility type II, 286
kyphoscoliotic type VI, 286
musculoskeletal pain in, 287
subtypes, 286–287
treatment, 287–292
type I or II, classic type, 286
vascular type IV, 286
Ehlers-Danlos vasculitis, 285
Elevated alkaline phosphatase and hypercalcemia
cholestatic liver injury, 406, 406*t*
granulomas, 407–408, 408*t*
hepatic sarcoidosis, 408–410, 409*t*
hepatocellular liver injury, 406–407, 407*t*
Elevated liver function tests (LFTs)
clinical monitoring, 325–326
differential diagnosis, 324–325, 325*t*
evaluation, 324–330
management, 328–330
serological workup, 325*t*
ELISA, 355
Endemic fungi, 393*b*
Endoscopic bronchial ultrasonography (EBUS), 525, 526*b*, 536
Endoscopic retrograde cholangiopancreatography (ERCP)
for biliary obstruction, 414–416, 415*b*
for cholangiocarcinoma (CCA), 416
choledocholithiasis, 311–312, 313*f*
Endoscopic ultrasound (EUS), 414–416, 525
Endothelin-1, 518–520
Endothelin receptor antagonists, 521
End-stage renal disease (ESRD), 22
Enlarged cardiac silhouette, 157*f*
Entecavir, for chronic hepatitis B (CHB), 320, 320*b*
Enterobacteriaceae, 492
Enthesitis, 252–254, 255*f*, 256*f*
Enzyme immunoassays (EIA), 366

Eosinophilic esophagitis (EoE), 332, 340*b*
Eosinophilic granulomatosis with polyangiitis (EGPA), 560
Ependymomas, 133
Epinephrine, in septic shock, 550*t*
Episodic cluster headache, 136
ERCP. *See* Endoscopic retrograde cholangiopancreatography (ERCP)
Erythrocyte sedimentation rate (ESR), 266, 269*f*, 282*b*, 295, 345–346
Esophageal candidiasis, 394–395, 394*f*
Esophageal dysphagia, 331
Esophageal manometry, 335*f*, 336–338, 337*t*
Esophagogastroduodenoscopy (EGD), 333, 334*f*, 336*b*
ESR. *See* Erythrocyte sedimentation rate (ESR)
Estrogen, 450–451
Ethacrynic acid, 30
European League Against Rheumatism (EULAR), classification criteria for polymyalgia rheumatica, 295, 298*t*
Expanded Gram-positive antibacterial therapy, 373, 373*t*
Extended-spectrum beta-lactamase (ESBL), 373
Extradural spinal tumors, 132
Extraintestinal involvement (EIM), 348–349

F

Falls, in older adults
- balance and gait assessment, 71–72
- evaluation, 70
- history, 70–71
- incidence, 68
- interventions, 72–73, 72*t*
- laboratory and diagnostic studies, 71
- medications, 71, 71*t*
- outcomes, 68–70
- risk factors, 68, 69*t*
- screening, 73–74

False hematuria, 19
Fanconi's syndrome, 35–36
Febrile neutropenia, 370*t*, 373
Fecal calprotectin, 345–346, 345*b*
Ferriman-Gallwey score, 464, 464*f*
Fever
- recurrent, 378–379
- returning traveler with, 378
  - differential diagnosis, 378, 379*t*, 380–382
  - Venn diagram of differential diagnoses, 380, 381*f*
- tests, 379

Fiberoptic bronchoscopy (FOB), 555–556
Fibrillin-1 gene, 285
Fick principle, 162
Fidaxomicin, for *C. difficile* infection, 367
Filaggrin, 118–119
Flapping tremor. *See* Asterixis
Fleischner Society guidelines, 534, 534*b*, 535*t*
Fluconazole, for cryptococcal meningoencephalitis, 356
Fluid resuscitation, 548–549
Fluorodeoxyglucose (FDG)-position emission tomography (PET) scan
- giant cell arteritis (GCA), 299, 300*f*
- pulmonary metastasis, 534–536, 535*f*

Focal necrotizing glomerulitis, 562*f*
Focal segmental glomerulosclerosis (FSGS), 36, 36*f*
Forced vital capacity (FVC), 506*b*, 507
Foreign body granulomas, 91
Fracture Risk Assessment Tool (FRAX), 449, 451*b*, 452*b*
Fresh frozen plasma (FFP), 52–53
Fungal biomarkers, role in neutropenic fever, 375
Fungal pneumonia, 398
Fungi, 381

G

Galactomannan assay, 375
Gallstones, 308*b*
Gamma glutamyl transpeptidase (GGT), 405
Gastroesophageal reflux disease (GERD), 307, 333, 538, 538*b*
GCA. *See* Giant cell arteritis (GCA)
GERD. *See* Gastroesophageal reflux disease (GERD)
Ghent nosology, 285
Giant cell arteritis (GCA), 297–298
- ACR classification criteria for, 298, 298*t*
- alternative therapy, 301–303
- aneurysm development in, 299, 300*f*
- characteristic pathology, 299
- cranial, 299–301
- diagnosis, 298–299
- extracranial, 299–301
- glucocorticoid-sparing treatments for, 302*t*
- inflammation of arterial wall, 299, 299*f*
- prednisone for, 301, 301*b*
- signs and symptoms, 299–301
- treatment, 301

Glomerular hematuria
- causes, 20–22, 21*t*
- *vs.* nonglomerular hematuria, 21*t*

Glucagon-like peptide 1 receptor agonists (GLP1 RAs), 425–426, 425*t*–426*t*
- cardiovascular and renal benefits, 427, 428*t*
- for diabetic ketoacidosis (DKA), 425*t*–426*t*, 426–427, 426*b*

Glucocorticoids
for CPPD arthritis, 275
for hepatic sarcoidosis, 410
side effects, 564*t*
Glutamate dehydrogenase (GDH), 366
Gonadotropin-releasing hormone (GnRH), 461
Gonococcal arthritis, 362*b*
Gout crystals, 276
GPCs. *See* Gram-positive cocci (GPCs)
G6PD deficiency, 383*b*
Gram-negative bacilli, 360
Gram-negative rods (GNR), 488
Gram-positive cocci (GPCs), 360, 361*f*, 486
Granulomas, 407
differential diagnosis, 90–91, 92*t*
hepatic, 407
causes, 407–408
differential diagnosis, 408*t*
histological variants, 408*t*
infectious, 530
Granulomatosis with polyangiitis (GPA), 560, 562–563

H

Haemophilus influenzae, 492
Hand eczema, 120
Hand hygiene, 365
Hand numbness
causes, 139
clinical diagnosis, 140–141
differential diagnosis, 139–140
evaluation, 142–143
Hand sanitizers, 365
Hantavirus, 9
HAP. *See* Hospital-acquired pneumonia (HAP)
Hashimoto's thyroiditis, 442–443
HBsAg. *See* Hepatitis B surface Ag (HBsAg)
HBV vaccine, 321–322
Headache, 353, 354*t*
Heart failure (HF)
classification, 172, 172*t*
diagnosis, 171–172
Heart failure with preserved ejection fraction (HFpEF)
counseling, 174–176
diagnosis, 170–172
hypertension, 173
kidneys and liver, 172
management, 173–174
volume removal, 173
Heart murmurs, 218, 219*t*
Hemangioblastomas, 133
Hematemesis, 553*t*
Hematocrit, 311
Hematopoietic stem-cell transplantation (HSCT), 372*b*, 373*b*
Hematoxylin and eosin (H&E) staining, 266–268
Hematuria
assessment, 20–24
causes, 19, 20*f*
diagnosis, 19–20
initial laboratory workup, 20
Hemoglobin A1c (HbA1c), 468
Hemolytic anemia, 379–380
Hemoptysis
bronchoalveolar lavage (BAL), 556, 558–560
causes, 554–555
classification, 553–554
defined, 553–554
early management, 554*t*
evaluation, 555–556
massive, 554*t*
Hemostasis, 234
Henoch-Schönlein purpura (HSP), 82–83
Hepatic sarcoidosis, 408
diagnosis, 408–409
imaging findings for, 409, 409*t*
Maddrey classification for, 408, 409*t*
management and treatment, 409–410
Hepatitis B core antibody (anti-HBc), 316–317
Hepatitis B immune globulin (HBIG), 321
Hepatitis B surface Ag (HBsAg), 316–317, 316*b*
Hepatitis B surface antibody (anti-HBs), 316–317
Hepatitis B virus (HBV)
prevalence, 316–317, 317*t*
screening tests for, 316–317, 318*t*
Hepatitis C virus (HCV)
associated cryoglobulinemic vasculitis, 269–270, 271*b*
infection, 325*b*
Hepatocellular carcinoma (HCC), 321–323
Hepatocellular liver injury, 406–407, 407*t*
Hepatocytes, 412
Hepatorenal syndrome (HRS)
vs. acute tubular necrosis (ATN), 18
biomarkers, 18
diagnosis, 16*t*, 17
treatment, 18
types, 18
Hermansky-Pudlak syndrome, 513*b*
High-resolution computed tomography (HRCT)
of chest, 507*b*, 508*f*
patterns of ILD, 508*t*
pulmonary nodules, 497, 499*f*, 500*b*
High-resolution manometry, 334–338, 335*f*
High-sensitivity CRP (hs-CRP), 266
Hirsutism
in female, 464
medications associated with, 464, 465*t*

Hirsutism *(Continued)*
prevalence, 464
treatment, 468
HIV. *See* Human immunodeficiency virus (HIV)
HIV-associated immune complex kidney disease (HIVICK), 33–34
HIV associated nephropathy (HIVAN), 34, 34*f*
HLA-B27, 254
Holosystolic murmur, 516
Homocysteine (HCY), 43
Honeycombing, 507
Hormone therapy (HT), for osteoporosis, 454*t*
Hospital-acquired pneumonia (HAP), 484–485
duration of treatment recommended for, 487
etiologies, 486
risk factors, 487–488
therapies for, 486–487
"Hot tub lung,", 543*b*
HRCT. *See* High-resolution computed tomography (HRCT)
HRS. *See* Hepatorenal syndrome (HRS)
Human chorionic gonadotropin (HCG), 444–445
Human immunodeficiency virus (HIV), 353
community-acquired pneumonia (CAP), 397
diagnostics, 396–397, 397*f*
and malaria, 385
Hydrocortisone, in septic shock, 550–551
Hydropneumothorax, 479*b*
Hydroxychloroquine (HCQ), for CPPD arthritis, 279–280
Hyperbilirubinemia, 311–312, 324
Hypercortisolemia, 461. *See also* Cushing disease
Hyperglycemia
differential diagnosis, 421–422, 422*t*
etiologies for, 421–429
risk factors, 421, 422*t*
Hyperosmolar hyperglycemic state (HHS), 429*b*
Hyperparasitemia, 383
Hyperprolactinemia, 436*b*, 461
Hypersensitivity, 382
Hypertension, 24, 173
Hypoglycemia, 383
defined, 424–425
symptoms, 424–425
Hypotension, 158–159
Hypothyroidism, 442–443
in pregnancy
changes in thyroid physiology, 444–445, 444*f*
incidence, 444
management, 446–447
postpartum management, 447
risks, 445
testing, 445
thyroid function tests, 444–445
signs and symptoms, 443, 443*t*
Hypoxemia, 158
causes, 475–483, 475*t*
defined, 475–477
differential diagnosis, 490
in patients on mechanical ventilation in ICU, 484–489
Hypoxia, 475–477

I

Ibandronate, for osteoporosis, 454*t*, 457
IBD. *See* Inflammatory bowel disease (IBD)
Idiopathic pulmonary fibrosis (IPF), 507
diagnosis, 509
gastroesophageal reflux, 511–512
incidence, 510–511
lung transplantation, 512–513, 512*t*, 513*t*
risk factors, 510–511
surgical lung biopsy, 509, 509*b*
treatment, 511
ILD. *See* Interstitial lung disease (ILD)
Immune reconstitution inflammatory syndrome (IRIS), 34, 357, 399
Implantable cardioverter-defibrillator (ICD), 157*f*
Incidental lung nodule
clinical significance, 530–537
management, 534, 535*t*
Inclusion body myositis (IBM), 260
Induction therapy, for microscopic polyangiitis (MPA), 563
Infectious arthritis, 360
Infectious Diseases Society of America (IDSA) Practice guidelines, 356, 390, 390*t*, 492
Inflammatory arthritis, 281*b*
Inflammatory back pain, 252
definition, 251–252
diagnosis, 252
Inflammatory bowel disease (IBD)
diagnosis, 346–348, 347*t*
extraintestinal manifestations, 348–349, 348*t*
treatment, 349–350, 349*t*
Inflammatory myositis, 260, 261*t*
Inflammatory polyarthritis, 251
Influenza, 397–398
Inorganic pyrophosphate (PPi), 279
Insulin-like growth factor 1 (IGF-1), 433, 436
Insulin resistance, 469
Interface hepatitis, 326*b*–327*b*
Interferon-alpha (IFN), 256
Interferon-gamma release assays (IGRA), 498*b*
International Agency for Research on Cancer (IARC), 503–504
International Classification of Ehlers-Danlos Syndromes, 285–286

International Society for Clinical Densitometry (ISCD), 452*b*
Interstitial edema, 157*f*
Interstitial lung disease (ILD), 505–506
  pulmonary function tests (PFTs), 507
  smoking-related, 511*b*
Intracranial hemorrhage (ICH), 201–202
Intracranial pressure (ICP), in AIDS patient
  antiretroviral therapy, 357
  causes, 353–357
  cerebrospinal fluid analysis, 354, 354*t*
  cryptococcal meningoencephalitis, 355–356
  cryptococcosis, 354–355
  etiologies, 354, 354*t*
  evaluation, 353–354
  management, 356
Intradural extramedullary spinal tumors, 132
Intramedullary spinal tumors, 132
IPF. *See* Idiopathic pulmonary fibrosis (IPF)
IRIS. *See* Immune reconstitution inflammatory syndrome (IRIS)
IV alteplase, 147–148

J

Jaundice, 383, 412
Joint hypermobility
  Beighton score, 282, 283*f*, 283*t*, 284*f*
  causes, 282–284
  differential diagnosis, 284–285
  evaluation, 282
  polyarticular pain, 281–282
Joint pain, 275
  differential diagnosis, 281, 282*t*, 294–295
  location and distribution, 293, 294*t*
  morning stiffness, 294
Jugular venous distention (JVD), 515–516

K

Keratinocyte necrosis, 109
Keratoconjunctivitis sicca, 242, 243*t*
Knee pain, 358

L

Laparoscopic appendectomy, 391
Laparoscopic or open Heller myotomy, for achalasia, 340–344
Lateral flow assay (LFA), 355
Latex agglutination, 355
LCV. *See* Leukocytoclastic vasculitis (LCV)
Leptospirosis, 9, 379*t*
LES. *See* Lower esophageal sphincter (LES)
Letrozole, for polycystic ovary syndrome (PCOS), 469–471
Leukocytoclastic vasculitis (LCV), 266*b*, 268, 268*f*
  clinical assessment, 81–82
  diagnosis, 79–80
  etiologies, 80–81
  histology, 80
  laboratory tests, 82
  signs and symptoms, 82
  treatments, 83–84
Levofloxacin
  for aspiration pneumonia, 490–491
  for hospital-acquired pneumonia (HAP), 487
  for neutropenic fever, 376–377
Levothyroxine, hypothyroidism in pregnancy, 446, 446*b*
LFTs. *See* Liver function tests (LFTs)
Life's Simple 7 approach, 152
Lipase, 309*b*
Liver biopsy, 326–328, 326*b*–327*b*
Liver function tests (LFTs), 324–330
Liver transplantation (LT), 416
Lobectomy, 525, 527
Lobular hepatitis with necrosis, 326*b*–327*b*, 327*f*
Loeys-Dietz syndrome, 285, 285*b*
Lower esophageal sphincter (LES), 338, 338*b*
Lower respiratory tract infection (LRTI), 394
Low molecular weight heparin (LMWH), 201–202
Lumbar puncture (LP), 353*b*, 384
Lung
  metastases in, 530, 532*f*
  rheumatoid nodules in, 530, 531*f*
Lung nodule
  characteristics, 532–534
  diagnosis, 532
  FDG-PET, 534–536, 535*f*
  incidental, 530–537
  malignancy, 532–534, 534*t*
  metastases in lung, 530, 532*f*
  rheumatoid nodules in lung, 530, 531*f*
  risk factors, 532
  solitary pulmonary, 530–532, 531*t*
  spiculated invasive adenocarcinoma, 532*f*
  tissue biopsy, 536–537
Lung transplant, 504*b*
Lyme disease, 362*b*

M

Macroaspiration, 491*b*
Macrolide, for community-acquired pneumonia (CAP), 487
Magnetic resonance angiography, 183*f*

Magnetic resonance cholangiopancreatography (MRCP)
for biliary obstruction, 414, 415*b*
for choledocholithiasis, 311–313, 313*f*
Magnetic resonance imaging (MRI)
sellar mass, 430, 431*f*
septic arthritis, 359
subdeltoid and trochanteric bursitis, 295, 296*f*–297*f*
Maintenance therapy, for microscopic polyangiitis (MPA), 563–565
Major adverse cardiovascular events (MACE), 458–459
Malaria, 379*t*, 383*b*
cerebral, 384
diagnosis, 383
HIV and, 385
prognosis, 383–384
treatment, 384–385
Malignancy, 382, 555*b*
MAP. *See* Mean arterial pressure (MAP)
Marfan's syndrome, 285, 285*b*
Marik Protocol, 551*b*
MASCC. *See* Multinational Association for Supportive Care in Cancer (MASCC) scoring system
McCune-Albright syndrome, 440
Mean arterial pressure (MAP), 158, 549, 549*b*, 550*b*
Mean corpuscular volume (MCV), 44, 44*f*
Medroxyprogesterone, for polycystic ovary syndrome (PCOS), 467
Megaloblastic anemia, 44
Meglitinides, 425–426, 425*t*–426*t*
Melanoma
ABCDEs, 102
diagnosis, 102
differential diagnosis, 100, 101*t*
follow-up, 105–106
physical examination, 100, 101*f*
prognostic factors, 103–105
risk factors, 102
skin of color, 102–103
staging system, 103, 103*t*–104*t*
subtypes, 100–102
treatment, 105
Membranoproliferative glomerulonephritis, 267*b*
Meningioma, 430
Menopausal hormone therapy (MHT)
for osteoporosis, 450–451
side effects, 459*t*
Meropenem, for hospital-acquired pneumonia (HAP), 487
Mesna (sodium 2-mercaptoethane sulfonate), 564*b*
Metastases, in lung, 530, 532*f*
Metastatic intramedullary tumors, 133
Metformin, 434*t*
for diabetic ketoacidosis, 424*b*
for hirsutism, 468
for polycystic ovary syndrome (PCOS), 467, 469–471
Methicillin-resistant *Staphylococcus aureus* (MRSA), 361*b*, 486
Methotrexate (MTX), 121
for giant cell arteritis (GCA), 301–302, 301*b*
for microscopic polyangiitis (MPA), 563–565
for polymyalgia rheumatica (PMR), 301–302, 301*b*
for pulmonary fibrosis, 509*b*
side effects, 301, 564*t*
Methyldopa, associated with hirsutism, 465*t*
Methylmalonic acid (MMA), 43
Metoclopramide, associated with hirsutism, 465*t*
Metronidazole
for aspiration pneumonia, 496
for *C. difficile* infection, 367
Microadenomas, 431
Microaspiration, 491*b*
Microscopic polyangiitis (MPA), 560
vs. anti-GBM (Goodpasture) disease, 563
clinical features, 562–563
diagnosis, 562
management, 563–565
Microvascular angina, 188
Migraine, 136, 138
Minoxidil, associated with hirsutism, 465*t*
Miscarriage, 445
Mitral regurgitation (MR)
acute and chronic presentations, 223
etiology, 224–225
hemodynamic compromise, 223
pharmacological and mechanical circulatory support device, 225
transcatheter, 225
treatment, 222–223
Mixed-picture liver disease, 405
Mohs micrographic surgery (MMS), 105
Monoarticular arthritis, 358
Moxifloxacin, for aspiration pneumonia, 496
MPA. *See* Microscopic polyangiitis (MPA)
MR. *See* Mitral regurgitation (MR)
MRCP. *See* Magnetic resonance cholangiopancreatography (MRCP)
MRI. *See* Magnetic resonance imaging (MRI)
MTX. *See* Methotrexate (MTX)
Multinational Association for Supportive Care in Cancer (MASCC) scoring system, 371–372, 372*b*, 372*t*
Murphy's sign, 307–308
Murphy's triad, 388

Muscle weakness
diagnostic workup, 262–263
differential diagnosis, 260–262, 261*t*
history, 259
laboratory tests, 260*t*
malignancy, 261
medications, 262
symptoms, 259–260
Myalgia, 260
Mycobacterium avium complex (MAC), 543*b*
Mycobacterium tuberculosis (MTB), 392
chest X-ray examination, 395–396, 395*f*
risk factors, 396*b*
Mycophenolate, for microscopic polyangiitis (MPA), 563–565
Myeloperoxidase (MPO), 269*b*, 560
Myonecrosis, 260
Myopathy, 260
Myositis, 260

N

Nasal retina, 432*b*
Nasogastric and postpyloric tubes
advantages and disadvantages, 496*t*
enteral feeding, placement for, 493–494, 495*f*
National Institutes of Health Stroke Scale (NIHSS) score, 146
National Osteoporosis Foundation, 449
Necrotizing myopathies, 260
Negative anti-*Saccharomyces cerevisiae* antibody, 345*b*
Neurological deficits, 146–147
Neutropenia
definition, 369*b*
febrile, 370*t*, 373
Neutropenic fever, 53
antimicrobials for, 373–375
differential diagnosis, 371
expanded Gram-positive antibacterial therapy, 373, 373*t*
fungal biomarkers, role of, 375
history and physical examination, 369–377
laboratory tests, 370–371, 371*t*
MASCC score, 372*b*, 372*t*
risk stratification in, 371–372, 372*t*
signs and symptoms, 369–370, 370*t*
Neutrophilic infiltration, of alveolar septa, 558*b*
New York Heart Association (NYHA) functional classification system, 172
Nine-Point Beighton Hypermobility Score, 283*t*
Nintedanib, for idiopathic pulmonary fibrosis (IPF), 511, 512*b*, 513*b*
Nitrates, 193, 201, 340
Nitric oxide, 518–520
Nitroglycerin, 194–195, 201
Noncardiogenic pulmonary edema, 383
Nonfunctioning pituitary macroadenoma
radiation therapy, 436
transsphenoidal surgery, 436
Nonglomerular hematuria, 21*t*
Noninflammatory polyarthritis, 251
Noninsulin antidiabetic drugs
side effects, 425*t*–426*t*, 427
for type 2 diabetes, 425–426, 425*t*–426*t*
Non-small-cell lung cancers (NSCLC), 524*b*
immunotherapy, 528
mutations, 528
palliative options, 528–529
stages, 526–527
surgery, 527
Non-ST-elevated myocardial infarction (NSTEMI), 196–197, 200
Nonsteroidal antiinflammatory drugs (NSAIDs), 4–6, 5*t*, 256*b*, 258, 275
Norepinephrine, in septic shock, 550*t*
Normocytic anemia, 295
NSAIDs. *See* Nonsteroidal antiinflammatory drugs (NSAIDs)
NSCLC. *See* Non-small-cell lung cancers (NSCLC)
Nucleic acid amplification tests (NAATs)
for *C. difficile* infection, 366–367
for PJP pneumonia, 398
Nucleoside/nucleotide analogs, for chronic hepatitis B (CHB), 320, 320*b*
Nummular lesions, 120

O

Obesity, 469
Obstructive sleep apnea (OSA), 468, 518*b*
Occupational lung disease, 497, 501*t*
differential diagnosis, 500–501
laboratory tests, 500*b*, 500*t*
perilymphatic nodules, 500*b*, 500*f*
pulmonary nodules, 497–504, 499*f*
silicosis, 502–504, 503*f*
OGTT. *See* Oral glucose tolerance test (OGTT)
Oligomenorrhea
diagnosis, 461–471, 462*t*
treatment, 467
Opioid therapy, for joint pain, 287
Oral glucose tolerance test (OGTT), 433, 468, 469*b*
Oropharyngeal dysphagia, 331, 493
Orthostatic vital sign measurements, 70
Oscillatory positive expiratory pressure (PEP) device, 543
Osteogenesis imperfecta, 284
Osteonecrosis of jaw (ONJ), 455

Osteoporosis
anabolic therapy, 459–460
bisphosphonate therapy
advantages and disadvantages, 457
side effects of, 455
bone architecture, 449, 450*f*
bone turnover markers (BTMs), 455, 457*b*
complications, 452–453
C-terminal telopeptide (CTX), 456
denosumab
risks and benefits of, 457
side effects, 459*t*
DEXA scan, 449, 455
diagnosis, 449–460
FRAX tool, 449
goal of therapy, 453
medications for high risk of fractures, 458–459
prognosis, 452–453
raloxifene, 457–458
recommended screening guidelines, 449–451
risk factors, 451–452
secondary, causes of, 452, 453*t*
SERM therapy, 457–458
treatment, 453, 454*t*

P

PAD. *See* Peripheral arterial disease (PAD)
Paget's disease, 86–87, 86*f*, 87*f*
of breast, 87–88
PAH. *See* Pulmonary arterial hypertension (PAH)
Palisading granulomas, 90
Palpable purpura, 77–79, 78*f*
Pancytopenia, 32, 50, 52*t*
Paracentesis-induced circulatory dysfunction, 18
Parasites, 382
Patent foramen ovale (PFO), 151
PCI. *See* Percutaneous coronary intervention (PCI)
PCOS. *See* Polycystic ovary syndrome (PCOS)
Penicillamine, associated with hirsutism, 465*t*
Penicillium, 393*b*
Peptic ulcer disease (PUD), 307–308
Percutaneous coronary intervention (PCI), 208, 212–213
Perilymphatic nodules, 500*b*, 500*f*
Peripheral arterial disease (PAD)
follow-up, 181
pharmacologic therapy, 181–182
risk factors, 178–179
screening, 179–180
treatment, 180–181
Peripheral edema, 231–232
Peripheral eosinophilia, 10*f*
Pernicious anemia, 45–47, 46*f*
Peroral endoscopic myotomy (POEM), for achalasia, 339*b*, 340–344
Petechiae, on lower extremity, 554*f*
PH. *See* Pulmonary hypertension (PH)
Phenothiazines, associated with hirsutism, 465*t*
Phenylephrine, in septic shock, 550*t*
Phenytoin, associated with hirsutism, 465*t*
Phosphodiesterase 5 (PDE-5) inhibitor
for achalasia, 340
for benign prostatic hyperplasia (BPH), 521*b*
for erectile dysfunction, 521*b*
side effects, 521
Physical therapy, for Ehlers-Danlos Syndromes (EDS), 287
Pigmented purpuric dermatoses. *See* Capillaritis
Pirfenidone, for idiopathic pulmonary fibrosis (IPF), 511, 513*b*
Pituitary adenomas, 430, 440
differential diagnosis, 435
functional, 432–435, 433*t*
monitoring after surgical resection, 439–440
nonfunctional, 432–435, 435*t*
sellar region, 431*t*
subtypes, 432
Pituitary macroadenoma, 430–431
endoscopic transsphenoidal craniotomy for, 438*b*
postoperative endocrine complications, 437
Pituitary microadenomas, 431
Pituitary stalk effect, 434*be*
Pituitary surgery
hyponatremia after, 438, 438*t*
postoperative considerations after, 437–438
PJP. *See Pneumocystis jiroveci* pneumonia (PJP)
Plasma exchange, 565
Plasmapheresis, 273–274
Plasmodium falciparum, 382, 382*f*
Platelet and vascular disorders, 49, 49*t*, 51*t*
Pulmonary nodules, attenuation in, 532, 533*f*
PMR. *See* Polymyalgia rheumatica (PMR)
Pneumatic dilation, for achalasia, 340–344
Pneumoconioses, 497, 502*b*, 504*b*
Pneumocystis jiroveci pneumonia (PJP), 301, 397
laboratory tests, 398
prophylaxis, 400*b*
treatment, 398–399, 399*t*
Pneumonia
aspiration, 490–491
community-acquired, 484–485
diagnosis, 485
duration of treatment recommended for, 487
etiologies, 486

Pneumonia *(Continued)*
hospital-acquired, 484–485
imaging in monitoring resolution of, 488–489
invasive and noninvasive sampling techniques, 485–486, 486*t*
right lower lobe (RLL) consolidation, 484, 484*b*
risk factors, 487–488
sputum cultures, role of, 485–486, 486*b*
therapies for, 486–487
ventilator-associated, 484–485
Pneumonitis, 490–491
Pneumothorax
chest X-ray, 477*b*, 477*f*
complications, 481–483, 482*t*
differential diagnosis, 479
needle aspiration, 481*b*, 481*f*
pigtail catheter placement, 481*b*, 482*f*
radiographic signs of, 477*b*
thoracostomy, 479–481, 480*t*
treatment, 479–481
types, 477–479, 478*t*
ultrasound, 476*b*, 476*f*
Polyarticular pain, 291
associated with hypermobility of joints, 281–282
causes of, 281–292
Polycystic ovary syndrome (PCOS), 442–443
abnormal hair growth, 464, 464*f*
biochemical testing in, 465–466, 466*t*
counseling, 469–471
diagnosis, 461*b*, 462–463, 462*t*, 468–469
elevation in testosterone and DHEA-S, 466
obesity and insulin resistance, first-line treatment for, 469
physical examination, 463–464
treatment, 467, 469–470
Polydipsia, 421
Polymerase chain reaction (PCR), 355, 366
Polymyalgia rheumatica (PMR), 295
alternative therapy, 301–303
classification criteria for, 295, 298*t*
differential diagnosis, 296, 298*t*
glucocorticoid-sparing treatments for, 302*t*
laboratory findings, 295
prednisone for, 301
treatment, 301
Polymyositis (PM), 260, 263–264
Polyuria, 421
Positive perinuclear antineutrophil cytoplasmic antibodies (p-ANCAs), 345*b*
Post-thrombectomy angiogram, 150*f*
Prednisone
for cryoglobulinemic vasculitis, 272*b*
for giant cell arteritis (GCA), 301, 301*b*
for polymyalgia rheumatica (PMR), 301
Pregnancy
chronic hepatitis B (CHB) during, 320–321, 321*b*
hypothyroidism in
changes in thyroid physiology, 444–445, 444*f*
incidence, 444
management, 446–447
postpartum management, 447
risks, 445
testing, 445
thyroid function tests, 444–445
thyroid autoimmunity in, 444
Premature ovarian failure, 461
Primaquine, 384*b*
Primary sclerosing cholangitis (PSC), 348*b*, 414, 416
Procalcitonin, 485, 548*b*
Progestin, 450–451, 467
Programmed death 1 (PD-1), 528
Progressive massive fibrosis (PMF), 502–503
Prolactinoma, 432–433, 433*t*
Prophylactic therapy, 137
Prostacyclin, 518–520, 520*b*
Proteinuria
clinical significance, 28
tests to evaluate, 27–28
Proton pump inhibitors, 365
Proximal renal tubular acidosis, 36
Pruritus, 412
PSC. *See* Primary sclerosing cholangitis (PSC)
Pseudo-claudication, 177
Pseudogout, 276
Pseudomembranous colitis, 363–364
Pseudomonas, 360, 486, 544
Pseudomonas aeruginosa, 374*b*, 492
Psoriatic arthritis
diagnosis, 254–255
HLA-B27, 254
joint involvement, 252, 253*t*
nail involvement, 252, 253*f*, 254*f*
symptoms, 253, 257–258
treatments, 255–258
X-ray findings, 255, 257*f*
Pulmonary arterial hypertension (PAH)
drugs associated with, 517*b*
pathophysiology, 518–520, 519*f*
therapies for, 520*t*
treatment, 520–521
Pulmonary capillaritis, 558*b*, 559*f*
Pulmonary capillary wedge pressure, 517
Pulmonary embolism (PE), 158
Pulmonary function tests (PFTs), 502, 506–507, 527, 539–540
diffuse alveolar hemorrhage (DAH), 560
restrictive pattern, 507

Pulmonary hypertension (PH), 504*b*
- diagnosis, 516–518
- etiology, 518
- groups, 517, 518*t*
- management, 520–521, 521*t*

Pulmonary metastasis, 535*f*
Pulmonary nodules
- evaluation, 497–504
- high-resolution computed tomography (HRCT), 497, 499*f*
- multiple, 497

Pulmonary tuberculosis, 395–396
Pulmonary vascular resistance (PVR), 517
Purified protein derivative (PPD) testing, 503–504, 504*b*
Purpura, 79
- differential diagnosis, 266–274, 267*t*
- laboratory tests, 266*b*, 268*t*
- nonpalpable, 266
- palpable, 266, 267*f*
- skin biopsy, 266–268

Purpuric macules, on lower extremity, 554*f*
Pyoderma gangrenosum, 348*t*, 349*f*

Q

qSOFA. *See* Quick sequential organ failure assessment (qSOFA)
Quadrants of abdomen, 387*f*
QuantiFERON Gold test, 498*b*
Quartz, 502
Quick sequential organ failure assessment (qSOFA), 546–548, 547*b*, 547*t*
Quinine, for malaria, 384

R

Radiation therapy, 436
Radiographs
- of joints and bones, 284
- of septic arthritis, 359

Raloxifene, for osteoporosis, 454*t*, 457–458
Range or motion (ROM), 293*b*
Ranolazine, 193–194
Ranson's criteria, 310–311
Rathke's cleft cyst, 430
Raynaud's phenomenon (RP), 272*b*
Receptor activator of nuclear factor kappa-B ligand (RANKL), 457
Regional lymph nodes, 526
Renal injury, 383
Renal papillary necrosis, 6*f*, 7*f*
Renal tubular acidosis (RTA), 35–37
Renin-angiotensin-aldosterone system (RAAS), 24
Respiratory bronchiolitis-interstitial lung disease (RB-ILD), 511*b*
Retroflexion, 333
R-factor chart, 406*t*
Rheumatoid arthritis, 295
Rheumatoid factor (RF), 295, 295*b*
Rheumatoid nodules, in lung, 530, 531*f*
Rickettsia, 379*t*
Rickettsia typhi, 381
Right-hand numbness. *See* Hand numbness
Right lower abdominal pain (RLQ), 388
Right ventricular hypertrophy, 516, 517*f*
Right ventricular systolic pressure (RVSP), 516, 517*b*
Risedronate, for osteoporosis, 454*t*
Rituximab
- for cryoglobulinemic vasculitis, 272*b*
- for microscopic polyangiitis (MPA), 563–565, 563*b*
- side effects, 273*b*, 564*t*

Romosozumab
- for osteoporosis, 454*t*, 458–459
- side effects, 459*t*

Rotterdam criteria, 462

S

Sarcoidal granulomas, 90
Sarcoidosis, 408
- cutaneous presentation, 94–95
- diagnosis, 93
- epidemiology, 92–93
- initial workup, 95–96, 95*t*
- organs involved, 93
- pathogenesis, 91–92
- serum ACE level, 96
- treatment, 96–98, 97*t*

SCAD. *See* Spontaneous coronary artery dissection (SCAD)
Schirmer's test, 244, 245*f*
Schistocytes, 51
Scintigraphy, 247
Secondary hemostasis, 234*f*
Secondary hypothyroidism, 435
Secondary spontaneous pneumothorax, 479, 479*t*
Secretion of antidiuretic hormone (SIADH), 437–438
Seizure, 484
Selective estrogen receptor modulator (SERM) therapy
- for osteoporosis, 450–451, 454*t*, 457–458
- side effects, 459*t*

Sellar mass, 430
- differential diagnosis, 430, 431*t*
- magnetic resonance imaging (MRI), 430, 431*f*

Sella turcica, 430
Senile purpura, 77, 78*f*
Sensorium, decreased, 383

Sepsis
corticosteroids in, 550–551
defined, 546
diagnosis, 546–551
early identification, 546–548
fluid resuscitation, 548–549
intravenous vasopressors, 550
management, 548
quick SOFA (qSOFA), 546–548, 547*b*, 547*t*
risk factors, 546*b*
sequential organ failure assessment (SOFA), 546–548, 547*b*
systemic inflammatory response syndrome (SIRS) criteria, 546–548, 547*t*
vasopressors in septic shock, 550*t*
Septic arthritis, 277, 358*b*
clinical findings and sensitivity for diagnosis, 358–359
diagnostic tests, 359
management, 361–362
synovial fluid analysis, 359*t*, 360
Septic shock, 158
distributive, 549*b*
hemodynamic pattern, 549
hydrocortisone in, 550–551
refractory, 551*b*
vasopressors in, 550*t*
Sequential organ failure assessment (SOFA), 546–548, 547*b*
Sex-hormone binding globulin (SHBG), 467
Shigella, 381
Shortness of breath, 259–260
causes, 515–522
diagnostic tests, 515–516
differential diagnosis, 231
pulmonary hypertension, 516–517
Sialometry, 247–248
Sigmoid esophagus, 337*f*
Silica, 502
Silicosis
complications, 503–504
diagnosis, 502
manifestations, 502–503
SIRS. *See* Systemic inflammatory response syndrome (SIRS) criteria
Sjögren's syndrome
arthritis, 248–249
classification criteria, 246–247, 246*t*
dry, fissured tongue, 244*f*
laboratory tests, 242–243
malignancy, 249–250
primary *vs.* secondary, 249
salivary gland involvement, 247–248
systemic manifestations, 248, 248*t*
treatment, 247
"SNOOP" mnemonic, 134
Sodium glucose cotransporter-2 (SGLT2) inhibitors, 425–426, 425*t*–426*t*
cardiovascular and renal benefits, 427, 428*t*
for diabetic ketoacidosis (DKA), 425*t*–426*t*, 426–427, 426*b*
SOFA. *See* Sequential organ failure assessment (SOFA)
Sofosbuvir-velpatasvir, for cryoglobulinemic vasculitis, 272*b*
Solitary pulmonary lung nodule, 530–532, 531*t*
Spiculated invasive adenocarcinoma, 532*f*
Spinal cord tumors
causes, 129–130
differential diagnosis, 130, 132*t*
initial workup, 130
lesion, location of, 130
management, 130–133
Spironolactone, for hirsutism, 468, 470
Spontaneous coronary artery dissection (SCAD), 209–210
clinical manifestations, 212
conditions and factors associated with, 211*t*, 215*f*
diagnosis, 210, 212
epidemiology, 210
prognosis, 213–216
risk factors, 210–212
treatment, 212–213, 216*f*
type 1, 213*f*
type 2, 214*f*
type 3, 214*f*
Sporicidal agents, 365
Sputum cultures, 485–486, 486*b*
Stable angina, 187
Staphylococcus aureus, 360, 492
Stasis dermatitis, 77
Statins, 192–193, 262
STEADI (Stopping Elderly Accidents, Deaths and Injuries) algorithm, 73–74
ST-elevated myocardial infarction (STEMI), 196–197, 199–204
Stevens-Johnson syndrome/toxic epidermal necrolysis (SJS/TEN)
clinical presentation, 112
diagnosis, 113–114
differential diagnosis, 111, 112*t*
drug culprits, 111
initial workup, 113
management, 114–115
medications, 111*t*
organ systems, 112–113
pathogenesis, 108–110
prognosis, 115–116
risk, 110–111

STOP-BANG questionnaire, 468
Streptococcus pneumoniae, 360, 486, 492
Streptococcus pyogenes, 360
Stroke
- IV alteplase administration, 147–148, 149*t*
- large *vs.* small infarct, 146*t*
- management, 148–152
- symptoms, 145–152

Subdeltoid bursitis, 295, 296*f*–297*f*
Subsolid nodules, 532
Sulfonylureas (SU), 425–426, 425*t*–426*t*
Suppurative granulomas, 91
Surgical lung biopsy, 509, 509*b*
Surgical resection, of nonfunctioning adenoma, 436
Symptomatology, 331
Synovial fluid
- analysis, 275–276, 277*t*, 359–360
- inflammatory *vs.* noninflammatory, 277, 277*t*

Systemic inflammatory response syndrome (SIRS) criteria, 546–548, 547*t*
Systemic lupus erythematous, 267*b*
Systemic vasculitis, 268–269
- antineutrophil cytoplasmic antibody (ANCA)-associated vasculitis, 269
- classification and clinical features, 270*f*, 270*t*
- differential diagnosis, 269–271
- immune complex small vessel vasculitis, 269
- large vessel vasculitis, 269
- small vessel vasculitis, 269–270

T

Talcosis, 501*t*
TEE. *See* Transesophageal echocardiography (TEE)
Tenofovir disoproxil fumarate (TDF), for chronic hepatitis B (CHB), 320, 320*b*
Teriparatide
- for osteoporosis, 454*t*, 458
- side effects, 459*t*

Terminal cleaning procedure, 365*b*
Terminal hair growth, 463–464, 463*f*
Thiazolidinedione (TZD), 425–426, 425*t*–426*t*
Thoracostomy, indications for, 480*t*
Thrombin, 234
Thrombocytopenia (TP), 380
Thrush, 394–395, 394*f*, 395*b*
Thunderclap headache, 134
Thyroid autoimmunity, 444–445
Thyroid-binding globulin (TBG), 444–445
Thyroid function tests, 444–445
Thyroid peroxidase antibody (TPO-Ab), 442–444
Thyroid stimulating hormone (TSH), 442–445
Thyroxine (T_4), 434, 442–445
Tibolone, for osteoporosis, 454*t*
Tissue biopsy, 536–537
TNM staging system, 526
Tobacco smoking, 532*b*
Tobramycin, for bronchiectasis, 544*b*
Tocilizumab
- for giant cell arteritis (GCA), 301–302
- for polymyalgia rheumatica (PMR), 301–302

Tofacitinib, for ulcerative colitis (UC), 350
Tolvaptan, 25
Tophi, 278
Total parenteral nutrition (TPN), 311
Traction bronchiectasis, 540*b*
Tram-track sign, 540
Tranexamic acid (TXA), for hemoptysis, 554*t*
Transesophageal echocardiography (TEE), 220, 223*f*, 515–516, 517*b*, 522*b*
Transforming growth factor-beta receptor gene (TGFBR), 285
Transjugular intrahepatic portosystemic shunt (TIPS), 18*b*
Transsphenoidal surgery, 436
Trigeminal autonomic cephalalgias (TACs), 135–136
Trigeminal neuralgia, 136*b*
Triiodothyronine (T_3), 434
Trimethoprim-sulfamethoxazole (TMP-SMX), for PJP pneumonia, 398
Triptans, 137
Trochanteric bursitis, 295, 296*f*–297*f*
Troponin, 515–516
True claudication, 177
TSH. *See* Thyroid stimulating hormone (TSH)
TSH-secreting tumor, 432–434, 433*t*
T-SPOT test, 498*b*
Tuberculoid granulomas, 90
Tuberculosis (TB), 497–498
Tubulointerstitial nephritis and uveitis (TINU), 9
Type 2 diabetes
- A1c target goals, 428–429
- noninsulin medications, 425–426, 425*t*–426*t*

Typhoid, 379*t*

U

UIP. *See* Usual interstitial pneumonia (UIP)
Ulcerative colitis (UC), 346, 347*t*
- 5-aminosalicylates (5-ASA) for, 349
- tofacitinib for, 350
- treatment for, 349–350, 349*t*

Ulcerative tongue lesions, 374, 374*f*
Ulnar neuropathy, 140
Ultrasound (US), 247
- appendicitis, 388–390, 389*f*
- cholelithiasis, 307*b*, 309*f*
- pneumothorax, 476*b*, 476*f*
- subdeltoid and trochanteric bursitis, 295, 296*f*–297*f*

Unfractionated heparin (UFH), 201–202
Unilateral nipple rash/lesion
differential diagnosis, 85
history, 85
management, 85–86
physical examination, 85
Unilateral peripheral edema, 231–232
United States Preventative Services Task Force (USPSTF), 449
Unstable angina (UA), 188, 196–197, 200
Up and Go Test, 71–72, 72*t*
Uremia/uremic syndrome
medical history and physical examination, 3–4
signs and symptoms, 3*t*, 5
Uremic bleeding, 4
Urinalysis
acute abdominal pain, 387
hematuria, 20–22, 20*b*
Urinary tract infection (UTI), 422*b*
Urine anion gap metabolic acidosis, 35
Ursodeoxycholic acid (UDCA), for hepatic sarcoidosis, 410
US National Institutes of Health (NIH) criteria, 462
Usual interstitial pneumonia (UIP), 507, 508*t*, 509–510, 510*t*

V

Valley fever, 393*b*
Valproic acid, associated with hirsutism, 465*t*
Valvular heart disease (VHD)
causes, 218, 219*t*
chest X-ray, 220, 221*f*
diagnosis, 219–222, 220*t*
differential diagnosis, 220–221
follow-up, 220
types, 218
Vancomycin
for *C. difficile* infection, 367
for infectious arthritis, 360*b*
for neutropenic fever, 373, 376*b*
Vancomycin-resistant enterococci (VRE), 373
VAP. *See* Ventilator-associated pneumonia (VAP)
Vasculitis, 560
classification, 553*t*
diagnosis, 560
leukocytoclastic, 266*b*, 268, 268*f*
systemic, 268–269
Vasopressors
intravenous, 550
in septic shock, 550*t*
VATS. *See* Video-assisted thoracoscopic surgery (VATS)
Velcro rales, 505
Venn diagram, 380
Ventilator-associated pneumonia (VAP), 484–485
duration of treatment recommended for, 487
etiologies, 486
risk factors, 487–488
therapies for, 486–487
Verapamil, 137
Vertebral fractures, 449
VHD. *See* Valvular heart disease (VHD)
Video-assisted thoracoscopic surgery (VATS), 525, 527, 536
Villefranche nosology, 286
Viruses, 381
Vitamin B_{12} deficiency
causes, 45, 45*t*
differential diagnosis, 45*t*
signs and symptoms, 44–45
treatment, 47–48
Vitamin D
for osteoporosis, 454*t*, 458
side effects, 459*t*
Volume overload
differential diagnosis, 169
initial workup, 169–170

W

Weight loss and fever, 392–400
Wellen's syndrome, 202
White blood cell urinary cast, 7, 7*f*
World Health Organization (WHO), 355*b*, 449

X

Xerostomia, 242, 243*t*, 247

Y

Yersinia enterocolitica 390

Z

Zoledronic acid, for osteoporosis, 454*t*, 457
Zosyn, for hospital-acquired pneumonia (HAP), 487